Household Safety Sourcebook

Hypertension Sourcebook

Immune System Disorders Sourcebook

Infant & Toddler Health Sourcebook

Infectious Diseases Sourcebook

Injury & Trauma Sourcebook

Kidney & Urinary Tract Diseases & Disorders Sourcebook

Learning Disabilities Sourcebook, 2nd Edition

Leukemia Sourcebook

Liver Disorders Sourcebook

Lung Disorders Sourcebook

Medical Tests Sourcebook, 2nd Edition

Men's Health Concerns Sourcebook, 2nd Edition

Mental Health Disorders Sourcebook, 3rd Edition

Mental Retardation Sourcebook

Movement Disorders Sourcebook

Muscular Dystrophy Sourcebook

Obesity Sourcebook

Osteoporosis Sourcebook

Pain Sourcebook, 2nd Edition

Pediatric Cancer Sourcebook

Physical & Mental Issues in Aging Sourcebook

Podiatry Sourcebook

Pregnancy & Birth Sourcebook, 2nd Edition

Prostate Cancer

Public Health Sourcebook

Reconstructive & Cosmetic Surgery Sourcebook

Rehabilitation Sourcebook

Respiratory Diseases & Disorders Sourcebook

Sexually Transmitted Diseases Sourcebook, 2nd Edition

Skin Disorders Sourcebook

Sleep Disorders Sourcebook, 2nd Edition

Smoking Concerns Sourcebook

Sports Injuries Sourcebook, 2nd Edition

Stress-Related Disorders Sourcebook

Stroke Sourcebook

Substance Abuse Sourcebook

Surgery Sourcebook

Thyroid Sourcebook

Transplantation Sourcebook

Traveler's Health Sourcebook

Vegetarian Sourcebook

Women's Health Concerns Sourcebook, 2nd Edition

Workplace Health & Safety Sourcebook

Worldwide Health Sourcebook

Teen Health Series

Alcohol Information for Teens

Asthma Information for Teens

Cancer Information for Teens

Diet Information for Teens

Drug Information for Teens

Eating Disorders Information for Teens

Fitness Information for Teens

Mental Health Information for Teens

Sexual Health Information for Teens

Skin Health Information for Teens

Sports Injuries Information for Teens

Suicide Information for Teens

Brain Disorders
SOURCEBOOK

Second Edition

Brain Disorders
SOURCEBOOK

*Basic Consumer Health Information about Acquired
and Traumatic Brain Injuries, Infections of the Brain,
Epilepsy and Seizure Disorders, Cerebral Palsy, and
Degenerative Neurological Disorders, Including
Amyotrophic Lateral Sclerosis (ALS), Dementias,
Multiple Sclerosis, and More*

*Along with Information on the Brain's Structure
and Function, Treatment and Rehabilitation
Options, Reports on Current Research Initiatives,
a Glossary of Terms Related to Brain Disorders
and Injuries, and a Directory of Sources for
Further Help and Information*

Edited by
Sandra J. Judd

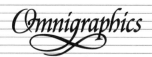

Omnigraphics

615 Griswold Street • Detroit, MI 48226

Bibliographic Note

Because this page cannot legibly accommodate all the copyright notices, the Bibliographic Note portion of the Preface constitutes an extension of the copyright notice.

Edited by Sandra J. Judd

Health Reference Series

Karen Bellenir, *Managing Editor*
David A. Cooke, M.D., *Medical Consultant*
Elizabeth Barbour, *Research and Permissions Coordinator*
Cherry Stockdale, *Permissions Assistant*
Dawn Matthews, *Verification Assistant*
Laura Pleva Nielsen, *Index Editor*
EdIndex, Services for Publishers, *Indexers*

* * *

Omnigraphics, Inc.

Matthew P. Barbour, *Senior Vice President*
Kay Gill, *Vice President—Directories*
Kevin Hayes, *Operations Manager*
Leif Gruenberg, *Development Manager*
David P. Bianco, *Marketing Director*

* * *

Peter E. Ruffner, *Publisher*

Frederick G. Ruffner, Jr., *Chairman*

Copyright © 2005 Omnigraphics, Inc.

ISBN 0-7808-0744-8

Library of Congress Cataloging-in-Publication Data

Brain disorders sourcebook : basic consumer health information about acquired and traumatic brain injuries, infections of the brain, epilepsy and seizure disorders, cerebral palsy, and degenerative neurological disorders, including amyotrophic lateral sclerosis (ALS), dementias, multiple sclerosis, and more; along with information on the brain's structure and function, treatment and rehabilitation options, reports on current research initiatives, a glossary of terms related to brain disorders and injuries, and a directory of sources for further help and information / edited by Sandra J. Judd.-- 2nd ed.
   p. cm. -- (Health reference series)
   Includes bibliographical references and index.
   ISBN 0-7808-0744-8 (hardcover : alk. paper)
   1. Brain--Diseases--Popular works. I. Judd, Sandra J. II. Health reference series (Unnumbered)
   RC351.B735 2005
   616.8--dc22
                                                              2005001822

Table of Contents

Visit www.healthreferenceseries.com to view *A Contents Guide to the Health Reference Series*, a listing of more than 10,000 topics and the volumes in which they are covered.

Preface ix

Part I: Understanding Brain Function

Chapter 1—Anatomy of the Brain 3

Chapter 2—Neurons, Brain Chemistry, and
 Neurotransmission 13

Chapter 3—Tests Used in Diagnosing
 Brain Disorders 23

 Section 3.1—Carotid Ultrasound 24

 Section 3.2—Cerebral Angiography 27

 Section 3.3—Cranial Computed Tomography
 (CT) Scan 31

 Section 3.4—Electroencephalogram (EEG) 35

 Section 3.5—Electromyography (EMG) 39

 Section 3.6—Nerve Conduction Velocity Test 42

 Section 3.7—Magnetic Resonance Imaging
 (MRI) 45

 Section 3.8—Positron Emission Tomography
 (PET) Scan 47

 Section 3.9—Spinal Tap (Lumbar Puncture) ... 51

Chapter 4—Recent Brain Research 53

    Section 4.1—Deep Brain Stimulation:
              Pacemakers for the Brain 54

    Section 4.2—The Women's Health
              Initiative Memory Study
              (WHIMS) 58

    Section 4.3—Bone Marrow Generates New
              Neurons in Human Brains 61

Chapter 5—Brain Death 65

Part II: Acquired and Traumatic Brain Injuries

Chapter 6—Stroke 71

    Section 6.1—Stroke: A Brain Attack 72

    Section 6.2—Recent Research on Stroke 108

Chapter 7—Brain Aneurysms 123

    Section 7.1—Understanding Brain
              Aneurysms 124

    Section 7.2—Treatment Options for
              Cerebral Aneurysms 129

Chapter 8—Brain Tumors 135

    Section 8.1—What You Need to Know
              about Brain Tumors 136

    Section 8.2—Metastatic Brain Tumors 154

Chapter 9—Infections of the Brain 159

    Section 9.1—Meningitis 160

    Section 9.2—Brain Abscess 170

    Section 9.3—Encephalitis 174

    Section 9.4—Cysticercosis 189

    Section 9.5—Trichinellosis 193

Chapter 10—Hypoxia 197

Chapter 11—Traumatic Brain Injuries 205

    Section 11.1—What You Need to Know
              about Traumatic Brain
              Injury 206

    Section 11.2—Concussion 226

    Section 11.3—Coma 229

    Section 11.4—Shaken Baby Syndrome 238

Part III: Epilepsy and Seizure Disorders

Chapter 12—Epilepsy 245

    Section 12.1—Seizures and Epilepsy 246

    Section 12.2—Epilepsy: Women's Concerns 274

    Section 12.3—Epilepsy in the Elderly 287

    Section 12.4—Understanding Vagus Nerve
                   Stimulation 293

    Section 12.5—Ketogenic Diet 300

Chapter 13—Nonepileptic Seizures 303

Chapter 14—First Aid for Seizures 309

Part IV: Degenerative Neurological Disorders

Chapter 15—Amyotrophic Lateral Sclerosis (ALS) 315

    Section 15.1—ALS: An Overview 316

    Section 15.2—Recent Research on ALS 325

Chapter 16—Dementias: Hope through Research 335

Chapter 17—Huntington Disease 367

    Section 17.1—Understanding Huntington
                   Disease 368

    Section 17.2—Recent Research on
                   Huntington Disease 387

Chapter 18—Multiple Sclerosis (MS) 393

    Section 18.1—MS: An Overview 394

    Section 18.2—MS Treatment: Some Safety
                   Issues 415

    Section 18.3—MS and Cooling 420

    Section 18.4—New Research on MS 426

Chapter 19—Parkinson Disease 433

    Section 19.1—Parkinson Disease: An
                   Overview 434

    Section 19.2—Recent Research on
                   Parkinson Disease 443

Part V: Other Brain Disorders

Chapter 20—Cerebral Palsy 461

Chapter 21—Headache 487

Chapter 22—Hydrocephalus 505

Chapter 23—Narcolepsy 511

Part VI: Additional Help and Information

Chapter 24—Glossary of Brain-Related Terms 525

Chapter 25—Brain Disorders: Resources for Information
and Support 557

Index 571

Preface

About This Book

Brain disorders, including acquired and traumatic injuries, degenerative neurological conditions, and other neurological diseases, comprise one of the most devastating classes of health conditions facing Americans today.

- According to the Centers for Disease Control and Prevention (CDC), 1.5 million people sustain a traumatic brain injury in the U.S. each year..

- The American Brain Tumor Association reports that more than 40,000 Americans are diagnosed with primary brain tumors each year, and an additional 100,000 cancer patients show symptoms of metastatic brain tumors.

- 250,000 Americans suffer from multiple sclerosis.

- Every year 5,000 Americans are diagnosed with amyotrophic lateral sclerosis (ALS, or Lou Gehrig's disease)

- 2 million Americans have experienced an unprovoked seizure or have been diagnosed with epilepsy.

- As many as 1.8 million Americans are severely affected by dementia.

Brain Disorders Sourcebook, Second Edition provides readers with updated health information about brain injuries, infections of the brain, epilepsy and seizure disorders, cerebral palsy, and degenerative neurological disorders, including amyotrophic lateral sclerosis (ALS), dementias, and multiple sclerosis. It also includes information on the brain's structure and function, treatment and rehabilitation options, reports on current research initiatives, a glossary of terms related to brain disorders and injuries, and a directory of sources for further help and information.

Readers seeking more in-depth information about some specific types of brain disorders and related issues may also wish to consult other books in the *Health Reference Series*:

- Alzheimer's Disease: *Alzheimer's Disease Sourcebook, Third Edition*
- Caregiving: *Caregiving Sourcebook*
- Genetic Disorders: *Genetic Disorders Sourcebook, Third Edition*
- Headache: *Headache Sourcebook*
- Movement Disorders: *Movement Disorders Sourcebook*
- Sleep Disorders: *Sleep Disorders Sourcebook, Second Edition*
- Stroke: *Stroke Sourcebook*

How to Use This Book

This book is divided into parts and chapters. Parts focus on broad areas of interest. Chapters are devoted to single topics within a part.

Part I: Understanding Brain Function begins with a look at the brain's anatomy and explains how it works. The types of tests used in diagnosing brain disorders are described, and the part concludes with an overview of recent research initiatives on brain function and a description of the criteria for determining brain death.

Part II: Acquired and Traumatic Brain Injuries looks at the most common types of brain injuries, including stroke, aneurysms, tumors, infections, hypoxia, and traumatic injuries. It offers a description of each of these types of brain injury and explains how it is diagnosed and treated.

Part III: Epilepsy and Seizure Disorders presents an in-depth look at epilepsy and other common seizure disorders, with detailed descriptions of the types of seizure disorders, their diagnosis and treatment, women's concerns about epilepsy, epilepsy in the elderly, vagus nerve stimulation, and the ketogenic diet.

Part IV: Degenerative Neurological Disorders describes the most common types of these devastating disorders, including amyotrophic lateral sclerosis (ALS or Lou Gehrig's disease), dementias, Huntington disease, multiple sclerosis, and Parkinson disease. Information about the prevalence of these disorders in the United States and their diagnosis and treatment is also included.

Part V: Other Brain Disorders provides a description of cerebral palsy, headache, hydrocephalus, and narcolepsy, including facts about how they are diagnosed and treated.

Part VI: Additional Help and Information offers a glossary of terms related to brain disorders and injuries and a directory of organizations that can provide further information and help in specific areas.

Bibliographic Note

This volume contains documents and excerpts from publications issued by the following U.S. government agencies: Centers for Disease Control and Prevention (CDC); National Cancer Institute (NCI); National Institute of Neurological Diseases and Disorders (NINDS); U.S. Food and Drug Administration (FDA); and the Women's Health Initiative (WHI).

In addition, this volume contains copyrighted documents from the following organizations and individuals: A.D.A.M., Inc.; American Association of Neurological Surgeons; American Heart Association; American Society of Interventional and Therapeutic Neuroradiology; Biological Sciences Curriculum Study; Brain Injury Association; Epilepsy Association of Australia; Epilepsy.com; Epilepsy Kingston and Area; Epilepsy Ontario; Epilepsy Toronto; Family Caregiver Alliance; Harvard Health Publications; Healthcommunities.com; International RadioSurgery Association; Lippincott Williams and Wilkins; Medtronic, Inc.; National Kidney Foundation; Nemours Foundation; Neurological Institute of New York at Columbia University Medical Center, Doppler Neurosonology Laboratory; New Mexico AIDS InfoNet; Parkinson's Disease Foundation; and University of Missouri-Columbia Health Care.

Full citation information is provided on the first page of each chapter. Every effort has been made to secure all necessary rights to reprint the copyrighted material. If any omissions have been made, please contact Omnigraphics to make corrections for future editions.

Acknowledgements

Thanks go to the many organizations, agencies, and individuals who have contributed materials for this *Sourcebook* and to medical consultant Dr. David Cooke, verification assistant Dawn Matthews, and document engineer Bruce Bellenir. Special thanks go to managing editor Karen Bellenir and permissions specialist Liz Barbour for their help and support.

About the Health Reference Series

The *Health Reference Series* is designed to provide basic medical information for patients, families, caregivers, and the general public. Each volume takes a particular topic and provides comprehensive coverage. This is especially important for people who may be dealing with a newly diagnosed disease or a chronic disorder in themselves or in a family member. People looking for preventive guidance, information about disease warning signs, medical statistics, and risk factors for health problems will also find answers to their questions in the *Health Reference Series*. The *Series*, however, is not intended to serve as a tool for diagnosing illness, in prescribing treatments, or as a substitute for the physician/patient relationship. All people concerned about medical symptoms or the possibility of disease are encouraged to seek professional care from an appropriate health care provider.

Locating Information within the Health Reference Series

The *Health Reference Series* contains a wealth of information about a wide variety of medical topics. Ensuring easy access to all the fact sheets, research reports, in-depth discussions, and other material contained within the individual books of the series remains one of our highest priorities. As the *Series* continues to grow in size and scope, however, locating the precise information needed by a reader may become more challenging.

A *Contents Guide to the Health Reference Series* was developed to direct readers to the specific volumes that address their concerns. It presents an extensive list of diseases, treatments, and other topics of general interest compiled from the Tables of Contents and major index headings. To access *A Contents Guide to the Health Reference Series*, visit www.healthreferenceseries.com.

xii

Medical Consultant

Medical consultation services are provided to the *Health Reference Series* editors by David A. Cooke, M.D. Dr. Cooke is a graduate of Brandeis University, and he received his M.D. degree from the University of Michigan. He completed residency training at the University of Wisconsin Hospital and Clinics. He is board-certified in Internal Medicine. Dr. Cooke currently works as part of the University of Michigan Health System and practices in Brighton, MI. In his free time, he enjoys writing, science fiction, and spending time with his family.

Our Advisory Board

We would like to thank the following board members for providing guidance to the development of this series:

Dr. Lynda Baker,
Associate Professor of Library and Information Science,
Wayne State University, Detroit, MI

Nancy Bulgarelli,
William Beaumont Hospital Library, Royal Oak, MI

Karen Imarisio,
Bloomfield Township Public Library, Bloomfield Township, MI

Karen Morgan,
Mardigian Library, University of Michigan-Dearborn,
Dearborn, MI

Rosemary Orlando,
St. Clair Shores Public Library, St. Clair Shores, MI

Health Reference Series *Update Policy*

The inaugural book in the *Health Reference Series* was the first edition of *Cancer Sourcebook* published in 1989. Since then, the *Series* has been enthusiastically received by librarians and in the medical community. In order to maintain the standard of providing high-quality health information for the layperson the editorial staff at Omnigraphics felt it was necessary to implement a policy of updating volumes when warranted.

Medical researchers have been making tremendous strides, and it is the purpose of the *Health Reference Series* to stay current with the most recent advances. Each decision to update a volume is made on an individual basis. Some of the considerations include how much new information is available and the feedback we receive from people who use the books. If there is a topic you would like to see added to the update list, or an area of medical concern you feel has not been adequately addressed, please write to:

Editor
Health Reference Series
Omnigraphics, Inc.
615 Griswold Street
Detroit, MI 48226
E-mail: editorial@omnigraphics.com

Part One

Understanding Brain Function

Chapter 1

Anatomy of the Brain

The brain serves many important functions. It gives meaning to things that happen in the world surrounding us.

We have five senses: sight, smell, hearing, touch, and taste. Through these senses, our brain receives messages, often many at one time. It puts together the messages in a way that has meaning for us, and can store that information in our memory. For example: An oven burner has been left on. By accident we touch the burner. Our brain receives a message from skin sensors on our hand. Instead of leaving our hand on the burner, our brain gives meaning to the signal and tells us to quickly remove our hand from the burner. Heat has been felt. If we were to leave our hand on the burner, pain and injury would result. As adults, we may have had a childhood memory of touching something hot that resulted in pain or watching someone else who has done so. Our brain uses that memory in a time of need and guides our actions and reactions in a harmful situation.

With the use of our senses: sight, smell, touch, taste, and hearing, the brain receives many messages at one time. It can select those that are most important. Our brain controls our thoughts, memory, and speech, the movements of our arms and legs, and the function of many organs within our body. It also determines how we respond to stressful situations (i.e., writing of an exam, loss of a job, birth of a child, illness, etc.) by regulating our heart and breathing rate. The brain is an organized structure, divided into many parts that serve specific and important functions.

Understanding the Nervous System

The nervous system is commonly divided into the central nervous system and the peripheral nervous system. The central nervous system is made up of the brain, its cranial nerves, and the spinal cord. The peripheral nervous system is composed of the spinal nerves that branch from the spinal cord and the autonomous nervous system (divided into the sympathetic and parasympathetic nervous system). It controls our response to stressful situations.

For the purpose of this chapter, we will speak specifically about some of the functions and parts of the brain. This is not to say that the brain functions alone. The central and peripheral nervous systems play many interconnected and complex roles.

A Microscopic View of the Brain

The brain is made up of two types of cells: neurons and neuroglia. The neuron is responsible for sending and receiving nerve impulses or signals. Try to picture electrical wiring in your home. An electrical circuit is made up of numerous wires connected in such a way that when a light switch is turned on, a light bulb will beam. A neuron that is excited will transmit its energy to neurons that are within its vicinity. Remember the sequence of events of drawing your hand away from a hot oven burner. A series of excited, interconnected neurons made you withdraw your hand.

Neuroglia provide neurons with nourishment, protection, and structural support. They are the most common types of cells involved in tumors that have originated in the brain. Astroglia or astrocytes, oligodendroglia, and ependymal cells are the types of glial cells commonly found in the brain. The name given a brain tumor may reflect the type of cell that is involved (e.g., astrocytoma, meaning astroglia or astrocyte cells are involved).

If you were to look under a microscope, you would be able to distinguish heart cells from brain cells. A neurosurgeon may remove tissue from a brain tumor to be studied by experts in the field of pathology. Pathologists, by identifying the type of cells that are present in brain tissue, will give brain tumor a particular name. Surgery, radiotherapy, or chemotherapy may be used to effectively treat the tumor.

The Meninges

The brain is found inside the bony covering called the cranium. The cranium protects the brain from injury. Together, the cranium and bones that protect our face are called the skull.

Meninges are three layers of tissue that cover and protect the brain and spinal cord. From the outermost layer inward they are: the dura mater, arachnoid, and pia mater.

In the brain, the dura mater is made up of two layers of whitish, inelastic (not stretchy) film or membrane. The outer layer is called the periosteum. An inner layer, the dura, lines the inside of the entire skull and creates little folds or compartments in which parts of the brain are neatly protected and secured. There are two special folds of the dura in the brain, the falx and the tentorium. The falx separates the right and left half of the brain and the tentorium separates the upper and lower parts of the brain.

The second layer of the meninges is the arachnoid. This membrane is thin and delicate and covers the entire brain. There is a space between the dura and the arachnoid membranes that is called the subdural space. The arachnoid is made up of delicate, elastic tissue and blood vessels of different sizes.

The layer of meninges closest to the surface of the brain is called the pia mater. The pia mater has many blood vessels that reach deep into the surface of the brain. The pia, which covers the entire surface of the brain, follows the folds of the brain. The major arteries supplying the brain provide the pia with its blood vessels. The space that separates the arachnoid and the pia is called the subarachnoid space. It is here where the cerebrospinal fluid (discussed next) will flow.

Cerebrospinal Fluid

Cerebrospinal fluid, also known as CSF, is found within the brain and surrounds the brain and the spinal cord. It is a clear, watery substance that helps to cushion the brain and spinal cord from injury. This fluid circulates through channels around the spinal cord and brain, constantly being absorbed and replenished. It is within hollow channels in the brain, called ventricles, where the fluid is produced. A specialized structure within each ventricle, called the choroid plexus, is responsible for the majority of CSF production. The brain normally maintains a balance between the amount of cerebrospinal fluid that is absorbed and the amount that is produced. Often, disruptions in the system occur.

The Ventricular System

The ventricular system is divided into four cavities called ventricles, which are connected by a series of holes (called foramen) and tubes.

Two ventricles enclosed in the cerebral hemispheres are called the lateral ventricles (first and second). They each communicate with the third ventricle through a separate opening called the Foramen of Munro.

The third ventricle is in the center of the brain, and its walls are made up of the thalamus and hypothalamus. The third ventricle connects with the fourth ventricle through a long tube called the Aqueduct of Sylvius.

Cerebrospinal fluid flowing through the fourth ventricle gets around the brain and spinal cord by passing through another series of openings. The condition hydrocephalus may occur when there is a blockage in the pathways through which the fluid normally travels. It may also arise from an overproduction of fluid or a difficulty in absorbing the fluid that is produced. Because the brain is enclosed within the bony skull, the extra fluid, trapped by blocked pathways, has no escape. This extra fluid within the brain will produce increased pressure symptoms: headaches, vomiting, drowsiness, and in some cases, confusion.

Brain tumors may block the channels of cerebrospinal fluid within the brain. Rare tumors involving the choroid plexus within the ventricles may affect the production and absorption of the fluid. Spinal cord tumors may block the fluid as it travels around the spinal cord. A surgical procedure of shunting extra fluid may be necessary.

Structures of the Brain

Cerebrum

The cerebrum, which forms the bulk of the brain, may be divided into two major parts: the right and left cerebral hemispheres. The cerebrum is often a term used to describe the entire brain. There is a fissure or groove that separates the two hemispheres, called the great longitudinal fissure (the falx of the dura is here). The two sides of the brain are joined at the bottom by the corpus callosum. The corpus callosum connects the two halves of the brain and delivers messages from one half of the brain to the other. The surface of the cerebrum (brain) contains billions of neurons and glia that together form the cerebral cortex.

The (cerebral) cortex appears grayish-brown in color and is called the "gray matter." The surface of the brain appears wrinkled. The cerebral cortex has small grooves (sulci), larger grooves (fissures), and bulges between the grooves called gyri. Scientists have specific names for the bulges and grooves on the surface of our brain. They serve as landmarks and are used to help isolate very specific regions of the brain. Decades of scientific research have revealed the specific functions of the various regions of the brain. Beneath the cerebral cortex or surface of the brain, connecting fibers between neurons form the "white matter" (appears white in color).

The cerebral hemispheres have several distinct fissures. By finding these landmarks on the surface of a brain, the brain can effectively be divided into pairs of "lobes." Lobes are simply broad regions of the brain. The cerebrum or brain may be divided into pairs of frontal, temporal, parietal, and occipital lobes. To state this in another way, each hemisphere has a frontal, temporal, parietal, and occipital lobe. Each lobe may be divided, once again, into areas that serve very specific functions. It must be remembered that each lobe of the brain does not function alone. There are very complex relationships between the lobes of the brain.

Messages within the brain are delivered in many ways. The signals are transported along routes called pathways. Any destruction of brain tissue by a tumor can disrupt the communication between different parts of the brain. The result will be a loss of function such as speech, ability to read, or ability to follow simple spoken commands. Messages can travel from one bulge on the brain to another (gyri to gyri), from one lobe to another, from one side of the brain to the other, from one lobe of the brain to structures that are found deep in the brain (e.g., the thalamus), or from the deep structures of the brain to another region in the central nervous system.

Researchers have stimulated the surface of the brain during surgery with an electrode that delivered a very weak electrical shock. It has been found that specific regions of the motor and sensory regions, when electrically stimulated, will cause movement or sensation to occur in a very specific part of the body. Touching one side of the brain sends the electrical signals to the other side of the body. If we touched the motor region on the right side of the brain, we would cause the opposite side or the left side of the body to move. Stimulating the left primary motor cortex would cause the right side of the body to move. The messages for movement and sensation will always cross to the other side of the brain and cause the opposite limb to move or feel a sensation. If your brain tumor is located on the right side of the brain in an area that controls the movement of your arm, your left arm may be weak or paralyzed. Each side of the brain controls the opposite side of the body.

Parts of the Brain and Their Functions

The following is a summary of the functions of the parts of the brain and their location.

Frontal Lobes

The areas that produce movement of parts of the body are found in the primary motor cortex or precentral gyrus. These regions are found in the frontal lobes.

The prefrontal cortex plays an important part in our memory, intelligence, concentration, temper, and personality. It helps us set goals, make plans, and judge our priorities.

The premotor cortex is a region found beside the primary motor cortex. It guides our eye and head movements and sense of orientation. Broca's area, important in language production, is found in the frontal lobe, usually on the left side.

Occipital Lobes

These lobes contain regions that contribute to our visual field or how our eyes see the world around us. They help us see light and objects and allow us to recognize and identify them. This region is called the visual cortex.

The occipital lobe on the right interprets visual signals from your left visual space, while the left occipital lobe does the same for your right visual space. Damage to one occipital lobe may result in loss of vision in the opposite visual field.

Temporal Lobes

The primary auditory cortex helps us hear sounds and gives sounds their meaning (e.g., the bark of a dog). The temporal lobes are the primary region responsible for memory. They contain Wernicke's area, which is involved in language and speech functions.

Parietal Lobes

The parietal lobes interpret, simultaneously, sensory signals received from other areas of the brain such as our vision, hearing, motor, sensory, and memory. Together, memory and the new information that is received give meaning to objects. A furry object touching your skin that purrs and appears to be your cat will have a different meaning than a furry object that barks and you see to be a dog.

Hypothalamus

The hypothalamus is a small structure that contains nerve connections that send messages to the pituitary gland. The hypothalamus handles information that comes from the autonomic nervous system. It plays a role in controlling our behavior, such as eating, sexual behavior, and sleeping, and regulates body temperature, emotions, secretion of hormones, and movement. The pituitary gland develops from an extension of the hypothalamus downward and from a second component extending upward from the roof of the mouth. These two components form the pituitary gland, which sits in a specialized bony container at the base of the skull called the pituitary fossa. It is involved in controlling a number of hormonal functions, including thyroid functions, functions of the adrenal glands, growth, and sexual maturation. The posterior part of the pituitary gland regulates the formation of urine.

Pineal Gland

The pineal gland is an outgrowth from the posterior or back portion of the third ventricle. In some mammals, it controls the response to darkness and light. In humans, it has some role in sexual maturation although the exact function of the pineal gland in humans is unclear.

Thalamus

The thalamus serves as a relay station for almost all information that comes from and goes to the cortex. It plays a role in pain sensation, attention, and alertness.

Cerebellum

The cerebellum is located at the back of the brain beneath the occipital lobes. It is separated from the cerebrum by the tentorium (fold of dura). The cerebellum fine-tunes our motor activity or movement (e.g., the fine movements of our fingers as they print a story or color a picture). It helps us maintain our posture and our sense of balance or equilibrium by controlling the tone of our muscles, and senses the position of our limbs. A tumor affecting the cerebellum may cause an individual to stagger and sway when he or she walks or have jerky movements of the arms and legs (a drunken appearance). An individual trying to reach an object may misjudge the distance and location of the object and fail to reach the object. The cerebellum is important in one's ability to perform rapid and repetitive actions, such as playing a video game. In the cerebellum, right-sided abnormalities produce symptoms on the same side of the body.

The brain stem is located in front of the cerebellum and may be considered as a "stem" or structure holding up the cerebrum. It consists of three structures: the midbrain, pons, and medulla oblongata. It serves as a relay station, passing messages back and forth between various parts of the body and the cerebral cortex. Many simple or primitive functions that are essential for survival are located here.

The midbrain is an important center for ocular motion, while the pons is involved with coordinating the eye and facial movements, facial sensation, hearing, and balance.

The medulla oblongata controls our breathing, blood pressure, heart rhythms, and swallowing. These functions are important to our survival. Messages from the cortex to the spinal cord and nerves that branch from the spinal cord are sent through the pons and the brain stem. Destruction of these regions of the brain will cause "brain death." The heart will no longer be able to beat on its own. Lungs will not be able to work on their own. Because we will be unable to breathe, oxygen will not be delivered to the brain. Brain cells, which require oxygen to survive, will die.

The reticular activating system is found in the midbrain, pons, medulla, and part of the thalamus. It controls our level of wakefulness, the attention we pay to what happens in the world that surrounds us and our pattern of sleep.

Originating in the brain stem are ten of the twelve cranial nerves that control hearing, eye movement, facial sensations, taste, swallowing, and movement of the face, neck, shoulder, and tongue muscles. The cranial nerves for smell and vision originate in the cerebrum. A tumor in this area may readily affect these nerves, causing, for example, one eye to "turn in" and the child to complain of double vision, or drooping of one side of the mouth with drooling.

10

Limbic System

This system is involved in our emotions. Included in this system are the hypothalamus, part of the thalamus, amygdala (active in producing aggressive behavior), and hippocampus (plays a role in our ability to remember new information).

Language and Speech Functions

In general, the left hemisphere or side of the brain is responsible for language and speech. Because of this, it has been called the "dominant" hemisphere. The right hemisphere plays a large part in interpreting visual information and spatial processing. In about one-third of individuals who are left-handed, speech function may be located on the right side of the brain. Left-handed individuals may need specialized testing to determine if their speech center is on the left or right side prior to any surgery in that area.

There is an area in the frontal lobe of the left hemisphere called Broca's area. It is beside the region that controls the movement of our facial muscles, tongue, jaw, and throat. If this area is destroyed, there is difficulty in producing the sounds of speech. One is unable to move the tongue or facial muscles in the appropriate way to make words. The individual can still read and understand spoken language but has difficulty in speaking and writing (i.e., forming letters and words, writing within lines). This problem is called Broca's aphasia.

There is a region in the left temporal lobe called Wernicke's area. Damage to this area causes Wernicke's aphasia. Words are heard but are meaningless (receptive aphasia). An individual can make speech sounds. These sounds, however, have no meaning, for the individual is unable to understand what is said by him or others.

Many neuroscientists believe that the left hemisphere and perhaps other portions of the brain are important in language. An aphasia is simply a disturbance of language. Certain parts of the brain are responsible for specific functions in language production. There are many types of aphasias, each depending upon the brain area that is affected, and the role that area plays in language production.

Cranial Nerves

There are twelve pairs of nerves that come from the brain itself. These are called the cranial nerves. These nerves are responsible for some very specialized features and they have traditionally been both named and numbered.

Table 1.1. Cranial Nerves and Their Function

Cranial Nerve	Function
I Olfactory	Smell
II Optic	Visual fields and ability to see
III Oculomotor	Eye movements; eyelid opening
IV Trochlear	Eye movements
V Trigeminal	Facial sensation
VI Abducens	Eye movements
VII Facial	Eyelid closing; facial expression; taste sensation
VIII Acoustic	Hearing; sense of balance
IX Glossopharyngeal	Taste sensation; swallowing
X Vagus	Swallowing; taste sensation
XI Accessory	Controls neck and shoulder muscles
XII Hypoglossal	Tongue movement

Chapter 2

Neurons, Brain Chemistry, and Neurotransmission

Communication between neurons is the foundation for brain function. Understanding how neurotransmission occurs is crucial to understanding how the brain processes and integrates information. Interruption of neural communication causes changes in cognitive processes and behavior.

The Brain Is Made Up of Nerve Cells and Glial Cells

The brain of an adult human weighs about three pounds and contains billions of cells. The two distinct classes of cells in the nervous system are neurons (nerve cells) and glia (glial cells).

The basic signaling unit of the nervous system is the neuron. The brain contains billions of neurons; the best estimates are that the adult human brain contains 10^{11} neurons. The interactions between neurons enable people to think, move, maintain homeostasis, and feel emotions. A neuron is a specialized cell that can produce different actions because of its precise connections with other neurons, sensory receptors, and muscle cells. A typical neuron has four morphologically defined regions: the cell body, dendrites, axons, and presynaptic terminals (see Figure 2.1).[1,2,3]

The cell body, also called the soma, is the metabolic center of the neuron. The nucleus is located in the cell body, and most of the cell's protein synthesis occurs in the cell body.

A neuron usually has multiple processes, or fibers, called dendrites that extend from the cell body. These processes usually branch out somewhat like tree branches and serve as the main apparatus for receiving input into the neuron from other nerve cells.

The cell body also gives rise to the axon. Axons can be very long processes; in some cases, they may be up to one meter in length. The axon is the part of the neuron that is specialized to carry messages away from the cell body and to relay messages to other cells. Some large axons are surrounded by a fatty insulating material called myelin, which enables the electrical signals to travel down the axon at higher speeds.

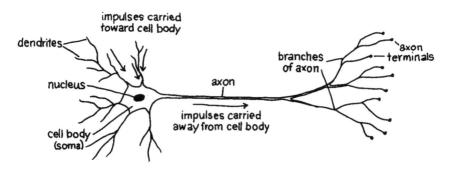

Figure 2.1. The neuron, or nerve cell, is the functional unit of the nervous system. The neuron has processes called dendrites that receive signals and an axon that transmits signals to another neuron.

Near its end, the axon divides into many fine branches that have specialized swellings called presynaptic terminals. These presynaptic terminals end in close proximity to the dendrites of another neuron. The dendrite of one neuron receives the message sent from the presynaptic terminal of another neuron (see Figure 2.2).

The site where a presynaptic terminal ends in close proximity to a receiving dendrite is called the synapse. The cell that sends out information is called the presynaptic neuron, and the cell that receives the information is called the postsynaptic neuron. It is important to note that the synapse is not a physical connection between the two neurons; there is no cytoplasmic continuity between the two neurons. The intercellular space between the presynaptic and postsynaptic neurons is called the synaptic space or synaptic cleft. An average neuron forms approximately one thousand synapses with other neurons. It

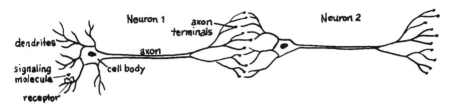

Figure 2.2. *Neurons transmit information to other neurons. Information passes from the axon of the presynaptic neuron to the dendrites of the postsynaptic neuron.*

has been estimated that there are more synapses in the human brain than there are stars in our galaxy. Furthermore, synaptic connections are not static. Neurons form new synapses or strengthen synaptic connections in response to life experiences. This dynamic change in neuronal connections is the basis of learning (see Figure 2.3).

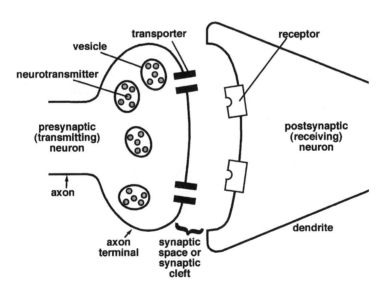

Figure 2.3. *The synapse is the site where chemical signals pass between neurons. Neurotransmitter is released from the presynaptic neuron terminals into the extracellular space, the synaptic cleft or synaptic space. The released neurotransmitter molecules can then bind to specific receptors on the postsynaptic neuron membrane to elicit a response.*

The brain contains another class of cells called glia. There are as many as ten to fifty times more glial cells than neurons in the central nervous system. Glial cells are categorized as microglia or macroglia. Microglia are phagocytic cells that are mobilized after injury, infection, or disease. They are derived from macrophages and are unrelated to other cell types in the nervous system. The three types of macroglia are oligodendrocytes, astrocytes, and Schwann cells. The oligodendrocytes and Schwann cells form the myelin sheaths that insulate axons and enhance conduction of electrical signals along the axons.

Scientists know less about the functions of glial cells than they do about the functions of neurons. Glial cells fulfill a variety of functions:

- Glial cells function as supporting elements in the nervous system to provide structure and to separate and insulate groups of neurons.

- Oligodendrocytes in the central nervous system and Schwann cells in the peripheral nervous system form myelin, the sheath that wraps around certain axons.

- Some glial cells are scavengers that remove debris after injury or neuronal death.

- Some glial cells buffer the potassium ion (K+) concentration in the extracellular space, and some glial cells take up and remove chemical neurotransmitters from the extracellular space after synaptic transmission.

- Some glial cells guide the migration of neurons and direct the outgrowth of axons during development.

- Some glial cells induce formation of impermeable tight junctions in endothelial cells that line the capillaries and venules of the brain to form the blood-brain barrier.

- Glial cells may serve nutritive functions for nerve cells.[3]

The Blood-Brain Barrier

The blood-brain barrier protects the neurons and glial cells in the brain from substances that could harm the cells. Endothelial cells that form the capillaries and venules make this barrier, forming impermeable tight junctions. Astrocytes surround the endothelial cells and induce them to form these junctions. Unlike blood vessels in other parts of the body that are relatively leaky to a variety of molecules, the blood-brain barrier keeps many substances, including toxins, away from the neurons and glia. Blood gases, such as oxygen, and small nutritional molecules do get into the brain.[3,4] In addition, drugs of abuse can penetrate the blood-brain barrier. Because most drugs are fat-soluble, they can pass through the barrier to reach the brain cells. The blood-brain barrier is important for maintaining the environment of neurons in the brain, but it also presents problems for scientists who are investigating new treatments for brain disorders. If a medication cannot get into the brain to the neurons, it cannot be effective. Researchers attempt to circumvent the problems in different ways. Some techniques attach potential therapeutic agents to molecules that pass through the blood-brain barrier, while others attempt to open the blood-brain barrier so that the therapeutic compounds can reach the brain's neurons.[5]

Neurons Use Electrical and Chemical Signals to Transmit Information

The billions of neurons that make up the brain coordinate thought, behavior, homeostasis, and more. How do all these neurons pass and receive information?

Neurons convey information by transmitting messages to other neurons or other types of cells, such as muscles. The following discussion focuses on how one neuron communicates with another neuron. Neurons employ electrical signals to relay information from one part of the neuron to another. The neuron converts the electrical signal to a chemical signal in order to pass the information to another neuron. The target neuron then converts the message back to an electrical impulse to continue the process.

Within a single neuron, information is conducted via electrical signaling. When a neuron is stimulated, an electrical impulse, called an action potential, moves along the neuron axon or dendrite.[6] Action potentials enable signals to travel very rapidly along the neuron fiber. Action potentials last less than 2 milliseconds (1 millisecond = 0.001 second), and the fastest action potentials can travel the length of a football field in 1 second. Action potentials result from the flow of ions across the neuronal cell membrane. Neurons, like all cells, maintain a balance of ions inside the cell that differs from the balance outside the cell. This uneven distribution of ions creates an electrical potential across the cell membrane. This is called the resting membrane potential. In humans, the resting membrane potential ranges from -40 millivolts (mV) to -80 mV, with -65 mV as an average resting membrane potential. The resting membrane potential is, by convention, assigned a negative number because the inside of the neuron is more negatively charged than the outside of the neuron. This negative charge results from the unequal distribution of sodium ions (Na+), potassium ions (K+), chloride ions (Cl-), and other organic ions. The resting membrane potential is maintained by an energy-dependent Na+-K+ pump that keeps Na+ levels low inside the neuron and K+ levels high inside the neuron. In addition, the neuronal membrane is more permeable to K+ than it is to Na+, so K+ tends to leak out of the cell more readily than Na+ diffuses into the cell.

A stimulus occurring at the end of a nerve fiber starts an electrical change that travels like a wave over the length of the neuron. This electrical change, the action potential, results from a change in the permeability of the neuronal membrane. Sodium ions rush into the neuron, and the inside of the cell becomes more positive. The Na+-K+ pump then restores the balance of sodium and potassium to resting levels. However, the influx of Na+ ions in one area of the neuron fiber starts a similar change in the adjoining segment, and the impulse moves from one end of the neuronal fiber to the other. Action potentials are an all-or-none phenomenon. Regardless of the stimuli, the amplitude and duration of an action potential are the same. The action potential either occurs or it doesn't. The response of the neuron to an action potential depends on how many action potentials it transmits and the time interval between them.

Electrical signals carry information within a single neuron. Communication between neurons (with a few exceptions in mammals) is a chemical process. When the neuron is stimulated, the electrical signal (action potential) travels down the axon to the axon terminals.

When the electrical signal reaches the end of the axon, it triggers a series of chemical changes in the neuron. Calcium ions (Ca++) flow into the neuron. The increased Ca++ in the axon terminal then initiates the release of neurotransmitter. A neurotransmitter is a molecule that is released from a neuron to relay information to another cell. Neurotransmitter molecules are stored in membranous sacs called vesicles in the axon terminal. Each vesicle contains thousands of molecules of a neurotransmitter. For neurons to release their neurotransmitter, the vesicles fuse with the neuronal membrane and then release their contents, the neurotransmitter, via exocytosis. The neurotransmitter molecules are released into the synaptic space and diffuse across the synaptic space to the postsynaptic neuron. A neurotransmitter molecule can then bind to a special receptor on the membrane of the postsynaptic neuron. Receptors are membrane proteins that are able to bind a specific chemical substance, such as a neurotransmitter. For example, the dopamine receptor binds the neurotransmitter dopamine, but does not bind other neurotransmitters such as serotonin. The interaction of a receptor and neurotransmitter can be thought of as a lock-and-key for regulating neuronal function. Just as a key fits only a specific lock, a neurotransmitter binds only to a specific receptor. The chemical binding of neurotransmitter and receptor initiates changes in the postsynaptic neuron that may generate an action potential in the postsynaptic neuron. If it does trigger an action potential, the communication process continues. After a neurotransmitter molecule binds to its receptor on the postsynaptic neuron, it comes off (is released from) the receptor and diffuses back into the synaptic space. The released neurotransmitter, as well as any neurotransmitter that did not bind to a receptor, is either degraded by enzymes in the synaptic cleft or taken back up into the presynaptic axon terminal by active transport through a transporter or reuptake pump. Once the neurotransmitter is back inside the axon terminal, it is either destroyed or repackaged into new vesicles that may be released the next time the neuron is stimulated. Different neurotransmitters are inactivated in different ways. (See Figures 2.4 and 2.5.)

Neurotransmitters Can Be Excitatory or Inhibitory

Different neurotransmitters fulfill different functions in the brain. Some neurotransmitters act to stimulate the firing of a postsynaptic neuron. Neurotransmitters that act this way are called excitatory neurotransmitters because they lead to changes that generate an action potential in the responding neuron.[1,7] Other neurotransmitters, called inhibitory neurotransmitters, tend to block the changes that cause an action potential to be generated in the responding cell. Table 2.1 lists some of the major neurotransmitters used in the body and their major functions. Each neuron generally synthesizes and releases a single type of neurotransmitter. (Neurons may contain other signaling chemicals, such as neurohormones, in addition to their neurotransmitter.)

The postsynaptic neuron often receives both excitatory and inhibitory messages. The response of the postsynaptic cell depends on which message is stronger. Keep in mind that a single neurotransmitter molecule cannot cause an action potential in the responding neuron. An action potential occurs when many neurotransmitter molecules bind to and activate their receptors. Each interaction contributes to the membrane permeability changes that generate the resultant action potential.

19

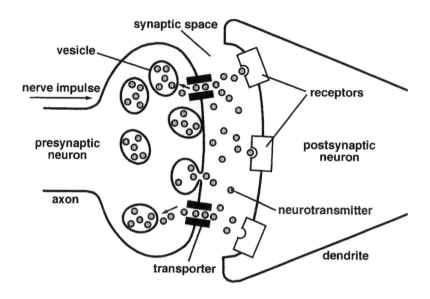

Figure 2.4. *Schematic diagram of a synapse. In response to an electrical impulse, neurotransmitter molecules released from the presynaptic axon terminal bind to the specific receptors for that neurotransmitter on the postsynaptic neuron. After binding to the receptor, the neurotransmitter molecules either may be taken back up into the presynaptic neuron through the transporter molecules for repackaging into vesicles or may be degraded by enzymes present in the synaptic cleft.*

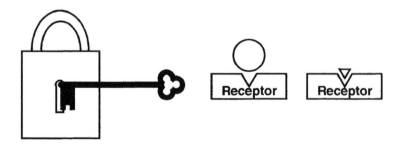

Figure 2.5. *Like a lock that will open only if the right key is used, a receptor will bind only a molecule that has the right chemical shape. Molecules that do not have the right "fit" will not bind to the receptor and will not cause a response.*

Table 2.1. Major Neurotransmitters in the Body

Neurotransmitter	Role in the body
Acetylcholine	A neurotransmitter used by spinal cord neurons to control muscles and by many neurons in the brain to regulate memory. In most instances, acetylcholine is excitatory.
Dopamine	The neurotransmitter that produces feelings of pleasure when released by the brain reward system. Dopamine has multiple functions depending on where in the brain it acts. It is usually inhibitory.
GABA (gamma-aminobutyric acid)	The major inhibitory neurotransmitter in the brain.
Glutamate	The most common excitatory neurotransmitter in the brain.
Glycine	A neurotransmitter used mainly by neurons in the spinal cord. It probably always acts as an inhibitory neurotransmitter.
Norepinephrine	Acts as a neurotransmitter and a hormone. In the peripheral nervous system, it is part of the fight-or-flight response. In the brain, it acts as a neurotransmitter regulating normal brain processes. Norepinephrine is usually excitatory, but is inhibitory in a few brain areas.
Serotonin	A neurotransmitter involved in many functions including mood, appetite, and sensory perception. In the spinal cord, serotonin is inhibitory in pain pathways.

Sources: D. P. Friedman and S. Rusche, *False Messengers: How Addictive Drugs Change the Brain* (Amsterdam: Harwood Academic Publishers, 1999); A. C. Guyton and J. E. Hall, "Organization of the Nervous System; Basic Functions of Synapses and Transmitter Substances," in *Textbook of Medical Physiology,* 9th ed. (Philadelphia: W. B. Saunders Company, 1996), 565–82; Society for Neuroscience *The Short Answer: Definitions for Common Neuroscience Terms,* 1999. Retrieved September 4, 2000, from the World Wide Web: http://apu.sfn.org/content/Publications/BrainBackgrounders/glossary.htm.

Resources

1. D. P. Friedman and S. Rusche. 1999. *False Messengers: How Addictive Drugs Change the Brain.* Amsterdam: Harwood Academic Publishers.

2. National Institute on Drug Abuse. 1997. *Mind over Matter: The Brain's Response to Drugs.* NIH Publication No. 98-3592. Retrieved August 21, 2000, from the World Wide Web: http://165.112.78.61/MOM/MOMIndex.html.

3. E. R. Kandel. 1991. "Nerve Cells and Behavior." In E. R. Kandel, J. H. Schwartz, and T. M. Jessell, eds., *Principles of Neural Science,* 3d ed., 18–32. Norwalk, CT: Appleton & Lange.

4. L. P. Rowland, M. E. Fink, and L. Rubin. 1991. "Cerebrospinal Fluid: Blood-Brain Barrier, Brain Edema, and Hydrocephalus." In E. R. Kandel, J. H. Schwartz, and T. M. Jessell, eds., *Principles of Neural Science,* 3d ed., 1050–60. Norwalk, CT: Appleton & Lange.

5. Society for Neuroscience. 1999. *Blood-Brain Barrier.* Retrieved August 21, 2000, from the World Wide Web: http://web.sfn.org/content/Publications/BrainBriefings/blood-brain.html.

6. J. Darnell, H. Lodish, and D. Baltimore. 1990. "Nerve Cells and the Electric Properties of Cell Membranes." In *Molecular Cell Biology,* 2d ed., 763–814. New York: Scientific American Books, W. H. Freeman and Company.

7. A. C. Guyton and J. E. Hall. 1996. "Organization of the Nervous System; Basic Functions of Synapses and Transmitter Substances." In *Textbook of Medical Physiology,* 9th ed., 565–82. Philadelphia: W. B. Saunders Company.

8. Society for Neuroscience. 1999. *The Short Answer: Definitions for Common Neuroscience Terms.* Retrieved September 4, 2000, from the World Wide Web: http://apu.sfn.org/content/Publications/BrainBackgrounders/glossary.htm.

Chapter 3

Tests Used in Diagnosing Brain Disorders

Chapter Contents

Section 3.1—Carotid Ultrasound 24
Section 3.2—Cerebral Angiography 27
Section 3.3—Cranial Computed Tomography (CT) Scan 31
Section 3.4—Electroencephalogram (EEG) 35
Section 3.5—Electromyography (EMG) 39
Section 3.6—Nerve Conduction Velocity Test 42
Section 3.7—Magnetic Resonance Imaging (MRI) 45
Section 3.8—Positron Emission Tomography (PET) Scan 47
Section 3.9—Spinal Tap (Lumbar Puncture) 51

Section 3.1

Carotid Ultrasound

What Is a Carotid Ultrasound?

A carotid ultrasound is a test that uses ultrasound waves to examine the arteries in the neck. These arteries are called carotid arteries and they are the major arteries that carry blood to the brain.

Carotid ultrasound is a noninvasive, safe, and painless procedure that helps doctors to detect hardening of the carotid arteries (atherosclerosis) or any blockage in the arteries.

How Does Carotid Ultrasound Work?

The Principles of Ultrasound

The probe (transducer) sends ultrasound waves and receives the reflected ultrasound waves from the arteries. A computer uses the information coming from the probe to construct ultrasound images of the neck arteries and compute blood flow velocities. The images are displayed on an ultrasound machine screen, printed on paper, and videotaped.

The Principles of Measuring Blood Flow Velocities within Arteries

To measure and calculate the velocities of the circulating blood within arteries of the neck an ultrasound machine uses the "Doppler principle" or "Doppler Effect," named after Christian Doppler (1803–53), the Austrian physicist who developed the famous principle. The Doppler principle is based on the fact that sound waves from a moving source are compressed or expanded, or that the frequency changes depending on whether the source is moving toward (compressed) or away (expanded) from the observer. The Doppler Effect was used to confirm that the universe is expanding.

In 1842, Doppler made an equation about the frequency and relative movement of sound source and observer. Doppler conducted a unique experiment to prove his theory. For two days, Doppler had a train pull repeatedly at different speeds a freight car with trumpeters playing on top of it. He then had a musician capable of determining the differences in sounds record the height of the notes played as the train moved closer (higher notes were recorded) or further away (lower notes were recorded). This effect proved Doppler's theory superbly.

What Does Carotid Ultrasound Show?

A carotid ultrasound test shows the walls of the carotid arteries and measures the blood flow velocities within arteries.

There are various abnormalities that can be detected by carotid ultrasound. These abnormalities can be mild, such as hardening or thickening of the wall of the carotid arteries, to severe, such as large plaques (large clots in the arteries) that obstruct the blood flow.

When the blood flow is severely obstructed by plaque in the carotid arteries, a stroke can occur. This process is similar to the buildup of plaque in the arteries to the heart that causes heart attacks. Since strokes occur in the brain, many doctors today refer to strokes as "brain attacks."

Stroke

Stroke is the third-leading cause of death in the United States today. Even stroke survivors are frequently left with permanent physical and mental disabilities. More than $70 billion are spent each year in this country to care for stroke and stroke survivors. The only way to save these lives, save the function of these limbs, and save the billions of dollars spent is to prevent stroke! Strokes due to carotid artery disease may be prevented. Severe carotid artery disease can be easily detected with this simple ultrasound examination that takes less than thirty minutes! You could nap right through this test and it might save your life!

Stroke Prevention

A simple ultrasound scan can quickly and easily tell if you have severe carotid disease. If you have a little bit of plaque the goal is to prevent it from becoming worse. When plaques grow to the point where they cause a 60–70 percent blockage or more, or if they cause symptoms of stroke, you may need treatment. This is where medical treatments and your own personal efforts can have a tremendous effect. Regular exercise, diet, and various medications may prevent stroke.

People with severe blockages in their carotid arteries should be considered for surgical treatment—called carotid endarterectomy. This procedure removes the plaque from inside the artery wall and restores the artery to normal. Recently, doctors specializing in the treatment of vascular problems started the use of balloon angioplasty and stent placement in the carotid arteries.

How Is Carotid Ultrasound Examination Performed?

You will be asked to lie on your back. An ultrasound transmission nonstaining gel and a probe will be placed on your neck.

How Long Does Carotid Ultrasound Take?

The entire test lasts from twenty to forty minutes, depending on the number of views, images, and Doppler velocity measurements.

Is Special Preparation for Carotid Ultrasound Necessary?

No special preparation is necessary for this test.

Is It Safe?

Carotid ultrasound is very safe. There are no risks from the ultrasound waves. Carotid ultrasound can be repeated many times without risks, complications, or side effects related to the ultrasound imaging.

What Are the Benefits?

A major benefit of the carotid ultrasound is that it provides information about the carotid arteries and blood flow to the brain without entering the body.

The information gained from the carotid ultrasound helps your doctor to make an accurate diagnosis and plan effective treatment that is best for you.

The Results

The results of the test will be reviewed and analyzed by a doctor after the test is performed. For the written results you may have to wait several days.

Section 3.2

Cerebral Angiography

Reprinted from "Cerebral Angiography," © 2003 A.D.A.M., Inc.
Reprinted with permission.

Alternative Names

Vertebral angiogram; Angiography—head; Carotid angiogram

Definition

The arteries are not normally seen in an x-ray, so a contrast dye is injected into one or more arteries to make them visible. For the cerebral angiography, the contrast dye is injected into one or both of the carotid or vertebral arteries that are in the neck.

How the Test Is Performed

This test is done in the hospital. You are asked to lie on the x-ray table. Your head is positioned and immobilized by using a strap, tape, or sandbags. Electrocardiogram (ECG) leads are taped to your arms and legs to monitor your heart during the test.

The area where the contrast dye will be injected is shaved and cleansed. The site is usually in the leg. You are given a local anesthetic, the artery is punctured, and a needle is inserted into the artery.

A catheter (a long, narrow, flexible tube) is inserted through the needle and into the artery. It is then threaded through the main vessels of the abdomen and chest until it is properly placed in the arteries of the neck. This procedure is monitored by a fluoroscope (a special x-ray that projects the images on a TV monitor).

27

The contrast dye is then injected into the neck area through the catheter, and the x-ray pictures are taken. The catheter is kept open by flushing it periodically with a saline solution containing heparin, which keeps the blood in the catheter from clotting. Your pulse, blood pressure, and breathing are monitored during the procedure.

After the x-rays are taken, the needle and catheter are withdrawn. Pressure is immediately applied on the leg at the site of insertion for ten to fifteen minutes to stop the bleeding. After that time, the area is checked and a tight bandage is applied. Your leg should be kept straight for twelve hours after the procedure.

Digital subtraction angiography (DSI) uses a computer to "subtract" out the bones and tissues in the region viewed such that only the vessels filled with contrast are seen.

How to Prepare for the Test

- Advise the health care provider if you are pregnant or if you have ever had any bleeding problems. Allergic reactions to x-ray contrast dye or any iodine substance and any other allergic reactions should be mentioned.

- You must sign a consent form.

- Routine blood tests will be done and an examination of the nervous system performed before the procedure.

- Food or fluid may be restricted four to eight hours before the procedure.

- You will be given a hospital gown to wear. You must remove all jewelry.

- A sedative or pain pill may be given to you before the procedure.

Infants and Children

The physical and psychological preparation you can provide for this or any test or procedure depends on your child's age, interests, previous experiences, and level of trust.

How the Test Will Feel

The x-ray table may be hard and cold, but you may ask for a blanket or pillow. There is a brief sting when the local anesthetic is given. This does not numb the artery, so there will be brief, sharp pain as the catheter is inserted into the artery. There is a slight feeling of pressure as the catheter is advanced.

As the dye is injected, there may be a warmth or burning sensation. You may experience a slight headache or feel flushed on the side of the face. There may be slight tenderness and bruising at the site of the injection after the test.

Why the Test Is Performed

The test is most frequently used to confirm cases of stroke, tumor, bulging of the artery walls, a clot, or a narrowing of the arteries, and to evaluate the arteries of the head and neck before a corrective surgery. It is used to get more exact information after something abnormal, such as bleeding within the brain, has been detected by an MRI or CT scan of the head.

What Abnormal Results Mean

If the contrast dye flows out of the blood vessel, it may indicate internal bleeding. Narrowed arteries may suggest cholesterol deposits, a spasm, or inherited disorders. If the vessels are displaced, this may be caused by tumors or bleeding within the skull, aneurysm (bulging of the artery walls), or malformation.

Additional Conditions under Which the Test May Be Performed

- arteriovenous malformation (cerebral)
- cerebral aneurysm
- hypertensive intracerebral hemorrhage
- intracerebral hemorrhage
- lobar intracerebral hemorrhage
- metastatic brain tumor
- neurosyphilis
- optic glioma
- pituitary tumor
- polycystic kidney disease
- primary brain tumor
- stroke secondary to carotid dissection
- stroke secondary to carotid stenosis

- stroke secondary to FMD [fibromuscular dysplasia]
- stroke secondary to syphilis
- syphilitic aseptic meningitis

What the Risks Are

There is the possibility of significant complications:

- A reaction to the contrast dye can occur.
- There is some risk of the catheter damaging the artery or knocking loose a piece of the artery wall, which can block blood flow and cause a stroke. This is rare, however.
- A clot or bleeding at the puncture site may result in a partial blockage of the blood to the leg.

Special Considerations

Notify your health care provider immediately if you have:

- facial weakness
- slurred speech
- visual trouble
- numbness in your leg during or after the procedure

Section 3.3

Cranial Computed Tomography (CT) Scan

Alternative Names

Head CT; CT scan—skull; CT scan—head; CT scan—orbits; CT scan—sinuses

Definition

A cranial CT scan involves computed tomography of the head, including the skull, brain, orbits (eyes), and sinuses.

How the Test Is Performed

A head CT will produce an image from the upper neck to the top of the head. If the patient cannot keep his or her head still, immobilization may be necessary. All jewelry, glasses, dentures, and other metal should be removed from the head and neck to prevent artifacts.

A contrast dye may be injected into a vein to further evaluate a mass. (The mass becomes brighter with contrast dye if it has a lot of blood vessels). Contrast dye is also used to produce an image of the blood vessels of the head and brain.

The total amount of time in the CT scanner is usually a few minutes.

How to Prepare for the Test

Generally, there is no preparation necessary.

Infants and Children

The physical and psychological preparation you can provide for this or any test or procedure depends on your child's age, interests, previous experiences, and level of trust.

31

How the Test Will Feel

As with any intravenous iodinated contrast injection, there may be a slight temporary burning sensation in the arm, metallic taste in the mouth, or whole body warmth. This is a normal occurrence and will subside in a few seconds.

Otherwise, the CT scan is painless.

Why the Test Is Performed

A CT scan is recommended to help:

- evaluate acute cranial-facial trauma
- determine acute stroke
- evaluate suspected subarachnoid or intracranial hemorrhage
- evaluate headache
- evaluate loss of sensory or motor function
- determine if there is abnormal development of the head and neck

CT scans are also used to view the facial bones, jaw, and sinus cavities.

What Abnormal Results Mean

There may be signs of:

- trauma
- bleeding (for example, chronic subdural hematoma or intracranial hemorrhage)
- stroke
- masses or tumors
- abnormal sinus drainage
- sensorineural hearing loss
- malformed bone or other tissues
- brain abscess
- cerebral atrophy (loss of brain tissue)
- brain tissue swelling
- hydrocephalus (fluid collecting in the skull)

Additional conditions under which the test may be performed:

- acoustic neuroma
- acoustic trauma
- acromegaly
- acute (subacute) subdural hematoma
- amyotrophic lateral sclerosis
- arteriovenous malformation (cerebral)
- benign positional vertigo
- throat cancer
- central pontine myelinolysis
- cerebral aneurysm
- Cushing's syndrome
- deep intracerebral hemorrhage
- delirium
- dementia
- dementia due to metabolic causes
- drug-induced tremor
- encephalitis
- epilepsy
- essential tremor
- extradural hemorrhage
- familial tremor
- general paresis
- generalized tonic-clonic seizure
- hemorrhagic stroke
- hepatic encephalopathy
- Huntington's disease
- hypertensive intracerebral hemorrhage
- hypopituitarism
- intracerebral hemorrhage
- juvenile angiofibroma
- labyrinthitis
- lobar intracerebral hemorrhage
- Ludwig's angina
- mastoiditis

- melanoma of the eye
- Ménière's disease
- meningitis
- metastatic brain tumor
- multi-infarct dementia
- multiple endocrine neoplasia (MEN) I
- neurosyphilis
- normal pressure hydrocephalus (NPH)
- occupational hearing loss
- optic glioma
- orbital cellulitis
- otitis media; chronic
- otosclerosis
- partial (focal) seizure
- partial complex seizure
- petit mal seizure
- pituitary tumor
- primary brain tumor
- primary lymphoma of the brain
- prolactinoma
- retinoblastoma
- Reye's syndrome
- schizophrenia
- senile dementia/Alzheimer's type
- acute sinusitis
- stroke secondary to atherosclerosis
- stroke secondary to cardiogenic embolism
- stroke secondary to FMD
- stroke secondary to syphilis
- subarachnoid hemorrhage
- syphilitic aseptic meningitis
- temporal lobe seizure
- toxoplasmosis
- transient ischemic attack (TIA)
- Wilson's disease

What the Risks Are

Iodine is the usual contrast dye. Some patients are allergic to iodine and may experience a reaction that may include hives, itching, nausea, breathing difficulty, or other symptoms.

As with any x-ray examination, radiation is potentially harmful. Consult your health care provider about the risks if multiple CT scans are needed over a period of time.

Special Considerations

A CT scan can decrease or eliminate the need for invasive procedures to diagnose problems in the skull. This is one of the safest means of studying the head and neck.

Section 3.4

Electroencephalogram (EEG)

Reprinted from "EEG," © 2004 A.D.A.M., Inc.
Reprinted with permission.

Alternative Names

Electroencephalogram; Brain wave test

Definition

An electroencephalogram (EEG) is a test to detect abnormalities in the electrical activity of the brain.

How the Test Is Performed

Brain cells communicate by producing tiny electrical impulses. In an EEG, electrodes are placed on the scalp over multiple areas of the brain to detect and record patterns of electrical activity and check for abnormalities.

The test is performed by an EEG technician in a specially designed room that may be in your health care provider's office or at a hospital. You will be asked to lie on your back on a table or in a reclining chair.

The technician will apply between sixteen and twenty-five flat metal discs (electrodes) in different positions on your scalp. The discs are held in place with a sticky paste. The electrodes are connected by wires to an amplifier and a recording machine.

The recording machine converts the electrical signals into a series of wavy lines that are drawn onto a moving piece of graph paper. You will need to lie still with your eyes closed because any movement can alter the results.

You may be asked to do certain things during the recording, such as breathe deeply and rapidly for several minutes or look at a bright flickering light.

How to Prepare for the Test

You will need to wash your hair the night before the test. Do not use any oils, sprays, or conditioner on your hair before this test.

Your health care provider may want you to discontinue some medications before the test. Do not change or stop medications without first consulting your health care provider.

You should avoid all foods containing caffeine for eight hours before the test.

Sometimes it is necessary to sleep during the test, so you may be asked to reduce your sleep time the night before.

Infants and Children

The preparation you can provide for this test depends on your child's age, previous experiences, and level of trust.

How the Test Will Feel

This test causes no discomfort. Although having electrodes pasted onto your skin may feel strange, they only record activity and do not produce any sensation.

Why the Test Is Performed

EEG is used to help diagnose the presence and type of seizure disorders, to look for causes of confusion, and to evaluate head injuries, tumors, infections, degenerative diseases, and metabolic disturbances that affect the brain.

It is also used to evaluate sleep disorders and to investigate periods of unconsciousness. The EEG may be done to confirm brain death in a comatose patient.

EEG cannot be used to "read the mind," measure intelligence, or diagnose mental illness.

Normal Values

Brain waves have normal frequency and amplitude, and other characteristics are typical.

What Abnormal Results Mean

Abnormal findings may indicate the following:

- Seizure disorders (such as epilepsy or convulsions)
- Structural brain abnormality (such as a brain tumor or brain abscess)
- Head injury, encephalitis (inflammation of the brain)
- Hemorrhage (abnormal bleeding caused by a ruptured blood vessel)
- Cerebral infarct (tissue that is dead because of a blockage of the blood supply)
- Sleep disorders (such as narcolepsy).

EEG may confirm brain death in someone who is in a coma. Additional conditions under which the test may be performed:

- Arteriovenous malformation (cerebral)
- Benign positional vertigo
- Cerebral aneurysm
- Complicated alcohol abstinence (delirium tremens)
- Creutzfeldt-Jacob disease
- Delirium
- Dementia
- Dementia due to metabolic causes
- Febrile seizure (children)
- Generalized tonic-clonic seizure

- Hepatic encephalopathy
- Hepatorenal syndrome
- Insomnia
- Labyrinthitis
- Ménière's disease
- Metastatic brain tumor
- Multiple sclerosis
- Optic glioma
- Partial (focal) seizure
- Partial complex seizure
- Petit mal seizure
- Pick's disease
- Senile dementia (Alzheimer's type)
- Shy-Drager syndrome
- Syphilitic aseptic meningitis
- Temporal lobe seizure

What the Risks Are

The procedure is very safe. If you have a seizure disorder, a seizure may be triggered by the flashing lights or hyperventilation. The health care provider performing the EEG is trained to take care of you if this happens.

Section 3.5

Electromyography (EMG)

Reprinted from "Electromyography," © 2004 A.D.A.M., Inc.
Reprinted with permission.

Alternative Names

EMG; Myogram

Definition

Electromyography is a test that measures the health of the muscles and the nerves controlling the muscles.

How the Test Is Performed

For an EMG, a needle electrode is inserted through the skin into the muscle. The electrical activity detected by this electrode is displayed on an oscilloscope, and may be heard through a speaker.

After placement of the electrode(s), you may be asked to contract the muscle (for example, by bending your arm). The presence, size, and shape of the wave form—the action potential—produced on the oscilloscope provide information about the ability of the muscle to respond when the nerves are stimulated.

A nerve conduction velocity test is usually performed in conjunction with an EMG.

How to Prepare for the Test

No special preparation is usually necessary. To ensure accurate readings, avoid using any creams or lotions on the day of the test.

Infants and Children

The preparation you can provide for this test depends on your child's age, previous experiences, and level of trust.

How the Test Will Feel

There may be some discomfort with insertion of the electrodes (similar to an intramuscular injection). Afterward, the muscle may feel tender or bruised for a few days.

Why the Test Is Performed

EMG is most often used when people have symptoms of weakness and examination shows impaired muscle strength. It can help to differentiate primary muscle conditions from muscle weakness caused by neurologic disorders.

Normal Values

Muscle tissue is normally electrically silent at rest. Once the insertion activity (caused by the trauma of needle insertion) quiets down, there should be no action potential on the oscilloscope. When the muscle is voluntarily contracted, action potentials begin to appear. As contraction is increased, more and more muscle fibers produce action potentials until a disorderly group of action potentials of varying rates and amplitudes (complete recruitment and interference pattern) appears with full contraction.

What Abnormal Results Mean

Disorders or conditions that cause abnormal results include the following:

- Polymyositis
- Denervation (reduced nervous stimulation)
- Carpal tunnel syndrome
- Amyotrophic lateral sclerosis (ALS)
- Myopathy (muscle degeneration, may be caused by a number of disorders, including muscular dystrophy)
- Myasthenia gravis
- Alcoholic neuropathy
- Axillary nerve dysfunction
- Becker's muscular dystrophy
- Brachial plexopathy
- Cervical spondylosis

- Common peroneal nerve dysfunction
- Dermatomyositis
- Distal median nerve dysfunction
- Duchenne's muscular dystrophy
- Facioscapulohumeral muscular dystrophy (Landouzy-Dejerine)
- Familial periodic paralysis
- Femoral nerve dysfunction
- Friedreich's ataxia
- Guillain-Barré
- Lambert-Eaton syndrome
- Mononeuritis multiplex
- Mononeuropathy
- Peripheral neuropathy
- Radial nerve dysfunction
- Sciatic nerve dysfunction
- Sensorimotor polyneuropathy
- Shy-Drager syndrome
- Thyrotoxic periodic paralysis
- Tibial nerve dysfunction
- Ulnar nerve dysfunction

What the Risks Are

- Bleeding (minimal)
- Infection at the electrode sites (minimal risk)

Special Considerations

Trauma to the muscle from EMG may cause false results on blood tests (such as creatine kinase), a muscle biopsy, or other tests.

Section 3.6

Nerve Conduction Velocity Test

Reprinted from "Nerve Conduction Velocity," © 2003 A.D.A.M., Inc.
Reprinted with permission.

Alternative Names

NCV

Definition

Nerve conduction velocity (NCV) is a test of the speed of conduction of impulses through a nerve.

How the Test Is Performed

The nerve is stimulated, usually with surface electrodes, which are patch-like electrodes (similar to those used for ECG) placed on the skin over the nerve at various locations. One electrode stimulates the nerve with a very mild electrical impulse.

The resulting electrical activity is recorded by the other electrodes. The distance between electrodes and the time it takes for electrical impulses to travel between electrodes are used to calculate the nerve conduction velocity.

Electromyography is often done at the same time as the NCV test.

How to Prepare for the Test

Normal body temperature must be maintained (low body temperature slows nerve conduction).

Infants and Children

The physical and psychological preparation you can provide for this or any test or procedure depends on your child's age, interests, previous experiences, and level of trust.

How the Test Will Feel

The impulse may feel like an electric shock. Depending on how strong the stimulus is, the patient will feel it to varying degrees. It may be uncomfortable for some patients during the actual test. There should be no residual pain once the test is finished.

Often the nerve conduction test is followed by electromyography (EMG), which involves needles being placed into the muscle and the patient contracting that muscle. This can be uncomfortable during the test, and muscle soreness at the site of the needles may be experienced afterward as well.

Why the Test Is Performed

This test is used to diagnose nerve damage or destruction.

Normal Values

NCV is related to the diameter of the nerve and the normal degree of myelination (the presence of a myelin sheath on the axon) of the nerve. Newborn infants have values that are approximately half that of adults, and adult values are normally reached by age three to four.

What Abnormal Results Mean

Most often, abnormal results are caused by some sort of neuropathy (nerve damage or destruction), including:

- Demyelination (destruction of the myelin sheath)
- Conduction block (the impulse is blocked somewhere along the nerve pathway)
- Axonopathy (damage to the nerve axon)

Some of the associated diseases or conditions include:

- Alcoholic neuropathy
- Diabetic neuropathy
- Nerve effects of uremia (from kidney failure)
- Traumatic injury to a nerve
- Guillain-Barré syndrome

- Diphtheria
- Carpal tunnel syndrome
- Brachial plexopathy
- Charcot-Marie-Tooth disease (hereditary)
- Chronic inflammatory polyneuropathy
- Common peroneal nerve dysfunction
- Distal median nerve dysfunction
- Femoral nerve dysfunction
- Friedreich's ataxia
- General paresis
- Lambert-Eaton syndrome
- Mononeuritis multiplex
- Primary amyloid
- Radial nerve dysfunction
- Sciatic nerve dysfunction
- Secondary systemic amyloid
- Sensorimotor polyneuropathy
- Tibial nerve dysfunction
- Ulnar nerve dysfunction

Any peripheral neuropathy can cause abnormal results, as can damage to the spinal cord and disc herniation (herniated nucleus pulposus) with nerve root compression.

What the Risks Are

There are essentially no risks.

Special Considerations

A NCV test reflects the status of the "best" surviving nerve fibers and may remain normal if even a few fibers are unaffected by a disease process. A normal NCV test result can occur despite extensive nerve damage.

Section 3.7

Magnetic Resonance Imaging (MRI)

Excerpted from the online companion to the *Harvard Medical School Family Health Guide*, © 2003 President and Fellows of Harvard College. www.health.harvard.edu. Reprinted with permission.

What is the test?

An MRI (Magnetic Resonance Imaging) scan is an excellent way to view the brain. This test provides your doctor with a collection of many black-and-white pictures, each showing a slightly different "slice" or cross-section of your brain. These "slices" are spaced close to ¼-inch apart, so your doctor can get a very good representative idea about how the different parts or "lobes" of the brain, the brain's balance center or "cerebellum," and the brain stem look.

The MRI scan machine uses a powerful magnet and carefully programmed radio signals to detect differences between types of tissues inside your skull. Then a computer uses this information to generate realistic pictures that represent your brain. The MRI can show the difference between brain tissue and tumors and can also show areas of brain that have been damaged by a stroke or by other neurological conditions.

How do I prepare for the test?

MRI cannot be performed on certain people, such as those who have cardiac pacemakers or certain other metal implants. For these patients, exposure to the powerful magnet in the MRI would be unsafe. If you have had any previous surgery (including eye surgery or brain surgery) or if you have a pacemaker, make sure that your doctor knows about it. Some patients who are obese are too large to fit in a standard MRI scan machine. For these patients, a few centers have machines that can accommodate a larger person.

Before the MRI scan, you may need to have an IV placed. Some MRI scans require a dye that gets put through the IV, so that areas of inflammation or abnormality are easier to detect. This dye is called

45

"gadolinium," and is different from the contrast dye used for x-rays or CT scans. You will be asked to remove metal objects such as belt buckles or watches.

What happens when the test is performed?

The MRI is a large machine that has a circular tunnel built through it, like a donut with a hole. You will lie on your back on a narrow table that can be moved back and forth into the MRI tunnel. When the MRI is taken, expect to hear some loud noises from the machine. Some MRI departments will offer you earplugs or a stereo headset to wear to block this noise. Your table will be moved by an automatic control operated by the technician. You will be asked to hold your breath for a few seconds for each picture that is taken. If you are a patient who needs to have dye injected through the IV, this is usually done halfway through the scanning and rarely causes any side effects.

The MRI scan typically takes between thirty and sixty minutes to complete. It is difficult for some who suffer from claustrophobia or who have trouble lying flat for that long a time. If you think you might be someone who would require an anti-anxiety medicine to get through the procedure, you should discuss this with your doctor ahead of time.

After the study, the IV will be removed and you can go about your normal activities.

What risks are there from the test?

There are no risks from the MRI scan, except for patients who have metal implants from previous surgeries or pacemakers. The MRI causes no side effects.

Must I do anything special after the test is over?

No.

How long is it before the result of the test is known?

It will take the MRI department at least an hour to develop the pictures from your scan and it will take additional time for a doctor to examine the MRI pictures and to decide how they look. Typically you can get a preliminary interpretation within a day or two of when the test was done; the formal reading of your MRI might take a bit longer.

Section 3.8

Positron Emission Tomography (PET) Scan

Reprinted from "Isotope Study," © 2003 A.D.A.M., Inc.
Reprinted with permission.

Alternative Names

Scintillation; Radionuclide organ imaging; Radioisotope; Radioactive uptake; Nuclear radiography; Nuclear medicine scan

Definition

Nuclear radiology is a subspecialty of radiology in which radioisotopes (compounds containing radioactive forms of atoms) are introduced into the body for the purpose of imaging, evaluating organ function, or localizing disease or tumors.

Unlike conventional or computed radiography (such as plain x-rays and CT scans) in which x-ray beams are generated within a machine and projected through the patient, in isotope studies the radiation (gamma rays) originates from within a radiopharmaceutical (material tagged with a radioisotope) in the body.

Special detector cameras are placed close against the area of interest for a period of time, and once enough gamma rays are "seen," a computer creates an image representing where the isotope localized within the organ or body.

Generally, nuclear medicine scans do not provide the level of anatomic detail seen on x-ray, ultrasound, CT, or MR images. However, correlation with other imaging, clinical information, and laboratory results helps identify and confirm disease.

How the Test Is Performed

A radioactive isotope needs to be introduced into the body. This may be done in several ways:

- Through a needle into a vein (usually the inside of the elbow).

- Through a catheter that is inserted into a vein or artery and is then guided to the organ being tested.

- Ingestion (for example, to test the thyroid, the patient drinks radioactive iodine).

- Subcutaneous injection (under the skin).

- Collecting a patient's own blood from a vein, adding the radio-isotope compound in a laboratory, and then injecting back into the patient.

After a certain period of time has passed (ranging from a few hours to a day or more for different exams), you will be placed on a table (called a gantry) under the scanner, which may rotate around the body.

It is imperative that you remain still to produce accurate and useful sets of images. For some tests, a counter is placed over the organ, and the amount of radioactivity or intensity of radioactivity is recorded.

A technician interprets the information as it is transmitted to the computer and can guide the camera to specific locations to improve the imaging.

How to Prepare for the Test

Inform the technician or physician of *all* medications you are currently and have recently been taking, since they may interfere with the isotopes given for the exam. Also be sure to mention any recent imaging studies involving injected contrast media (dye) and oral or rectal contrast (such as from gastrointestinal studies) since they may also interfere.

You must sign a consent form before the radioactive compound is given. You may need to fast overnight before the test. Depending on the region being scanned, you may need to wear a hospital gown. Remove jewelry, dentures, and other metal that may affect the scan by blocking the gamma rays from the detectors.

For Infants and Children

The preparation you can provide for this test depends on your child's age and experience.

How the Test Will Feel

If the isotope is injected, there will be a sharp prick when the needle is inserted. If a catheter is inserted, the site of insertion is usually numbed with an anesthetic. You will first feel a prick when the needle is inserted, but you will feel little more than slight pressure or tugging during the injection of the isotope. If the isotope is ingested, the flavor of the liquid may be unpleasant, but no pain is involved.

For patients who are extremely sensitive to the isotope, there may be nausea, headache, or vomiting. Discuss allergies with the health care provider or technician before the test.

Why the Test Is Performed

Nuclear radiography shows the size, shape, position, and some function of the target organs specific for a particular radioisotope molecule. If another test has indicated cancer or abscess, this test can help support that diagnosis and indicate the location. Repeat examinations can be used to gauge response to therapies.

What Abnormal Results Mean

- abnormal size, shape, or position of an organ
- change in organ function
- stones
- cancer
- arthritis
- bone fractures
- acute infection
- growths
- abscesses
- embolism
- cysts
- intrauterine bleeding
- spinal fluid leak
- spleen injury
- swelling of the testicles
- blood clots

Additional conditions under which the test may be performed:

- anaplastic carcinoma of the thyroid
- autonomic neuropathy

- gastroparesis
- Huntington's disease
- unilateral hydronephrosis

What the Risks Are

Generally, the energy of emitted radiation in nuclear radiography is similar to that of x-rays used in plain films and CT scans. There is potential for cell damage and mutations in egg or sperm cells.

The target organs of the isotope in the examination may receive the majority of the radiation dose, however, the amounts used are strictly controlled and regulated to use the least amount necessary for the purpose of imaging.

The radiation doses used for *treatment* of certain disorders (for instance, iodine for thyroid disease) are many times greater and will require additional instructions to protect others during treatment.

For radiation, the greatest concern is with pregnant or nursing women. Infants and fetuses are more sensitive to the effects of radiation because they are still undergoing organ development.

Higher doses of radiation and repeated exposures to radiation increase the risk. Radioactive materials decay (release energy and then transform into nonradioactive atoms) at specific rates as the body continuously removes them (usually filtered by the lungs, kidneys, or liver, depending on the compound used). Thus, all radioisotope activity eventually ceases, usually within a few days.

Risks related to injections and allergic reactions to the radioisotope exist, but are rare.

Special Considerations

The benefits of conducting an isotope study to diagnose a potentially serious condition usually outweigh concerns about radiation or other side effects.

Section 3.9

Spinal Tap (Lumbar Puncture)

Excerpted from the online companion to the *Harvard Medical School Family Health Guide.* © 2003 President and Fellows of Harvard College. www.health.harvard.edu. Reprinted with permission.

What is the test?

A lumbar puncture, also known as a "spinal tap," removes a sample of fluid through a needle from the space surrounding the spinal cord. This fluid is known as "cerebrospinal fluid," or "CSF." The test is used to diagnose meningitis infections and some neurological conditions.

How do I prepare for the test?

No advanced preparation is needed, except for the signing of a consent form, which is generally required when the procedure is done outside of an emergency situation. Lumbar puncture does not require hospitalization. Tell your doctor ahead of time if you have ever had an allergic reaction to the medicine lidocaine or the numbing medicine used at the dentist's office.

What happens when the test is performed?

Most patients will be asked to wear a hospital gown. In most cases, you will be asked to lie on your side with your knees curled up against your chest. In some cases, the doctor will ask you to sit on the bed or a table instead, leaning forward against some pillows.

The doctor will feel your back to know where your lower vertebrae are and will feel the bones in the back of your pelvis. An area on your lower back will be cleaned with soap. Medicine given through a small needle is used to numb the skin and the tissue underneath the skin in the area from which the sample will be removed. This causes some very brief stinging.

A different needle is then placed in the same area and moved forward until fluid can be obtained through it from the spinal canal. Because the needle must be placed through a small opening in between two bones, it is sometimes necessary for the doctor to move the needle in and out several times to locate the opening. Because of the numbing medicine used in this area, most patients experience only a sense of pressure from this movement. Occasionally some patients do get a sharp feeling in the back or (rarely) in the leg. Let your doctor know if you feel anything painful.

Sometimes the doctor will measure the pressure of the fluid before taking a sample. The pressure is measured with a tube that looks like a large thermometer held against the needle. The fluid sample collected is usually less than three tablespoons. You will not feel any discomfort when it is removed. After this, the needle is taken out. Usually a Band-Aid is the only dressing necessary.

The whole lumbar puncture, including set-up time, takes between thirty and forty-five minutes. The needle is in place for close to one minute.

What risks are there from the test?

The most significant risk from a lumbar puncture is that it can cause a temporary headache. Lying down for a few hours after the test can make a headache less likely to occur. Other problems are rare, but can include infection or bleeding. Because the volume of fluid is small, a lumbar puncture almost never causes movement of the brain or spinal cord.

Doctors routinely do a physical examination and in some cases order a brain scan before recommending a lumbar puncture, to make sure you do not have a medical condition that could put you at risk for movement of the brain during the procedure, a very rare but serious complication.

Must I do anything special after the test is over?

Many patients are asked to lie flat for a while after the test, sometimes for a few hours.

How long is it before the result of the test is known?

Depending on the tests being done on the fluid sample, results take between a few hours and a few days to return.

Chapter 4

Recent Brain Research

Chapter Contents

Section 4.1—Deep Brain Stimulation: Pacemakers for
the Brain 54
Section 4.2—The Women's Health Initiative Memory
Study (WHIMS) 58
Section 4.3—Bone Marrow Generates New Neurons in
Human Brains 61

Section 4.1

Deep Brain Stimulation: Pacemakers for the Brain

What is deep brain stimulation?

Deep brain stimulation (DBS) is a surgical option for patients with Parkinson's disease, Essential Tremor, dystonia, and tremor due to multiple sclerosis. During DBS surgery electrodes are implanted within the brain to deliver electrical impulses. The stimulation offers patients relief from tremors, rigidity, slowness of movement, and stiffness, and may help balance problems associated with their conditions. The stimulation can be adjusted as a patient's condition changes over time.

Deep brain stimulation is a new and improved variation of an old surgery. The old surgery involved destroying small parts of the brain within structures called the thalamus or globus pallidus. Today, it is no longer necessary to destroy even small parts of the brain.

How does deep brain stimulation work?

An electrode implanted in the brain emits pulses of energy to block the abnormal activity in the brain that causes the symptoms. The success of deep brain stimulation surgery is directly related to finding the specific area in the brain for stimulation.

Who is a candidate for this surgery?

Any patient who:

- Is not satisfied with his or her level of control
- Exhibits Parkinson's disease symptoms causing a decline in the quality of life
- Has had an adequate and reasonable trial of medications

How is deep brain stimulation surgery done?

It is important to note that surgical techniques can vary among centers and surgeons. The surgical methods described here are used at the Cleveland Clinic Foundation in Cleveland, Ohio.

Deep brain stimulation involves the implantation of a very thin lead containing four electrode contacts into a specific target area in the brain. The lead extends through a small opening in the skull and is connected to an extension wire. The extension wire is connected to an impulse generator or "pacemaker," which is implanted under the skin over the chest. Programming of the stimulation is easy and painless.

The surgeon is aided by computerized brain-mapping technology to find the precise location in the brain where nerve signals generate the tremors and other symptoms. Highly sophisticated imaging and recording equipment are used to map both the physical structure and the functioning of the brain.

The patient is awake during surgery to allow the surgical team to assess the patient's brain functions. While the electrode is being advanced through the brain, the patient does not feel any pain because of the unique nature of the human brain and its inability to generate pain signals. When the surgeon makes the small opening in the skull a local anesthetic is administered. The anesthetic used is similar to those used during a dental procedure to numb an area of the mouth.

Most patients are in the hospital for about three days. The stimulators are implanted below the collarbone either at the time of electrode implantation or later. The patient is placed under general anesthesia for this part of the procedure. The stimulators are turned on for the first time within a few weeks after implantation.

How effective is deep brain stimulation?

In properly selected patients, deep brain stimulation is remarkably safe and effective, although not completely without risk. Beneficial effects have been demonstrated to last for several years. Patients who initially responded well to medications, but over time have developed sides effects, can experience between 60 and 80 percent improvement in such symptoms as tremor and slowness of movement. Patients on average report a 50 percent improvement in their walking and balance. Similarly, patients with involuntary movements (dyskinesia) due to their medications, experience over 80 percent reduction in their involuntary movements. Most patients are able to significantly reduce their medications following deep brain stimulation.

Regarding Parkinson disease in particular, an important indicator of the effectiveness of any treatment is the duration of "on-time" without dyskinesia. This means the patient is mobile and can perform everyday tasks without experiencing the involuntary movements. On average, deep brain stimulation doubles the amount of "on-time" without dyskinesia.

What risks are associated with deep brain stimulation?

As with any surgery, the procedure is not entirely risk free. There is approximately a 2 to 3 percent chance of brain hemorrhage that may be of no significance, or may cause paralysis, stroke, speech impairment, or other major problems. This means that for every one hundred patients who undergo surgery, two or three will experience a permanent or severe complication. However, this also means that many patients will have no complications. There is a 15 percent chance of a minor or temporary problem. Rarely, infections can occur. While treatment of infection may require removal of the electrode, the infections themselves have not caused lasting damage.

The electrode that is implanted in the brain, and the electrical systems that provide stimulation, are generally very well tolerated with no significant changes in brain tissue around the electrodes.

Who can be evaluated for deep brain stimulation?

Patients with Parkinson disease, essential tremor, dystonia, or tremor due to multiple sclerosis, with movement-related symptoms that cannot be controlled by medications can be evaluated as possible candidates for deep brain stimulation. In addition, patients who experience intolerable side effects from medication may also be candidates.

Deep brain stimulation has been successful in treating patients as young as thirteen years of age. In general, surgery is performed on those under seventy-five years of age. However, each patient must be assessed individually concerning his or her stamina and overall health.

Does Medicare cover deep brain stimulation?

This FDA-approved procedure is covered by Medicare for the treatment of Parkinson disease and essential tremor. However, this is not the case in all states. Some states' programs do not cover DBS surgery. Outside of Medicare, most insurance companies are also covering the costs of DBS surgery. To determine if Medicare in your state, or your individual insurance policy, covers all or a portion of the costs, you would need to contact your benefit representative directly.

Has deep brain stimulation been approved by the Food and Drug Administration?

Yes. In January of 2002 the FDA approved deep brain stimulation for the treatment of Parkinson disease. It had previously been approved for the treatment of essential tremor.

What happens after deep brain stimulation surgery?

A series of adjustments in the electrical pulse will be made over the next weeks or months. It is necessary for patients to be able to travel to a location where the stimulation of their implanted pacemakers can be adjusted following surgery. The first few follow-up visits should be to the center where the surgery was performed, but subsequent electrical programming can take place at another medical center.

Section 4.2

The Women's Health Initiative Memory Study (WHIMS)

Reprinted from "Frequently Asked Questions about the Women's Health Initiative Memory Study (WHIMS)," June 2004. The Women's Health Initiative (WHI) was established by National Institutes of Health (NIH) to address the most common causes of death, disability, and impaired quality of life in postmenopausal women. The WHI Program Office is located within the Office of the Director of the National Heart, Lung, and Blood Institute (NHLBI). The WHI website, coordinated by the Fred Hutchinson Cancer Research Center (FHCRC), is available online at www.whi.org.

What is WHIMS?

WHIMS is a sub-study within the Women's Health Initiative (WHI). In the past, some studies reported a positive association between use of hormone therapy and cognitive protection, while others failed to find protective effects. Because of these inconsistent results, a large, controlled randomized clinical trial of hormone treatment was needed. Only women who joined the Hormone Program and were sixty-five years of age and older when they joined were invited to participate in WHIMS. The purpose of WHIMS was to find out if taking hormones (estrogen alone or estrogen plus progestin) would prevent dementia or slow the decline of cognitive function in postmenopausal women.

What is cognitive function?

Cognitive function includes brain-related abilities like attention, concentration, memory, language, abstract reasoning, and calculation.

What is dementia?

When cognitive function declines to the point that it interferes a great deal with day-to-day activities, and other medical conditions have been ruled out, a diagnosis of dementia might be given. Different brain diseases can cause dementia. The most well known is Alzheimer's disease. Other diseases that block the normal flow of blood in the brain can also cause dementia. What causes these diseases and how they progress is not well understood at this time. However, much research is being done to find treatments that can decrease the effects of these diseases on everyday functioning.

What were the main findings about estrogen plus progestin and cognition?

For women age sixty-five and older who took active estrogen plus progestin pills:

- More developed dementia compared to women taking placebo (inactive) pills.

- They had worse scores, on average, on screening tests for dementia compared to women taking placebo.

What is the increased risk for women taking estrogen plus progestin?

A woman is more likely to develop dementia if she is taking estrogen plus progestin. However, the number of women who actually do develop dementia is relatively modest—45 out of 10,000 women taking estrogen plus progestin each year, compared to 22 out of 10,000 women taking placebo each year. While this difference in rates is important, the overall risk remains small.

What are the conclusions from these findings?

Overall, in women age sixty-five and older, estrogen plus progestin treatment is harmful to cognitive function. For some women, their decline in cognitive function will be so serious that they will be diagnosed as having dementia. Therefore, we recommend that health care providers should not prescribe estrogen plus progestin to enhance or improve cognitive function in postmenopausal women who do not have dementia.

If you are age sixty-five or older and are having severe menopausal symptoms, you should talk with your health care provider. Your provider can recommend an appropriate treatment based on your personal risk for breast cancer, cardiovascular disease, and dementia.

What type of hormone treatment did women in the Estrogen Plus Progestin Study take?

Women who were randomized to receive active hormones in this study were taking conjugated equine estrogens 0.625 mg each day and medroxyprogesterone acetate 2.5 mg each day (Prempro™). When WHI first began, this was the most commonly prescribed hormonal therapy in the United States for postmenopausal women with a uterus.

Is there an increased risk of dementia in women taking estrogen alone (without progestin)?

WHIMS includes a study of estrogen alone (without progestin) for women who did not have a uterus before they joined WHI. Final results from the Estrogen-Alone Study remain uncertain. Participants in the Estrogen-Alone Study are asked to continue to take their study pills and to come in for their regular clinical visits. The National Heart, Lung, and Blood Institute, which oversees the WHI, continues to review the study of women receiving estrogen alone and will provide investigators and participants with any new information about the study that might affect their participation.

Should I discuss this new information with my health care provider?

Yes. Your WHI clinic has a letter that you may take to your health care provider. Your provider may also want to read the WHIMS scientific paper in the May 28, 2003, *Journal of the American Medical Association*. Your health care provider may also want to speak with your local WHIMS principal investigator about the results.

I am taking prescription hormones. What should I do?

Talk with your health care provider about your individual health risk profile and the hormones you are currently taking.

What if I am under age sixty-five?

Currently, it is not known if the WHIMS findings about cognitive function in women who take estrogen plus progestin apply to women younger than sixty-five years of age. This question may be answered by future research studies on hormone therapy in younger women.

Section 4.3

Bone Marrow Generates New Neurons in Human Brains

Reprinted from "Bone Marrow Generates New Neurons in Human Brains," National Institute of Neurological Disorders and Stroke, January 20, 2003.

A new study strongly suggests that some cells from bone marrow can enter the human brain and generate new neurons and other types of brain cells. If researchers can find a way to control these cells and direct them to damaged areas of the brain, this finding may lead to new treatments for stroke, Parkinson disease, and other neurological disorders.

"This study shows that some kind of cell in bone marrow, most likely a stem cell, has the capacity to enter the brain and form neurons," says Éva Mezey, M.D., Ph.D., from the National Institute of Neurological Disorders and Stroke (NINDS), who led the study. Earlier work by Dr. Mezey and others has shown that bone marrow cells can enter the mouse brain and produce new neurons. However, the new study is the first to show that this phenomenon can occur in the human brain. The study was supported in part by the NINDS and appears in the January 20, 2003, online early edition of the *Proceedings of the National Academy of Sciences*.[1] The NINDS is a component of the National Institutes of Health, which is part of the U.S. Department of Health and Human Services.

In the study, Dr. Mezey and colleagues examined brain tissue taken at autopsy from four female patients—two adults and two children—who had received bone marrow transplants from male donors. The bone marrow transplants had been performed to treat leukemia and other non-neurological diseases, and the patients survived from one to nine months after their transplants. The investigators searched the autopsied brain tissue for male cells, which contain a Y chromosome. The Y chromosomes in these cells served as a useful way of distinguishing donor-derived cells from those of the female transplant recipients. The researchers found cells with Y chromosomes in brain tissue from all four of the patients.

Most of the bone marrow–derived cells in the brain tissue were glia (support cells) and other non-neuronal cells. However, a small number of neurons from each brain also contained Y chromosomes, showing that those cells had developed from the transplanted male bone marrow. Most of these neurons were found in the cerebral cortex—the outer layer of the brain, which is responsible for conscious thought—and in the hippocampus, a region that helps with memory and other functions.

The Y chromosome–positive cells within each patient's brain appeared in clusters, rather than being randomly dispersed throughout the brain tissue. The clusters sometimes contained both neuronal and non-neuronal cells. This suggests that a single bone marrow–derived stem cell may migrate into an "area of need" within the brain and then change, or differentiate, into several other kinds of cells, Dr. Mezey says. The clusters also might result from a large number of marrow cells that are "called" to specific parts of the brain. Previous studies have suggested that stem cells can respond to signals from within the brain that guide them to damaged regions.

The brain sections with the largest number of marrow-derived neurons came from the youngest of the four patients, who had her transplant at nine months of age. That patient also survived for nine months after the transplant—much longer than the other patients in this study. The researchers do not know if the number of marrow-derived neurons in this patient was due to her young age or to the length of time she survived after receiving the transplant. The brains of young people usually undergo more changes than those of older people, and this might have encouraged the development of new neurons, Dr. Mezey notes. However, it is also possible that new cells enter the brain at a steady rate over time, regardless of a person's age.

It is possible that irradiation or other treatments that the four patients received might have increased the ability of marrow cells to enter the brain. However, other studies have suggested that bone marrow cells circulating in the blood enter the brain even in healthy subjects who have never received a bone marrow transplant, and there is no reason to think that a transplant is necessary for stem cells to enter the nervous system, Dr. Mezey says.

The numbers of marrow-derived neurons identified in the human brain tissue were very low—much lower than the numbers identified in a previous mouse study, says Dr. Mezey. However, the numbers might be greater in patients who survive for longer periods after transplant, she suggests.

Bone marrow contains at least two kinds of stem cells: hematopoietic stem cells, which usually differentiate into blood cells, and mesenchymal stem cells, which can differentiate into many kinds of cells in the body. The researchers do not yet know which type of cell differentiates into the neurons and other marrow-derived cells they identified in the brain.

Recent studies have shown that instead of developing into new cell types, adult stem cells sometimes fuse with mature cells from existing tissues that have already undergone differentiation. The resulting cells carry four sex chromosomes (X and Y chromosomes) instead of the usual two. While Dr. Mezey and her colleagues cannot exclude the possibility that fusion accounts for their results, they looked at several hundred donor-derived cells from one of the patients and did not see doubled sex chromosomes in any of the cells they examined.

Previous studies have found some cells with Y chromosomes in adult women who had not received any transplants. Researchers believe these Y cells may have come from a past pregnancy with a male fetus. However, two of the subjects in this study were children, and the male cells in those individuals could not have come from a pregnancy, says Dr. Mezey.

Scientists must now determine what growth factors or other signals prompt the bone marrow cells to enter the brain and develop into neurons. This may lead to new ways of treating Parkinson disease or other disorders where neurons lost to disease are not normally replaced. Researchers might also be able to discover factors that can increase the number of cells entering the brain or prompt the cells to find useful targets.

"These studies are very much the beginning, but scientists should start to look down this road and find out if and how we can go further," says Dr. Mezey. She cautions that it is too early to know if this finding will lead to useful treatments for neurological disorders. She and her colleagues are now planning to study brain tissue from people who survived for longer periods after receiving a bone marrow transplant in order to see if the number of marrow-derived neurons increases with time. They also plan to study mice to determine which cells in the bone marrow develop into neurons.

Resources

1. Mezey, É., Key, S., Vogelsang, G., Szalayova, I., Lange, G. D., Crain, B. "Transplanted bone marrow generates new neurons in human brains." *Proceedings of the National Academy of Sciences*, Online Early Edition, January 20, 2003.

Chapter 5

Brain Death

The diagnosis of brain death is defined as "death based on the absence of all neurologic function." Families who have had a loved one declared brain dead may have questions about what the term really means.

What does "brain death" mean?

Brain death is a legal definition of death. It is the complete and irreversible cessation (stopping) of all brain function. It means that, as a result of severe trauma or injury to the brain, the body's blood supply to the brain is blocked and the brain dies. Brain death is death. It is permanent and irreversible.

How is it decided that an individual is brain dead?

A physician conducts the required medical tests to make the diagnosis of brain death. These tests are based on sound and legally accepted medical guidelines. Among other things, tests include a clinical examination to show that an individual has no brain reflexes and cannot breathe on his or her own.

In some situations, other testing may be needed. You can ask your doctor to explain or show you how brain death was determined for your loved one.

Possibly, an individual may exhibit spinal activity or reflexes such as twitching or muscle contractions. Spinal reflexes are caused by electrical impulses that remain in the spinal column. These reflexes may occur even though the brain is dead.

What happens to an individual while these tests are being done?

The individual is placed on a machine that breathes for him or her, called a ventilator, because the brain can no longer send signals telling the body to breathe. Special medications to help maintain blood pressure and other body functions may also be given.

During the brain death testing, the ventilator and medications continue but they do not interfere with the brain death determination.

Aren't there drugs that can stop the brain from working and give a false diagnosis?

Certain drugs, such as muscle relaxants and sedatives, can mask brain function. When the tests are performed, the individual can have only low levels of these drugs in the body. It may be necessary to wait for these levels to go down. The physician can then accurately measure brain activity. Often other tests are done to confirm brain death if certain drugs are present in the body.

If brain death is confirmed, why does an individual's heart continue beating?

As long as the heart has oxygen, it can continue to work. The ventilator provides enough oxygen to keep the heart beating for several hours. Without this artificial help, the heart would stop beating.

Is it possible that an individual is in a coma?

No. A patient in a coma continues to have brain activity and function. When brain death occurs, all brain function ceases and there is no chance of recovery.

Is there anything else that can be done?

Before brain death is declared, everything possible to save an individual's life is done. After the diagnosis of brain death is made there is no chance of recovery.

The individual may appear to be only sleeping. The ventilator fills the lungs with air. The heart monitors may indicate that the heart is sill beating. The individual's body may be warm to the touch and there may still be color in his or her face. But, in fact, the individual is dead.

What happens when an individual is declared brain dead?

Once the diagnosis of brain death is made, an individual is pronounced legally dead. This is the time that should appear on the death certificate. The time of death is not the time when the ventilator is removed.

Does an individual feel any pain or suffer after brain death is declared?

No. When someone is dead, there is no feeling of pain or suffering.

After brain death is declared, what happens next?

In many cases brain death results from a sudden accident or injury. A health care professional will talk with you about certain decisions you need to make at this time. Among those decisions could be removing the ventilator and the possibility of organ or tissue donation.

Remember, the individual is already legally dead and removing the ventilator does not cause death.

Part Two

Acquired and Traumatic Brain Injuries

Chapter 6

Stroke

Chapter Contents

Section 6.1—Stroke: A Brain Attack 72
Section 6.2—Recent Research on Stroke 108

Section 6.1

Stroke: A Brain Attack

Reprinted from "Stroke: Hope through Research," National Institute of
Neurological Disorders and Stroke, updated November 2004.

Introduction

More than 2,400 years ago the father of medicine, Hippocrates,
recognized and described stroke—the sudden onset of paralysis. Until recently, modern medicine has had very little power over this disease, but the world of stroke medicine is changing and new and better
therapies are being developed every day. Today, some people who have
a stroke can walk away from the attack with no or few disabilities if
they are treated promptly. Doctors can finally offer stroke patients
and their families the one thing that until now has been so hard to
give: hope.

In ancient times stroke was called apoplexy, a general term that
physicians applied to anyone suddenly struck down with paralysis.
Because many conditions can lead to sudden paralysis, the term apoplexy did not indicate a specific diagnosis or cause. Physicians knew
very little about the cause of stroke, and the only established therapy
was to feed and care for the patient until the attack ran its course.

The first person to investigate the pathological signs of apoplexy
was Johann Jacob Wepfer. Born in Schaffhausen, Switzerland, in 1620,
Wepfer studied medicine and was the first to identify postmortem
signs of bleeding in the brains of patients who died of apoplexy. From
autopsy studies he gained knowledge of the carotid and vertebral arteries that supply the brain with blood. He also was the first person
to suggest that apoplexy, in addition to being caused by bleeding in
the brain, could be caused by a blockage of one of the main arteries
supplying blood to the brain; thus stroke became known as a cerebrovascular disease ("cerebro" refers to a part of the brain; "vascular"
refers to the blood vessels and arteries).

Medical science would eventually confirm Wepfer's hypotheses, but
until very recently doctors could offer little in the area of therapy. Over
the last two decades basic and clinical investigators, many of them

sponsored and funded in part by the National Institute of Neurological Disorders and Stroke (NINDS), have learned a great deal about stroke. They have identified major risk factors for the disease and have developed surgical techniques and drug treatments for the prevention of stroke. Yet perhaps the most exciting new development in the field of stroke research is the recent approval of a drug treatment that can reverse the course of stroke if given during the first few hours after the onset of symptoms.

Studies with animals have shown that brain injury occurs within minutes of a stroke and can become irreversible within as little as an hour. In humans, brain damage begins from the moment the stroke starts and often continues for days afterward. Scientists now know that there is a very short window of opportunity for treatment of the most common form of stroke. Because of these and other advances in the field of cerebrovascular disease, stroke patients now have a chance for survival and recovery.

Cost of Stroke to the United States

- total cost of stroke to the United States: estimated at about $43 billion/year
- direct costs for medical care and therapy: estimated at about $28 billion/year
- indirect costs from lost productivity and other factors: estimated at about $15 million/year
- average cost of care for a patient up to ninety days after a stroke: $15,000[1]
- for 10 percent of patients, cost of care for the first ninety days after a stroke: $35,000[1]
- percentage of direct cost of care for the first ninety days[1]:
  - initial hospitalization = 43 percent
  - rehabilitation = 16 percent
  - physician costs = 14 percent
  - hospital readmission = 14 percent
  - medications and other expenses = 13 percent

What Is Stroke?

A stroke occurs when the blood supply to part of the brain is suddenly interrupted or when a blood vessel in the brain bursts, spilling blood into the spaces surrounding brain cells. In the same way that a person suffering a loss of blood flow to the heart is said to be having a heart attack, a person with a loss of blood flow to the brain or sudden bleeding in the brain can be said to be having a "brain attack."

Brain cells die when they no longer receive oxygen and nutrients from the blood or when they are damaged by sudden bleeding into or around the brain. Ischemia is the term used to describe the loss of oxygen and nutrients for brain cells when there is inadequate blood flow. Ischemia ultimately leads to infarction, the death of brain cells, which are eventually replaced by a fluid-filled cavity (or infarct) in the injured brain.

When blood flow to the brain is interrupted, some brain cells die immediately, while others remain at risk for death. These damaged cells make up the ischemic penumbra and can linger in a compromised state for several hours. With timely treatment these cells can be saved. The ischemic penumbra is discussed in more detail in the Appendix [at the end of this section of this chapter].

Even though a stroke occurs in the unseen reaches of the brain, the symptoms of a stroke are easy to spot. They include sudden numbness or weakness, especially on one side of the body; sudden confusion or trouble speaking or understanding speech; sudden trouble seeing in one or both eyes; sudden trouble walking, dizziness, or loss of balance or coordination; or sudden severe headache with no known cause. All of the symptoms of stroke appear suddenly, and often there is more than one symptom at the same time. Therefore stroke can usually be distinguished from other causes of dizziness or headache. These symptoms may indicate that a stroke has occurred and that medical attention is needed immediately.

There are two forms of stroke: ischemic, which is blockage of a blood vessel supplying the brain, and hemorrhagic, which is bleeding into or around the brain. The following sections describe these forms in detail.

Ischemic Stroke

An ischemic stroke occurs when an artery supplying the brain with blood becomes blocked, suddenly decreasing or stopping blood flow and ultimately causing a brain infarction. This type of stroke accounts for approximately 80 percent of all strokes. Blood clots are the most common cause of artery blockage and brain infarction. The process of clotting is necessary and beneficial throughout the body because it stops bleeding and allows repair of damaged areas of arteries or veins.

However, when blood clots develop in the wrong place within an artery they can cause devastating injury by interfering with the normal flow of blood. Problems with clotting become more frequent as people age.

Blood clots can cause ischemia and infarction in two ways. A clot that forms in a part of the body other than the brain can travel through blood vessels and become wedged in a brain artery. This free-roaming clot is called an embolus and often forms in the heart. A stroke caused by an embolus is called an embolic stroke. The second kind of ischemic stroke, called a thrombotic stroke, is caused by thrombosis, the formation of a blood clot in one of the cerebral arteries that stays attached to the artery wall until it grows large enough to block blood flow.

Ischemic strokes can also be caused by stenosis, or a narrowing of the artery due to the buildup of plaque (a mixture of fatty substances, including cholesterol and other lipids) and blood clots along the artery wall. Stenosis can occur in large arteries and small arteries and is therefore called large vessel disease or small vessel disease, respectively. When a stroke occurs due to small vessel disease, a very small infarction results, sometimes called a lacunar infarction, from the French word "lacune" meaning "gap" or "cavity."

The most common blood vessel disease that causes stenosis is atherosclerosis. In atherosclerosis, deposits of plaque build up along the inner walls of large and medium-sized arteries, causing thickening, hardening, and loss of elasticity of artery walls and decreased blood flow. The role of cholesterol and blood lipids with respect to stroke risk is discussed in the section on cholesterol under "Who Is at Risk for Stroke?"

Hemorrhagic Stroke

In a healthy, functioning brain, neurons do not come into direct contact with blood. The vital oxygen and nutrients the neurons need from the blood come to the neurons across the thin walls of the cerebral capillaries. The glia (nervous system cells that support and protect neurons) form a blood-brain barrier, an elaborate meshwork that surrounds blood vessels and capillaries and regulates which elements of the blood can pass through to the neurons.

When an artery in the brain bursts, blood spews out into the surrounding tissue and upsets not only the blood supply but the delicate chemical balance neurons require to function. This is called a hemorrhagic stroke. Such strokes account for approximately 20 percent of all strokes.

Hemorrhage can occur in several ways. One common cause is a bleeding aneurysm, a weak or thin spot on an artery wall. Over time, these weak spots stretch or balloon out under high arterial pressure. The thin walls of these ballooning aneurysms can rupture and spill blood into the space surrounding brain cells.

Hemorrhage also occurs when arterial walls break open. Plaque-encrusted artery walls eventually lose their elasticity and become brittle and thin, prone to cracking. Hypertension, or high blood pressure, increases the risk that a brittle artery wall will give way and release blood into the surrounding brain tissue.

A person with an arteriovenous malformation (AVM) also has an increased risk of hemorrhagic stroke. AVMs are a tangle of defective blood vessels and capillaries within the brain that have thin walls and can therefore rupture.

Bleeding from ruptured brain arteries can either go into the substance of the brain or into the various spaces surrounding the brain. Intracerebral hemorrhage occurs when a vessel within the brain leaks blood into the brain itself. Subarachnoid hemorrhage is bleeding under the meninges, or outer membranes, of the brain into the thin fluid-filled space that surrounds the brain.

The subarachnoid space separates the arachnoid membrane from the underlying pia mater membrane. It contains a clear fluid (cerebrospinal fluid or CSF) as well as the small blood vessels that supply the outer surface of the brain. In a subarachnoid hemorrhage, one of the small arteries within the subarachnoid space bursts, flooding the area with blood and contaminating the cerebrospinal fluid. Since the CSF flows throughout the cranium, within the spaces of the brain, subarachnoid hemorrhage can lead to extensive damage throughout the brain. In fact, subarachnoid hemorrhage is the most deadly of all strokes.

Transient Ischemic Attacks

A transient ischemic attack (TIA), sometimes called a mini-stroke, starts just like a stroke but then resolves, leaving no noticeable symptoms or deficits. The occurrence of a TIA is a warning that the person is at risk for a more serious and debilitating stroke. Of the approximately fifty thousand Americans who have a TIA each year, about one-third will have an acute stroke sometime in the future. The addition of other risk factors compounds a person's risk for a recurrent stroke. The average duration of a TIA is a few minutes. For almost all TIAs, the symptoms go away within an hour. There is no way to tell whether symptoms will be just a TIA or persist and lead to death or disability. The patient should assume that all stroke symptoms signal an emergency and should not wait to see if they go away.

Recurrent Stroke

Recurrent stroke is frequent; about 25 percent of people who recover from their first stroke will have another stroke within five years. Recurrent stroke is a major contributor to stroke disability and death, with the risk of severe disability or death from stroke increasing with each stroke recurrence. The risk of a recurrent stroke is greatest right after a stroke, with the risk decreasing with time. About 3 percent of stroke patients will have another stroke within thirty days of their first stroke, and one-third of recurrent strokes take place within two years of the first stroke.

How Do You Recognize Stroke?

Symptoms of stroke appear suddenly. Watch for these symptoms and be prepared to act quickly for yourself or on behalf of someone you are with:

- Sudden numbness or weakness of the face, arm, or leg, especially on one side of the body.
- Sudden confusion, trouble talking, or understanding speech.
- Sudden trouble seeing in one or both eyes.
- Sudden trouble walking, dizziness, or loss of balance or coordination.
- Sudden severe headache with no known cause.

If you suspect you or someone you know is experiencing any of these symptoms indicative of a stroke, do not wait. Call 911 emergency immediately. There are now effective therapies for stroke that must be administered at a hospital, but they lose their effectiveness if not given within the first three hours after stroke symptoms appear. Every minute counts!

How Is the Cause of Stroke Determined?

Physicians have several diagnostic techniques and imaging tools to help diagnose the cause of stroke quickly and accurately. The first step in diagnosis is a short neurological examination. When a possible stroke patient arrives at a hospital, a health care professional, usually a doctor or nurse, will ask the patient or a companion what happened and when the symptoms began. Blood tests, an electrocardiogram, and CT scans will often be done. One test that helps doctors judge the severity of a stroke is the standardized NIH Stroke Scale, developed by the NINDS. Health care professionals use the NIH Stroke Scale to measure a patient's neurological deficits by asking the patient to answer questions and to perform several physical and mental tests. Other scales include the Glasgow Coma Scale, the Hunt and Hess Scale, the Modified Rankin Scale, and the Barthel Index.

Imaging for the Diagnosis of Acute Stroke

Health care professionals also use a variety of imaging devices to evaluate stroke patients. The most widely used imaging procedure is the computed tomography (CT) scan. Also known as a CAT scan or computed axial tomography, CT creates a series of cross-sectional images of the head and brain. Because it is readily available at all hours at most major hospitals and produces images quickly, CT is the preferred diagnostic technique for acute stroke. CT also has unique diagnostic benefits. It will quickly rule out a hemorrhage, can occasionally show a tumor that might mimic a stroke, and may even show evidence of early infarction. Infarctions generally show up on a CT scan about six to eight hours after the start of stroke symptoms.

If a stroke is caused by hemorrhage, a CT can show evidence of bleeding into the brain almost immediately after stroke symptoms appear. Hemorrhage is the primary reason for avoiding certain drug treatments for stroke, such as thrombolytic therapy, the only proven acute stroke therapy for ischemic stroke (see section on "What Stroke Therapies Are Available?"). Thrombolytic therapy cannot be used until the doctor can confidently diagnose the patient as suffering from an ischemic stroke, because this treatment might increase bleeding and could make a hemorrhagic stroke worse.

Another imaging device used for stroke patients is the magnetic resonance imaging (MRI) scan. MRI uses magnetic fields to detect subtle changes in brain tissue content. One effect of stroke is an increase of water content in the cells of brain tissue, a condition called cytotoxic edema. MRI can detect edema as soon as a few hours after the onset of stroke. The benefit of MRI over CT imaging is that MRI is better able to detect small infarcts soon after stroke onset. Unfortunately, not every hospital has access to an MRI device and the procedure is time-consuming and expensive. It also is not as accurate in determining when hemorrhage is present. Finally, because MRI takes longer to perform than CT, it should not be used if it delays treatment. Other types of MRI scans, often used for the diagnosis of cerebrovascular disease and to predict the risk of stroke, are magnetic resonance angiography (MRA) and functional magnetic resonance imaging (fMRI). Neurosurgeons use MRA to detect stenosis (blockage) of the brain arteries inside the skull by mapping flowing blood. Functional MRI uses a magnet to pick up signals from oxygenated blood and can show brain activity through increases in local blood flow. Duplex Doppler ultrasound and arteriography are two diagnostic imaging techniques used to decide if an individual would benefit from a surgical procedure called carotid endarterectomy. This surgery is used to remove fatty deposits from the carotid arteries and can help prevent stroke.

Doppler ultrasound is a painless, noninvasive test in which sound waves above the range of human hearing are sent into the neck. Echoes bounce off the moving blood and the tissue in the artery and can be formed into an image. Ultrasound is fast, painless, risk-free, and relatively inexpensive compared to MRA and arteriography, but it is not considered to be as accurate as arteriography. Arteriography is an x-ray of the carotid artery taken when a special dye is injected into the artery. The procedure carries its own small risk of causing a stroke and is costly to perform. The benefits of arteriography over MR techniques and ultrasound are that it is extremely reliable and still the best way to measure stenosis of the carotid arteries. Even so, significant advances are being made every day involving noninvasive imaging techniques such as fMRI (see section on surgery in "What Stroke Therapies Are Available?").

Who Is at Risk for Stroke?

Some people are at a higher risk for stroke than others. Unmodifiable risk factors include age, gender, race/ethnicity, and stroke family history. In contrast, other risk factors for stroke, like high blood pressure or cigarette smoking, can be changed or controlled by the person at risk.

Unmodifiable Risk Factors

It is a myth that stroke occurs only in elderly adults. In actuality, stroke strikes all age groups, from fetuses still in the womb to centenarians. It is true, however, that older people have a higher risk for stroke than the general population and that the risk for stroke increases with age. For every decade after the age of fifty-five, the risk of stroke doubles, and two-thirds of all strokes occur in people over sixty-five years old. People over sixty-five also have a sevenfold greater risk of dying from stroke than the general population, and the incidence of stroke is increasing proportionately with the increase in the elderly population. When the baby boomers move into the over-sixty-five age group, stroke and other diseases will take on even greater significance in the health care field.

Gender also plays a role in risk for stroke. Men have a higher risk for stroke, but more women die from stroke. The stroke risk for men is 1.25 times that for women, but men do not live as long as women, so men are usually younger when they have their strokes and therefore have a higher rate of survival than women. In other words, even though women have fewer strokes than men, women are generally older when they have their strokes and are more likely to die from them.

Stroke seems to run in some families. Several factors might contribute to familial stroke risk. Members of a family might have a genetic tendency for stroke risk factors, such as an inherited predisposition for hypertension or diabetes. The influence of a common lifestyle among family members could also contribute to familial stroke.

The risk for stroke varies among different ethnic and racial groups. The incidence of stroke among African Americans is almost double that of white Americans, and twice as many African Americans who have a stroke die from the event, compared to white Americans. African Americans between the ages of forty-five and fifty-five have four to five times the stroke death rate of whites. After age fifty-five the stroke mortality rate for whites increases and is equal to that of African Americans.

Compared to white Americans, African Americans have a higher incidence of stroke risk factors, including high blood pressure and cigarette smoking. African Americans also have a higher incidence and prevalence of some genetic diseases, such as diabetes and sickle cell anemia, that predispose them to stroke.

Hispanics and Native Americans have stroke incidence and mortality rates more similar to those of white Americans. In Asian Americans stroke incidence and mortality rates are also similar to those in white Americans, even though Asians in Japan, China, and other countries of the Far East have significantly higher stroke incidence and mortality rates than white Americans. This suggests that environment and lifestyle factors play a large role in stroke risk.

The "Stroke Belt"

Several decades ago, scientists and statisticians noticed that people in the southeastern United States had the highest stroke mortality rate in the country. They named this region the stroke belt. For many years, researchers believed that the increased risk was due to the higher percentage of African Americans and an overall lower socioeconomic status (SES) in the southern states. A low SES is associated with an overall lower standard of living, leading to a lower standard of health care and therefore an increased risk of stroke. Yet researchers now know that the higher percentage of African Americans and the overall lower SES in the southern states do not adequately account for the higher incidence of, and mortality from, stroke in those states. This means that other factors must be contributing to the higher incidence of and mortality from stroke in this region.

Recent studies have also shown that there is a stroke buckle in the stroke belt. Three southeastern states, North Carolina, South Carolina, and Georgia, have an extremely high stroke mortality rates, higher than the rates in other stroke belt states and up to two times the stroke mortality rate of the United States overall. The increased risk could be due to geographic or environmental factors or to regional differences in lifestyle, including higher rates of cigarette smoking and a regional preference for salty, high-fat foods.

Other Risk Factors

The most important risk factors for stroke are hypertension, heart disease, diabetes, and cigarette smoking. Others include heavy alcohol consumption, high blood cholesterol levels, illicit drug use, and genetic or congenital conditions, particularly vascular abnormalities. People with more than one risk factor have what is called "amplification of risk." This means that the multiple risk factors compound their destructive effects and create an overall risk greater than the simple cumulative effect of the individual risk factors.

Hypertension

Of all the risk factors that contribute to stroke, the most powerful is hypertension, or high blood pressure. People with hypertension have a risk for stroke that is four to six times higher than the risk for those without hypertension. One-third of the adult U.S. population, about fifty million people (including 40 to 70 percent of those over age sixty-five) have high blood pressure. Forty to 90 percent of stroke patients have high blood pressure before their stroke event.

A systolic pressure of 120 mm of Hg over a diastolic pressure of 80 mm of Hg is generally considered normal. Persistently high blood pressure greater than 140 over 90 leads to the diagnosis of the disease called hypertension. The impact of hypertension on the total risk for stroke decreases with increasing age; therefore factors other than hypertension play a greater role in the overall stroke risk in elderly adults. For people without hypertension, the absolute risk of stroke increases over time until around the age of ninety, when the absolute risk becomes the same as that for people with hypertension.

As with stroke, there is a gender difference in the prevalence of hypertension. In younger people, hypertension is more common among men than among women. With increasing age, however, more women than men have hypertension. This hypertension gender-age difference probably has an impact on the incidence and prevalence of stroke in these populations.

Antihypertensive medication can decrease a person's risk for stroke. Recent studies suggest that treatment can decrease the stroke incidence rate by 38 percent and decrease the stroke fatality rate by 40 percent. Common hypertensive agents include adrenergic agents, beta-blockers, angiotensin converting enzyme inhibitors, calcium channel blockers, diuretics, and vasodilators.

Heart Disease

After hypertension, the second most powerful risk factor for stroke is heart disease, especially a condition known as atrial fibrillation. Atrial fibrillation is irregular beating of the left atrium, or left upper chamber, of the heart. In people with atrial fibrillation, the left atrium beats up to four times faster than the rest of the heart. This leads to an irregular flow of blood and the occasional formation of blood clots that can leave the heart and travel to the brain, causing a stroke.

Atrial fibrillation, which affects as many as 2.2 million Americans, increases an individual's risk of stroke by 4 to 6 percent, and about 15 percent of stroke patients have atrial fibrillation before they experience a stroke. The condition is more prevalent in the upper age groups, which means that the prevalence of atrial fibrillation in the United States will increase proportionately with the growth of the elderly population. Unlike hypertension and other risk factors that have a lesser impact on the ever-rising absolute risk of stroke that comes with advancing age, the influence of atrial fibrillation on total risk for stroke increases powerfully with age. In people over eighty years old, atrial fibrillation is the direct cause of one in four strokes.

Other forms of heart disease that increase stroke risk include malformations of the heart valves or the heart muscle. Some valve diseases, like mitral valve stenosis or mitral annular calcification, can double the risk for stroke, independent of other risk factors.

Heart muscle malformations can also increase the risk for stroke. Patent foramen ovale (PFO) is a passage or a hole (sometimes called a "shunt") in the heart wall separating the two atria, or upper chambers, of the heart. Clots in the blood are usually filtered out by the lungs, but PFO could allow emboli or blood clots to bypass the lungs and go directly through the arteries to the brain, potentially causing a stroke. Research is currently under way to determine how important PFO is as a cause for stroke. Atrial septal aneurysm (ASA), a congenital (present from birth) malformation of the heart tissue, is a bulging of the septum or heart wall into one of the atria of the heart. Researchers do not know why this malformation increases the risk for stroke. PFO and ASA frequently occur together and therefore amplify the risk for stroke. Two other heart malformations that seem to increase the risk for stroke for unknown reasons are left atrial enlargement and left ventricular hypertrophy. People with left atrial enlargement have a larger than normal left atrium of the heart; those with left ventricular hypertrophy have a thickening of the wall of the left ventricle.

Another risk factor for stroke is cardiac surgery to correct heart malformations or reverse the effects of heart disease. Strokes occurring in this situation are usually the result of surgically dislodged plaques from the aorta that travel through the bloodstream to the arteries in the neck and head, causing stroke. Cardiac surgery increases a person's risk of stroke by about 1 percent. Other types of surgery can also increase the risk of stroke.

Blood Cholesterol Levels

Most people know that high cholesterol levels contribute to heart disease. Yet many don't realize that a high cholesterol level also contributes to stroke risk. Cholesterol, a waxy substance produced by the liver, is a vital body product. It contributes to the production of hormones and vitamin D and is an integral component of cell membranes. The liver makes enough cholesterol to fuel the body's needs and this natural production of cholesterol alone is not a large contributing factor to atherosclerosis, heart disease, and stroke. Research has shown that the danger from cholesterol comes from a dietary intake of foods that contain high levels of cholesterol. Foods high in saturated fat and cholesterol, like meats, eggs, and dairy products, can increase the amount of total cholesterol in the body to alarming levels, contributing to the risk of atherosclerosis and thickening of the arteries.

Cholesterol is classified as a lipid, meaning that it is fat-soluble rather than water-soluble. Other lipids include fatty acids, glycerides, alcohol, waxes, steroids, and fat-soluble vitamins A, D, and E. Lipids and water, like oil and water, do not mix. Blood is a water-based liquid; therefore cholesterol does not mix with blood. In order to travel through the blood without clumping together, cholesterol needs to be covered by a layer of protein. The cholesterol and protein together are called a lipoprotein.

There are two kinds of cholesterol, commonly called the "good" and the "bad." Good cholesterol is high-density lipoprotein, or HDL; bad cholesterol is low-density lipoprotein, or LDL. Together, these two forms of cholesterol make up a person's total serum cholesterol level. Most cholesterol tests measure the level of total cholesterol in the blood and don't distinguish between good and bad cholesterol. For these total serum cholesterol tests, a level of less than 200 mg/dL is considered safe, while a level of more than 240 is considered dangerous and places a person at risk for heart disease and stroke. (mg/dL describes the weight of cholesterol in milligrams in a deciliter of blood. This is the standard way of measuring blood cholesterol levels.)

Most cholesterol in the body is in the form of LDL. LDLs circulate through the bloodstream, picking up excess cholesterol and depositing cholesterol where it is needed (for example, for the production and maintenance of cell membranes). Yet when too much cholesterol is circulating in the blood, the body cannot handle the excessive LDLs, that build up along the inside of the arterial walls. The buildup of LDL coating on the inside of the artery walls hardens and turns into arterial plaque, leading to stenosis and atherosclerosis. This plaque blocks blood vessels and contributes to the formation of blood clots. A person's LDL level should be less than 130 mg/dL to be safe. LDL levels between 130 and 159 put a person at a slightly higher risk for atherosclerosis, heart disease, and stroke. A score over 160 puts a person at great risk for a heart attack or stroke.

The other form of cholesterol, HDL, is beneficial and contributes to stroke prevention. HDL carries a small percentage of the cholesterol in the blood, but instead of depositing its cholesterol on the inside of artery walls, HDL returns to the liver to unload its cholesterol. The liver then eliminates the excess cholesterol by passing it along to the kidneys. Currently, any HDL score higher than 35 is considered desirable. Recent studies have shown that high levels of HDL are associated with a reduced risk for heart disease and stroke and that low levels (less than 35 mg/dL), even in people with normal levels of LDL, lead to an increased risk for heart disease and stroke.

A person may lower his or her risk for atherosclerosis and stroke by improving his or her cholesterol levels. A healthy diet and regular exercise are the best ways to lower total cholesterol levels. In some cases, physicians may prescribe cholesterol-lowering medication, and recent studies have shown that the newest types of these drugs, called reductase inhibitors or statin drugs, significantly reduce the risk for stroke in most patients with high cholesterol. Scientists believe that statins may work by reducing the amount of bad cholesterol the body produces and by reducing the body's inflammatory immune reaction to cholesterol plaque associated with atherosclerosis and stroke.

Diabetes

Diabetes is another disease that increases a person's risk for stroke. People with diabetes have three times the risk of stroke compared to people without diabetes. The relative risk of stroke from diabetes is highest in the fifth and sixth decades of life and decreases after that. Like hypertension, the relative risk of stroke from diabetes is highest for men at an earlier age and highest for women at an older age. People with diabetes may also have other contributing risk factors that can amplify the overall risk for stroke. For example, the prevalence of hypertension is 40 percent higher in the diabetic population compared to the general population.

Modifiable Lifestyle Risk Factors

Cigarette smoking is the most powerful modifiable stroke risk factor. Smoking almost doubles a person's risk for ischemic stroke, independent of other risk factors, and it increases a person's risk for subarachnoid hemorrhage by up to 3.5 percent. Smoking is directly responsible for a greater percentage of the total number of strokes in young adults than in older adults. Risk factors other than smoking—like hypertension, heart disease, and diabetes—account for more of the total number of strokes in older adults.

Heavy smokers are at greater risk for stroke than light smokers. The relative risk of stroke decreases immediately after quitting smoking, with a major reduction of risk seen after two to four years.

Unfortunately, it may take several decades for a former smoker's risk to drop to the level of someone who never smoked.

Smoking increases the risk of stroke by promoting atherosclerosis and increasing the levels of blood-clotting factors, such as fibrinogen. In addition to promoting conditions linked to stroke, smoking also increases the damage that results from stroke by weakening the endothelial wall of the cerebrovascular system. This leads to greater damage to the brain from events that occur in the secondary stage of stroke. (The secondary effects of stroke are discussed in greater detail in the Appendix.)

High alcohol consumption is another modifiable risk factor for stroke. Generally, an increase in alcohol consumption leads to an increase in blood pressure. While scientists agree that heavy drinking is a risk for both hemorrhagic and ischemic stroke, in several research studies daily consumption of smaller amounts of alcohol has been found to provide a protective influence against ischemic stroke, perhaps because alcohol decreases the clotting ability of platelets in the blood. Moderate alcohol consumption may act in the same way as aspirin to decrease blood clotting and prevent ischemic stroke. Heavy alcohol consumption, though, may seriously deplete platelet numbers and compromise blood clotting and blood viscosity, leading to hemorrhage. In addition, heavy drinking or binge drinking can lead to a rebound effect after the alcohol is purged from the body. The consequences of this rebound effect are that blood viscosity (thickness) and platelet levels skyrocket after heavy drinking, increasing the risk for ischemic stroke.

The use of illicit drugs, such as cocaine and crack cocaine, can cause stroke. Cocaine may act on other risk factors, such as hypertension, heart disease, and vascular disease, to trigger a stroke. It decreases relative cerebrovascular blood flow by up to 30 percent, causes vascular constriction, and inhibits vascular relaxation, leading to narrowing of the arteries. Cocaine also affects the heart, causing arrhythmias and rapid heart rate that can lead to the formation of blood clots.

Marijuana smoking may also be a risk factor for stroke. Marijuana decreases blood pressure and may interact with other risk factors, such as hypertension and cigarette smoking, to cause rapidly fluctuating blood pressure levels, damaging blood vessels.

Other drugs of abuse, such as amphetamines, heroin, and anabolic steroids (and even some common, legal drugs, such as caffeine and L-asparaginase and pseudoephedrine found in over-the-counter decongestants), have been suspected of increasing stroke risk. Many of these drugs are vasoconstrictors, meaning that they cause blood vessels to constrict and blood pressure to rise.

Head and Neck Injuries

Injuries to the head or neck may damage the cerebrovascular system and cause a small number of strokes. Head injury or traumatic brain injury may cause bleeding within the brain, leading to damage akin to that caused by a hemorrhagic stroke. Neck injury, when associated with spontaneous tearing of the vertebral or carotid arteries caused by sudden and severe extension of the neck, neck rotation, or pressure on the artery, is a contributing cause of stroke, especially in young adults. This type of stroke is often called "beauty-parlor syndrome," which refers to the practice of extending the neck backward over a sink for hair washing in beauty parlors. Neck calisthenics, "bottoms-up" drinking, and improperly performed chiropractic manipulation of the neck can also put strain on the vertebral and carotid arteries, possibly leading to ischemic stroke.

Infections

Recent viral and bacterial infections may act with other risk factors to add a small risk for stroke. The immune system responds to infection by increasing inflammation and increasing the infection-fighting properties of the blood. Unfortunately, this immune response increases the number of clotting factors in the blood, leading to an increased risk of embolic-ischemic stroke.

Genetic Risk Factors

Although there may not be a single genetic factor associated with stroke, genes do play a large role in the expression of stroke risk factors such as hypertension, heart disease, diabetes, and vascular malformations. It is also possible that an increased risk for stroke within a family is due to environmental factors, such as a common sedentary lifestyle or poor eating habits, rather than hereditary factors.

Vascular malformations that cause stroke may have the strongest genetic link of all stroke risk factors. A vascular malformation is an abnormally formed blood vessel or group of blood vessels. One genetic vascular disease is called CADASIL, which stands for cerebral autosomal dominant arteriopathy with subcortical infarcts and leukoencephalopathy. CADASIL is a rare, genetically inherited, congenital vascular disease of the brain that causes strokes, subcortical dementia, migraine-like headaches, and psychiatric disturbances. CADASIL is very debilitating, and symptoms usually surface around the age of forty-five. Although CADASIL can be treated with surgery to repair the defective blood vessels, patients often die by the age of sixty-five. The exact incidence of CADASIL in the United States is unknown.

What Stroke Therapies Are Available?

Physicians have a wide range of therapies to choose from when determining a stroke patient's best therapeutic plan. The type of stroke therapy a patient should receive depends upon the stage of disease. Generally there are three treatment stages for stroke: prevention, therapy immediately after stroke, and post-stroke rehabilitation. Therapies to prevent a first or recurrent stroke are based on treating an individual's underlying risk factors for stroke, such as hypertension, atrial fibrillation, and diabetes, or preventing the widespread formation of blood clots that can cause ischemic stroke in everyone, whether or not risk factors are present. Acute stroke therapies try to stop a stroke while it is happening by quickly dissolving a blood clot causing the stroke or by stopping the bleeding of a hemorrhagic stroke. The purpose of post-stroke rehabilitation is to overcome disabilities that result from stroke damage.

Therapies for stroke include medications, surgery, or rehabilitation.

Medications

Medication or drug therapy is the most common treatment for stroke. The most popular classes of drugs used to prevent or treat stroke are antithrombotics (antiplatelet agents and anticoagulants), thrombolytics, and neuroprotective agents.

Antithrombotics prevent the formation of blood clots that can become lodged in a cerebral artery and cause strokes. Antiplatelet drugs prevent clotting by decreasing the activity of platelets, blood cells that contribute to the clotting property of blood. These drugs reduce the risk of blood-clot formation, thus reducing the risk of ischemic stroke. In the context of stroke, physicians prescribe antiplatelet drugs mainly for prevention. The most widely known and used antiplatelet drug is aspirin. Other antiplatelet drugs include clopidogrel and ticlopidine. The NINDS sponsors a wide range of clinical trials to determine the effectiveness of antiplatelet drugs for stroke prevention.

Anticoagulants reduce stroke risk by reducing the clotting property of the blood. The most commonly used anticoagulants include warfarin (also known as Coumadin®) and heparin. The NINDS has sponsored several trials to test the efficacy of anticoagulants versus antiplatelet drugs. The Stroke Prevention in Atrial Fibrillation (SPAF) trial found that, although aspirin is an effective therapy for the prevention of a second stroke in most patients with atrial fibrillation, some patients with additional risk factors do better on warfarin therapy. Another study, the Trial of Org 10127 in Acute Stroke Treatment (TOAST), tested the effectiveness of low-molecular weight heparin (Org 10172) in stroke prevention. TOAST showed that heparin anticoagulants are not generally effective in preventing recurrent stroke or improving outcome.

Thrombolytic agents are used to treat an ongoing, acute ischemic stroke caused by an artery blockage. These drugs halt the stroke by dissolving the blood clot that is blocking blood flow to the brain. Recombinant tissue plasminogen activator (rt-PA) is a genetically engineered form of t-PA, a thrombolytic substance made naturally by the body. It can be effective if given intravenously within three hours of stroke symptom onset, but it should be used only after a physician has confirmed that the patient has suffered an ischemic stroke. Thrombolytic agents can increase bleeding and therefore must be used only after careful patient screening. The NINDS rt-PA Stroke Study showed the efficacy of t-PA and in 1996 led to the first FDA-approved treatment for acute ischemic stroke. Other thrombolytics are currently being tested in clinical trials.

Neuroprotectants are medications that protect the brain from secondary injury caused by stroke (see Appendix). Although only a few neuroprotectants are FDA-approved for use at this time, many are in clinical trials. There are several different classes of neuroprotectants that show promise for future therapy, including calcium antagonists, glutamate antagonists, opiate antagonists, antioxidants, apoptosis inhibitors, and many others. One of the calcium antagonists, nimodipine, also called a calcium channel blocker, has been shown to decrease the risk of the neurological damage that results from subarachnoid hemorrhage. Calcium channel blockers, such as nimodipine, act by reducing the risk of cerebral vasospasm, a dangerous side effect of subarachnoid hemorrhage in which the blood vessels in the subarachnoid space constrict erratically, cutting off blood flow.

Surgery

Surgery can be used to prevent stroke, to treat acute stroke, or to repair vascular damage or malformations in and around the brain. There are two prominent types of surgery for stroke prevention and treatment: carotid endarterectomy and extracranial/intracranial (EC/IC) bypass.

Carotid endarterectomy is a surgical procedure in which a doctor removes fatty deposits (plaque) from the inside of one of the carotid arteries, which are located in the neck and are the main suppliers of blood to the brain. As mentioned earlier, the disease atherosclerosis is characterized by the buildup of plaque on the inside of large arteries, and the blockage of an artery by this fatty material is called stenosis. The NINDS has sponsored two large clinical trials to test the efficacy of carotid endarterectomy: the North American Symptomatic Carotid Endarterectomy Trial (NASCET) and the Asymptomatic Carotid Atherosclerosis Trial (ACAS). These trials showed that carotid endarterectomy is a safe and effective stroke prevention therapy for most people with greater than 50 percent stenosis of the carotid arteries when performed by a qualified and experienced neurosurgeon or vascular surgeon.

Currently, the NINDS is sponsoring the Carotid Revascularization Endarterectomy vs. Stenting Trial (CREST), a large clinical trial designed to test the effectiveness of carotid endarterectomy versus a newer surgical procedure for carotid stenosis called stenting. The procedure involves inserting a long, thin catheter tube into an artery in the leg and threading the catheter through the vascular system into the narrow stenosis of the carotid artery in the neck. Once the catheter is in place in the carotid artery, the radiologist expands the stent with a balloon on the tip of the catheter. The CREST trial will test the effectiveness of the new surgical technique versus the established standard technique of carotid endarterectomy surgery.

EC/IC bypass surgery is a procedure that restores blood flow to a blood-deprived area of brain tissue by rerouting a healthy artery in the scalp to the area of brain tissue affected by a blocked artery. The NINDS-sponsored EC/IC Bypass Study tested the ability of this surgery to prevent recurrent strokes in stroke patients with atherosclerosis. The study showed that, in the long run, EC/IC does not seem to benefit these patients. The surgery is still performed occasionally for patients with aneurysms, some types of small artery disease, and certain vascular abnormalities.

One useful surgical procedure for treatment of brain aneurysms that cause subarachnoid hemorrhage is a technique called "clipping." Clipping involves clamping off the aneurysm from the blood vessel, which reduces the chance that it will burst and bleed.

A new therapy that is gaining wide attention is the detachable coil technique for the treatment of high-risk intracranial aneurysms. A small platinum coil is inserted through an artery in the thigh and threaded through the arteries to the site of the aneurysm. The coil is then released into the aneurysm, where it evokes an immune response from the body. The body produces a blood clot inside the aneurysm, strengthening the artery walls and reducing the risk of rupture. Once the aneurysm is stabilized, a neurosurgeon can clip the aneurysm with less risk of hemorrhage and death to the patient.

Rehabilitation Therapy

Stroke is the number one cause of serious adult disability in the United States. Stroke disability is devastating to the stroke patient and family, but therapies are available to help rehabilitate post-stroke patients.

For most stroke patients, physical therapy (PT) is the cornerstone of the rehabilitation process. A physical therapist uses training, exercises, and physical manipulation of the stroke patient's body with the intent of restoring movement, balance, and coordination. The aim of PT is to have the stroke patient relearn simple motor activities such as walking, sitting, standing, lying down, and the process of switching from one type of movement to another.

Another type of therapy involving relearning daily activities is occupational therapy (OT). OT also involves exercise and training to help the stroke patient relearn everyday activities such as eating, drinking and swallowing, dressing, bathing, cooking, reading and writing, and toileting. The goal of OT is to help the patient become independent or semi-independent.

Speech and language problems arise when brain damage occurs in the language centers of the brain. Due to the brain's great ability to learn and change (called brain plasticity), other areas can adapt to take over some of the lost functions. Speech therapy helps stroke

Table 6.1. Post-Stroke Rehabilitation

Type	Goal
Physical Therapy (PT)	Relearn walking, sitting, lying down, switching from one type of movement to another
Occupational Therapy (OT)	Relearn eating, drinking, swallowing, dressing, bathing, cooking, reading, writing, toileting
Speech Therapy	Relearn language and communications skills
Psychological/Psychiatric Therapy	Alleviate some mental and emotional problems

patients relearn language and speaking skills, or learn other forms of communication. Speech therapy is appropriate for patients who have no deficits in cognition or thinking, but have problems understanding speech or written words, or problems forming speech. A speech therapist helps stroke patients help themselves by working to improve language skills, develop alternative ways of communicating, and develop coping skills to deal with the frustration of not being able to communicate fully. With time and patience, a stroke survivor should be able to regain some, and sometimes all, language and speaking abilities.

Many stroke patients require psychological or psychiatric help after a stroke. Psychological problems, such as depression, anxiety, frustration, and anger, are common post-stroke disabilities. Talk therapy, along with appropriate medication, can help alleviate some of the mental and emotional problems that result from stroke. Sometimes it is also beneficial for family members of the stroke patient to seek psychological help as well.

What Disabilities Can Result from a Stroke?

Although stroke is a disease of the brain, it can affect the entire body. Some of the disabilities that can result from a stroke include paralysis, cognitive deficits, speech problems, emotional difficulties, daily living problems, and pain.

Paralysis

A common disability that results from stroke is paralysis on one side of the body, called hemiplegia. A related disability that is not as debilitating as paralysis is one-sided weakness or hemiparesis. The paralysis or weakness may affect only the face, an arm, or a leg or may affect one entire side of the body and face. A person who suffers a stroke in the left hemisphere of the brain will show right-sided paralysis or paresis. Conversely, a person with a stroke in the right hemisphere of the brain will show deficits on the left side of the body. A stroke patient may have problems with the simplest of daily activities, such as walking, dressing, eating, and using the bathroom. Motor deficits can result from damage to the motor cortex in the frontal lobes of the brain or from damage to the lower parts of the brain, such as the cerebellum, which controls balance and coordination. Some stroke patients also have trouble eating and swallowing, called dysphagia.

Cognitive Deficits

Stroke may cause problems with thinking, awareness, attention, learning, judgment, and memory. If the cognitive problems are severe, the stroke patient may be said to have apraxia, agnosia, or "neglect." In the context of stroke, neglect means that a stroke patient has no knowledge of one side of his or her body, or one side of the visual field, and is unaware of the deficit. A stroke patient may be unaware of his or her surroundings, or may be unaware of the mental deficits that resulted from the stroke.

Language Deficits

Stroke victims often have problems understanding or forming speech. A deficit in understanding speech is called aphasia. Trouble speaking or forming words is called dysarthria. Language problems usually result from damage to the left temporal and parietal lobes of the brain.

Emotional Deficits

A stroke can lead to emotional problems. Stroke patients may have difficulty controlling their emotions or may express inappropriate emotions in certain situations. One common disability that occurs with many stroke patients is depression. Post-stroke depression may be more than a general sadness resulting from the stroke incident. It is a clinical behavioral problem that can hamper recovery and rehabilitation and may even lead to suicide. Post-stroke depression is treated as any depression is treated, with antidepressant medications and therapy.

Pain

Stroke patients may experience pain, uncomfortable numbness, or strange sensations after a stroke. These sensations may be due to many factors including damage to the sensory regions of the brain, stiff joints, or a disabled limb. An uncommon type of pain resulting from stroke is called central stroke pain or central pain syndrome (CPS). CPS results from damage to an area in the mid-brain called the thalamus. The pain is a mixture of sensations, including heat and cold, burning, tingling, numbness, and sharp stabbing and underlying aching pain. The pain is often worse in the extremities—the hands and feet—and is made worse by movement and temperature changes, especially cold temperatures. Unfortunately, since most pain medications provide little relief from these sensations, very few treatments or therapies exist to combat CPS.

What Special Risks Do Women Face?

Some risk factors for stroke apply only to women. Primary among these are pregnancy, childbirth, and menopause. These risk factors are tied to hormonal fluctuations and changes that affect a woman in different stages of life. Research in the past few decades has shown that high-dose oral contraceptives, the kind used in the 1960s and 1970s, can increase the risk of stroke in women. Fortunately, oral contraceptives with high doses of estrogen are no longer used and have been replaced with safer and more effective oral contraceptives with lower doses of estrogen. Some studies have shown the newer low-dose oral contraceptives may not significantly increase the risk of stroke in women.

Other studies have demonstrated that pregnancy and childbirth can put a woman at an increased risk for stroke. Pregnancy increases the risk of stroke as much as three to thirteen times. Of course, the risk of stroke in young women of childbearing years is very small to begin with, so a moderate increase in risk during pregnancy is still a relatively small risk. Pregnancy and childbirth cause strokes in approximately eight in one hundred thousand women. Unfortunately, 25 percent of strokes during pregnancy end in death, and hemorrhagic strokes, although rare, are still the leading cause of maternal death in the United States. Subarachnoid hemorrhage, in particular, causes one to five maternal deaths per ten thousand pregnancies.

A study sponsored by the NINDS showed that the risk of stroke during pregnancy is greatest in the postpartum period—the six weeks following childbirth. The risk of ischemic stroke after pregnancy is about nine times higher, and the risk of hemorrhagic stroke is more than twenty-eight times higher for postpartum women than for women who are not pregnant or postpartum. The cause is unknown.

In the same way that the hormonal changes during pregnancy and childbirth are associated with increased risk of stroke, hormonal changes at the end of the childbearing years can increase the risk of stroke. Several studies have shown that menopause, the end of a woman's reproductive ability marked by the termination of her menstrual cycle, can increase a woman's risk of stroke. Fortunately, some studies have suggested that hormone replacement therapy can reduce some of the effects of menopause and decrease stroke risk. Currently, the NINDS is sponsoring the Women's Estrogen for Stroke Trial (WEST), a randomized, placebo-controlled, double-blind trial, to determine whether estrogen therapy can reduce the risk of death or recurrent stroke in postmenopausal women who have a history of a recent TIA or nondisabling stroke. The mechanism by which estrogen can prove beneficial to postmenopausal women could include its role in cholesterol control. Studies have shown that estrogen acts to increase levels of HDL while decreasing LDL levels.

Are Children at Risk for Stroke?

The young have several risk factors unique to them. Young people seem to suffer from hemorrhagic strokes more than ischemic strokes, a significant difference from older age groups, where ischemic strokes make up the majority of stroke cases. Hemorrhagic strokes represent 20 percent of all strokes in the United States, and young people account for many of these.

Clinicians often separate the "young" into two categories: those younger than fifteen years of age, and those between fifteen and forty-four years of age. People fifteen to forty-four years of age are generally considered young adults and have many of the risk factors mentioned previously, such as drug use, alcohol abuse, pregnancy, head and neck injuries, heart disease or heart malformations, and infections. Some other causes of stroke in the young are linked to genetic diseases.

Medical complications that can lead to stroke in children include intracranial infection, brain injury, vascular malformations such as moyamoya syndrome, occlusive vascular disease, and genetic disorders such as sickle cell anemia, tuberous sclerosis, and Marfan's syndrome.

The symptoms of stroke in children are different from those in adults and young adults. A child experiencing a stroke may have seizures, a sudden loss of speech, a loss of expressive language (including body language and gestures), hemiparesis (weakness on one side of the body), hemiplegia (paralysis on one side of the body), dysarthria (impairment of speech), convulsions, headache, or fever. It is a medical emergency when a child shows any of these symptoms.

In children with stroke the underlying conditions that led to the stroke should be determined and managed to prevent future strokes. For example, a recent clinical study sponsored by the National Heart, Lung, and Blood Institute found that giving blood transfusions to young children with sickle cell anemia greatly reduces the risk of stroke. The institute even suggests attempting to prevent stroke in high-risk children by giving them blood transfusions before they experience a stroke.

Most children who experience a stroke will do better than most adults after treatment and rehabilitation. This is due in part to the immature brain's great plasticity, the ability to adapt to deficits and injury. Children who experience seizures along with stroke do not recover as well as children who do not have seizures. Some children may experience residual hemiplegia, though most will eventually learn how to walk.

What Research Is Being Done by the NINDS?

The NINDS is the leading supporter of stroke research in the United States and sponsors a wide range of experimental research studies, from investigations of basic biological mechanisms to studies with animal models and clinical trials.

Currently, NINDS researchers are studying the mechanisms of stroke risk factors and the process of brain damage that results from stroke. Some of this brain damage may be secondary to the initial death of brain cells caused by the lack of blood flow to the brain tissue. This secondary wave of brain injury is a result of a toxic reaction to the primary damage and mainly involves the excitatory neurochemical glutamate. Glutamate in the normal brain functions as a chemical messenger between brain cells, allowing them to communicate. Yet an excess amount of glutamate in the brain causes too much activity and brain cells quickly "burn out" from too much excitement, releasing more toxic chemicals, such as caspases, cytokines, monocytes, and oxygen-free radicals. These substances poison the chemical environment of surrounding cells, initiating a cascade of degeneration and programmed cell death, called apoptosis. NINDS researchers are studying the mechanisms underlying this secondary insult, which consists mainly of inflammation, toxicity, and a breakdown of the blood vessels that provide blood to the brain. Researchers are also looking for ways to prevent secondary injury to the brain by providing different types of neuroprotection for salvageable cells that prevent inflammation and block some of the toxic chemicals created by dying brain cells. From this research, scientists hope to develop neuroprotective agents to prevent secondary damage. For more information on excitotoxicity, neuroprotection, and the ischemic cascade, please refer to the Appendix.

Another area of research involves experiments with vasodilators, medications that expand or dilate blood vessels and thus increase blood flow to the brain. Vasodilators have long been used to treat many disorders, including heart disease. Researchers hope that vasodilators may aid in the rehabilitation of stroke victims by increasing blood flow to the brain. So far, unfortunately, they have shown limited success, possibly because they have not been given soon enough after the onset of stroke.

Basic research has also focused on the genetics of stroke and stroke risk factors. One area of research involving genetics is gene therapy. Gene therapy involves putting a gene for a desired protein in certain cells of the body. The inserted gene will then "program" the cell to produce the desired protein. If enough cells in the right areas produce enough protein, then the protein could be therapeutic. Scientists must find ways to deliver the therapeutic DNA to the appropriate cells and must learn how to deliver enough DNA to enough cells so that the tissues produce a therapeutic amount of protein. Gene therapy is in the very early stages of development and there are many problems to overcome, including learning how to penetrate the highly impermeable blood-brain barrier and how to halt the host's immune reaction to the virus that carries the gene to the cells. Some of the proteins used for stroke therapy could include neuroprotective proteins, antiinflammatory proteins, and DNA/cellular repair proteins, among others.

The NINDS supports and conducts a wide variety of studies in animals, from genetics research on zebra fish to rehabilitation research on primates. Much of the institute's animal research involves rodents, specifically mice and rats. For example, one study of hypertension and stroke uses rats that have been bred to be hypertensive and therefore stroke-prone. By studying stroke in rats, scientists hope to get a better picture of what might be happening in human stroke patients. Scientists can also use animal models to test promising therapeutic interventions for stroke. If a therapy proves to be beneficial to animals, then scientists can consider testing the therapy in human subjects.

One promising area of stroke animal research involves hibernation. The dramatic decrease of blood flow to the brain in hibernating animals is extensive—extensive enough that it would kill a nonhibernating animal. During hibernation, an animal's metabolism slows down, body temperature drops, and energy and oxygen requirements of brain cells decrease. If scientists can discover how animals hibernate without experiencing brain damage, then maybe they can discover ways to stop the brain damage associated with decreased blood flow in stroke patients. Other studies are looking at the role of hypothermia, or decreased body temperature, on metabolism and neuroprotection.

Both hibernation and hypothermia have a relationship to hypoxia and edema. Hypoxia, or anoxia, occurs when there is not enough oxygen available for brain cells to function properly. Since brain cells require large amounts of oxygen for energy requirements, they are especially vulnerable to hypoxia. Edema occurs when the chemical balance of brain tissue is disturbed and water or fluids flow into the brain cells, making them swell and burst, releasing their toxic contents into the surrounding tissues. Edema is one cause of general brain tissue swelling and contributes to the secondary injury associated with stroke.

The basic and animal studies discussed previously do not involve people and fall under the category of preclinical research; clinical research involves people. One area of investigation that has made the transition from animal models to clinical research is the study of the mechanisms underlying brain plasticity and the neuronal rewiring that occurs after a stroke.

New advances in imaging and rehabilitation have shown that the brain can compensate for function lost as a result of stroke. When cells in an area of the brain responsible for a particular function die after a stroke, the patient becomes unable to perform that function. For example, a stroke patient with an infarct in the area of the brain responsible for facial recognition becomes unable to recognize faces, a syndrome called facial agnosia. Yet, in time, the person may come to recognize faces again, even though the area of the brain originally programmed to perform that function remains dead. The plasticity of the brain and the rewiring of the neural connections make it possible for one part of the brain to change functions and take up the more important functions of a disabled part. This rewiring of the brain and restoration of function, which the brain tries to do automatically, can be helped with therapy. Scientists are working to develop new and better ways to help the brain repair itself to restore important functions to the stroke patient.

One example of a therapy resulting from this research is the use of transcranial magnetic stimulation (TMS) in stroke rehabilitation. Some evidence suggests that TMS, in which a small magnetic current is delivered to an area of the brain, may possibly increase brain plasticity and speed up recovery of function after a stroke. The TMS device is a small coil that is held outside of the head, over the part of the brain needing stimulation. Currently, several studies at the NINDS are testing whether TMS has any value in increasing motor function and improving functional recovery.

Clinical Trials

Clinical research is usually conducted in a series of trials that become progressively larger. A phase I clinical trial is directly built upon the lessons learned from basic and animal research and is used to test the safety of therapy for a particular disease and to estimate possible efficacy in a few human subjects. A phase II clinical trial usually involves many subjects at several different centers and is used to test safety and possible efficacy on a broader scale, to test different dosing for medications or to perfect techniques for surgery, and to determine the best methodology and outcome measures for the bigger phase III clinical trial to come.

A phase III clinical trial is the largest endeavor in clinical research. This type of trial often involves many centers and many subjects. The trial usually has two patient groups who receive different treatments, but all other standard care is the same and represents the best care available. The trial may compare two treatments, or, if there is only one treatment to test, patients who do not receive the test therapy receive instead a placebo. The patients are told that the additional treatment they are receiving may be either the active treatment or a placebo. Many phase III trials are called double-blind, randomized clinical trials. Double-blind means that neither the subjects nor the doctors and nurses who are treating the subjects and determining the response to the therapy know which treatment a subject receives. Randomization refers to the placing of subjects into one of the treatment groups in a way that can't be predicted by the patients or investigators. These clinical trials usually involve many investigators and take many years to complete. The hypothesis and methods of the trial are very precise and well thought out. Clinical trial designs, as well as the concepts of blinding and randomization, have developed over years of experimentation, trial, and error. At the present time, researchers are developing new designs to maximize the opportunity for all subjects to receive therapy.

Most treatments for general use come out of phase III clinical trials. After one or more phase III trials are finished, and if the results are positive for the treatment, the investigators can petition the FDA for government approval to use the drug or procedure to treat patients. Once the treatment is approved by the FDA, it can be used by qualified doctors throughout the country.

NINDS-Sponsored Stroke Clinical Trials: April 2004

Clinical trials give researchers a way to test new treatments in human subjects. Clinical trials test surgical devices and procedures, medications, rehabilitation therapies, and lifestyle and psychosocial interventions to determine how safe and effective they are and to establish the proper amount or level of treatment. Because of their scope and the need for careful analysis of data and outcomes, clinical trials are usually conducted in three phases and can take several years or more to complete.

- *Phase I* clinical trials are small (involving fewer than one hundred people) and are designed to define side effects and tolerance of the medication or therapy.

- *Phase II* trials are conducted with a larger group of subjects and seek to measure the effects of a therapy and establish its proper dosage or level of treatment.

- *Phase III* trials often involve hundreds (sometimes thousands) of volunteer patients who are assigned to treatment and nontreatment groups to test how well the treatment works and how safe it is at the recommended dosage or level of therapy. Many of these trials use a controlled, randomized, double-blind study design. This means that patients are randomly assigned to groups and neither the subject nor the study staff knows to which group a patient belongs. Phase III randomized clinical trials are often called the gold standard of clinical trials.

NINDS conducts clinical trials at the NIH Clinical Center and also provides funding for clinical trials at hospitals and universities across the United States and Canada. Following are findings from some of the largest and most significant recent clinical trials, as well as summaries of some of the most promising clinical trials in progress.

Findings from Recently Completed Clinical Trials

Warfarin vs. Aspirin Recurrent Stroke Study (WARSS)

WARSS was a seven-year double-blind randomized clinical trial that enrolled more than two hundred patients at forty-eight participating centers. It was the largest clinical trial ever to compare the benefits of aspirin to warfarin for the prevention of recurrent stroke. Findings from the study were published in the *New England Journal of Medicine* (November 15, 2001), which showed that aspirin works as well as warfarin in helping to prevent recurrent strokes in most patients. Whether warfarin was superior to aspirin for stroke prevention was unclear prior to WARSS. Most clinicians believed that warfarin was a better blood thinner than aspirin, although it had three drawbacks: it was more expensive, it required monthly blood tests for proper monitoring, and it had a greater risk for side effects. The WARSS trial demonstrated that aspirin was not only cheaper and safer than warfarin for preventing stroke, it was just as effective—without the additional costs of monthly monitoring.

African American Antiplatelet Stroke Prevention Study (AAASPS)

The AAASPS study was a randomized double-blind trial that enrolled 1,800 African American stroke patients at more than sixty sites to compare the benefits of ticlopidine to aspirin in preventing recurrent stroke. A previous clinical trial of ticlopidine had indicated that the antiplatelet drug might be particularly effective for stroke reduction among nonwhites, primarily African Americans. The trial ended early when data analysis suggested that there was less than a 1 percent chance that ticlopidine would be shown to be superior to aspirin if the study were carried to completion. Results showed that 650 mg of aspirin per day is just as effective as ticlopidine in preventing recurrent stroke and has the added benefit of easy availability, lower cost, and less risk for side effects. The findings were published in the *Journal of the American Medical Association* (June 11, 2003).

Women's Estrogen for Stroke Trial (WEST)

WEST was the first clinical trial to test the benefits of estrogen therapy for prevention of recurrent cerebrovascular disease in women. The randomized double-blind placebo-controlled trial recruited 664 postmenopausal women from twenty-one hospitals across the United States. Findings from the study, published in the *New England Journal of Medicine* (October 2001), demonstrated that hormone replacement therapy with estrogen did not reduce the risk of stroke or death in postmenopausal women who had already had one stroke or transient ischemic attack (TIA, also called mini-stroke). The data also suggested that women who received estrogen were more likely to have a fatal stroke during the first six months of treatment, and that their nonfatal strokes were more severe. Based on these findings, the WEST investigators recommended against prescribing estrogen therapy for the purpose of preventing future recurrent stroke in postmenopausal women.

Ongoing Clinical Trials

The Family Intervention in Recovery from Stroke Trial (FIRST)

This study is testing whether or not the daily involvement and support of family, friends, and neighbors can improve the functional abilities of elderly stroke patients. An intervention has been designed to mobilize the social networks of stroke patients to provide effective emotional and practical support. Close to three hundred patients from two large city hospitals have been randomly assigned to two groups: one that receives the intervention, and one that receives the usual care. At three months and six months, members of each group are being assessed for functional ability based both on how well they think they are doing and on their performance on tests that measure functional abilities. A number of previous studies have indicated that psychosocial interventions can improve emotional adjustment in stroke patients and promote longer survival rates in patients with chronic illnesses. This is the first study to focus specifically on the impact of such psychosocial interventions on physical function in stroke survivors.

The Carotid Revascularization Endarterectomy vs. Stenting Trial (CREST)

The use of dilation and stenting techniques similar to those used to unclog and open heart arteries has been proposed as a less invasive alternative to carotid endarterectomy (a surgical procedure that opens and widens blocked carotid arteries on either side of the neck). This trial is comparing the two techniques for safety and effectiveness. The standard carotid endarterectomy surgical procedure is being used on one set of patients. A procedure that inserts an expanding metal scaffold (stent) into the neck artery after widening it with balloon dilation is being tested on another group. If stenting is shown to be safe, effective, and durable, this less invasive procedure is likely to have a wider application in medical practice. A small add-on study to CREST is using genetic sampling and screening techniques to identify specific genes that could increase the risk for stroke.

Carotid Occlusion Surgery Study (COSS)

The goal of this multicenter randomized clinical trial is to determine if extracranial bypass surgery can reduce the risk of subsequent stroke for a subgroup of people who have a blocked carotid artery and an increased oxygen extraction fraction (OEF, which indicates how hard the brain has to work to pull oxygen out of the blood supply). An increased OEF has been shown to be a powerful and independent risk factor for subsequent stroke—increasing the odds by 25 to 50 percent. Participants have been randomly assigned to medical care with antiplatelet therapy, or antiplatelet therapy in combination with extracranial bypass surgery, which increases blood flow to the brain by using a healthy blood vessel to bypass the blocked artery. The participants are being followed for an average of two years to monitor incidence of stroke.

Warfarin vs. Aspirin for Intracranial Arterial Stenosis (WASID)

The goal of this trial is to compare the effectiveness of warfarin to aspirin in preventing subsequent strokes or other vascular-related events, such as heart attacks, in patients with clogged arteries in the brain (intracranial arterial stenosis). This is a randomized multicenter trial that is following two groups of patients who have had a transient ischemic attack (TIA, commonly called a mini-stroke), or a minor stroke caused by blocked or narrowed arteries in the brain. One group is receiving warfarin; the other is taking aspirin. Patients are being followed for four years to compare the rates of death due to stroke and vascular-related diseases. This study hopes to show which treatment is better for patients with intracranial arterial stenosis.

Intraoperative Hypothermia for Aneurysm Surgery Trial (IHAST)

Aneurysmal subarachnoid hemorrhage (SAH), in which a bulging artery ruptures and bleeds into the area between the skull and the brain, accounts for only 5 percent of all strokes but has a high rate of mortality and high levels of disability in those who survive. The usual course of treatment is to clip and seal the area around the ruptured artery to end the bleeding and establish normal circulation. The trial investigators believe that this surgical procedure often causes additional neurological damage that can lead to death or substantial disability after surgery. IHAST is a randomized clinical trial designed to evaluate the safety and effectiveness of hypothermia (lowering body temperature to 33 degrees centigrade) to prevent neurological damage during surgery. Patients are being tested three months following surgery to establish whether or not there is an improvement in neurological outcome if hypothermia is used during surgery.

Extremity Constraint-Induced Therapy Evaluation (EXCITE)

Impaired movement in the arms and legs is a major consequence of stroke. Therapeutic interventions to improve motor function and promote independent use of arms and hands are limited. One technique that has been shown to be successful in basic research studies with animal and human subjects is constraint-induced (CI) movement therapy (also called forced use). The CI technique involves restriction of the less affected arm, while the more affected arm is forced to perform repetitive motions. This trial has randomized stroke patients with at least minimal ability in their arms to two groups—one that receives customary care and one that receives CI therapy. A year after the trial begins, the customary care group will cross over to also receive CI therapy, in order to test whether or not delayed therapy can be effective. Changes in both groups in terms of increased motor function and psychosocial function will be measured.

Warfarin vs. Aspirin in Reduced Cardiac Ejection Fraction (WARCEF)

The purpose of this study is to determine which of two treatments—warfarin or aspirin—is better for preventing death from stroke in patients with low ejection fraction (EF) and heart failure. EF is a measurement that indicates the amount of blood pumped (ejected) from the heart with each beat. Low EF is a known risk factor for stroke in people with heart failure, because the lower the EF, the less blood is being pumped out of the heart. This multicenter (70 sites) study has enrolled thousands of patients with low EF and randomly assigned them to be treated with warfarin or aspirin. Telephone reports and physical exams every four months over the course of three years have been recording their health status and the occurrence of stroke or other cardiovascular events. Data is also being analyzed for differences in therapy response among men and women, and African Americans and other racial groups. The study will define the optimal stroke prevention therapy for patients with cardiac failure and low EF.

Secondary Prevention of Small Subcortical Strokes (SPS3)

This trial is testing the benefits of combined antiplatelet therapy (aspirin and clopidogrel) compared to intensive blood pressure control to prevent recurring stroke in people who have small subcortical strokes (S3). S3, in which the threadlike arteries within cerebral tissue become blocked and halt blood flow to the brain, is the most frequent type of stroke in Hispanic Americans. For those who survive S3, there is a high risk for additional strokes, vascular dementia, and cognitive decline. The trial is enrolling 2,500 patients (20 percent of whom will be Hispanic Americans) who will then be assigned to two interventions: treatment with aspirin and clopidogrel, or intensive blood pressure control. Patients are being followed every three months for three years. There have been no previous clinical trials focused on the use of combined antiplatelet therapy after S3, on optimal target levels of blood pressure control after stroke, or on prevention of stroke and dementia in Hispanic Americans. The results of this trial will help establish optimal stroke prevention treatment levels for those with S3 and determine if those levels are different for Hispanic Americans.

Field Administration of Stroke Therapy Magnesium Trial (FAST-MAG)

This is a three-phase trial to develop and test methods that can quickly deliver neuroprotective therapies to prevent further damage to brain tissue after stroke. While a number of neuroprotective drugs have been shown to reduce stroke damage to brain tissue in animals, there have been no Phase III clinical trials in humans, mostly because of difficulties in administering the drugs quickly enough. In the first phase of this project, paramedics will immediately administer a neuroprotective agent (magnesium sulfate) to patients with symptoms of acute stroke and the outcomes will be evaluated for safety, practicality, and timesaving over hospital treatment. The second phase is a standard, Phase III clinical trial that randomizes patients to receive either treatment with magnesium sulfate or placebo. The last phase will test differences in outcomes between early treatment before patients reach the hospital versus later treatment in the hospital. If early treatment is shown to be practical as well as more beneficial, a larger multicenter trial can be launched to demonstrate the advantages of administering therapy before patients arrive at the hospital. The results from such a trial could potentially set a new standard of care.

Appendix

The Ischemic Cascade

The brain is the most complex organ in the human body. It contains hundreds of billions of cells that interconnect to form a complex network of communication. The brain has several different types of cells, the most important of which are neurons. The organization of neurons in the brain and the communication that occurs among them lead to thought, memory, cognition, and awareness. Other types of brain cells are generally called glia (from the Greek word meaning "glue"). These supportive cells of the nervous system provide scaffolding and support for the vital neurons, protecting them from infection, toxins, and trauma. Glia make up the blood-brain barrier between blood vessels and the substance of the brain.

Stroke is the sudden onset of paralysis caused by injury to brain cells from disruption in blood flow. The injury caused by a blocked blood vessel can occur within several minutes and progress for hours as the result of a chain of chemical reactions that is set off after the start of stroke symptoms. Physicians and researchers often call this chain of chemical reactions that lead to the permanent brain injury of stroke the ischemic cascade.

Primary Cell Death

In the first stage of the ischemic cascade, blood flow is cut off from a part of the brain (ischemia). This leads to a lack of oxygen (anoxia) and lack of nutrients in the cells of this core area. When the lack of oxygen becomes extreme, the mitochondria, the energy-producing structures within the cell, can no longer produce enough energy to keep the cell functioning. The mitochondria break down, releasing toxic chemicals called oxygen-free radicals into the cytoplasm of the cell. These toxins poison the cell from the inside out, causing destruction of other cell structures, including the nucleus.

The lack of energy in the cell causes the gated channels of the cell membrane that normally maintain homeostasis to open and allow toxic amounts of calcium, sodium, and potassium ions to flow into the cell. At the same time, the injured ischemic cell releases excitatory amino acids, such as glutamate, into the space between neurons, leading to overexcitation and injury to nearby cells. With the loss of homeostasis, water rushes into the cell, making it swell (called cytotoxic edema) until the cell membrane bursts under the internal pressure. At this point the nerve cell is essentially permanently injured and for all purposes dead (necrosis and infarction). After a stroke starts, the first cells that are going to die may die within four to five minutes. The response to the treatment that restores blood flow as late as two hours after stroke onset would suggest that, in most cases, the process is not over for at least two to three hours. After that, with rare exceptions, most of the injury that has occurred is essentially permanent.

Secondary Cell Death

Due to exposure to excessive amounts of glutamate, nitric oxide, free radicals, and excitatory amino acids released into the intercellular space by necrotic cells, nearby cells have a more difficult time surviving. They are receiving just enough oxygen from cerebral blood flow (CBF) to stay alive. A compromised cell can survive for several hours in a low-energy state. If blood flow is restored within this narrow window of opportunity, at present thought to be about two hours, then some of these cells can be salvaged and become functional again. Researchers funded by the NINDS have learned that restoring blood flow to these cells can be achieved by administrating the clot-dissolving thrombolytic agent t-PA within three hours of the start of the stroke.

Inflammation and the Immune Response

While anoxic and necrotic brain cells are doing damage to still viable brain tissue the immune system of the body is injuring the brain through an inflammatory reaction mediated by the vascular system. Damage to the blood vessel at the site of a blood clot or hemorrhage attracts inflammatory blood elements to that site. Among the first blood elements to arrive are leukocytes, white blood cells that are covered with immune system proteins that attach to the blood vessel wall at the site of the injury. After they attach, the leukocytes penetrate the endothelial wall, move through the blood-brain barrier, and invade the substance of the brain, causing further injury and brain cell death. Leukocytes called monocytes and macrophages release inflammatory chemicals (cytokines, interleukins, and tissue necrosis factors) at the site of the injury. These chemicals make it harder for the body to naturally dissolve a clot that has caused a stroke by inactivating anti-clotting factors and inhibiting the release of natural tissue plasminogen activator. NINDS researchers are currently working to create interventional therapies that will inhibit the effects of cytokines and other chemicals in the inflammatory process during stroke.

These brain cells that survive the loss of blood flow (ischemia) but are not able to function make up the ischemic penumbra. These areas of still-viable brain cells exist in a patchwork pattern within and around the area of dead brain tissue (also called an infarct).

Resources

1. "The Stroke/Brain Attack Reporter's Handbook," National Stroke Association, Englewood, Colorado, 1997

Section 6.2

Recent Research on Stroke

This section begins with "Angioplasty Clears Clogged Brain Arteries," February 5, 2004, reproduced with permission from www. americanheart.org. © 2004, American Heart Association. Additional press releases from the American Heart Association are cited separately within the text.

Angioplasty Clears Clogged Brain Arteries

Angioplasty opened narrowed brain arteries, preventing strokes in patients for whom standard medication had failed, according to a study presented at the American Stroke Association's 29th International Stroke Conference.

"Angioplasty improves the outcome over what we would expect to see with medication alone," said study author Michael P. Marks, M.D., associate professor of radiology and neurosurgery and chief of interventional neuroradiology at Stanford University Medical Center in Palo Alto, California. Additionally, "Stent treatment may not be necessary."

The study was not a head-to-head comparison of angioplasty and medical therapy. Researchers used data from other studies to make risk comparisons.

Angioplasty uses a tiny balloon threaded into the area of blockage. Once in this area, the balloon is inflated. As it expands, it forces the fatty plaque against the artery wall, opening the vessel. Balloon angioplasty is widely used to open blocked heart arteries but is not as commonly used for clearing neck and brain arteries. In some cases, a miniature wire tube called a stent is left behind after angioplasty to keep the artery propped open.

Blood thinners such as aspirin and anticoagulants such as warfarin are standard medical therapy for clogged brain vessels. Anticoagulants interfere with the blood's ability to clot.

The study examined both the overall rate of stroke and the rate of stroke in areas supplied by the treated vessel in patients with symptomatic intracranial stenosis (narrowing of a brain blood vessel) undergoing angioplasty.

Researchers studied thirty-six patients with significant intracranial stenosis, all of whom had unsuccessful medical therapy. Before angioplasty stenosis averaged 84.2 percent. After angioplasty, stenosis averaged 43.3 percent.

One ischemic stroke occurred during angioplasty but the patient recovered. No other ischemic strokes occurred within one month of angioplasty, the periprocedural period.

Two deaths occurred in the periprocedural period, one due to reperfusion hemorrhage and one due to vessel perforation. Follow-up was available in thirty-four patients and varied between 4 and 128 months (average follow-up 53 months) with twenty-nine patients (or 85.3 percent) having greater than 24 months follow-up. The annual stroke rate in the area of the angioplasty was 3.36 percent. The annual rate for all strokes was 5.38 percent.

"One would expect 8 percent to 10 percent of these patients to have suffered a stroke in the territory of angioplasty annually had they been treated with medication," Marks said.

The researchers then looked at the subgroup of patients at high risk of stroke after angioplasty, which "has been used as an argument to use stents," he said. High-risk patients include those who still have significant vessel narrowing (residual stenosis) after angioplasty and those in whom the angioplasty caused a small tear, or dissection, in the vessel.

For patients with residual stenoses, some argue that the stent will open the vessel wider, Marks said. Some also believe stenting can help repair tears.

The subgroup of eighteen patients with moderate but significant residual stenosis (50 percent to 75 percent) had an annual stroke rate of 3 percent—just as low as when there was no residual stenosis, Marks said. "So by opening the vessel even a small amount, we had a favorable effect on clinical outcome."

There does not appear to be any advantage to adding a stent to help prop the artery open after angioplasty for patients with symptomatic intracranial stenosis compared to angioplasty alone, he said.

Also, none of the eleven patients with evidence of a tear in their vessel after angioplasty had a stroke at follow-up. "The tear heals itself. Stenting is not necessary for these patients either," he said.

Co-authors are Mary L. Marcellus, R.N.; Huy M. Do, M.D.; Gary K. Steinberg, M.D., Ph.D.; David C. Tong, M.D.; and Gregory A. Albers, M.D.

Cooling Helmets May Provide Innovative Stroke Treatment

February 5, 2004, reproduced with permission from www.american heart.org. © 2004, American Heart Association.

Helmets that cool the brain may minimize stroke damage, according to two small studies presented at the American Heart Association's 29th International Stroke Conference.

In a Japanese study, a "helmet-type cooling apparatus" was tested on seventeen patients with severe ischemic stroke. An American study tested a "NASA-spinoff" helmet on six patients with severe ischemic stroke.

Ischemic strokes are caused by blood clots in blood vessels of the brain or leading to it.

The helmets may improve patient outcomes and lengthen the time treatment window for ischemic strokes.

Hypothermia—low temperature—is known to protect the brain from ischemic injury. However, overall surface cooling is associated with various adverse effects, said Kentaro Yamada, M.D., of the National Cardiovascular Center in Osaka, Japan.

"The largest problem of systemic surface cooling is the requirement of general anesthesia, which increases risks of respiratory and circulatory diseases," he said. "Systemic surface cooling is commonly associated with severe infections, arrhythmia, hypopotassemia (low potassium), or decrease of platelet counts, which may countervail protective effects of hypothermia."

He also noted that "in our experience of hypothermia therapy in acute stroke patients using systemic surface cooling, excellent functional recovery was obtained in 83 percent of younger patients under age sixty but only in 20 percent of elderly patients."

Scientists have tried various methods to cool the brain, including cooling the entire body, using dry ice, and blowing cool air on the head. However, methods were unable to selectively cool the brain rapidly and maintain such preferential cooling over the rest of the body, said Huan Wang, M.D., assistant and resident of neurosurgery at the University of Illinois, College of Medicine, Peoria, Illinois.

He said it is well known that "brains like to be cold." Stroke and head trauma patients fare worse when they are running fevers. However, the same is not true for the rest of the body, including the heart and immune system, which do better at normal temperatures, Wang said.

Yamada and colleagues tested the helmet on patients (average age sixty-eight) three to twelve hours after stroke onset. The helmet was attached to the head and neck. The cooling of the head continued nonstop for three to seven days without anesthesia.

Researchers evaluated functional outcome three to ten months after stroke. The surface cooling was performed successfully in all patients.

Tympanic temperature, which measures surface brain temperature, was lowered 4.0 degrees Fahrenheit, and jugular temperature, which reflects deep brain temperature, was lowered 1.4 degrees Fahrenheit. In hypothermia with a helmet, such a temperature gradient in the brain results because of the local nature of the cooling method, Yamada said. Some patients experienced mild shivering, elevated potassium levels, mild skin damage, and infections, but none had serious adverse effects.

After ten months of follow-up, only one patient (6 percent) had died. Six patients (35 percent) had "good" functional outcome three to ten months after stroke.

The American study evaluated patients average age sixty-eight and used liquid cooling technology developed by NASA scientist William Elkins, "father of the American spacesuit," Wang said.

In animal studies, researchers have determined that cooling the brain can reduce the damage that stroke does to the brain tissue by as much as 70 percent, Wang said. "The goal with this therapy, therefore, is to try to improve neurological outcomes by minimizing stroke's effect," Wang said. "The first step in that direction was to find a therapy that effectively cooled the brain and, judging by this study, we have."

In this study, researchers gauged brain temperature via tiny fiberoptic probes inserted in the brain. These probes are often used to monitor vital brain functions of stroke patients in intensive care. The patients had neurological deterioration despite being treated for brain swelling.

Researchers took patients' brain temperatures at the start of the study (before patients put on the helmets) and throughout the next forty-eight to seventy-two hours. They found that the helmet preferentially cools the brain much more rapidly and profoundly than it does the body. The patients' brains cooled an average of 6 degrees Fahrenheit the first hour, without dropping body temperature significantly. Then, the helmet continued cooling the brain, while cooling body temperature at a much slower rate. Researchers were able to use the technology an average of six to eight hours before body temperature dropped below 97 degrees F. Five patients tolerated the helmet cooling well. One eighty-five-year-old woman with a previous heart arrhythmia experienced an abnormal heart rate but responded promptly to treatment.

The study did not report patient outcomes, but Wang said the treatment has great potential. If EMS personnel can use the helmet in the field, they theoretically can lengthen the time that a stroke patient is eligible for clot-busting therapy. "We believe that if you keep the brain tissue cool, you will have a longer tissue survival time. Then, when we open the artery, we could salvage much more brain tissue and hopefully avoid adverse neurological effects," Wang said.

"Rapid and selective brain cooling is a simple but elegant strategy that has been shown to limit injury in stroke, brain trauma, and cardiac arrest," said Vinay Nadkarni, M.D., immediate past chair of the American Heart Association's emergency cardiovascular care committee. "Building upon space-age technology, this novel technique is a good example of how bright scientists and innovative industry technologists can collaborate to speed the delivery of emergency cardiovascular care interventions. This device, and others like it, may have wide applicability in the field."

Yamada's co-authors are Hiroshi Moriwaki, M.D.; Hiroshi Oe, M.D.; Takemori Yamawaki, M.D.; Kazuyuki Nagatsuka, M.D.; Masahiro Oomura, M.D.; Kenichi Todo, M.D.; Kotoro Miyashita, M.D.; and Hiroaki Naritomi, M.D.

Wang's co-authors are David Wang, D.O.; William Olivero, M.D.; Giuseppe Lanzino, M.D.; Debra Honings, R.N.; Mary Rodde, R.N.; Janet Burnham, R.N.; Joe Milbrandt, Ph.D.: and Jean Rose, R.N., M.S.

Corkscrew Device Retrieves Clots, Quickly Reverses Stroke Damage

February 5, 2004, reproduced with permission from www.american heart.org. © 2004, American Heart Association.

A revolutionary tiny corkscrew that captures blood clots from vessels deep inside the brain can "almost instantly" reverse damage caused by ischemic stroke, according to the first report on the safety and efficacy of the device presented at the American Stroke Association's 29th International Stroke Conference.

Ischemic strokes are caused by a blood clot that blocks blood supply to the brain. Each year, about seven hundred thousand Americans suffer a stroke and 88 percent of those strokes are ischemic, according to the American Stroke Association.

Blood clots causing stroke can be dissolved using the FDA-approved clot-busting drug tissue plasminogen activator (tPA) as standard therapy. But, it must be initiated intravenously within three hours (the earlier the better) of stroke onset to be effective. Moreover, it "typically takes one to two hours for tPA to dissolve a clot and open a vessel, if at all," said Sidney Starkman, M.D., professor of emergency medicine and neurology at the University of California, Los Angeles and co-director of the UCLA Stroke Center.

The investigational device, the Concentric MERCI® Retrieval System, restored blood flow in 61 of 114 patients (54 percent) in Phase I and II of the Mechanical Embolus Removal in Cerebral Ischemia (MERCI I /II) trials, which studied patients up to eight hours after initial stroke symptoms who were not eligible for standard tPA therapy, said principal investigator Starkman.

Restoring blood flow in these trials reversed paralysis and other stroke symptoms, Starkman said.

"How often do we get a chance to reverse a patient's stroke on the table? We have had patients completely paralyzed on one side of their body, who were made normal almost instantaneously when the clot was retrieved," he said.

Of the sixty-one patients whose arteries were unblocked with the device, "twenty-three have no disability or have minor disability, such as handwriting problems," Starkman said.

The MERCI® Retrieval System is inserted into an artery in the groin, and then carefully guided via standard angiography into the brain until it reaches the blood clots. The device is made from a combination of nickel and titanium, "which is unique in that it allows the device to have a 'memory.' So in this case, when it is deployed, it 'remembers' to form itself into a helical shape, like a corkscrew," Starkman said.

Starkman says the corkscrew-shaped MERCI Retriever is the only device specifically designed to remove clots from all major cerebral vessels.

Once the device "captures" the blood clot, the device and clot are withdrawn into a larger catheter with a balloon. During the evacuation process, the balloon is briefly inflated to momentarily stop blood flow so the clots can be safely removed. Starkman added that the retrieval procedure can be performed only by a highly trained team at specialized centers.

The results presented today are based on 114 patients from twenty-five centers, (average age seventy, 46 percent women), whose average National Institutes of Health baseline stroke score was 19, which indicates severe impairment.

"Thus far, we have seen that the MERCI® Retrieval System is quite safe and we believe it holds great promise, but more research is needed to refine the device and study its effectiveness," Starkman said.

Concentric Medical, Inc., of Mountain View, California, funded the studies. The Food and Drug Administration is reviewing the device.

Blood-Diverting Catheter Holds Promise for Stroke Treatment

February 5, 2004, reproduced with permission from www.american heart.org. © 2004, American Heart Association.

A new catheter device that diverts some blood from the lower body to the brain appears safe for treating acute stroke and may significantly reduce stroke complications—even after a critical treatment window has lapsed.

The results of this experimental study were reported at the American Stroke Association's 29th International Stroke Conference.

"The device treats stroke by a unique approach that increases blood flow to the brain," said lead author Morgan S. Campbell III, M.D., director of interventional neurology at the Alabama Neurological Institute, in Birmingham. "Ten of the fifteen patients who were conscious when they arrived at the hospital improved during the procedure, which is very impressive."

Campbell and his colleagues tested the safety and effectiveness of the device, called NeuroFlo, on patients who suffered ischemic strokes. Ischemic strokes occur when a blood clot blocks an artery, reducing blood flow and oxygen to part of the brain. Using two balloons attached to a catheter, NeuroFlo diverts some blood from the lower extremities and sends it to the upper body.

Not all the brain cells affected by an ischemic stroke die immediately, Campbell said. A large number of cells in the stroke area initially have the potential to recover if their blood supply is restored. In theory, increasing the volume of blood to these damaged brain cells should preserve some of them even more than three hours after a stroke onset.

Ischemic stroke patients who arrive within three hours of symptom onset can often be treated with clot-busting drugs. However, these clot busters are not recommended for use more than three hours after stroke onset.

"The blood volume theory has been studied before but no one had really shown that it actually works and makes a difference," Campbell said. "So it is very encouraging that the device can divert more oxygenated blood to the brain and that patients get better."

Campbell conducted the study while he was an assistant professor of neurology and radiology at the University of Texas Health Science Center at Houston. He and colleagues at eight medical centers in the United States, Turkey, Germany, and Argentina studied seventeen patients whose strokes had been in progress for 3 to 12 hours. The average time between stroke onset and the beginning of treatment was 7.5 hours.

Each patient had a NeuroFlo device inserted into an artery in the groin. The device was then threaded up to the abdominal aorta and positioned with collapsed balloons above and below the renal arteries. The balloons were then inflated to partially obstruct the aorta. The device was left in place for one hour.

"By blowing up these balloons and limiting the blood flow to the lower extremities, we shifted more of the blood flow up to the head," Campbell explained.

This greater volume of blood increased collateral flow, the flow of blood through smaller vessels in the brain. The collateral flow bypassed the blocked section of the artery that was causing the patient's stroke, and brought needed oxygen to the cells downstream from the blockage.

The study's primary intent was to test the device's safety. Although two study participants died, their deaths were attributed to their strokes and not adverse effects of the device. Nor did people treated with the device suffer damage to their kidneys, heart, or blood vessels.

The research team also evaluated the patients' treatment response.

Twelve of sixteen patients monitored with ultrasound had a 15 percent increase or more of their cerebral blood flow velocity, with an average boost of 25 percent. Ultrasound waves passing into the skull can measure blood flow velocity. Velocity is an indirect measure of blood flow volume.

The blood pressure in the arteries increased an average of only 6 percent overall and did not increase in five patients. "This shows the increased blood flow did not simply result from an increase in blood pressure but from an increase in blood volume," Campbell said. "This is the desired effect of the device."

The researchers also assessed the degree of deficit of the stroke patients. While undergoing their hour-long treatment, ten of the fifteen conscious patients (67 percent) showed significantly higher scores on the National Institutes of Health Stroke Scale, the most commonly used assessment tool in acute stroke. Thirty days after treatment, six of the fifteen survivors had "good" physical function, on the modified Rankin scale, which rates disability.

The second phase of the study has begun enrollment. CoAxia, Inc., the device's maker, will seek approval from the U.S. Food and Drug Administration to conduct a larger clinical trial.

Co-authors are James C. Grotta, M.D.; Camilo R. Gomez, M.D.; and Gazi Ozdemir, M.D.

Cholesterol Drugs May Lower Risk for Mental Impairment after Stroke

February 6, 2004, reproduced with permission from www.american heart.org. © 2004, American Heart Association.

High cholesterol may increase the risk of stroke, but cholesterol-lowering drugs might reduce the risk of impaired brain function after a stroke, according to a study presented at the American Stroke Association's 29th International Stroke Conference.

Patients with a history of high cholesterol had a lower risk of cognitive impairment three to six months after stroke. However, the finding likely relates to high cholesterol treatment, rather than a protective or helpful effect of cholesterol. About 45 percent of the patients were being treated with cholesterol-lowering drugs known as statins before their stroke, said Eugenia Gencheva, M.D., a research fellow at the University of Illinois at Chicago (UIC) Center for Stroke Research. The research was conducted at Rush Medical College in Chicago.

"We're certainly not saying that the high cholesterol itself is protective," added David Nyenhuis, Ph.D., associate professor of neurology and rehabilitation at UIC. "Patients who had elevated cholesterol levels were more likely to be treated with statin drugs. We believe that perhaps statins were exerting the protective effect."

Elevated cholesterol is a risk factor for atherosclerotic vascular disease. In this observational study, hypercholesterolemia was determined by self-report and verification of current medication. Participants taking cholesterol-lowering drugs were defined as hypercholesterolemic, although their cholesterol levels might have been within acceptable limits as a result of their treatment.

Several observational studies have indicated that statin therapy is associated with a reduced risk of Alzheimer's disease and vascular dementia. However, the precise mechanisms by which statins might affect cognitive impairment are poorly understood, Gencheva said.

"Other research has shown that the effect of statins might be mediated by direct cholesterol-lowering properties, causing a reduction in cholesterol production and turnover in the brain," she said. "Statins also might reduce the concentration of proteins linked with dementia that accumulate in the brain in Alzheimer's patients."

Cognitive impairment—or loss of memory or other aspects of brain function—often occurs after stroke. Cardiovascular risk factors such as hypertension, diabetes, and obesity are widely assumed to influence cognitive impairment after stroke. But, the assumption hasn't been documented in medical literature, Gencheva said.

At the UIC Center for Stroke Research, an ongoing study led by Philip B. Gorelick, M.D, M.P.H., focuses on identifying markers for dementia after stroke through brain scans with magnetic resonance imaging. As an extension of that research, investigators evaluated demographic factors and cardiovascular risk factors as potential predictors of stroke-related cognitive impairment.

Ischemic strokes, which are caused by clots that disrupt blood flow to the brain, can result in various brain disorders known collectively as vascular cognitive impairment. The mildest disorder is vascular cognitive impairment-no dementia (VCIND); at the opposite end of the spectrum is vascular dementia, the most severe form of stroke-related brain dysfunction. The prevalence of VCIND is not known but vascular dementia may occur in up to one-third of stroke survivors, researchers said.

This study focused on VCIND. Researchers studied 103 consecutive ischemic stroke patients—41 diagnosed with VCIND and 62 who had no evidence of cognitive impairment after their strokes. All patients completed interviews that included questions about potential risk factors for cognitive impairment, and underwent neuropsychological testing. Information about cholesterol levels, blood pressure, and other vascular risk factors was self-reported and not based on actual measurement when patients were evaluated.

An initial analysis of different variables identified three statistically significant predictors of cognitive impairment: the patient's level of education, the presence of heart disease (defined as a history of heart attack, heart failure, disease of the heart muscle, disease of the heart valve, and abnormal heart rhythm), and a history of high cholesterol (hypercholesterolemia).

In a second analysis, heart disease and hypercholesterolemia remained significant predictors of cognitive impairment when results were not adjusted for education level. Increased education and hypercholesterolemia were associated with a reduced risk of cognitive impairment after stroke. When the researchers performed an analysis that controlled for the confounding effects of education, only hypercholesterolemia remained as a statistically significant predictor of the risk for cognitive impairment.

"Education is a well-known protective factor for cognitive impairment, and after adjusting for the effects of education, only hypercholesterolemia as defined in the study was statistically significant in the multivariate model," Gencheva said.

A major strength of the main study is that patients are being followed over time, including annual neurocognitive testing and MRI scans, Nyenhuis said. Continued evaluation of the patients eventually could lead to identification of changes in brain regions or structures that predict cognitive impairment.

Co-authors are Gorelick and Sally Freels, Ph.D. The National Institutes of Health supported the study.

Metabolic Syndrome May Be an Important Link to Stroke

February 6, 2004, reproduced with permission from www.american heart.org. © 2004, American Heart Association.

Metabolic syndrome—the simultaneous occurrence of multiple cardiovascular risk factors—may almost double the risk of stroke, researchers reported at the American Stroke Association's 29th International Stroke Conference.

The findings suggest that treating the risk-factor components of metabolic syndrome might reduce stroke risk before the onset of Type 2 diabetes.

"Before it becomes necessary to begin aggressive treatment of diabetes and other predisposing factors for stroke, it might be possible to take steps that can prevent these serious conditions from developing," said the study's lead author, Robert M. Najarian, a third-year medical student at Boston University School of Medicine.

The U.S. National Cholesterol Education Program (NCEP) and the World Health Organization define the metabolic syndrome as the simultaneous presence of at least three of five metabolic abnormalities: abdominal obesity, high fasting levels of blood sugar, high triglycerides levels, low levels of HDL ("good" cholesterol) and high blood pressure.

This study found that compared to people without metabolic syndrome, men with the condition have a 78 percent greater risk of stroke, and women affected by the condition have more than double the stroke risk of women who do not have the syndrome. But, the overall stroke risk associated with metabolic syndrome remained below that of people with diabetes.

Metabolic syndrome greatly increases a person's chances of developing Type 2 diabetes. Because of its strong association with diabetes, metabolic syndrome often is considered a prediabetic condition. Both conditions increase the risk of coronary heart disease, and diabetes is a potent risk factor for stroke. However, the relative effect of metabolic syndrome and diabetes on stroke risk has not been studied extensively.

Najarian and his co-investigators compared the impact of metabolic syndrome and diabetes on the ten-year risk of stroke and transient ischemic attack (TIA), a temporary interruption in blood flow to the brain that often precedes a stroke. The study involved 1,881 diabetes-free participants (average age fifty-nine) of the offspring cohort in the Framingham Heart Study.

Men and women were evaluated for a current diagnosis of diabetes and the five metabolic syndrome components: abdominal obesity (waist circumference greater than thirty-five inches in women and greater than forty inches in men); low HDL (less than 40 mg/dL in men and less than 50 mg/dL in women); blood pressure 130/85 mm Hg or greater, or current treatment with antihypertensive medication; triglycerides 150 mg/dL or greater; and fasting blood glucose of 110–26 mg/dL (the definition of impaired fasting glucose). Participants were considered to have the metabolic syndrome if they met at least three of the five criteria.

Najarian found that 27.6 percent of the men and 21.5 percent of the women met the criteria for a diagnosis of metabolic syndrome without including diabetes. When the additional 216 participants with diabetes were included in the analysis, 30.3 percent of men and 24.7 percent of women met diagnosis criteria.

During a maximum follow-up of fourteen years, 5.6 percent of the men in the study and 4.3 percent of the women had a stroke or TIA. Diabetic patients had a significantly higher ten-year risk of stroke compared to people with metabolic syndrome: 14 percent vs. 8 percent in men and 10 percent vs. 6 percent in women.

Although metabolic syndrome is a less potent risk factor for stroke than diabetes, the condition occurs more often than diabetes, making it a major consideration for stroke risk and prevention, Najarian said. Interventions aimed at preventing or treating metabolic syndrome could have a major impact on overall stroke risk.

"Metabolic syndrome looks like the precursor for a number of health problems," Najarian said. "Because the prevalence of the syndrome is so high, we need to start thinking about how to prevent the condition, particularly since it appears to be a factor in the continuum that leads to outright diabetes and cardiovascular disease. The end result is a higher death rate from all causes, a higher death rate from vascular causes, and higher rates of cardiovascular disease."

Co-authors are Lisa M. Sullivan, Ph.D.; Ralph B. D'Agostino, Ph.D.; Peter F. Wilson, M.D.; William B. Kannel, M.D.; and Philip A. Wolf, M.D.

Najarian is a recipient of an American Stroke Association 2003 Student Scholarship in Cerebrovascular Disease.

Editor's note: The American Heart Association's The Heart Of Diabetes: Understanding Insulin Resistance is a free twelve-month program designed to educate people about the association between cardiovascular disease, diabetes, and insulin resistance. People with Type 2 diabetes are encouraged to control their heart disease risk through physical activity, nutrition and cholesterol management. To register for the program, call 1-800-AHA-USA1 or visit www.americanheart .org/diabetes.

Statins May Provide Better Outcomes in People with Stroke

April 8, 2004, reproduced with permission from www.americanheart .org. © 2004, American Heart Association.

People who are taking cholesterol-lowering drugs when they have an ischemic stroke appear to regain greater functional independence than stroke survivors who aren't taking the drugs, according to a small study published in the April 8, 2004, rapid access issue of *Stroke: Journal of the American Heart Association.*

Cholesterol-lowering drugs—called statins—reduce the risk of heart disease, but this research indicates that they may also protect against damage caused by ischemic stroke. Ischemic strokes result from a blood clot that blocks blood flow to the brain.

In a study of 167 stroke patients (average age seventy), those taking statins at the time of an ischemic stroke were better able to care for themselves and be functionally independent three months later than those not taking that class of drugs, said study lead author, Joan Martí-Fabregas, M.D., Ph.D., of Servei de Neurologia at the Hospital de la Santa Creu i Sant Pau in Barcelona, Spain.

Thirty patients had been treated with statins and 137 had not. Symptoms of neurological deficits were essentially the same between both groups at the time of admission. All patients had a computed tomography or magnetic resonance imaging of their brain to determine the presence of an ischemic stroke.

Three months after stroke, recovery was significantly higher among patients who had been taking statins. Using the neurological functioning scale called the Barthel Index, 76.7 percent of survivors who had been taking statins were living without significant disability, compared to 51.8 percent of those not taking statins.

Marti-Fabregas cautions that this is an observational study and not a therapeutic trial. "At this moment, we don't recommend beginning statin therapy at the onset of stroke. However, our study points to the need for a randomized controlled trial with statins in the acute stages of ischemic stroke. We really are convinced that statins do benefit patients with ischemic stroke, and statins appear to be safe," she said.

Co-authors are Meritxell Gomis, M.D.; Adriá Arboix, M.D., Ph.D.; Aitziber Aleu, M.D.; Javier Pagonabarraga, M.D.; Robert Belvís, M.D.; Dolores Cocho, M.D.; Jaume Roquer, M.D., Ph.D.; Ana Rodríguez, M.D.; Maria Dolores Garcia, M.D.; Laura Molina-Porcel, M.D.; Jordi Díaz-Manera, M.D.; and Josep-Lluis Martí-Vilalta, M.D., Ph.D.

Antioxidants in Fruits and Vegetables May Decrease Stroke Risk

June 3, 2004, reproduced with permission from www.americanheart .org. © 2004, American Heart Association.

Sufficient blood levels of carotenoids, a family of antioxidants in fruits and vegetables, might reduce the risk of ischemic stroke, according to a study published in the June 3, 2004, rapid access issue of *Stroke: Journal of the American Heart Association.*

An ischemic stroke is caused by a blood clot and is the most common type of stroke.

Fruit and vegetable intake has long been associated with a lower risk of ischemic stroke, said study author Jing Ma, M.D., Ph.D., assistant professor of medicine, Brigham and Women's Hospital, Harvard Medical School, Boston. Researchers investigated which antioxidants in fruits and vegetables might have this positive effect.

The Physicians' Health Study involved 22,071 U.S. male physicians, 68 percent of whom provided blood samples at the start of the study in 1982. Among the 15,000 who didn't have cardiovascular disease at the beginning of the study, 297 had an ischemic stroke during the study's thirteen-year follow-up.

Analyzing blood samples among stroke patients, researchers measured levels of antioxidants, including carotenoids (vitamin A family, including alpha-carotene, beta-carotene, lycopene, lutein, and beta-cryptoxanthin) and tocopherols (vitamin E). They then compared their findings to the blood levels of an equal number of men who did not have stroke.

They found that men who were in the lowest 20 percent quintile (bottom fifth) for carotenoid levels of alpha-carotene, beta-carotene, and lycopene had the highest risk of ischemic stroke.

Men who were above the second through fifth quintiles were at a 40 percent lower risk of developing ischemic stroke during the thirteen years than men in the lowest quintile, Ma said.

Once blood levels moved beyond that 20 percent threshold of carotene, the stroke protection benefit did not seem to increase with higher levels, Ma said.

The carotenoid level could have been the result of these men eating fruits and vegetables or taking antioxidant supplements.

The observational study shows an association between fruit and vegetable intake and stroke risk, but did not prove that eating fruits and vegetables caused the lower risk.

The results of this study support a diet high in fruits and vegetables to reduce ischemic stroke risk, she said.

The American Heart Association recommends a total well-balanced nutritious diet consisting of a variety of foods: fruits, vegetables, whole grain cereals and bread, nonfat and low-fat dairy products, lean meat, fish and poultry, and the use of monounsaturated and polyunsaturated fats for saturated fat.

Co-authors are A. Elizabeth Hak, M.D., Ph.D.; Calpurnyia B. Powell, B.S.; Hannia Campos, Ph.D.; J. Michael Gaziano, M.D.; Walter Willett, M.D., Dr.P.H.; and Meir J. Stampfer, M.D., Dr.P.H.

Chapter 7

Brain Aneurysms

Chapter Contents

Section 7.1—Understanding Brain Aneurysms 124
Section 7.2—Treatment Options for Cerebral Aneurysms 129

Section 7.1

Understanding Brain Aneurysms

What Is a Brain Aneurysm?

A brain aneurysm, also called a cerebral or intracranial aneurysm, is an abnormal bulging outward of one of the arteries in the brain. It is estimated that up to one in fifteen people in the United States will develop a brain aneurysm during their lifetime.

Brain aneurysms are often discovered when they rupture, causing bleeding into the brain or the space closely surrounding the brain called the subarachnoid space, causing a subarachnoid hemorrhage. Subarachnoid hemorrhage from a ruptured brain aneurysm can lead to a hemorrhagic stroke, brain damage, and death.

The main goals of treatment once an aneurysm has ruptured are to stop the bleeding and potential permanent damage to the brain and to reduce the risk of recurrence. Unruptured brain aneurysms are sometimes treated to prevent rupture.

Incidence Rates of Brain Aneurysms

- Approximately 0.2 to 3 percent of people with a brain aneurysm may suffer from bleeding per year

- The annual incidence of aneurysmal subarachnoid hemorrhage in the United States exceeds thirty thousand people. Between 10 and 15 percent of these patients will die before reaching the hospital, and over 50 percent will die within the first thirty days after rupture. Of those who survive, about half suffer some permanent neurological deficit

- Brain aneurysms can occur in people of all ages, but are most commonly detected in those ages thirty-five to sixty

- Women are actually more likely to get a brain aneurysm than men, with a ratio of 3:2

Symptoms of Brain Aneurysms

Ruptured Cerebral Aneurysm Symptoms

Sometimes patients describing "the worst headache in my life" are actually experiencing one of the symptoms of brain aneurysms related to having a rupture. Other ruptured cerebral aneurysm symptoms include:

- Nausea and vomiting
- Stiff neck or neck pain
- Blurred vision or double vision
- Pain above and behind the eye
- Dilated pupils
- Sensitivity to light
- Loss of sensation

Unruptured Cerebral Aneurysm Symptoms

Before an aneurysm ruptures, patients often experience no symptoms of brain aneurysms. In about 40 percent of cases, people with unruptured aneurysms will experience some or all of the following cerebral aneurysm symptoms:

- Peripheral vision deficits
- Thinking or processing problems
- Speech complications
- Perceptual problems
- Sudden changes in behavior
- Loss of balance and coordination
- Decreased concentration
- Short-term memory difficulty
- Fatigue

Because the symptoms of brain aneurysms can also be associated with other medical conditions, diagnostic neuroradiology is regularly used to identify both ruptured and unruptured brain aneurysms.

Diagnosis of Brain Aneurysms

Diagnosis of a ruptured cerebral aneurysm is commonly made by finding signs of subarachnoid hemorrhage on a CT scan (computerized tomography, sometimes called a CAT scan). The CT scan is a computerized test that rapidly x-rays the body in cross-sections, or slices, as the body is moved through a large, circular machine. If the CT scan is negative but a ruptured aneurysm is still suspected, a lumbar puncture is performed to detect blood in the cerebrospinal fluid (CSF) that surrounds the brain and spinal cord.

To determine the exact location, size, and shape of an aneurysm (ruptured or unruptured), neuroradiologists will use either cerebral angiography or tomographic angiography.

Cerebral angiography, the traditional method, involves introducing a catheter (small plastic tube) into an artery (usually in the leg) and steering it through the blood vessels of the body to the artery involved by the aneurysm. A special dye, called a contract agent, is injected into the patient's artery and its distribution is shown on x-ray projections. This method may not detect some aneurysms due to overlapping structures or spasm.

Computed tomographic angiography (CTA) is an alternative to the traditional method and can be performed without the need for arterial catheterization. This test combines a regular CT scan with a contrast dye injected into a vein. Once the dye is injected into a vein, it travels to the brain arteries, and images are created using a CT scan. These images show exactly how blood flows into the brain arteries.

Treatment of Brain Aneurysms

Surgery or minimally invasive endovascular coiling techniques can be used in the treatment of brain aneurysms. It is important to note, however, that not all aneurysms are treated at the time of diagnosis or are amenable to both forms of treatment. Patients need to consult a neurovascular specialist to determine if they are candidates for either treatment.

Surgical Treatment

To get to the aneurysm, surgeons must first remove a section of the skull, a procedure called a craniotomy. The surgeon then spreads the brain tissue apart and places a tiny metal clip across the neck to stop blood flow into the aneurysm. After clipping the aneurysm, the surgeon secures the bone in its original place and the wound is closed.

Minimally Invasive Treatment: Coil Embolization or Endovascular Coiling

Endovascular therapy is a minimally invasive procedure that accesses the treatment area from within the blood vessel. In the case of aneurysms, this treatment is called coil embolization, or "coiling." In contrast to surgery, endovascular coiling does not require open surgery. Instead, physicians use real-time x-ray technology, called fluoroscopic imaging, to visualize the patient's vascular system and treat the disease from inside the blood vessel.

Endovascular treatment of brain aneurysms involves insertion of a catheter (small plastic tube) into the femoral artery in the patient's leg and navigating it through the vascular system, into the head and into the aneurysm. Tiny platinum coils are threaded through the catheter and deployed into the aneurysm, blocking blood flow into the aneurysm and preventing rupture. The coils are made of platinum so that they can be visible via x-ray and be flexible enough to conform to the aneurysm shape. This endovascular coiling, or filling, of the aneurysm is called embolization and can be performed under general anesthesia or light sedation. More than 125,000 patients worldwide have been treated with detachable platinum coils.

Endovascular Coiling vs. Surgical Clipping

Treatment of Ruptured Aneurysms

Until recently, most studies on the surgical clipping and endovascular treatment of brain aneurysms were either small-scale studies or were retrospective studies that relied on analyzing historical case records. The only multicenter prospective randomized clinical trial—considered the gold standard in study design—comparing surgical clipping and endovascular coiling of ruptured aneurysm is the International Subarachnoid Aneurysm Trial (ISAT).[1]

The study found that, in patients equally suited for both treatment options, endovascular coiling treatment produces substantially better patient outcomes than surgery in terms of survival free of disability at one year. The relative risk of death or significant disability at one year for patients treated with coils was 22.6 percent lower than in surgically treated patients.

The study results were so compelling that the trial was halted early after enrolling 2,143 of the planned 2,500 patients because the trial steering committee determined it was no longer ethical to randomize patients to neurosurgical clipping. Long-term follow-up will be essential to assess the durability of the substantial early advantage of endovascular coiling over conventional neurosurgical clipping for the treatment of brain aneurysms.

It is important to note that patients enrolled in the ISAT were evaluated by both a neurosurgeon and an endovascular coiling specialist, and both physicians had to agree that the aneurysm was treatable by either technique. This study provides compelling evidence that, if medically possible, all patients with ruptured brain aneurysms should receive an endovascular consultation as part of the protocol for the treatment of brain aneurysms.

Treatment of Unruptured Aneurysms

Although no multicenter randomized clinical trial comparing endovascular coiling and surgical treatment of unruptured aneurysms has yet been conducted, retrospective analyses have found that endovascular coiling is associated with less risk of bad outcomes, shorter hospital stays, and shorter recovery times compared with surgery.

Studies have shown that:

- Average hospital stays are more than twice as long with surgery as compared to endovascular coiling treatment[2]

- Four times as many surgical patients report new symptoms or disability after treatment as compared to coiled patients[3]

- There can be a dramatic difference in recovery times. One study showed that surgically treated patients had an average recovery time of one year, compared to coiled patients, who recovered in twenty-seven days[3]

Resources

1. Molyneux A, Kerr R, Stratton I, Sandercock P, Clarke M, Shrimpton J, Holman R. International Subarachnoid Aneurysm Trial (ISAT) of Neurosurgical Clipping versus Endovascular Coiling in 2,143 Patients with Ruptured Intracranial Aneurysms: A Randomised Trial. *Lancet.* 360 (2002): 1267–74.

2. Johnston SC, et al. Surgical and Endovascular Treatment of Unruptured Cerebral Aneurysms at University Hospitals. *Neurology.* 52 (1999): 1799–1805.

3. Johnston SC, et al. Endovascular and Surgical Treatment of Unruptured Cerebral Aneurysms: Comparison of Risks. *Ann Neurology.* 48 (2000): 11–19.

Section 7.2

Treatment Options for Cerebral Aneurysms

What Is an Aneurysm?

A cerebral or intracranial aneurysm is a dilation of an artery in the brain that results from a weakening of the inner muscular layer (the intima) of a blood vessel wall. The vessel develops a "blister-like" dilation that can become thin and rupture without warning. The resultant bleeding into the space around the brain is called a subarachnoid hemorrhage (SAH). This kind of hemorrhage can lead to a stroke, coma, and death.

The exact mechanisms by which cerebral aneurysms develop are unknown. However, a number of factors are believed to contribute to the formation of cerebral aneurysms. These include: (1) hypertension (high blood pressure); (2) cigarette smoking; (3) congenital (genetic) predisposition; (4) injury or trauma to blood vessels; and (5) complication from some types of blood infections.

Types of Aneurysms

An unruptured aneurysm is one whose sac has not previously leaked. An aneurysm ruptures when a hole develops in the sac of the aneurysm. The hole can be small, in which case only a small amount of blood leaks, or large, leading to a major hemorrhage. Every year approximately thirty thousand patients in the United States suffer from a ruptured cerebral aneurysm, and up to 6 percent of the population may have an unruptured cerebral aneurysm. The management of both ruptured and unruptured cerebral aneurysms poses a significant challenge for patients and their treating physicians.

Treatment Options

Today there are three treatment options for people with the diagnosis of cerebral aneurysm: (1) medical (nonsurgical) therapy; (2) surgical therapy or clipping; and (3) endovascular therapy or coiling.

Medical Therapy

Medical therapy is an option for the treatment of only unruptured intracranial aneurysms. Strategies include smoking cessation and blood pressure control. These are the only factors that have been shown to have a significant effect on aneurysm formation, growth, or rupture. You and your doctor can work together to design an individualized smoking cessation program that is both practical and feasible for your lifestyle. In addition, if you suffer from high blood pressure, your doctor may choose to start you on an antihypertensive (blood pressure lowering) medication or diet and exercise program. Finally, periodic radiographic imaging (either MRA, CT Scan, or conventional angiography) at regular intervals will likely be recommended to monitor the size and growth of the aneurysm.

Surgical Clipping

Victor Horsley, M.D., in 1855 was the first to surgically treat a brain aneurysm. In 1937, Walter Dandy, M.D., introduced the method of "clipping" an aneurysm when he applied a V-shaped, silver clip to the neck of an internal carotid artery aneurysm. Since that time, aneurysm clips have evolved into hundreds of varieties, shapes, and sizes. The mechanical sophistication of available clips, along with the advent of the operating microscope in the 1960s have made surgical clipping the gold standard in the treatment of both ruptured and unruptured cerebral aneurysms. In spite of these advances, surgical clipping remains an invasive and technically challenging procedure.

How Is an Aneurysm Surgically Clipped?

An aneurysm is clipped through a craniotomy, which is a surgical procedure in which the brain and the blood vessels are accessed through an opening in the skull. After the aneurysm is identified, it is carefully dissected (separated) from the surrounding brain tissue. A small metal clip (usually made from titanium) is then applied to the neck (base) of the aneurysm. Aneurysm clips come in all different shapes and sizes, and the choice of a particular clip is based on the size and location of an aneurysm. The clip has a spring mechanism that allows the two "jaws" of the clip to close around either side of the aneurysm, thus occluding (separating) the aneurysm from the parent (origin) blood vessel.

Endovascular Coiling

Endovascular techniques for treating aneurysms date back to the 1970s with the introduction of proximal balloon occlusion by Fjodor A. Serbinenko, M.D. During the 1980s endovascular treatment of aneurysms with balloon angioplasty was associated with high procedural rate of rupture and complications. The development of Guglielmi detachable coils (GDCs), and their FDA approval in 1995, revolutionized endovascular treatment of cerebral aneurysms.

The common goal of both surgical clipping and endovascular coiling is obliteration (destruction) of the aneurysm. Efficacy (long-term success or effectiveness of the treatment) is measured by evidence of aneurysm obliteration (destruction), without evidence of recanalization (reformation of a blood channel through the blockage), or evidence of recurrence (aneurysm regrowth) when assessed on follow-up radiographic imaging (MRA, CTA, or conventional angiography).

How Is an Aneurysm Endovascularly Coiled?

Guglielmi detachable coils, known as GDCs, are soft wire spirals made out of platinum. These coils are deployed (released) into an aneurysm via a catheter that is inserted into an artery in the groin and carefully advanced into the brain. Once the coils are released into the aneurysm, the blood flow pattern within the aneurysm is altered, and the slow or sluggish remaining blood flow leads to a thrombosis (clot) of the aneurysm. A thrombosed aneurysm is obliterated and, therefore, cannot rupture. Endovascular coiling is an attractive option for treating aneurysms because it is less invasive. The long-term durability of coiling, however, is still unknown, and not all aneurysms are suitable for coiling. As experience with coiling grows, the indications and pitfalls continue to be refined.

Who Performs the Procedure?

Surgical clipping of a cerebral aneurysm is always performed by a neurosurgeon, often one with expertise in cerebrovascular disease. Most cerebrovascular neurosurgeons have had five to seven years of general neurosurgery training and an additional one to two years of special cerebrovascular training.

Endovascular coiling is done either by a neurosurgeon or by an interventional neuroradiologist. An interventional radiologist has undergone extensive training (three to five years) in both radiology and interventional (invasive) procedures involving the brain and spinal cord. All neurosurgeons who perform endovascular coiling have undergone additional training in endovascular techniques in addition to full neurosurgery training (five to seven years of residency).

Safety and Common Complications.

Although the frequencies of certain complications vary according to the intervention, both clipping and coiling share the same complications. Rupture of the aneurysm is one of the most serious complications seen in either procedure. Exact frequencies of ruptures are not well documented, but reported rupture rates range from 2 percent to 3 percent for both coiling and clipping. Rupture can cause massive intracerebral hemorrhage (hemorrhagic stroke, or bleeding into the brain) and subsequent coma or death. Although rupture can have catastrophic consequences during either procedure, surgery probably provides a better opportunity to control hemorrhage because of direct access to the ruptured aneurysm and the supplying vessels.

Ischemic stroke (stroke secondary to a decreased blood oxygen) is another serious complication frequently encountered in both clipping and coiling. The pattern and distribution of strokes varies according to the aneurysm location and procedure type.

The actual length of the procedure, the associated risks, the projected recovery time, and the expected prognosis (outcome) depend on both the location of the aneurysm, the presence and severity of hemorrhage, and the patient's underlying medical condition. Therefore, each individual's case should be discussed with the treating neurosurgeon or physician.

Review of Current Literature

Comparing the safety, effectiveness, and long-term outcome of endovascular coiling to surgical clipping of cerebral aneurysms is a major research initiative in neurosurgery today. A randomized, controlled trial is needed to compare the safety and long-term outcome of surgical clipping to endovascular coiling for the treatment of cerebral aneurysms.

Results from the International Subarachnoid Aneurysm Trial (ISAT), a randomized control trial that compared surgical clipping to endovascular coiling in the treatment of ruptured aneurysms, were recently published in the *Lancet*. The results indicate that endovascular coiling is slightly less risky (6.9 percent) than surgical clipping. These results are informative, but they must be interpreted with caution because this study was the first of its kind, and the follow-up period for the patients was short (one year). The durability or long-term permanence of endovascular coiling has yet to be established. As far as the safety of clipping or coiling, the study showed no difference in the mortality (death) rate between clipping and coiling. Therefore, no definite conclusions can be made regarding the superiority of one treatment over the other. Additional study is needed.

How Do I Decide Which Procedure to Have If I Have a Cerebral Aneurysm?

The treatment of choice for an intracranial aneurysm, like all medical decisions, should be agreed upon by both the physician and the patient. In the case of either ruptured or unruptured intracranial aneurysms, the treating physician should discuss the risks and benefits of each available treatment option. The physician will usually make recommendations for one treatment over another, depending on the facts of each individual case.

Although unresolved controversies remain as to the best treatment option for an individual patient, both surgical clipping and endovascular coiling are considered to be viable treatment options in the management of cerebral aneurysms today.

Chapter 8

Brain Tumors

Chapter Contents

Section 8.1—What You Need to Know about Brain
                Tumors 136
Section 8.2—Metastatic Brain Tumors 154

Section 8.1

What You Need to Know about Brain Tumors

Excerpted from "What You Need to Know about Brain Tumors,"
National Cancer Institute, National Institutes of Health, July 2002,
NIH Publication No. 02-1558.

Introduction

This chapter has important information about brain tumors. It discusses possible causes, symptoms, diagnosis, treatment, and follow-up care. It also has information to help patients cope with brain tumors.

Primary and Secondary Brain Tumors

A tumor that begins in the brain is called a primary brain tumor. In children, most brain tumors are primary tumors. In adults, most tumors in the brain have spread there from the lung, breast, or other parts of the body. When this happens, the disease is not brain cancer. The tumor in the brain is a secondary tumor. It is named for the organ or the tissue in which it began.

Treatment for secondary brain tumors depends on where the cancer started and the extent of the disease.

The Brain

The brain is a soft, spongy mass of tissue. It is protected by the bones of the skull and three thin membranes called meninges. Watery fluid called cerebrospinal fluid cushions the brain. This fluid flows through spaces between the meninges and through spaces within the brain called ventricles.

A network of nerves carries messages back and forth between the brain and the rest of the body. Some nerves go directly from the brain to the eyes, ears, and other parts of the head. Other nerves run through the spinal cord to connect the brain with the other parts of the body. Within the brain and spinal cord, glial cells surround nerve cells and hold them in place.

The brain directs the things we choose to do (like walking and talking) and the things our body does without thinking (like breathing). The brain is also in charge of our senses (sight, hearing, touch, taste, and smell), memory, emotions, and personality.

The three major parts of the brain control different activities.

Cerebrum

The cerebrum is the largest part of the brain. It is at the top of the brain. It uses information from our senses to tell us what is going on around us and tells our body how to respond. It controls reading, thinking, learning, speech, and emotions.

The cerebrum is divided into the left and right cerebral hemispheres, which control separate activities. The right hemisphere controls the muscles on the left side of the body. The left hemisphere controls the muscles on the right side of the body.

Cerebellum

The cerebellum is under the cerebrum at the back of the brain. The cerebellum controls balance and complex actions like walking and talking.

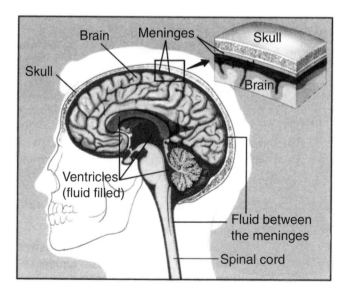

Figure 8.1. *The brain and nearby structures*

Brain Stem

The brain stem connects the brain with the spinal cord. It controls hunger and thirst. It also controls breathing, body temperature, blood pressure, and other basic body functions.

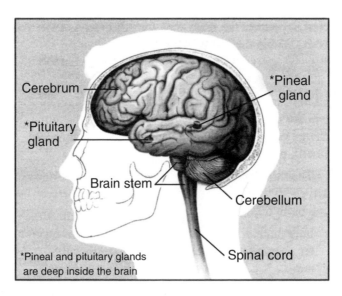

Figure 8.2. *Major parts of the brain*

Understanding Cancer

Cancer begins in cells, the building blocks that make up tissues. Tissues make up the organs of the body.

Normally, cells grow and divide to form new cells as the body needs them. When cells grow old, they die, and new cells take their place.

Sometimes this orderly process goes wrong. New cells form when the body does not need them, and old cells do not die when they should. These extra cells can form a mass of tissue called a growth or tumor.

Benign and Malignant Brain Tumors

Brain tumors can be benign or malignant.

Benign brain tumors do not contain cancer cells.

- Usually, benign tumors can be removed, and they seldom grow back.

- The border or edge of a benign brain tumor can be clearly seen. Cells from benign tumors do not invade tissues around them or spread to other parts of the body. However, benign tumors can press on sensitive areas of the brain and cause serious health problems.

- Unlike benign tumors in most other parts of the body, benign brain tumors are sometimes life threatening.

- Very rarely, a benign brain tumor may become malignant.

Malignant brain tumors contain cancer cells.

- Malignant brain tumors are generally more serious and often are life threatening.

- They are likely to grow rapidly and crowd or invade the surrounding healthy brain tissue.

- Very rarely, cancer cells may break away from a malignant brain tumor and spread to other parts of the brain, to the spinal cord, or even to other parts of the body. The spread of cancer is called metastasis.

- Sometimes, a malignant tumor does not extend into healthy tissue. The tumor may be contained within a layer of tissue. Or the bones of the skull or another structure in the head may confine it. This kind of tumor is called encapsulated.

Tumor Grade

Doctors sometimes group brain tumors by grade—from low grade (grade I) to high grade (grade IV). The grade of a tumor refers to the way the cells look under a microscope. Cells from high-grade tumors look more abnormal and generally grow faster than cells from low-grade tumors.

Primary Brain Tumors

Tumors that begin in brain tissue are known as primary tumors of the brain. (Information about secondary brain tumors appears in the following section.) Primary brain tumors are named according to the type of cells or the part of the brain in which they begin.

Gliomas

The most common primary brain tumors are gliomas. They begin in glial cells. There are many types of gliomas.

- **Astrocytoma:** The tumor arises from star-shaped glial cells called astrocytes. In adults, astrocytomas most often arise in the cerebrum. In children, they occur in the brain stem, the cerebrum, and the cerebellum. A grade III astrocytoma is sometimes called an anaplastic astrocytoma. A grade IV astrocytoma is usually called a glioblastoma multiforme.

- **Brain Stem Glioma:** The tumor occurs in the lowest part of the brain. Brain stem gliomas most often are diagnosed in young children and middle-aged adults.

- **Ependymoma:** The tumor arises from cells that line the ventricles or the central canal of the spinal cord. They are most commonly found in children and young adults.

- **Oligodendroglioma:** This rare tumor arises from cells that make the fatty substance that covers and protects nerves. These tumors usually occur in the cerebrum. They grow slowly and usually do not spread into surrounding brain tissue. They are most common in middle-aged adults.

Other Types of Primary Brain Tumors

Some types of brain tumors do not begin in glial cells. The most common of these are medulloblastomas, meningiomas, Schwannomas, craniopharyngiomas, germ cell tumors, and pineal region tumors.

- **Medulloblastoma:** This tumor usually arises in the cerebellum. It is the most common brain tumor in children. It is sometimes called a primitive neuroectodermal tumor.

- **Meningioma:** This tumor arises in the meninges. It usually grows slowly.

- **Schwannoma:** A tumor that arises from a Schwann cell. These cells line the nerve that controls balance and hearing. This nerve is in the inner ear. The tumor is also called an acoustic neuroma. It occurs most often in adults.

- **Craniopharyngioma:** The tumor grows at the base of the brain, near the pituitary gland. This type of tumor most often occurs in children.

- **Germ Cell Tumor of the Brain:** The tumor arises from a germ cell. Most germ cell tumors that arise in the brain occur in people younger than thirty. The most common type of germ cell tumor of the brain is a germinoma.

- **Pineal Region Tumor:** This rare brain tumor arises in or near the pineal gland. The pineal gland is located between the cerebrum and the cerebellum.

Secondary Brain Tumors

When cancer spreads from its original place to another part of the body, the new tumor has the same kind of abnormal cells and the same name as the primary tumor. Cancer that spreads to the brain from another part of the body is different from a primary brain tumor. When cancer cells spread to the brain from another organ (such as the lung or breast), doctors may call the tumor in the brain a secondary tumor or metastatic tumor. Secondary tumors in the brain are far more common than primary brain tumors.

Brain Tumors: Who's at Risk?

No one knows the exact causes of brain tumors. Doctors can seldom explain why one person develops a brain tumor and another does not. However, it is clear that brain tumors are not contagious. No one can "catch" the disease from another person.

Research has shown that people with certain risk factors are more likely than others to develop a brain tumor. A risk factor is anything that increases a person's chance of developing a disease.

The following risk factors are associated with an increased chance of developing a primary brain tumor:

- **Being male:** In general, brain tumors are more common in males than females. However, meningiomas are more common in females.

- **Race:** Brain tumors occur more often among white people than among people of other races.

- **Age:** Most brain tumors are detected in people who are seventy years old or older. However, brain tumors are the second most common cancer in children. (Leukemia is the most common childhood cancer.) Brain tumors are more common in children younger than eight years old than in older children.

141

- **Family history:** People with family members who have gliomas may be more likely to develop this disease.

- **Environmental exposure:** Being exposed to radiation or certain chemicals at work can also increase the risk of developing a primary brain tumor.

  - *Radiation:* Workers in the nuclear industry have an increased risk of developing a brain tumor.

  - *Formaldehyde:* Pathologists and embalmers who work with formaldehyde have an increased risk of developing brain cancer. Scientists have not found an increased risk of brain cancer among other types of workers exposed to formaldehyde.

  - *Vinyl chloride:* Workers who make plastics may be exposed to vinyl chloride. This chemical may increase the risk of brain tumors.

  - *Acrylonitrile:* People who make textiles and plastics may be exposed to acrylonitrile. This exposure may increase the risk of brain cancer.

Scientists are investigating whether cell phones may cause brain tumors. Studies thus far have not found an increased risk of brain tumors among people who use cell phones.

Scientists also continue to study whether head injuries are a risk factor for brain tumors. So far, these studies have not found an increased risk among people who have had head injuries.

Most people who have known risk factors do not get brain cancer. On the other hand, many who do get the disease have none of these risk factors. People who think they may be at risk should discuss this concern with their doctor. The doctor may be able to suggest ways to reduce the risk and can plan an appropriate schedule for checkups.

Symptoms

The symptoms of brain tumors depend on tumor size, type, and location. Symptoms may be caused when a tumor presses on a nerve or damages a certain area of the brain. They also may be caused when the brain swells or fluid builds up within the skull.

These are the most common symptoms of brain tumors:

- Headaches (usually worse in the morning)
- Nausea or vomiting

- Changes in speech, vision, or hearing
- Problems balancing or walking
- Changes in mood, personality, or ability to concentrate
- Problems with memory
- Muscle jerking or twitching (seizures or convulsions)
- Numbness or tingling in the arms or legs

These symptoms are not sure signs of a brain tumor. Other conditions also could cause these problems. Anyone with these symptoms should see a doctor as soon as possible. Only a doctor can diagnose and treat the problem.

Diagnosis

If a person has symptoms that suggest a brain tumor, the doctor may perform one or more of the following procedures:

- **Physical exam:** The doctor checks general signs of health.

- **Neurologic exam:** The doctor checks for alertness, muscle strength, coordination, reflexes, and response to pain. The doctor also examines the eyes to look for swelling caused by a tumor pressing on the nerve that connects the eye and brain.

- **CT scan:** An x-ray machine linked to a computer takes a series of detailed pictures of the head. The patient may receive an injection of a special dye so the brain shows up clearly in the pictures. The pictures can show tumors in the brain.

- **MRI:** A powerful magnet linked to a computer makes detailed pictures of areas inside the body. These pictures are viewed on a monitor and can also be printed. Sometimes a special dye is injected to help show differences in the tissues of the brain. The pictures can show a tumor or other problem in the brain.

The doctor may ask for other tests:

- **Angiogram:** Dye injected into the bloodstream flows into the blood vessels in the brain to make them show up on an x-ray. If a tumor is present, the doctor may be able to see it on the x-ray.

- **Skull x-ray:** Some types of brain tumors cause calcium deposits in the brain or changes in the bones of the skull. With an x-ray, the doctor can check for these changes.

- **Spinal tap:** The doctor may remove a sample of cerebrospinal fluid (the fluid that fills the spaces in and around the brain and spinal cord). This procedure is performed with local anesthesia. The doctor uses a long, thin needle to remove fluid from the spinal column. A spinal tap takes about thirty minutes. The patient must lie flat for several hours afterward to keep from getting a headache. A laboratory checks the fluid for cancer cells or other signs of problems.

- **Myelogram:** This is an x-ray of the spine. A spinal tap is performed to inject a special dye into the cerebrospinal fluid. The patient is tilted to allow the dye to mix with the fluid. This test helps the doctor detect a tumor in the spinal cord.

- **Biopsy:** The removal of tissue to look for tumor cells is called a biopsy. A pathologist looks at the cells under a microscope to check for abnormal cells. A biopsy can show cancer, tissue changes that may lead to cancer, and other conditions. A biopsy is the only sure way to diagnose a brain tumor. Surgeons can obtain tissue to look for tumor cells in three ways:

  - *Needle biopsy:* The surgeon makes a small incision in the scalp and drills a small hole into the skull. This is called a burr hole. The doctor passes a needle through the burr hole and removes a sample of tissue from the brain tumor.

  - *Stereotactic biopsy:* An imaging device, such as CT or MRI, guides the needle through the burr hole to the location of the tumor. The surgeon withdraws a sample of tissue with the needle.

  - *Biopsy at the same time as treatment:* Sometimes the surgeon takes a tissue sample when the patient has surgery to remove the tumor.

Sometimes a biopsy is not possible. If the tumor is in the brain stem or certain other areas, the surgeon may not be able to remove tissue from the tumor without damaging normal brain tissue. The doctor uses MRI, CT, or other imaging tests instead.

Questions to Ask Your Doctor about Biopsy

A person who needs a biopsy may want to ask the doctor the following questions:

- Why do I need a biopsy? How will the biopsy affect my treatment plan?

- What kind of biopsy will I have?

- How long will it take? Will I be awake? Will it hurt?

- What are the chances of infection or bleeding after the biopsy? Are there any other risks?

- How soon will I know the results?

- If I do have a brain tumor, who will talk to me about treatment? When?

Treatment

Many people with brain tumors want to take an active part in making decisions about their medical care. They want to learn all they can about their disease and their treatment choices. However, shock and stress after a diagnosis of a brain tumor can make it hard to think of everything to ask the doctor. It often helps to make a list of questions before an appointment. To help remember what the doctor says, patients may take notes or ask whether they may use a tape recorder. Some also want to have a family member or friend with them when they talk to the doctor—to take part in the discussion, to take notes, or just listen.

The doctor may refer the patient to a specialist, or the patient may ask for a referral. Specialists who treat brain tumors include neurosurgeons, neurooncologists, medical oncologists, and radiation oncologists. The patient may be referred to other health care professionals who work together as a team. The medical team may include a nurse, dietitian, mental health counselor, social worker, physical therapist, occupational therapist, and speech therapist. Children may need tutors to help with schoolwork.

Getting a Second Opinion

Before starting treatment, the patient might want a second opinion about the diagnosis and the treatment plan. Some insurance companies require a second opinion; others may cover a second opinion if the patient or doctor requests it.

There are a number of ways to find a doctor for a second opinion:

- The patient's doctor may refer the patient to one or more specialists. At cancer centers, several specialists often work together as a team.

- A local or state medical society, a nearby hospital, or a medical school can usually provide the names of specialists.

- The American Board of Medical Specialties (ABMS) has a list of doctors who have met certain education and training requirements and have passed specialty examinations. The Official ABMS Directory of Board Certified Medical Specialists lists doctors' names along with their specialty and their educational background. The directory is available in most public libraries. Also, ABMS offers this information on the Internet at http://www.abms.org.

Preparing for Treatment

The doctor can describe treatment choices and discuss the results expected with each treatment option. The doctor and patient can work together to develop a treatment plan that fits the patient's needs.

Treatment depends on a number of factors, including the type, location, size, and grade of the tumor. For some types of brain cancer, the doctor also needs to know whether cancer cells were found in the cerebrospinal fluid.

These are some questions a person may want to ask the doctor before treatment begins:

- What type of brain tumor do I have?
- Is it benign or malignant?
- What is the grade of the tumor?
- What are my treatment choices? Which do you recommend for me? Why?
- What are the benefits of each kind of treatment?
- What are the risks and possible side effects of each treatment?
- What is the treatment likely to cost?
- How will treatment affect my normal activities?
- Would a clinical trial (research study) be appropriate for me? Can you help me find one?

People do not need to ask all of their questions or understand all of the answers at one time. They will have other chances to ask the doctor to explain things that are not clear and to ask for more information.

Methods of Treatment

People with brain tumors have several treatment options. Depending on the tumor type and stage, patients may be treated with surgery, radiation therapy, or chemotherapy. Some patients receive a combination of treatments.

In addition, at any stage of disease, patients may have treatment to control pain and other symptoms of the cancer, to relieve the side effects of therapy, and to ease emotional problems. This kind of treatment is called symptom management, supportive care, or palliative care.

The doctor is the best person to describe the treatment choices and discuss the expected results.

A patient may want to talk to the doctor about taking part in a clinical trial, which is a research study of new treatment methods. The section on "The Promise of Cancer Research" has more information about clinical trials.

Surgery

Surgery is the usual treatment for most brain tumors. Surgery to open the skull is called a craniotomy. It is performed under general anesthesia. Before surgery begins, the scalp is shaved. The surgeon then makes an incision in the scalp and uses a special type of saw to remove a piece of bone from the skull. After removing part or all of the tumor, the surgeon covers the opening in the skull with that piece of bone or with a piece of metal or fabric. The surgeon then closes the incision in the scalp.

These are some questions a person may want to ask the doctor before having surgery:

- How will I feel after the operation?

- What will you do for me if I have pain?

- How long will I be in the hospital?

- Will I have any long-term effects? Will my hair grow back? Are there any side effects from using metal or fabric to replace the bone in the skull?

- When can I get back to my normal activities?

- What is my chance of a full recovery?

Sometimes surgery is not possible. If the tumor is in the brain stem or certain other areas, the surgeon may not be able to remove the tumor without damaging normal brain tissue. Patients who cannot have surgery may receive radiation or other treatment.

Radiation Therapy

Radiation therapy (also called radiotherapy) uses high-energy rays to kill tumor cells. The radiation may come from x-rays, gamma rays, or protons. A large machine aims radiation at the tumor and the tissue close to it. Sometimes the radiation may be directed to the entire brain or to the spinal cord.

Radiation therapy usually follows surgery. The radiation kills tumor cells that may remain in the area. Sometimes, patients who cannot have surgery have radiation therapy instead.

The patient goes to a hospital or clinic for radiation therapy. The treatment schedule depends on the type and size of the tumor and the age of the patient. Each treatment lasts only a few minutes.

Doctors take steps to protect the healthy tissue around the brain tumor:

- **Fractionation:** Radiation therapy usually is given five days a week for several weeks. Giving the total dose of radiation over an extended period helps to protect healthy tissue in the area of the tumor.

- **Hyperfractionation:** The patient gets smaller doses of radiation two or three times a day instead of a larger amount once a day.

- **Stereotactic radiation therapy:** Narrow beams of radiation are directed at the tumor from different angles. For this procedure, the patient wears a rigid head frame. An MRI or CT scan creates pictures of the tumor's exact location. The doctor uses a computer to decide on the dose of radiation needed, as well as the sizes and angles of the radiation beams. The therapy may be given during a single visit or over several visits.

- **Three-dimensional conformal radiation therapy:** A computer creates a three-dimensional image of the tumor and nearby brain tissue. The doctor aims multiple radiation beams to the exact shape of the tumor. The precise focus of the radiation beams protects normal brain tissue.

- **Proton beam radiation therapy:** The source of radiation is protons rather than x-rays. The doctor aims the proton beams at the tumor. Protons can pass through healthy tissue without damaging it.

These are some questions a person may want to ask the doctor before having radiation therapy:

- Why do I need this treatment?
- When will the treatments begin? When will they end?
- How will I feel during therapy? Are there side effects?
- What can I do to take care of myself during therapy?
- How will we know if the radiation is working?
- Will I be able to continue my normal activities during treatment?

Chemotherapy

Chemotherapy, the use of drugs to kill cancer cells, is sometimes used to treat brain tumors. The drugs may be given by mouth or by injection. Either way, the drugs enter the bloodstream and travel throughout the body. The drugs are usually given in cycles so that a recovery period follows each treatment period.

Chemotherapy may be given in an outpatient part of the hospital, at the doctor's office, or at home. Rarely, the patient may need to stay in the hospital.

Children are more likely than adults to have chemotherapy. However, adults may have chemotherapy after surgery and radiation therapy.

For some patients with recurrent cancer of the brain, the surgeon removes the tumor and implants several wafers that contain chemotherapy. Each wafer is about the size of a dime. Over several weeks, the wafers dissolve, releasing the drug into the brain. The drug kills cancer cells.

Patients may want to ask these questions about chemotherapy:

- Why do I need this treatment?
- What will it do?
- Will I have side effects? What can I do about them?
- When will treatment start? When will it end?
- How often will I need checkups?

Side Effects of Treatment

Because treatment may damage healthy cells and tissues, unwanted side effects are common. These side effects depend on many factors, including the location of the tumor and the type and extent of the treatment. Side effects may not be the same for each person, and they may even change from one treatment session to the next. Before treatment starts, the health care team will explain possible side effects and suggest ways to help the patient manage them.

Surgery

Patients often have a headache or are uncomfortable for the first few days after surgery. However, medicine can usually control their pain. Patients should feel free to discuss pain relief with the doctor or nurse.

It is also common for patients to feel tired or weak. The length of time it takes to recover from an operation varies for each patient.

Other, less common, problems may occur. Cerebrospinal fluid or blood may build up in the brain. This swelling is called edema. The health care team monitors the patient for signs of these problems. The patient may receive steroids to help relieve swelling. A second surgery may be needed to drain the fluid. The surgeon may place a long, thin tube (shunt) in a ventricle of the brain. The tube is threaded under the skin to another part of the body, usually the abdomen. Excess fluid is carried from the brain and drained into the abdomen. Sometimes the fluid is drained into the heart instead.

Infection is another problem that may develop after surgery. If this happens, the health care team gives the patient an antibiotic.

Brain surgery may damage normal tissue. Brain damage can be a serious problem. The patient may have problems thinking, seeing, or speaking. The patient also may have personality changes or seizures. Most of these problems lessen or disappear with time, but sometimes damage to the brain is permanent. The patient may need physical therapy, speech therapy, or occupational therapy.

Radiation Therapy

Some patients have nausea for several hours after treatment. The health care team can suggest ways to help patients cope with this problem. Radiation therapy also may cause patients to become very tired as treatment continues. Resting is important, but doctors usually advise patients to try to stay as active as they can.

In addition, radiation therapy commonly causes hair loss. Hair usually grows back within a few months. Radiation therapy also may affect the skin in the treated area. The scalp and ears may become red, dry, and tender. The health care team can suggest ways to relieve these problems.

Sometimes radiation therapy causes brain tissue to swell. Patients may get a headache or feel pressure. The health care team watches for signs of this problem. They can provide medicine to reduce the discomfort.

Radiation sometimes kills healthy brain tissue. This side effect is called radiation necrosis. Necrosis can cause headaches, seizures, or even the patient's death.

In children, radiation may damage the pituitary gland and other areas of the brain. This could cause learning problems or slow down growth and development. In addition, radiation during childhood increases the risk of secondary tumors later in life. Researchers are studying whether chemotherapy may be used instead of radiation therapy in young children with brain tumors.

Side effects may be worse if chemotherapy and radiation therapy are given at the same time. The doctor can suggest ways to ease these problems.

Chemotherapy

The side effects of chemotherapy depend mainly on the drugs that are used. The most common side effects include fever and chills, nausea and vomiting, loss of appetite, and weakness. Some side effects may be relieved with medicine.

Patients who receive an implant (a wafer) that contains a drug are monitored by the health care team for signs of infection after surgery. An infection can be treated with an antibiotic.

Supportive Care

At any stage of disease, people with brain tumors receive supportive care to prevent or control problems and to improve their comfort and quality of life during treatment. Patients may have treatment to control pain and other symptoms of a brain tumor, to relieve the side effects of therapy, and to ease emotional problems.

These are common types of supportive care for people with brain tumors:

- **Steroids:** Most patients with brain tumors need steroids to help relieve swelling of the brain.

- **Anticonvulsant medicine:** Brain tumors can cause seizures. Patients may take an anticonvulsant medicine to prevent or control seizures.

- **Shunt:** If fluid builds up in the brain, the surgeon may place a shunt to drain the fluid. Information about shunts is under "Surgery" in the "Side Effects" section.

Many people with brain tumors receive supportive care along with treatments intended to slow the progress of the disease. Some decide not to have antitumor treatment and receive only supportive care to manage their symptoms.

Rehabilitation

Rehabilitation can be a very important part of the treatment plan. The goals of rehabilitation depend on the person's needs and how the tumor has affected daily activities. The health care team makes every effort to help the patient return to normal activities as soon as possible. Several types of therapists can help:

- **Physical therapists:** Brain tumors and their treatment may cause paralysis. They may also cause weakness and problems with balance. Physical therapists help patients regain strength and balance.

- **Speech therapists:** Speech therapists help patients who have trouble speaking, expressing thoughts, or swallowing.

- **Occupational therapists:** Occupational therapists help patients learn to manage activities of daily living, such as eating, using the toilet, bathing, and dressing.

Children with brain tumors may have special needs. Sometimes children have tutors in the hospital or at home. Children who have problems learning or remembering what they learn may need tutors or special classes when they return to school.

Follow-Up Care

Regular follow-up is very important after treatment for a brain tumor. The doctor checks closely to make sure that the tumor has not returned. Checkups may include careful physical and neurologic exams. From time to time, the patient may have MRI or CT scans. If the patient has a shunt, the doctor checks to see that it is working well. The doctor can explain the follow-up plan—how often the patient must visit the doctor and what tests will be needed.

Support for People with Brain Tumors

Living with a serious disease such as a brain tumor is not easy. Some people find they need help coping with the emotional and practical aspects of their disease. Support groups can help. In these groups, patients or their family members get together to share what they have learned about coping with the disease and the effects of treatment. Patients may want to talk with a member of their health care team about finding a support group. Groups may offer support in person, over the telephone, or on the Internet.

People living with a brain tumor may worry about caring for their families, keeping their jobs, or continuing daily activities. Concerns about treatments and managing side effects, hospital stays, and medical bills are also common. Doctors, nurses, and other members of the health care team can answer questions about treatment, working, or other activities. Meeting with a social worker, counselor, or member of the clergy can be helpful to those who want to talk about their feelings or discuss their concerns. Often, a social worker can suggest resources for financial aid, transportation, home care, or emotional support.

The Promise of Cancer Research

Doctors all over the country are conducting many types of clinical trials. These are research studies in which people take part voluntarily. Studies include new ways to treat brain tumors. Research has already led to advances, and researchers continue to search for more effective approaches.

Patients who join these studies have the first chance to benefit from treatments that have shown promise in earlier research. They also make an important contribution to medical science by helping doctors learn more about the disease. Although clinical trials may pose some risks, researchers take very careful steps to protect their patients.

Researchers are testing new anticancer drugs, doses, and treatment schedules. They are working with various drugs and drug combinations, as well as combinations of drugs and radiation therapy. They also are testing new methods and schedules of radiation therapy.

Patients who are interested in being part of a clinical trial should talk with their doctor.

Section 8.2

Metastatic Brain Tumors

Brain metastases are the most common type of brain tumors, with the total number diagnosed annually outnumbering all other intracranial tumors combined. With the increasing survival of patients with systemic (extracranial) disease, the incidence of the most common cancers (lung, breast, melanoma, renal, and colon) is thought to be rising. Autopsy data show that the frequency of brain metastases in patients dying from cancer varies from 20 to 50 percent, and may be higher if dural, leptomeningeal, or spinal metastases are taken into account. As the incidence of brain metastases rises due to improved cancer therapy for systemic disease, it is imperative that improved intracranial therapy be developed as well.

The most common source of brain metastases in males is lung cancer and in females is breast cancer, but with the increasing frequency of lung cancer in females, it is expected that for females this too will be the primary cause of metastatic brain tumors.

How Do Tumors Metastasize?

The mechanisms by which primary tumors produce brain metastases is thought to be hematogenous spread from primary or secondary sites in the lung. Since the brain has no lymphatic system, all tumors metastasizing to the brain do so by spreading through the bloodstream. Arterial blood passes through the lungs before entering the brain, and collects tumor cells filtered out in capillaries, which subsequently embolize to the brain. This is correlated with sites of localization: the cerebrum is involved in 80 to 85 percent of all brain metastases, the cerebellum in 10 to 15 percent, and the brainstem in 3 to 5 percent. The overall distribution corresponds roughly to the relative size of blood flow regions in the brain.

Different types of primary tumors have different relative frequencies of single versus multiple metastases. Melanoma has the highest tendency to produce multiple lesions, followed by lung and breast cancers. Though many studies have indicated that 37 to 50 percent of patients present with a single metastasis, recent studies have shown that patients with one lesion detected by CT may demonstrate multiple lesions detected by MRI. These findings clearly agree with our data in which the majority of patients presented with multiple lesions upon contrast dye with MRI.

Common Symptoms

Metastatic brain tumors present with the usual signs and symptoms of any expanding intracranial mass lesion. These include increased intracranial pressure and focal neurological deficits with focal irritations. Such symptoms include headaches, focal weakness, mental status changes, seizures, ataxia (inability to coordinate voluntary muscular movements) and sensory and visual changes. Though most of these symptoms are of gradual onset, acute episodes may occur due to hemorrhages into a metastasis. When such an event occurs, either choroid carcinoma or melanoma must be considered, because these have the greatest tendency to hemorrhage. Because of the greater incidence of bronchogenic metastasis, these lesions represent the most common source of a hemorrhagic lesion.

Whole Brain Radiation Therapy (WBRT)

Brain metastases carry an ominous prognosis regardless of primary status or treatment given. The median survival of untreated patients, or those treated with corticosteroids alone to reduce brain edema, is about one month. Whole brain radiation therapy (WBRT) is the most widely used method of treating brain metastasis, despite the fact that patients treated this way have an expected survival of only three to four months. Death from recurrent or persistent tumors occurs in about 50 percent of the patients.

The radiosensitivity of the tumor itself is not taken into account when these patients are being treated. Most tumors that metastasize to the brain, such as non–small cell lung, renal, colon, and melanoma, are radioresistant (resistant to radiation therapy). Worse yet, many treating facilities continue to use prophylactic cranial radiation despite the fact that only one study has ever demonstrated a statistically significant increase in life span. (Prophylactic radiation therapy is treatment given before lesions have appeared within the brain.)

Significant neurotoxicity has been reported with the use of WBRT. Acute effects include hair loss (alopecia), nausea, vomiting, lethargy, otitis media, and severe cerebral edema. Though some of these effects can be transient, dermatitis, alopecia, and otitis media can persist for months after irradiation. Chronic effects are even more serious, and these include atrophy, leukoencephalopathy, radiation necrosis, neurological deterioration, and dementia. Reports of development of severe radiation-induced dementia have varied between 11 percent in one-year survivors to 50 percent in those surviving two years. The time involved in this therapeutic intervention frequently is over two weeks, in itself a burden to many patients.

Surgery and WBRT

Surgical removal of solitary and occasionally multiple lesions has been reported to enhance survival, with several reports indicating improvement of neurological function. Recently, the concept of multiple craniotomies for multiple lesions has been promoted, though only in those patients with "accessible locations" and "good clinical condition." The risks of postoperative morbidity in "eloquent" areas must also be considered when contemplating surgical intervention. The complications of the surgery itself include hemorrhages and wound infection.

Pseudomeningoceles form in 8 to 9 percent of patients, and an estimated 10 percent of patients develop clinically evident thromboembolic complications such as deep vein thrombosis or pulmonary embolisms. Recent reports have also indicated an operative mortality of approximately 3 percent. Though adjunct WBRT has been prescribed in the past, and Patchell et al. showed that a subset of patients with favorable prognosis and a single brain metastasis that had surgery followed by adjunct WBRT had a median survival of ten months, other subsequent randomized trials failed to show a benefit to surgical resection.

Radiosurgery

Radiosurgery is a technique that allows the delivery of a single high dose of radiation in a highly accurate manner. The gamma knife (a dedicated neurosurgical instrument) allows numerous beams of radiation to converge on a target site, resulting in a high dose of radiation delivered to the target site with a sharp dose gradient at the target edge. A recent report by Somaza et al. revealed that even in patients with radioresistant tumors (such as melanoma), local tumor control was achieved in 97 percent of patients and neurological improvement occurred in 53 percent of affected patients.

Median survival with radiosurgery alone improved from two to three months to nine months in patients with single or multiple metastatic melanoma lesions to the brain. Despite such results, radiosurgery has not been considered a primary therapy. In the recent past most treatment centers treat only unresectable tumors or recurrent tumors with this modality.

Multiple Metastases

The issue of multiple metastases has become important, as has the issue of lesion size. From our perspective, neither number of lesions nor the size of the lesions has been shown scientifically to be a limiting factor in single session gamma knife treatment. Multiple metastases may be more of an issue in terms of the equipment itself not allowing multiple lesions to be treated in a single sitting. At the Miami Neuroscience Center, at Health South Doctor's Hospital in Coral Gables, Florida, we have treated 460 patients (261 females and 199 males) with a mean of four lesions per treatment. The patients had the following types of cancers: 111 males and 111 females had lung cancer, thirty-two males and sixteen females had melanoma, seven males and twenty females had colon cancer, and eight males and sixteen females had renal cancer.

When we looked specifically at the outcome of metastatic breast carcinoma, we found the following results: sixty-eight women were treated, ranging in age from twenty-five to eighty-three years, and the median age was fifty-two. Thirty-eight patients had previously received conventional modalities, including WBRT. A total of 110 treatments were given to the sixty-eight women with an average of eight tumor sites per patient. Twenty-seven (40 percent) of sixty-eight survived one year, seven (10 percent) survived two years, and two (3 percent) survived more than three years. Twenty-six patients with one to three lesions were treated, eighteen with four to seven lesions, and twenty-four with more than eight lesions. Their overall local control rate was 94 percent, with thirty-nine (91 percent) of the forty-three patients expiring, dying of causes unrelated to their brain metastases. There was no significant difference in survival and local control based on the number of lesions treated. Survival was clearly found to be independent of the number of lesions treated.

Similarly, when we looked at our renal cell carcinoma patients, we found similar results. Twenty-two patients were treated: eight females and fourteen males. The range of lesions was between 1 and 21, with a median of 3.4 per patient. Twelve of twenty-two (55 percent) had

WBRT. Age ranged from thirty-eight to eighty, with a median age of sixty. The median survival was 8.7 months (3 to 55 months), with local control in twenty of twenty-two patients (91 percent). Eight patients (36 percent) required re-treatment for new lesions. Survival at one year was 24 percent in patients older than sixty, but 54 percent in those younger than sixty. Once again, the number of sites or prior WBRT did not have statistically significant effects on survival.

In our study, gamma knife radiosurgery shifted the question of survival to that of systemic control. Previous whole brain radiation therapy results have yielded no survival advantage to the treatment. The overall complication rate with one-session gamma knife has been 1.2 percent, in which patients having biopsy proven radiation necrosis required treatment with stereotactic aspiration and corticosteroids. This is a very low rate of complications.

Conclusion

In conclusion, we believe that one-session gamma knife radiosurgery for brain metastases is a superior mode of treatment for either single or multiple metastases. Survival rates match or exceed those previously reported for surgery with whole brain radiation or whole brain radiation alone. Radiosurgery yields added advantages: outpatient treatment, lower morbidity, greater flexibility in terms of local and number of tumors treated, and the ability to treat the patient over multiple periods of time for the development of new lesions.

We have not found that WBRT leads to a survival benefit nor that it prevents later onset of remote metastases in other brain locations. In our opinion, radiosurgery alone is the primary mode of therapy for brain metastases, unless the patient presents with neurological deficits resulting from mass effect, thus requiring surgical intervention. Radiosurgery clearly provides a very high rate of local control and preservation of neurological function with minimum effort and morbidity to the patient.

Chapter 9

Infections of the Brain

Chapter Contents

Section 9.1—Meningitis 160
Section 9.2—Brain Abscess 170
Section 9.3—Encephalitis 174
Section 9.4—Cysticercosis 189
Section 9.5—Trichinellosis 193

Section 9.1

Meningitis

"Meningococcal Disease" is reprinted from "Meningococcal Disease," Centers for Disease Control and Prevention (CDC), National Center for Infectious Diseases, Division of Bacterial and Mycotic Diseases, April 2003. "Cochlear Implants and Bacterial Meningitis" is reprinted from "Cochlear Implants and Bacterial Meningitis," U.S. Food and Drug Administration, *FDA Consumer Magazine*, November–December 2003. "Cryptococcal Meningitis" is reprinted with permission from the New Mexico AIDS Education and Training Center at the University of New Mexico Health Sciences Center. Revised May 2004. New Mexico AIDS InfoNet fact sheets are regularly updated. To find the most current information, visit www.aidsinfonet .org. "Meningococcal Vaccine: What You Need to Know" is reprinted from "Meningococcal Vaccine: What You Need to Know," CDC, National Immunization Program, Vaccine Information Statement: Meningococcal, July 2003.

Meningococcal Disease

What is meningitis?

Meningitis is an infection of the fluid of a person's spinal cord and the fluid that surrounds the brain. People sometimes refer to it as spinal meningitis. Meningitis is usually caused by a viral or bacterial infection. Knowing whether meningitis is caused by a virus or bacterium is important because the severity of illness and the treatment differ. Viral meningitis is generally less severe and resolves without specific treatment, while bacterial meningitis can be quite severe and may result in brain damage, hearing loss, or learning disability. For bacterial meningitis, it is also important to know which type of bacteria is causing the meningitis because antibiotics can prevent some types from spreading and infecting other people. Before the 1990s, *Haemophilus influenzae* type b (Hib) was the leading cause of bacterial meningitis, but new vaccines being given to all children as part of their routine immunizations have reduced the occurrence of invasive disease due to *H. influenzae*. Today, *Streptococcus pneumoniae* and *Neisseria meningitidis* are the leading causes of bacterial meningitis.

What are the signs and symptoms of meningitis?

High fever, headache, and stiff neck are common symptoms of meningitis in anyone over the age of two years. These symptoms can develop over several hours, or they may take one to two days. Other symptoms may include nausea, vomiting, discomfort looking into bright lights, confusion, and sleepiness. In newborns and small infants, the classic symptoms of fever, headache, and neck stiffness may be absent or difficult to detect, and the infant may only appear slow or inactive, or be irritable, have vomiting, or be feeding poorly. As the disease progresses, patients of any age may have seizures.

How is meningitis diagnosed?

Early diagnosis and treatment are very important. If symptoms occur, the patient should see a doctor immediately. The diagnosis is usually made by growing bacteria from a sample of spinal fluid. The spinal fluid is obtained by performing a spinal tap, in which a needle is inserted into an area in the lower back where fluid in the spinal canal is readily accessible. Identification of the type of bacteria responsible is important for selection of correct antibiotics.

Can meningitis be treated?

Bacterial meningitis can be treated with a number of effective antibiotics. It is important, however, that treatment be started early in the course of the disease. Appropriate antibiotic treatment of most common types of bacterial meningitis should reduce the risk of dying from meningitis to below 15 percent, although the risk is higher among the elderly.

Is meningitis contagious?

Yes, some forms of bacterial meningitis are contagious. The bacteria are spread through the exchange of respiratory and throat secretions (i.e., coughing, kissing). Fortunately, none of the bacteria that cause meningitis are as contagious as things like the common cold or the flu, and they are not spread by casual contact or by simply breathing the air where a person with meningitis has been.

However, sometimes the bacteria that cause meningitis have spread to other people who have had close or prolonged contact with a patient with meningitis caused by *Neisseria meningitidis* (also called meningococcal meningitis) or Hib. People in the same household or daycare center, or anyone with direct contact with a patient's oral secretions (such as a boyfriend or girlfriend) would be considered at increased risk of acquiring the infection. People who qualify as close contacts of a person with meningitis caused by *N. meningitidis* should receive antibiotics to prevent them from getting the disease. Antibiotics for contacts of a person with Hib meningitis disease are no longer recommended if all contacts four years of age or younger are fully vaccinated against Hib disease.

Are there vaccines against meningitis?

Yes, there are vaccines against Hib and against some strains of *N. meningitidis* and many types of *Streptococcus pneumoniae*. The vaccines against Hib are very safe and highly effective.

There is also a vaccine that protects against four strains of *N. meningitidis*, but it is not routinely used in the United States. The vaccine against *N. meningitidis* is sometimes used to control outbreaks of some types of meningococcal meningitis in the United States. Meningitis cases should be reported to state or local health departments to assure follow-up of close contacts and recognize outbreaks. College freshman, especially those who live in dormitories, are at higher risk for meningococcal disease and should be educated about the availability of a safe and effective vaccine that can decrease their risk. Although large epidemics of meningococcal meningitis do not occur in the United States, some countries experience large, periodic epidemics. Overseas travelers should check to see if meningococcal vaccine is recommended for their destination. Travelers should receive the vaccine at least one week before departure, if possible. Information on areas for which meningococcal vaccine is recommended can be obtained by calling the Centers for Disease Control and Prevention at (404)-332-4565.

There are vaccines to prevent meningitis due to *S. pneumoniae* (also called pneumococcal meningitis) that can also prevent other forms of infection due to *S. pneumoniae*. The pneumococcal polysaccharide vaccine is recommended for all persons over sixty-five years of age and younger persons at least two years old with certain chronic medical problems. There is a newly licensed vaccine (pneumococcal conjugate vaccine) that appears to be effective in infants for the prevention of pneumococcal infections and is routinely recommended for all children greater than two years of age.

Cochlear Implants and Bacterial Meningitis

Children with a cochlear implant to treat hearing loss have a greater risk of developing bacterial meningitis compared to children in the general population, according to a study conducted by the Centers for Disease Control and Prevention (CDC), the Food and Drug Administration, and state and local health departments.

The study, published in the July 31, 2003, issue of the *New England Journal of Medicine*, also found that children with a specific type of cochlear implant that had an extra piece called a "positioner" had 4.5 times the risk of developing meningitis compared to those who had other cochlear implant types. However, the study authors note that individuals who are candidates for cochlear implants may have factors that increase their risk of meningitis compared to the general population even prior to being implanted with the device. The study was not able to determine whether the implant, the preexisting risk factors, or perhaps a combination of both caused the increased occurrence of meningitis in the cochlear implant population studied.

Meningitis is an infection in the fluid that surrounds the brain and spinal cord. Of the two types of meningitis—viral and bacterial—bacterial is the more serious of the two and is the type that has been reported in people with cochlear implants.

The FDA and the CDC began investigating this possible link between cochlear implants and meningitis in July 2002 after receiving reports of bacterial meningitis among children who had received the implants. As soon as the FDA became aware of a possible association between the implants and bacterial meningitis, the agency issued a public health Web notice and began working with manufacturers of cochlear implants to determine the nature and extent of the problem. Because early available information suggested that more cases of meningitis occurred in children with the implant that had the positioner than with other devices, the manufacturer of this implant voluntarily withdrew it from the market in July 2002.

"Working closely with CDC's network for monitoring infection outbreaks is an important part of how we monitor the safety of medical products in use in the population," says FDA commissioner Mark B. McClellan, M.D., Ph.D. "In this case, we identified a heightened risk of meningitis that demanded prompt action, and the FDA was able to take it."

Nearly ten thousand children and thirteen thousand adults in the United States with severe to profound hearing loss have a cochlear implant. The implant is an electronic device containing electrodes that are surgically inserted into one of the structures of the inner ear, the cochlea, to activate nerve fibers and allow sound signals to be transmitted to the brain. It can help children with hearing loss perceive sounds and learn to speak.

The study group involved 4,264 children who received a cochlear implant in the United States between January 1, 1997, and August 6, 2002, and who were younger than six at the time of the implant. Bacterial meningitis was found in 26 children, and 15 of these children had meningitis caused by the bacterium *Streptococcus pneumoniae.* Less than one case of the disease would be ordinarily seen in a group this size during the same time period, based on the rates in the general population.

The FDA and the CDC continue to track new cases of meningitis in the United States that occur in people who have cochlear implants.

Advice for Parents

- Make sure your child is up to date on vaccines at least two weeks before having a cochlear implant. If your child has already received an implant, check with the child's doctor to ensure that all vaccinations are up to date. (Current vaccines protect against the most common strains of bacteria causing meningitis, but they do not protect against all strains.)

- Watch for possible signs and symptoms of meningitis: high fever, headache, stiff neck, nausea or vomiting, discomfort looking into bright lights, and sleepiness or confusion. A young child or infant with meningitis might be sleepy, cranky, or eat less. Contact a doctor promptly if your child shows any of these symptoms.

- Watch for signs and symptoms of an ear infection, which can include ear pain, fever, and decreased appetite. Seek prompt medical attention for any possible ear infections.

- Talk about the risks and benefits of cochlear implants with your child's doctor and discuss whether your child has certain medical conditions that might make him or her more likely to get meningitis.

Cryptococcal Meningitis

What Is Cryptococcal Meningitis?

Cryptococcus is a fungus. It is very common in the soil. It can get into your body when you breathe in dust or dried bird droppings. It does not seem to spread from person to person.

Meningitis is the most common illness caused by Cryptococcus. Meningitis is an infection of the lining of the spinal cord and brain.

It can cause coma and death. Cryptococcus can also infect the skin, lungs, or other parts of the body. The risk of cryptococcal infection is highest when your T-cell (CD4+) counts are below 100.

The first signs of meningitis include fever, fatigue, a stiff neck, headache, nausea and vomiting, confusion, and blurred vision or sensitivity to bright lights. The symptoms may come on slowly.

HIV disease or medications can also cause these symptoms. Therefore, laboratory tests are used to confirm that you have meningitis.

The tests use spinal fluid. Doctors get the fluid by doing a spinal tap. A needle is inserted into the middle of your back just above your hips. The needle removes a sample of spinal fluid. The test is safe and usually not too painful. However, after a spinal tap, some people get headaches that can last a few days.

The spinal fluid can be tested for cryptococcus in two ways. A *CRAG test* looks for an antigen (a protein) produced by cryptococcus. A *culture* is a way to see if the cryptococcus fungus can be grown from the sample of spinal fluid. CRAG tests are quick and can produce same-day results. A culture can take a week or more to show a positive result.

How Is Meningitis Treated?

Meningitis is treated with anti-fungal drugs. Some physicians use fluconazole. It is available in pill form or as an intravenous drug. Fluconazole is fairly effective, and is generally easy to tolerate. Other doctors prefer to use a combination of amphotericin B and flucytosine capsules. Amphotericin B is a very strong drug. It is given as an injection or a slow intravenous infusion. Both of these drugs can have serious side effects. In a newer form of amphotericin, the medication is encased in fat bubbles (liposomes). This form may have fewer side effects.

Cryptococcal meningitis comes back after the first time in about half of the people who get it. Repeat cases are reduced if people keep taking antifungal drugs.

How Do I Choose a Treatment for Meningitis?

If you have meningitis, you will be treated with anti-fungal drugs such as amphotericin B, fluconazole, and flucytosine. Amphotericin B is the strongest, but it can damage your kidneys. The other drugs have less serious side effects, but they are less effective at clearing out the cryptococcus.

If meningitis is diagnosed early enough, it can be treated without using amphotericin B. The usual treatment, however, is two weeks of amphotericin B followed by oral fluconazole. The fluconazole is continued for life. Without it, the meningitis is likely to come back.

Can Meningitis Be Prevented?

Taking fluconazole when your T-cell count is below 50 can help prevent cryptococcal meningitis. But there are several reasons why most doctors don't use it:

• Most fungal infections are easy to treat.

• Fluconazole is a very expensive drug.

• Taking fluconazole for a long period of time can lead to yeast infections (such as thrush, vaginitis, or severe candida infection of the throat) that are resistant to fluconazole. These resistant infections can be treated only with amphotericin B.

The Bottom Line

Cryptococcal meningitis occurs most often in people with T-cell counts below 100. Although antifungal drugs can prevent cryptococcal meningitis, they are usually not used because of their high cost and the risk of developing drug-resistant yeast infections.

If you get meningitis, early diagnosis might allow treatment with less toxic drugs. Contact your physician if you have headaches, a stiff neck, vision problems, confusion, nausea, or vomiting.

If you develop meningitis, you will have to continue taking antifungal drugs to prevent the disease from coming back.

Meningococcal Vaccine: What You Need to Know

What is meningococcal disease?

Meningococcal disease is a serious illness, caused by a bacteria. It is the leading cause of bacterial meningitis in children two to eighteen years old in the United States. Meningitis is an infection of the brain and spinal cord coverings. Meningococcal disease can also cause blood infections.

About 2,600 people get meningococcal disease each year in the United States. Between 10 and 15 percent of these people die, in spite of treatment with antibiotics. Of those who live, another 10 percent lose their arms or legs, become deaf, have problems with their nervous systems, become mentally retarded, or suffer seizures or strokes.

Anyone can get meningococcal disease, but it is most common in infants less than one year of age, international travelers, and people with certain medical conditions. College freshmen, particularly those who live in dormitories, have a slightly increased risk of getting meningococcal disease.

Meningococcal vaccine can prevent four types of meningococcal disease. These include two of the three types most common in the United States and a type that is the main cause of epidemics in Africa. Meningococcal vaccine cannot prevent all types of the disease, but it does help to protect many people who might become sick if they didn't get the vaccine.

Drugs such as penicillin can be used to treat meningococcal infection. Still, about one out of every ten people who get the disease die from it, and many others are affected for life. This is why it is important that people with the highest risk for meningococcal disease get the vaccine.

Who should get meningococcal vaccine and when?

Meningococcal vaccine is not routinely recommended for most people. People who should get the vaccine include:

- U.S. military recruits
- People who might be affected during an outbreak of certain types of meningococcal disease.
- Anyone traveling to, or living in, a part of the world where meningococcal disease is common, such as West Africa.
- Anyone who has a damaged spleen, or whose spleen has been removed.
- Anyone who has terminal complement component deficiency (an immune system disorder).

The vaccine should also be considered for:

- Some laboratory workers who are routinely exposed to the meningococcal bacteria.

The vaccine may also be given to college students who choose to be vaccinated. College freshmen, especially those who live in dormitories, and their parents should discuss the risks and benefits of vaccination with their health care providers.

Meningococcal vaccine is usually not recommended for children under two years of age, but under special circumstances it may be given to infants as young as three months (the vaccine does not work as well in very young children). Ask your health care provider for details.

How many doses?

- For people two years of age and over: one dose (Sometimes an additional dose is recommended for people who continue to be at high risk. Ask your provider.)

- For children three months to two years of age who need the vaccine: two doses, three months apart

Who should not get meningococcal vaccine or should wait?

People should not get meningococcal vaccine if they have ever had a serious allergic reaction to a previous dose of the vaccine.

People who are mildly ill at the time the shot is scheduled can still get meningococcal vaccine. People with moderate or severe illnesses should usually wait until they recover. Your provider can advise you.

Meningococcal vaccine may be given to pregnant women.

What are the risks from meningococcal vaccine?

A vaccine, like any medicine, is capable of causing serious problems, such as severe allergic reactions. The risk of the meningococcal vaccine causing serious harm, or death, is extremely small.

Getting meningococcal vaccine is much safer than getting the disease.

Some people who get meningococcal vaccine have mild side effects, such as redness or pain where the shot was given. These symptoms usually last for one to two days. A small percentage of people who receive the vaccine develop a fever.

What if there is a serious reaction?

What should I look for?

Look for any unusual condition, such as a severe allergic reaction, high fever, or unusual behavior. If a serious allergic reaction occurred, it would happen within a few minutes to a few hours after the shot. Signs of a serious allergic reaction can include difficulty breathing, weakness, hoarseness or wheezing, a fast heartbeat, hives, dizziness, paleness, or swelling of the throat.

What should I do?

- Call a doctor, or get the person to a doctor right away.
- Tell your doctor what happened, the date and time it happened, and when the vaccination was given.
- Ask your health care provider to file a Vaccine Adverse Events Reporting System (VAERS) form. Or call VAERS yourself at 800-822-7967 or visit their website at www.vaers.org.

How can I learn more?

Ask your doctor or nurse. They can give you the vaccine package insert or suggest other sources of information. You can also call your local or state health department's immunization program.

Section 9.2

Brain Abscess

Alternative Names

Abscess—brain; cerebral abscess; CNS abscess

Definition

A brain abscess is a mass of immune cells, pus, and other material that can occur when the brain is infected by bacteria or fungus.

Causes, Incidence, and Risk Factors

Brain abscesses commonly occur when bacteria or fungi infect part of the brain. Inflammation develops in response. Infected brain cells, white blood cells, and live and dead microorganisms collect in a limited area of the brain. This area becomes enclosed by a membrane that forms around it and creates a mass.

While this immune response can protect the brain by isolating the infection, it can also do more harm than good. The brain swells in response to the inflammation, and the mass may put pressure on delicate brain tissue. Infected material can block the blood vessels of the brain, further damaging tissues by causing cell death and swelling of additional cells. Multiple abscesses are uncommon except in immuno-compromised patients.

Infectious agents gain access to the brain in several ways. The most common way is through infected blood. Ear and sinus infections may also spread directly to the brain because of their close proximity.

Symptoms may develop gradually or suddenly. There may be little or no sign of general infection throughout the body. Early symptoms are usually headache, muscle weakness, visual changes, difficulty with balance or coordination, or seizures.

People at higher risk include those with congenital heart diseases, such as tetralogy of Fallot, and people with congenital blood vessel abnormalities of the lungs, such as Osler-Weber-Rendu disease. These disorders carry a high risk of infection of the heart or lungs, which can then spread to the brain. People with HIV infection or other conditions that compromise the immune system are also at higher risk.

Symptoms

- Headache
- Stiff neck, shoulders, or back
- Aching of neck, shoulders, or back
- Vomiting
- Changes in mental status
  - Drowsiness
  - Confusion
  - Inattention
  - Irritability
  - Slow thought processes
  - Decreasing responsiveness
  - Eventual coma
- Seizures
- Fever and chills
- Localized loss of nerve functions (focal neurologic deficits)
  - Vision changes
  - Muscle function/feeling loss
  - Decreased sensation
  - Decreased movement
  - Weakness
  - Decreased speech (aphasia)
  - Other language difficulties
  - Loss of coordination

Note: Symptoms may develop gradually, over a period of two weeks, or they may develop suddenly. Once symptoms occur, they progressively worsen.

Signs and Tests

A neurologic examination will usually reveal increased intracranial pressure and problems with brain function causing confusion or other problems. The problems will relate to the area of the brain where the abscess is located. The physician will look for the possible source of the infection.

- CBC may indicate infection or inflammation.
- Blood cultures will reveal any bacteria in the bloodstream.
- Chest x-ray will reveal lung infections (one of the more common sources of infection).
- EEG may be abnormal if seizures or focal neurologic deficits are present.
- Cranial CT scan or MRI of head shows the abscess and its exact location.

Treatment

Cerebral abscess is a medical emergency. Intracranial pressure may become high enough to cause death. Hospitalization is required until the condition is stabilized. Life support may be required in some cases.

Medication, not surgery, is advised for multiple abscesses, a small abscess (less than 2 cm), an abscess deep within the brain, an abscess accompanied by meningitis, the presence of shunts in the brain (for hydrocephalus), or an underlying disease that makes surgery dangerous (debilitating disease).

Antimicrobials are given, initially through a vein, then by mouth. Antibiotics that work against a number of different bacteria (broad-spectrum antibiotics) are the most common antimicrobial prescribed. It is not uncommon for multiple antibiotic medications to be used in order to ensure effective treatment of the infection. Antifungal medications may also be prescribed if fungal infection is likely.

The presence of a compressive lesion (which is injuring brain tissue by pressing on it) or a large abscess with a high degree of swelling around it can raise intracranial pressure to the point where immediate treatment is needed.

Surgery is required if there is persistent or progressive increase in intracranial pressure, if the mass does not reduce after use of antimicrobial medications, or if the mass contains gas (produced by some types of bacteria). Surgery may also be needed if there are signs of impending rupture of the abscess into the fluid-containing system of the brain (the ventricles).

Surgery consists of opening and draining the abscess and is usually accompanied by cultures of the fluid. This allows antimicrobial treatment to be adjusted so that it is specific to the causative micro-organism. The specific surgical procedure depends on the size and depth of the mass. The entire mass may be removed (excised) if it is near the surface and completely encapsulated. Needle aspiration guided by CT scan or MRI scan may be needed for a deep abscess. This may also include injecting antimicrobials directly into the mass.

Osmotic diuretics and steroids may also be used to reduce swelling of the brain.

Expectations (Prognosis)

If untreated, the disorder is almost always fatal. The outcome is usually improved with the use of CT and MRI scans for accurate diagnosis and by the administration of broad-spectrum antimicrobials.

The death rate is around 10 percent with treatment. Neurologic changes may be chronic or may resolve over time. Seizures or neurologic losses (inability to move, speak, see) may occur after surgery.

Complications

- Meningitis, severe and life threatening
- Epilepsy
- Permanent neurologic losses (vision, speech, movement)
- Recurrence of infection

Calling Your Health Care Provider

Go to the emergency room or call the local emergency number (such as 911) if symptoms suggestive of brain abscess occur. Cerebral abscess is a medical emergency!

Prevention

The risk of developing a cerebral abscess may be reduced by treating any disorders that can cause them. Such treatment should include a follow-up examination after infections are treated.

Preventive antibiotics given for people with congenital or rheumatic heart disorders prior to dental or urologic procedures may reduce the risk.

Section 9.3

Encephalitis

Encephalitis

Overview

Encephalitis is irritation and swelling (inflammation) of the brain.
It often coexists with inflammation of the covering of the brain and
spinal cord (meningitis) and most cases are caused by viral infection.
Encephalitis ranges from mild to severe and may result in permanent
neurological damage and death.

Types

Primary Encephalitis: This type results from viral infection of
the brain and spinal cord. Primary encephalitis may occur in isolated
cases (sporadic) or occur in many people at the same time in the same
area (epidemic).

The most common type of sporadic infection is *herpes simplex encephalitis*, which is caused by the herpesvirus. This type carries a high
risk for serious neurological damage and death and can occur in newborns if the virus is passed from the mother to the infant during birth.

Arthropod-borne viruses (transmitted through the bite of insects
and ticks) may cause *arboviral encephalitis*. Mosquitoes are the most
common agents of transmission and most cases occur during warmer
weather, when the insects are more active. Arboviral encephalitis and
rabies encephalitis (usually transmitted through the bite of an infected animal) may be sporadic or epidemic.

In the United States, the most common types of arboviral encephalitis are St. Louis, La Crosse, western equine, and eastern equine.
Recent outbreaks of West Nile encephalitis (transmitted by mosquitoes, commonly infects birds) have occurred in eastern, southeastern,

and midwestern regions of the United States, following bird migration.

Other types of arboviral encephalitis include the following:

- Japanese (widespread in Asia)
- Murray Valley (endemic in Australia)
- Powassan (transmitted by ticks; occurs in Canada and the northern United States)
- Tick-borne (occurs throughout Europe; vaccine available)
- Venezuelan equine (common in Central and South America)

Secondary Encephalitis: This type develops as a complication of a viral infection or reactivation of a latent virus. Viruses can become reactive when the immune system is suppressed by other conditions (e.g., malnutrition, stress, disease). Infections that may cause secondary encephalitis include influenza, chickenpox (varicella-zoster), measles (rubeola), mumps, and German measles (rubella).

Secondary encephalitis that develops as a result of a variola virus infection following smallpox vaccination or reactivation of another viral infection (called acute disseminated encephalitis) is often fatal.

Incidence and Prevalence

Incidence of encephalitis throughout the world is difficult to determine because the disease is often underreported. Approximately 150 to 3,000 cases, most of which are mild, may occur each year in the United States. Herpesvirus accounts for most cases of encephalitis in the United States.

Arboviral encephalitis is more prevalent in warm climates, and incidence varies considerably from area to area and from year to year. St. Louis encephalitis is the most prevalent type of arboviral encephalitis in the United States, and Japanese encephalitis is the most prevalent type in other parts of the world.

Encephalitis is more common in children and young adults.

Causes and Risk Factors

Encephalitis is caused by several types of viral infections. Herpesvirus is the most common cause, and encephalitis can also result from infection following smallpox vaccination and reactivation of viral infection such as influenza, chickenpox, measles, mumps, and rabies (usually in undeveloped countries).

Arthropod-borne viruses, which are usually transmitted by mosquitoes, cause arboviral encephalitis. People who live in warm, moist climates are at higher risk for this type.

Signs and Symptoms

Primary symptoms of encephalitis include sudden fever, stiff neck, malaise, sensitivity to light (photosensitivity), and headache. Infants may develop bulging of the soft spots (fontanels) of the skull. Other early symptoms include the following:

- Abnormal sleep patterns
- Behavioral changes (e.g., lethargy, confusion)
- Exhaustion
- Nausea
- Muscle stiffness
- Sore throat
- Upper respiratory tract infection (coughing, sneezing, congestion)

Neurological complications that may be permanent or improve as the infection runs its course include the following:

- Altered mental state (e.g., disorientation, personality changes)
- Convulsions
- Drooping eyelids (ptosis), double vision (diplopia), crossed eyes (strabismus)
- Hyperactive deep tendon reflexes
- Increased intracranial pressure
- Loss of consciousness
- Mental retardation
- Motor dysfunction
- Partial paralysis (paresis) of the extremities
- Projectile vomiting
- Pupil irregularities
- Restlessness
- Seizures
- Tremor

Most people infected with an arthropod-borne virus do not develop encephalitis. Infection usually does not produce symptoms (called asymptomatic) or causes flu-like symptoms such as fever, headache, and malaise.

Diagnosis

Diagnosis of encephalitis is based on the following:

- Medical history (including recent exposure to insects, travel, personality changes, and contact with unusual animals or illnesses)
- Neurological examination
- Blood and urine tests
- Imaging tests (e.g., CT scan, MRI scan, EEG)
- Spinal tap

A neurological exam is performed to evaluate mental status, detect neurological problems such as motor dysfunction and seizures, and help determine which area of the brain is affected.

Blood and urine tests are used to isolate and identify viruses. Enzyme-linked immunosorbent assays (ELISA), including IgM-capture ELISA (MAC-ELISA) and IgG ELISA, can identify viruses that cause encephalitis soon after infection. Polymerase chain reaction (PCR) can identify small amounts of viral DNA.

Computed tomography (CT scan) and magnetic resonance imaging (MRI scan) produce computer images of the brain and are used to detect abnormalities such as swelling (edema) and bleeding (hemorrhage). MRI is able to detect abnormalities earlier in the course of the infection. Electroencephalogram (EEG) involves placing electrodes on the scalp to record and analyze electrical activity in the brain. Wave patterns can suggest seizure disorder or a specific viral infection, such as herpesvirus.

Spinal tap, or lumbar puncture, is performed to detect signs of infection in cerebrospinal fluid and help make a diagnosis. In this procedure, a needle is inserted between two lower spine (lumbar) vertebrae, cerebrospinal fluid is collected, and the fluid is analyzed for elevated white blood cell counts, blood, and the presence of virus.

Treatment

Treatment for encephalitis depends on the cause. Some cases of viral encephalitis can be treated successfully if medication is started as soon as possible.

If herpes simplex encephalitis is suspected, antiviral medication such as acyclovir (Zovirax®) or ribavirin (Virazole®) is often administered immediately to improve chances for recovery and prevent complications. Side effects of these medications include nausea, vomiting, and headache. Treatment for viral encephalitis also includes palliative care.

There is no cure for arboviral encephalitis, and the goal of treatment is to relieve symptoms (palliative). Palliative care may include intravenous fluids (to prevent dehydration), antibiotics (to prevent secondary infections), and other medications (to prevent complications). Diuretics (e.g., furosemide, mannitol) may be administered to reduce intracranial pressure, and benzodiazepines (e.g., lorazepam [Ativan®]) may be administered to prevent seizures.

Prognosis

Prognosis depends on the type of encephalitis, the patient's age, overall health, and status of the immune system. Encephalitis caused by rabies, eastern equine encephalitis, Japanese encephalitis, and untreated viral encephalitis caused by herpesvirus carry a high risk for serious neurological damage and death. The prognosis is worse in very young patients, elderly patients, and patients with compromised immune systems. Acute disseminated encephalitis and encephalitis caused by rabies infection are often fatal. Rabies is transmitted through the bite of an infected animal, and there is no cure once symptoms have developed.

Prevention

In areas where arboviral encephalitis is prevalent, insecticide spraying may be used to control outbreaks. Wearing insect repellent and avoiding outdoor activities when mosquitoes are active may also be helpful.

A vaccine for Japanese encephalitis is available in the United States. People traveling to areas of the world where this disease is prevalent should be vaccinated. A vaccine for tick-borne encephalitis is available in Europe.

Administering antiviral medication (e.g., acyclovir) as soon as possible when encephalitis caused by herpesvirus is suspected may prevent serious neurological complications.

Information on Arboviral Encephalitides

Perspectives

Arthropod-borne viruses (i.e., arboviruses) are viruses that are maintained in nature through biological transmission between susceptible vertebrate hosts by blood feeding arthropods (mosquitoes, psychodids, ceratopogonids, and ticks). Vertebrate infection occurs when the infected arthropod takes a blood meal. The term "arbovirus" has no taxonomic significance. Arboviruses that cause human encephalitis are members of three virus families: the *Togaviridae* (genus Alphavirus), *Flaviviridae*, and *Bunyaviridae*.

All arboviral encephalitides are zoonotic [they originate in animals], being maintained in complex life cycles involving a nonhuman primary vertebrate host and a primary arthropod vector. These cycles usually remain undetected until humans encroach on a natural focus, or the virus escapes this focus via a secondary vector or vertebrate host as the result of some ecologic change. Humans and domestic animals can develop clinical illness but usually are "dead-end" hosts because they do not produce significant viremia, and do not contribute to the transmission cycle. Many arboviruses that cause encephalitis have a variety of different vertebrate hosts, and some are transmitted by more than one vector. Maintenance of the viruses in nature may be facilitated by vertical transmission (e.g., the virus is transmitted from the female through the eggs to the offspring).

Arboviral encephalitides have a global distribution, but there are four main virus agents of encephalitis in the United States: eastern equine encephalitis (EEE), western equine encephalitis (WEE), St. Louis encephalitis (SLE), and La Crosse (LAC) encephalitis, all of which are transmitted by mosquitoes. Another virus, Powassan, is a minor cause of encephalitis in the northern United States and is transmitted by ticks. A new Powassan-like virus has recently been isolated from deer ticks. Its relatedness to Powassan virus and its ability to cause disease has not been well documented. Most cases of arboviral encephalitis occur from June through September, when arthropods are most active. In milder (i.e., warmer) parts of the country, where arthropods are active late into the year, cases can occur into the winter months.

The majority of human infections are asymptomatic or may result in a nonspecific flu-like syndrome. Onset may be insidious or sudden with fever, headache, myalgias, malaise and occasionally prostration. Infection may, however, lead to encephalitis, with a fatal outcome or permanent neurologic sequelae [aftereffects]. Fortunately, only a small proportion of infected persons progress to frank encephalitis.

Experimental studies have shown that invasion of the central nervous system (CNS) generally follows initial virus replication in various peripheral sites and a period of viremia. Viral transfer from the blood to the CNS through the olfactory tract has been suggested. Because the arboviral encephalitides are viral diseases, antibiotics are not effective for treatment and no effective antiviral drugs have yet been discovered. Treatment is supportive, attempting to deal with problems such as swelling of the brain, loss of the automatic breathing activity of the brain, and other treatable complications like bacterial pneumonia.

There are no commercially available human vaccines for these U.S. diseases. There is a Japanese encephalitis vaccine available in the United States. A tick-borne encephalitis vaccine is available in Europe. An equine vaccine is available for EEE, WEE, and Venezuelan equine encephalitis (VEE). Arboviral encephalitis can be prevented in two major ways: personal protective measures and public health measures to reduce the population of infected mosquitoes. Personal measures include reducing time outdoors, particularly in early evening hours, wearing long pants and long-sleeved shirts, and applying mosquito repellent to exposed skin areas. Public health measures often require spraying of insecticides to kill juvenile (larvae) and adult mosquitoes.

Selection of mosquito control methods depends on what needs to be achieved, but in most emergency situations the preferred method to achieve maximum results over a wide area is aerial spraying. In many states aerial spraying may be available in certain locations as a means to control nuisance mosquitoes. Such resources can be redirected to areas of virus activity. When aerial spraying is not routinely used, such services are usually contracted for a given time period.

Financing of aerial spraying costs during large outbreaks is usually provided by state emergency contingency funds. Federal funding of emergency spraying is rare and almost always requires a federal disaster declaration. Such disaster declarations usually occur when the vector-borne disease has the potential to infect large numbers of people, when a large population is at risk, and when the area requiring treatment is extensive. Special large planes maintained by the United States Air Force can be called upon to deliver the insecticide(s) chosen for such emergencies. Federal disaster declarations have relied heavily on risk assessment by the CDC.

Laboratory diagnosis of human arboviral encephalitis has changed greatly over the last few years. In the past, identification of antibody relied on four tests: hemagglutination-inhibition, complement fixation, plaque reduction neutralization test, and the indirect fluorescent antibody (IFA) test. Positive identification using these immunoglobulin M (IgM)- and IgG-based assays requires a fourfold increase in titer between acute and convalescent serum samples. With the advent of solid-phase antibody-binding assays, such as enzyme-linked immunosorbent assay (ELISA), the diagnostic algorithm for identification of viral activity has changed. Rapid serologic assays such as IgM-capture ELISA (MAC-ELISA) and IgG ELISA may now be employed soon after infection. Early in infection, IgM antibody is more specific, while later in infection, IgG antibody is more reactive. Inclusion of monoclonal antibodies (MAbs) with defined virus specificities in these solid-phase assays has allowed for a level of standardization that was not previously possible.

Virus isolation and identification have also been useful in defining viral agents in serum, cerebrospinal fluid, and mosquito vectors. While virus isolation still depends upon growth of an unknown virus in cell culture or neonatal mice, virus identification has also been greatly facilitated by the availability of virus-specific MAbs for use in IFA assays. Similarly, MAbs with avidities sufficiently high to allow for specific binding to virus antigens in a complex protein mixture (e.g., mosquito pool suspensions) have enhanced our ability to rapidly identify virus agents in situ. While polymerase chain reaction (PCR) has been developed to identify a number of viral agents, such tests have not yet been validated for routine rapid identification in the clinical setting.

Mosquito-borne encephalitis offers a rare opportunity in public health to detect the risk of a disease before it occurs and to intervene to reduce that risk substantially. The surveillance required to detect risk is being increasingly refined by the potential utilization of these new technologies, which allows for rapid identification of dangerous viruses in mosquito populations. These rapid diagnostic techniques used in threat recognition can shorten public health response time and reduce the geographic spread of infected vectors and thereby the cost of containing them. The Arbovirus Diseases Branch of the National Center for Infectious Diseases (NCID)'s Division of Vector-Borne Infectious Diseases has responsibility for CDC's programs in surveillance, diagnosis, research, and control of arboviral encephalitides.

La Crosse Encephalitis

La Crosse (LAC) encephalitis was discovered in La Crosse, Wisconsin, in 1963. Since then, the virus has been identified in several Midwestern and Mid-Atlantic states. During an average year, about seventy-five cases of LAC encephalitis are reported to the CDC. Most cases of LAC encephalitis occur in children under sixteen years of age. LAC virus is a Bunyavirus and is a zoonotic pathogen cycled between the daytime-biting treehole mosquito, *Aedes triseriatus*, and vertebrate amplifier hosts (chipmunks, tree squirrels) in deciduous forest habitats. The virus is maintained over the winter by transovarial transmission in mosquito eggs. If the female mosquito is infected, she may lay eggs that carry the virus, and the adults coming from those eggs may be able to transmit the virus to chipmunks and to humans.

Historically, most cases of LAC encephalitis occur in the upper Midwestern states (Minnesota, Wisconsin, Iowa, Illinois, Indiana, and Ohio). Recently, more cases are being reported from states in the Mid-Atlantic (West Virginia, Virginia, and North Carolina) and southeastern (Alabama and Mississippi) regions of the country. It has long been suspected that LAC encephalitis has a broader distribution and a higher incidence in the eastern United States, but is under-reported because the etiologic agent is often not specifically identified.

LAC encephalitis initially presents as a nonspecific summertime illness with fever, headache, nausea, vomiting, and lethargy. Severe disease occurs most commonly in children under the age of sixteen and is characterized by seizures, coma, paralysis, and a variety of neurological sequelae after recovery. Death from LAC encephalitis occurs in less than 1 percent of clinical cases. In many clinical settings, pediatric cases presenting with CNS involvement are routinely screened for herpes or enteroviral etiologies. Since there is no specific treatment for LAC encephalitis, physicians often do not request the tests required to specifically identify LAC virus, and the cases are reported as aseptic meningitis or viral encephalitis of unknown etiology.

Also found in the United States, Jamestown Canyon and Cache Valley viruses are related to LAC, but rarely cause encephalitis.

Eastern Equine Encephalitis

Eastern equine encephalitis (EEE) is also caused by a virus transmitted to humans and equines by the bite of an infected mosquito. EEE virus is an alphavirus that was first identified in the 1930s and currently occurs in focal locations along the eastern seaboard, the Gulf Coast, and some inland Midwestern locations of the United States. While small outbreaks of human disease have occurred in the United States, equine epizootics [outbreaks] can be a common occurrence during the summer and fall.

It takes from four to ten days after the bite of an infected mosquito for an individual to develop symptoms of EEE. These symptoms begin with a sudden onset of fever, general muscle pains, and a headache of increasing severity. Many individuals will progress to more severe symptoms such as seizures and coma. Approximately one-third of all people with clinical encephalitis caused by EEE will die from the disease, and of those who recover, many will suffer permanent brain damage, with many of those requiring permanent institutional care.

In addition to humans, EEE virus can produce severe disease in horses, some birds, such as pheasants, quail, ostriches, and emus, and even puppies. Because horses are outdoors and attract hordes of biting mosquitoes, they are at high risk of contracting EEE when the virus is present in mosquitoes. Human cases are usually preceded by those in horses and exceeded in numbers by horse cases, which may be used as a surveillance tool.

EEE virus occurs in natural cycles involving birds and *Culiseta melanura*, in some swampy areas nearly every year during the warm months. Where the virus resides or how it survives in the winter is unknown. It may be introduced by migratory birds in the spring or it may remain dormant in some yet undiscovered part of its life cycle. With the onset of spring, the virus reappears in the birds (native bird species do not seem to be affected by the virus) and mosquitoes of the swamp. In this usual cycle of transmission, virus does not escape from these areas because the mosquito involved prefers to feed upon birds and does not usually bite humans or other mammals.

For reasons not fully understood, the virus may escape from enzootic foci in swamp areas in birds or bridge vectors such as *Coquilletidia perturbans* and *Aedes sollicitans*. These species feed on both birds and mammals and can transmit the virus to humans, horses, and other hosts. Other mosquito species, such as *Ae. vexans* and *Culex nigripalpus*, can also transmit EEE virus. When health officials maintain surveillance for EEE virus activity, this movement out of the swamp can be detected, and if the level of activity is sufficiently high, can recommend and undertake measures to reduce the risk to humans.

Western Equine Encephalitis

The alphavirus western equine encephalitis (WEE) was first isolated in California in 1930 from the brain of a horse with encephalitis, and remains an important cause of encephalitis in horses and humans in North America, mainly in western parts of the United States and Canada. In the western United States, the enzootic cycle of WEE involves passerine birds, in which the infection is inapparent, and culicine mosquitoes, principally *Cx. tarsalis*, a species that is associated with irrigated agriculture and stream drainages. The virus has also been isolated from a variety of mammal species. Other important mosquito vector species include *Aedes melanimon* in California, *Ae. dorsalis* in Utah and New Mexico, and *Ae. campestris* in New Mexico. WEE virus was isolated from field-collected larvae of *Ae. dorsalis*, providing evidence that vertical transmission may play an important role in the maintenance cycle of an alphavirus.

Expansion of irrigated agriculture in the North Platte River Valley during the past several decades has created habitats and conditions favorable for increases in populations of granivorous birds such as the house sparrow, *Passer domesticus*, and mosquitoes such as *Cx. tarsalis, Aedes dorsalis*, and *Aedes melanimon*. All of these species may play a role in WEE virus transmission in irrigated areas. In addition to *Cx. tarsalis, Ae. dorsalis*, and *Ae. melanimon*, WEE virus also has been isolated occasionally from some other mosquito species present in the area. Two confirmed and several suspect cases of WEE were reported from Wyoming in 1994. In 1995, two strains of WEE virus were isolated from *Culex tarsalis*, and neutralizing antibody to WEE virus was demonstrated in sera from pheasants and house sparrows. During 1997, thirty-five strains of WEE virus were isolated from mosquitoes collected in Scotts Bluff County, Nebraska.

Human WEE cases are usually first seen in June or July. Most WEE infections are asymptomatic or present as mild, nonspecific illness. Patients with clinically apparent illness usually have a sudden onset with fever, headache, nausea, vomiting, anorexia, and malaise, followed by altered mental status, weakness, and signs of meningeal irritation. Children, especially those under one year old, are affected more severely than adults and may be left with permanent sequelae [aftereffects], which is seen in 5 to 30 percent of young patients. The mortality rate is about 3 percent.

St. Louis Encephalitis

In the United States, the leading cause of epidemic flaviviral encephalitis is St. Louis encephalitis (SLE) virus. SLE is the most common mosquito-transmitted human pathogen in the United States. While periodic SLE epidemics have occurred only in the Midwest and southeast, SLE virus is distributed throughout the lower forty-eight states. Since 1964, there have been 4,437 confirmed cases of SLE with an average of 193 cases per year (range 4–1,967). However, less than 1 percent of SLE viral infections are clinically apparent, and the vast majority of infections remain undiagnosed. Illness ranges in severity from a simple febrile headache to meningoencephalitis, with an overall case-fatality ratio of 5 to 15 percent. The disease is generally milder in children than in adults, but in those children who do have disease, there is a high rate of encephalitis. The elderly are at highest risk for severe disease and death. During the summer season, SLE virus is maintained in a mosquito-bird-mosquito cycle, with periodic amplification by peridomestic birds and *Culex* mosquitoes. In Florida, the principal vector is *Cx. nigripalpus*, in the Midwest, *Cx. pipiens pipiens* and *Cx. p. quinquefasciatus*, and in the western United States, *Cx. tarsalis* and members of the *Cx. pipiens* complex.

Powassan Encephalitis

Powassan (POW) virus is a flavivirus and currently the only well-documented tick-borne transmitted arbovirus occurring in the United States and Canada. Recently a Powassan-like virus was isolated from the deer tick, *Ixodes scapularis*. Its relationship to POW and its ability to cause human disease has not been fully elucidated. POW's range in the United States is primarily in the upper tier states. In addition to isolations from man, the virus has been recovered from ticks (*Ixodes marxi, I. Cookie*, and *Dermacentor andersoni*) and from the tissues of a skunk (*Spilogale putorius*). It is a rare cause of acute viral encephalitis. POW virus was first isolated from the brain of a five-year-old child who died in Ontario in 1958. Patients who recover may have residual neurological problems.

Venezuelan Equine Encephalitis

Like EEE and WEE viruses, Venezuelan equine encephalitis (VEE) is an alphavirus and causes encephalitis in horses and humans and is an important veterinary and public health problem in Central and South America. Occasionally, large regional epizootics and epidemics can occur, resulting in thousands of equine and human infections. Epizootic strains of VEE virus can infect and be transmitted by a large number of mosquito species. The natural reservoir host for the epizootic strains is not known. A large epizootic that began in South America in 1969 reached Texas in 1971. It was estimated that over two hundred thousand horses died in that outbreak, which was controlled by a massive equine vaccination program using an experimental live attenuated VEE vaccine. There were several thousand human infections. A more recent VEE epidemic occurred in the fall of 1995 in Venezuela and Colombia with an estimated ninety thousand human infections. Infection of man with VEE virus is less severe than with EEE and WEE viruses, and fatalities are rare. Adults usually develop only an influenza-like illness, and overt encephalitis is usually confined to children. Effective VEE virus vaccines are available for equines.

Enzootic strains of VEE virus have a wide geographic distribution in the Americas. These viruses are maintained in cycles involving forest-dwelling rodents and mosquito vectors, mainly *Culex* (*Melanoconion*) species. Occasional cases or small outbreaks of human disease are associated with these viruses; the most recent outbreaks were in Venezuela in 1992, Peru in 1994, and Mexico in 1995–96.

Other Arboviral Encephalitides

Many other arboviral encephalitides occur throughout the world. Most of these diseases are problems only for those individuals traveling to countries where the viruses are endemic.

Japanese Encephalitis

Japanese encephalitis (JE) virus is a flavivirus, related to SLE, and is widespread throughout Asia. Worldwide, it is the most important cause of arboviral encephalitis, with over forty-five thousand cases reported annually. In recent years, JE virus has expanded its geographic distribution, with outbreaks in the Pacific. Epidemics occur in late summer in temperate regions, but the infection is enzootic and occurs throughout the year in many tropical areas of Asia. The virus is maintained in a cycle involving culicine mosquitoes and water birds. The virus is transmitted to man by *Culex* mosquitoes, primarily *Cx. tritaeniorhynchus*, which breed in rice fields. Pigs are the main amplifying hosts of JE virus in peridomestic environments.

The incubation period of JE is five to fourteen days. Onset of symptoms is usually sudden, with fever, headache, and vomiting. The illness resolves in five to seven days if there is no CNS involvement. The mortality in most outbreaks is less than 10 percent, but is higher in children and can exceed 30 percent. Neurologic sequelae in patients who recover are reported in up to 30 percent of cases. A formalin-inactivated vaccine prepared in mice is used widely in Japan, China, India, Korea, Taiwan, and Thailand. This vaccine is currently available for human use in the United States, for individuals who might be traveling to endemic countries.

Tick-Borne Encephalitis

Tick-borne encephalitis (TBE) is caused by two closely related flaviviruses that are distinct biologically. The eastern subtype causes

Russian spring–summer encephalitis (RSSE) and is transmitted by *Ixodes persulcatus*, whereas the western subtype is transmitted by *Ixodes ricinus* and causes Central European encephalitis (CEE). The name CEE is somewhat misleading, since the condition can occur throughout much of Europe. Of the two subtypes, RSSE is the more severe infection, having a mortality of up to 25 percent in some outbreaks, whereas mortality in CEE seldom exceeds 5 percent.

The incubation period is seven to fourteen days. Infection usually presents as a mild, influenza-type illness or as benign, aseptic meningitis, but may result in fatal meningoencephalitis. Fever is often biphasic, and there may be severe headache and neck rigidity, with transient paralysis of the limbs, shoulders, or less commonly the respiratory musculature. A few patients are left with residual paralysis. Although the great majority of TBE infections follow exposure to ticks, infection has occurred through the ingestion of infected cows' or goats' milk. An inactivated TBE vaccine is currently available in Europe and Russia.

West Nile Encephalitis

West Nile virus (WNV) is a flavivirus belonging taxonomically to the Japanese encephalitis serocomplex that includes the closely related St. Louis encephalitis (SLE) virus, Kunjin and Murray Valley encephalitis viruses, as well as others. WNV was first isolated in the West Nile Province of Uganda in 1937. The first recorded epidemics occurred in Israel during 1951–54 and in 1957. Epidemics have been reported in Europe in the Rhone delta of France in 1962 and in Romania in 1996. The largest recorded epidemic occurred in South Africa in 1974.

An outbreak of arboviral encephalitis in New York City and neighboring counties in New York state in late August and September 1999 was initially attributed to St. Louis encephalitis virus based on positive serologic findings in cerebrospinal fluid (CSF) and serum samples using a virus-specific IgM-capture enzyme-linked immunosorbent assay (ELISA). The outbreak has been subsequently confirmed as caused by West Nile virus based on the identification of virus in human, avian, and mosquito samples. See also these *MMWR* articles: "Outbreak of West Nile-Like Viral Encephalitis—New York, 1999," *MMWR* 48, no. 38 (1999): 845–49 and "Update: West Nile-Like Viral Encephalitis—New York, 1999," *MMWR* 48, no. 39 (1999): 890–92. A recent outbreak of West Nile (WN) encephalitis occurred in Bucharest, Romania, in 1996.

The virus that caused the New York area outbreak has been definitively identified as a strain of WNV. The genomic sequences identified to date from human brain and virus isolates from zoo birds, dead crows, and mosquito pools are identical. SLE and West Nile viruses are antigenically related, and cross-reactions are observed in most serologic tests. The isolation of viruses and genomic sequences from birds, mosquitoes, and human brain tissue permitted the discovery of West Nile virus in North America and prompted more specific testing. The limitations of serologic assays emphasize the importance of isolating the virus from entomologic, clinical, or veterinary material.

Although it is not known when and how West Nile virus was introduced into North America, international travel of infected persons to New York or transport by imported infected birds may have played a role. WNV can infect a wide range of vertebrates; in humans it usually produces either asymptomatic infection or mild febrile disease, but can cause severe and fatal infection in a small percentage of patients. Within its normal geographic distribution of Africa, the Middle East, western Asia, and Europe, WNV has not been documented to cause epizootics in birds; crows and other birds with antibodies to WNV are common, suggesting that asymptomatic or mild infection usually occurs among birds in those regions. Similarly, substantial bird virulence of SLE virus has not been reported. Therefore, an epizootic producing high mortality in crows and other bird species is unusual for either WNV or SLE virus. For both viruses, migratory birds may play an important role in the natural transmission cycles and spread. Like SLE virus, WNV is transmitted principally by *Culex* species mosquitoes, but also can be transmitted by *Aedes, Anopheles*, and other species. The predominance of urban *Culex pipiens* mosquitoes trapped during this outbreak suggests an important role for this species. Enhanced surveillance for early detection of virus activity in birds and mosquitoes will be crucial to guide control measures.

Murray Valley Encephalitis

Murray Valley encephalitis (MVE) is endemic in New Guinea and in parts of Australia and is related to SLE, WN, and JE viruses. Inapparent infections are common, and the small number of fatalities have mostly been in children.

Section 9.4

Cysticercosis

Reprinted from "Cysticercosis Fact Sheet," Centers for Disease Control and Prevention, Division of Parasitic Diseases, October 2003.

What is cysticercosis?

Cysticercosis is an infection caused by the pork tapeworm, *Taenia solium*. Infection occurs when the tapeworm larvae enter the body and form cysticerci (cysts). When cysticerci are found in the brain, the condition is called neurocysticercosis.

Where is cysticercosis found?

The tapeworm that causes cysticercosis is found worldwide. Infection is found most often in rural, developing countries with poor hygiene where pigs are allowed to roam freely and eat human feces. This allows the tapeworm infection to be completed and the cycle to continue. Infection can occur, though rarely, if you have never traveled outside of the United States. Taeniasis and cysticercosis are very rare in Muslim countries where eating pork is forbidden.

How can I get cysticercosis?

By accidentally swallowing pork tapeworm eggs. Tapeworm eggs are passed in the bowel movement of a person who is infected. These tapeworm eggs are spread through food, water, or surfaces contaminated with feces. This can happen by ingesting contaminated water or food, or by putting contaminated fingers to your mouth. A person who has a tapeworm infection can reinfect him- or herself (autoinfection). Once inside the stomach, the tapeworm egg hatches, penetrates the intestine, travels through the bloodstream, and may develop into cysticerci in the muscles, brain, or eyes.

What are the signs and symptoms of cysticercosis?

Signs and symptoms will depend on the location and number of cysticerci in your body.

- **Cysticerci in the Muscles:** Cysticerci in the muscles generally do not cause symptoms. However, you may be able to feel lumps under your skin.

- **Cysticerci in the Eyes:** Although rare, cysticerci may float in the eye and cause blurry or disturbed vision. Infection in the eyes may cause swelling or detachment of the retina.

- **Neurocysticercosis (Cysticerci in the Brain or Spinal Cord):** Symptoms of neurocysticercosis depend upon where and how many cysticerci (often called lesions) are found in the brain. Seizures and headaches are the most common symptoms. However, confusion, lack of attention to people and surroundings, difficulty with balance, and swelling of the brain (called hydrocephalus) may also occur. Death can occur suddenly with heavy infections.

How long will I be infected before symptoms begin?

Symptoms can occur months to years after infection, usually when the cysts are in the process of dying. When this happens, the brain can swell. The pressure caused by swelling is what causes most of the symptoms of neurocysticercosis. Most people with cysticerci in muscles won't have symptoms of infection.

How is cysticercosis diagnosed?

Diagnosis can be difficult and may require several testing methods. Your health care provider will ask you about where you have traveled and your eating habits. Diagnosis of neurocysticercosis is usually made by MRI or CT brain scans. Blood tests are available to help diagnose an infection, but may not always be accurate. If surgery is necessary, confirmation of the diagnosis can be made by the laboratory.

What should I do if I think I have cysticercosis?

See your health care provider.

Is there treatment for cysticercosis?

Yes. Infections are generally treated with anti-parasitic drugs in combination with anti-inflammatory drugs. Surgery is sometimes necessary to treat cases in the eyes, to treat cases that are not responsive to drug treatment, or to reduce brain edema (swelling). Not all cases of cysticercosis are treated.

I have been diagnosed with neurocysticercosis. My health care provider has decided not to treat me. How was this decision made?

Often, the decision of whether or not to treat neurocysticercosis is based upon the number of lesions found in the brain and the symptoms you have. When only one lesion is found, often treatment is not given. If you have more than one lesion, specific anti-parasitic treatment is generally recommended.

If the brain lesion is considered calcified (this means that a hard shell has formed around the tapeworm larvae), the cysticerci is considered dead and specific anti-parasitic treatment is not beneficial.

As the cysticerci die, the lesion will shrink. The swelling will go down, and often symptoms (such as seizures) will go away.

Can infection be spread from person to person?

No. Cysticercosis is not spread from person to person. However, a person infected with the intestinal tapeworm stage of the infection (*T. solium*) will shed tapeworm eggs in his or her bowel movements. Tapeworm eggs that are accidentally swallowed by another person can cause infection.

Should I be tested for an intestinal tapeworm infection?

Yes. Family members may also be tested. Because the tapeworm infection can be difficult to diagnose, your health care provider may ask you to submit several stool specimens over several days or to examine your stools for evidence of a tapeworm.

How can I prevent cysticercosis and other disease-causing germs?

- Avoid eating raw or undercooked pork and other meats.
- Don't eat meat of pigs that are likely to be infected with the tapeworm.
- Wash hands with soap and water after using the toilet and before handling food, especially when traveling in developing countries.

- Wash and peel all raw vegetables and fruits before eating. Avoid food that may be contaminated with feces.

- Drink only bottled or boiled (1 minute) water or carbonated (bubbly) drinks in cans or bottles. Do not drink fountain drinks or any drinks with ice cubes. Another way to make water safe is by filtering it through an "absolute 1 micron or less" filter *and* dissolving iodine tablets in the filtered water. "Absolute 1 micron" filters can be found in camping and outdoor supply stores.

For More Information

1. Del Brutto OH, Rajshekhar V, White AC, Tsang VCW, Nash TE, Takayanugi OM, Schantz PM, Evans CAW, Flisser A, Correa D, Boero OD, Allan JC, Sarti E, Gonzalez AE, Gilman RH, Garcia HH. Proposed diagnostic criteria for neurocysticercosis. *Neurol* 57 (2001): 177–83.

2. Garcia HH, Evans CAW, Nash TE, Takayanagui O, White AC, Botero DV, Tsang VCW, Schantz P, Allan J, Flisser A, Correra D, Sarti E, Friedland J, Martinez SM, Gonzalez AE, Gilman RH, Del Brutto OH. Consensus: Current Guidelines for the Treatment of Neurocysticercosis. *Clin Microbiol Rev* 15 (2003): 747–56.

3. Schantz PM, Taenia solium Cysticercosis: An Overview of Global Distribution and Transmission. Chapter in *Taenia solium Cysticercosis. From Basic to Clinical Science,* CABI Publishing, 2002, 63–74.

4. Shandera WX, Schantz PM, White AC. Taenia solium cysticercosis: The special case of the United States. Chapter in *Taenia solium Cysticercosis. From Basic to Clinical Science*, CABI Publishing, 2002, 139–44.

Section 9.5

Trichinellosis

Reprinted from "Trichinellosis Fact Sheet," Centers for Disease Control
and Prevention, Division of Parasitic Diseases, July 2004.

What is trichinellosis?

Trichinellosis, also called trichinosis, is caused by eating raw or
undercooked pork and wild game products infected with the larvae
of a species of worm called *Trichinella*. Infection occurs worldwide, but
is most common in areas where raw or undercooked pork, such as ham
or sausage, is eaten.

What are the symptoms of a trichinellosis infection?

Nausea, diarrhea, vomiting, fatigue, fever, and abdominal discomfort are the first symptoms of trichinellosis. Headaches, fevers, chills,
cough, eye swelling, aching joints and muscle pains, itchy skin, diarrhea,
or constipation follow the first symptoms. If the infection is heavy,
patients may experience difficulty coordinating movements, and have
heart and breathing problems. In severe cases, death can occur.

For mild to moderate infections, most symptoms subside within a
few months. Fatigue, weakness, and diarrhea may last for months.

How soon after infection will symptoms appear?

Abdominal symptoms can occur one to two days after infection.
Further symptoms usually start two to eight weeks after eating contaminated meat. Symptoms may range from very mild to severe and
relate to the number of infectious worms consumed in meat. Often,
mild cases of trichinellosis are never specifically diagnosed and are
assumed to be the flu or other common illnesses.

How does infection occur in humans and animals?

When a human or animal eats meat that contains infective *Trichinella* cysts, the acid in the stomach dissolves the hard covering of the cyst and releases the worms. The worms pass into the small intestine and, in one to two days, become mature. After mating, adult females lay eggs. Eggs develop into immature worms, travel through the arteries, and are transported to muscles. Within the muscles, the worms curl into a ball and encyst (become enclosed in a capsule). Infection occurs when these encysted worms are consumed in meat.

Am I at risk for trichinellosis?

If you eat raw or undercooked meats, particularly pork, bear, wild feline (such as a cougar), fox, dog, wolf, horse, seal, or walrus, you are at risk for trichinellosis.

Can I spread trichinellosis to others?

No. Infection can occur only by eating raw or undercooked meat containing *Trichinella* worms.

What should I do if I think I have trichinellosis?

See your health care provider, who can order tests and treat symptoms of trichinellosis infection. If you have eaten raw or undercooked meat, you should tell your health care provider.

How is trichinellosis infection diagnosed?

A blood test or muscle biopsy can show if you have trichinellosis.

How is trichinellosis infection treated?

Several safe and effective prescription drugs are available to treat trichinellosis. Treatment should begin as soon as possible and the decision to treat is based upon symptoms, exposure to raw or undercooked meat, and laboratory test results.

Is trichinellosis common in the United States?

Infection was once very common and usually caused by ingestion of undercooked pork. However, infection is now relatively rare. During 1997–2001, an average of 12 cases per year were reported. The number of cases has decreased because of legislation prohibiting the feeding of raw meat garbage to hogs, commercial and home freezing of pork, and the public awareness of the danger of eating raw or undercooked pork products. Cases are less commonly associated with pork products and more often associated with eating raw or undercooked wild game meats.

How can I prevent trichinellosis?

- Cook meat products until the juices run clear or to an internal temperature of 170 degrees Fahrenheit.

- Freeze pork less than six inches thick for twenty days at 5 degrees Fahrenheit to kill any worms.

- Cook wild game meat thoroughly. Freezing wild game meats, unlike freezing pork products, even for long periods of time, may not effectively kill all worms.

- Cook all meat fed to pigs or other wild animals.

- Do not allow hogs to eat uncooked carcasses of other animals, including rats, which may be infected with trichinellosis.

- Clean meat grinders thoroughly if you prepare your own ground meats.

Curing (salting), drying, smoking, or microwaving meat does not consistently kill infective worms.

For More Information

1. CDC. Trichinellosis surveillance, United States, 1997–2001. In: CDC Surveillance Summaries (July 25). *MMWR* 2003; 52 (no. SS-6): 1–8.

2. Moorhead A, Grunenwald PE, Dietz VJ, Schantz PM. Trichinellosis in the United States, 1991–1996: Declining but not gone. *Am J Trop Med Hyg* 60 (1999): 66–69.

Chapter 10

Hypoxia

Introduction and Definition

The brain requires a constant flow of oxygen to function normally. A hypoxic-anoxic injury, also known as HAI, occurs when that flow is disrupted, essentially starving the brain and preventing it from performing vital biochemical processes. Hypoxic refers to a partial lack of oxygen; anoxic means a total lack. In general, the more complete the deprivation, the more severe the harm to the brain and the greater the consequences.

The diminished oxygen supply can cause serious impairments in cognitive skills, as well as in physical, psychological, and other functions. Recovery can occur in many cases, but it depends largely on the parts of the brain affected, and its pace and extent are unpredictable.

As a result, HAI can have a catastrophic impact on the lives not only of those injured but their families, friends, and caregivers as well. Treatment can be costly and complicated, especially because HAI patients frequently need substantial medical and rehabilitative help and may suffer from significant long-term disabilities. A shortage of easy-to-understand, accessible information about HAI can make the situation even more stressful for affected individuals and their families. This chapter will help answer your questions about this condition.

Causes of Hypoxic-Anoxic Injury

Why is oxygen important to us? Our bodies require oxygen in order to metabolize glucose. This process provides energy for the cells. The brain consumes about a fifth of the body's total oxygen supply, and needs energy to transmit electrochemical impulses between cells and to maintain the ability of neurons to receive and respond to these signals.

Cells of the brain will start to die within a few minutes if they are deprived of oxygen. The result is a cascade of problems. In particular, the disruption of the transmission of electrochemical impulses impacts the production and activity of important substances called neurotransmitters, which regulate many cognitive, physiological, and emotional processes.

There are many neurotransmitters, and they perform a wide variety of important functions, although the specific ways neurotransmitters work are not fully understood. Some, such as serotonin, dopamine, and norepinephrine, play an important role in regulating moods. Endorphins are critical for controlling pain and enhancing pleasure, while acetylcholine is important for memory functions.

A variety of disease processes and injuries can cause HAI. The most common is called hypoxic-ischemic injury, also known as HII or stagnant anoxia. This occurs when some internal event prevents enough oxygen-rich blood from reaching the brain. While strokes and cardiac arrhythmia can both result in HII, the most frequent cause is cardiac arrest.

Anesthesia accidents and cardiovascular disease each account for just under a third of cardiac arrests, according to a 1989 study. Other possible causes are asphyxia, generally caused by suicide attempts or near-drownings (16 percent), chest trauma (10 percent), electrocution (6.5 percent), severe bronchial asthma (3 percent), and barbiturate poisoning (3 percent).

Occasionally, HAI is caused by anoxic anoxia, which is when the air itself does not contain enough oxygen to be absorbed and used by the body. This can occur at high altitudes, where the air is thinner than at sea level, but is extremely unusual otherwise. Another syndrome, toxic anoxia, involves the presence in the body of toxins or other substances that may interfere with the way an individual processes oxygen.

Another occasional cause of HAI is anemic anoxia, which can occur when someone does not have enough blood or hemoglobin, a chemical in the red blood cells, which carry oxygen throughout the body.

Acute hemorrhage, chronic anemia, and carbon monoxide poisoning are conditions that can result in anemic anoxia.

Acute hemorrhage is essentially massive bleeding, caused, for example, by a gunshot or other wound. Chronic anemia is an ailment in which a person suffers from persistently low levels of red blood cells or hemoglobin. Carbon monoxide poisoning, which appears to damage parts of the brain controlling movement, occurs in suicide attempts using automobile exhaust, but can also happen due to malfunctioning furnaces and other accidents involving machinery and industrial equipment.

Symptoms

HAI is generally marked by an initial loss of consciousness or coma, a condition that looks like sleep but from which a person cannot be awakened. The period of unconsciousness, whether short or long, might be followed by a persistent vegetative state, in which a person is neither comatose nor responsive to external stimuli. This state is frequently referred to as "wakeful unresponsiveness."

Even when a person has fully recovered consciousness, he or she might suffer from a long list of symptoms. In many ways, these symptoms are similar to those commonly seen after a blow to the head. The effects can vary widely depending upon the part of the brain that has been injured and the extent of the damage. Some of the major cognitive (thought) problems are:

- **Short-term memory loss.** This is the most common cognitive symptom, especially among those who have HII. The reason is that the part of the brain that is believed to be responsible for learning new information, called the hippocampus, has neurons that are highly sensitive to oxygen deprivation.

- **Decline in executive functions.** Disruption of such critical tasks as reasoning, making judgments, and synthesizing information. This can lead to impulsive behavior, poor decision making, and inability to direct, divide, or switch attention.

- **Difficulty with words, also known as anomia.** These linguistic problems include not being able to remember the right word, selecting the wrong word, confusing similar words, not understanding commonly used words, and so on.

- **Visual disturbances.** Difficulty processing visual information can occur in some cases. One rare disorder is called cortical blindness, in which the area of the brain responsible for vision becomes disconnected from the rest of the brain. Because the brain cannot tell that this part is damaged, people may appear to act as though they can see even though they display no ability to identify or recognize objects, shapes, or colors.

Some common physical deficits are:

- **Ataxia, or a lack of coordination.** This often expresses itself as a sort of bobbing or weaving, similar to what is seen in people who are drunk.

- **Apraxia,** or an inability to execute a familiar sequence of physical movements such as brushing teeth, combing hair, using eating utensils, and so on.

- **Spasticity, rigidity, and myoclonus,** disorders that can include a tendency toward jerky motions, trembling of the extremities, or other abnormal movements.

- **Quadriparesis,** a weakness of the arms and legs.

Other symptoms can include hallucinations and delusions; increased agitation and confusion; depression and other mood disorders; personality changes, such as irritability and a reduced threshold for frustration; and an inability to focus or concentrate.

Predicting the Outcome

Because people with HAI have often suffered extensive damage, complete recovery is not assured. In fact, predicting the outcome of HAI is a bit like estimating how high a rocket will go. There are some general factors that are helpful in making initial forecasts, but the actual course of the rocket is also dependent upon real-world conditions and many unforeseeable variables.

Studies that have been done suggest that recovery may be more limited than in cases where a person has suffered a traumatic brain injury of comparable severity. Nonetheless, there are some clues that can clearly offer a bit of guidance in judging the likelihood of at least a partial recovery. These include:

- **Length of coma.** As you might expect, the longer a person is in a coma, the less promising the outcome, although individual cases can vary dramatically from the norm. One study suggested that if a coma lasts less than twelve hours, there is likely to be little long-term damage. Another study indicated that 21 percent of HAI patients who remained in a coma for four weeks or less experienced a good recovery, while the recovery for others was poor. Many patients come out of a coma but remain in what is called a persistent vegetative state, a sort of wakeful unresponsiveness in which some brain functions continue to operate but with no apparent consciousness. Some doctors believe that if the persistent vegetative state in a patient with HAI continues for more than three months, there is virtually no chance of further recovery.

- **Visual cues.** If both eyes have fixed or dilated pupils, the prognosis is generally poor. Since this can indicate significant damage to the brain stem, the area of the brain responsible for regulating such basic functions as breathing, the outcome is not promising. Neurologists can also conduct tests to measure some standard eye-movement responses to determine what kind of damage has been suffered.

- **Age.** Some studies suggest that patients younger than twenty-five have a better rate of recovery than those who are older.

- **Brain imaging tests,** such as MRI or CT scans. Acute brain damage that has occurred in the immediate past does not typically show up on this type of scan. However, imaging tests conducted several months down the line may indicate the atrophy or loss of some brain matter.

- **Electroencephalography (EEG) and evoked potentials (EPs).** An EEG that reveals continued cortical activity is a positive sign. An EP, which charts electrical activity arising in response to outside stimuli, can also give some indication of the state of the brain after HAI.

Treatment

Unfortunately, direct treatment of anoxia is limited. Some studies have suggested that the use of barbiturates, which slow down the brain's activity, may be helpful in the first two or three days after the onset of the injury. Otherwise, the general medical approach is to maintain the body's status.

Once a person's condition has been stabilized, the next question is to what extent he or she can recover. Recovery can take many months and even years, and in many cases the person never regains his or her prior level of functioning. In general, the sooner rehabilitation starts, the better.

During rehabilitation, the individual and family members may interact with a variety of professionals as the need for constant medical attention from a doctor decreases. Such professionals may include a physical therapist, who aids in improving motor skills such as walking; an occupational therapist, who assists in retraining the person to perform skills of daily living, such as dressing and going to the bathroom; a speech therapist, who may help address cognitive problems as well as language disorders; and a neuropsychologist, who may assess the level and type of cognitive impairment, collaborate on retraining, and assist both the individual and family members with behavior and emotional issues.

Advice for Caregivers

As recovery may take months and even years, it is important for both the patient and family members involved in rehabilitation efforts to establish a good working relationship with the various specialists. It's important to understand that rehab often proceeds in an unpredictable way, with progress measured in small steps rather than giant leaps.

Patients and family caregivers, therefore, often experience intense bouts of frustration at what they perceive to be the slow pace of recovery. Expectations and hope may at times outstrip the person's actual level of progress, and the potential for disappointment and misunderstanding—between patient and family, or caregivers and rehabilitation professionals—can be significant.

While the process will never be easy, the following tips may help to minimize possible tension and conflict:

- Find out as early as possible who will be part of the rehab team. Get to know the professionals as soon as they begin working with the patient. Ask them for a realistic assessment of the situation. What can you and the patient expect? What is the bare minimum they hope to achieve? What is the likely outcome? What is the most optimistic forecast? This way, you will understand the range of possibilities and can gauge your expectations accordingly.

- Learn as much as possible about the role of each of the rehabilitation specialists. Ask them how you can make their jobs easier.

Are there steps you need to take to prepare the patient for them each day? Are there exercises you can help with? Are there times you would be better off staying out of the way?

- Stay informed and involved. Family members and friends can play a critical role in monitoring care, charting progress, providing support to both the patient and the professionals, and answering any questions that may arise. Working as a team is one way to help maximize the recovery potential.

- Plan regular meetings for family members and friends involved in the caregiving process. This will give everyone a chance to exchange information, voice concerns, and stay on top of the changing situation. If possible, invite one or more of the rehabilitation professionals so they can fill in the group as a whole rather than having to repeat information to every individual.

- Recovery can be completely unpredictable, and the love of those around a patient can play a key role in stimulating progress. Motivation is an important factor, and someone who feels supported in his or her efforts may well find greater reserves of internal strength to press forward with the rehabilitation process.

- Celebrate every success, not just the big ones. The first time the patient takes a step unaided, handles a fork properly, or remembers someone's name should be considered a major victory. Hopefully, more will follow, but it is important to take joy in every advance, small or large.

Resources

National Institute of Neurological Disorders and Stroke Cerebral Hypoxia Information Page, www.ninds.nih.gov/health_and_medical/disorders/anoxia_doc.htm

Zasler, Nathan. Ask the Doctor. *Brain Injury Source* (magazine of the Brain Injury Association of America) 3, no. 3 (Summer 1999); www.biausa.org/Pages/askthedoctor.html

Groswasser, Ze'ev, Cohen, M., & Costeff, H. Rehabilitation outcome after anoxic brain damage. *Archives of Physical Medicine & Rehabilitation* 70 (1989): 186–88.

Chapter 11

Traumatic Brain Injuries

Chapter Contents

Section 11.1—What You Need to Know about
                    Traumatic Brain Injury 206
Section 11.2—Concussion 226
Section 11.3—Coma 229
Section 11.4—Shaken Baby Syndrome 238

Section 11.1

What You Need to Know about Traumatic Brain Injury

Reprinted from "Traumatic Brain Injury: Hope through Research," National Institute of Neurological Disorders and Stroke, National Institutes of Health, NIH Publication Number 02-158, updated November 2004.

Introduction

Traumatic brain injury (TBI) is a major public health problem, especially among male adolescents and young adults ages fifteen to twenty-four, and among elderly people of both sexes seventy-five years and older. Children aged five and younger are also at high risk for TBI.

Perhaps the most famous TBI patient in the history of medicine was Phineas Gage. In 1848, Gage was a twenty-five-year-old railway construction foreman working on the Rutland and Burlington Railroad in Vermont. In the nineteenth century, little was understood about the brain and even less was known about how to treat injury to it. Most serious injuries to the brain resulted in death due to bleeding or infection. Gage was working with explosive powder and a packing rod, called a tamping iron, when a spark caused an explosion that propelled the three-foot long, pointed rod through his head. It penetrated his skull at the top of his head, passed through his brain, and exited the skull by his temple. Amazingly, he survived the accident with the help of physician John Harlow, who treated Gage for seventy-three days. Before the accident Gage was a quiet, mild-mannered man; after his injuries he became an obscene, obstinate, self-absorbed man. He continued to suffer personality and behavioral problems until his death in 1861.

Today, we understand a great deal more about the healthy brain and its response to trauma, although science still has much to learn about how to reverse damage resulting from head injuries.

TBI costs the country more than $48 billion a year, and between 2.5 and 6.5 million Americans alive today have had a TBI. Survivors of TBI are often left with significant cognitive, behavioral, and communicative disabilities, and some patients develop long-term medical complications, such as epilepsy.

Other statistics dramatically tell the story of head injury in the United States. Each year:

- approximately 270,000 people experience a moderate or severe TBI,
- approximately 70,000 people die from head injury,
- approximately 1 million head-injured people are treated in hospital emergency rooms,
- approximately 60,000 new cases of epilepsy occur as a result of head trauma,
- approximately 230,000 people are hospitalized for TBI and survive, and
- approximately 80,000 of these survivors live with significant disabilities as a result of the injury.

What Is a Traumatic Brain Injury?

TBI, also called acquired brain injury or simply head injury, occurs when a sudden trauma causes damage to the brain. The damage can be focal—confined to one area of the brain—or diffuse—involving more than one area of the brain. TBI can result from a closed head injury or a penetrating head injury. A closed injury occurs when the head suddenly and violently hits an object but the object does not break through the skull. A penetrating injury occurs when an object pierces the skull and enters brain tissue.

What Are the Signs and Symptoms of TBI?

Symptoms of a TBI can be mild, moderate, or severe, depending on the extent of the damage to the brain. Some symptoms are evident immediately, while others do not surface until several days or weeks after the injury. A person with a mild TBI may remain conscious or may experience a loss of consciousness for a few seconds or minutes. The person may also feel dazed or not like him- or herself for several days or weeks after the initial injury. Other symptoms of mild TBI include headache, confusion, lightheadedness, dizziness, blurred vision or tired eyes, ringing in the ears, bad taste in the mouth, fatigue or lethargy, a change in sleep patterns, behavioral or mood changes, and trouble with memory, concentration, attention, or thinking.

A person with a moderate or severe TBI may show these same symptoms, but may also have a headache that gets worse or does not go away, repeated vomiting or nausea, convulsions or seizures, inability to awaken from sleep, dilation of one or both pupils of the eyes, slurred speech, weakness or numbness in the extremities, loss of coordination, and increased confusion, restlessness, or agitation. Small children with moderate to severe TBI may show some of these signs as well as signs specific to young children, such as persistent crying, inability to be consoled, and refusal to nurse or eat. Anyone with signs of moderate or severe TBI should receive medical attention as soon as possible.

What Are the Causes of and Risk Factors for TBI

Half of all TBIs are due to transportation accidents involving automobiles, motorcycles, bicycles, and pedestrians. These accidents are the major cause of TBI in people under age seventy-five. For those seventy-five and older, falls cause the majority of TBIs. Approximately 20 percent of TBIs are due to violence, such as firearm assaults and child abuse, and about 3 percent are due to sports injuries. Fully half of TBI incidents involve alcohol use.

The cause of the TBI plays a role in determining the patient's outcome. For example, approximately 91 percent of firearm TBIs (two-thirds of which may be suicidal in intent) result in death, while only 11 percent of TBIs from falls result in death.

What Are the Different Types of TBI?

Concussion is the most minor and the most common type of TBI. Technically, a concussion is a short loss of consciousness in response to a head injury, but in common language the term has come to mean any minor injury to the head or brain.

Other injuries are more severe. As the first line of defense, the skull is particularly vulnerable to injury. Skull fractures occur when the bone of the skull cracks or breaks. A depressed skull fracture occurs when pieces of the broken skull press into the tissue of the brain. A penetrating skull fracture occurs when something pierces the skull, such as a bullet, leaving a distinct and localized injury to brain tissue.

Skull fractures can cause bruising of brain tissue called a contusion. A contusion is a distinct area of swollen brain tissue mixed with blood released from broken blood vessels. A contusion can also occur in response to shaking of the brain back and forth within the confines of the skull, an injury called contrecoup. This injury often occurs in car accidents after high-speed stops and in shaken baby syndrome, a severe form of head injury that occurs when a baby is shaken forcibly enough to cause the brain to bounce against the skull. In addition, contrecoup can cause diffuse axonal injury, also called shearing, which involves damage to individual nerve cells (neurons) and loss of connections among neurons. This can lead to a breakdown of overall communication among neurons in the brain.

Damage to a major blood vessel in the head can cause a hematoma, or heavy bleeding into or around the brain. Three types of hematomas can cause brain damage. An epidural hematoma involves bleeding into the area between the skull and the dura. With a subdural hematoma, bleeding is confined to the area between the dura and the arachnoid membrane. Bleeding within the brain itself is called intracerebral hematoma.

Another insult to the brain that can cause injury is anoxia. Anoxia is a condition in which there is an absence of oxygen supply to an organ's tissues, even if there is adequate blood flow to the tissue. Hypoxia refers to a decrease in oxygen supply rather than a complete absence of oxygen. Without oxygen, the cells of the brain die within several minutes. This type of injury is often seen in near-drowning victims, in heart attack patients, or in people who suffer significant blood loss from other injuries that decrease blood flow to the brain.

What Medical Care Should a TBI Patient Receive?

Medical care usually begins when paramedics or emergency medical technicians arrive on the scene of an accident or when a TBI patient arrives at the emergency department of a hospital. Because little can be done to reverse the initial brain damage caused by trauma, medical personnel try to stabilize the patient and focus on preventing further injury. Primary concerns include insuring proper oxygen supply to the brain and the rest of the body, maintaining adequate blood flow, and controlling blood pressure. Emergency medical personnel may have to open the patient's airway or perform other procedures to make sure the patient is breathing. They may also perform CPR to help the heart pump blood to the body, and they may treat other injuries to control or stop bleeding. Because many head-injured patients may also have spinal cord injuries, medical professionals take great care in moving and transporting the patient. Ideally, the patient is placed on a backboard and in a neck restraint. These devices immobilize the patient and prevent further injury to the head and spinal cord.

As soon as medical personnel have stabilized the head-injured patient, they assess the patient's condition by measuring vital signs and reflexes and by performing a neurological examination. They check the patient's temperature, blood pressure, pulse, breathing rate, and pupil size in response to light. They assess the patient's level of consciousness and neurological functioning using the Glasgow Coma Scale, a standardized, fifteen-point test that uses three measures—eye opening, best verbal response, and best motor response—to determine the severity of the patient's brain injury.

Glasgow Coma Scale

The eye opening part of the Glasgow Coma Scale has four scores:

- 4 indicates that the patient can open his eyes spontaneously.
- 3 is given if the patient can open his eyes on verbal command.
- 2 indicates that the patient opens his eyes only in response to painful stimuli.
- 1 is given if the patient does not open his eyes in response to any stimulus.

The best verbal response part of the test has five scores:

- 5 is given if the patient is oriented and can speak coherently.
- 4 indicates that the patient is disoriented but can speak coherently.
- 3 means the patient uses inappropriate words or incoherent language.
- 2 is given if the patient makes incomprehensible sounds.
- 1 indicates that the patient gives no verbal response at all.

The best motor response test has six scores:

- 6 means the patient can move his arms and legs in response to verbal commands.
- A score between 5 and 2 is given if the patient shows movement in response to a variety of stimuli, including pain.
- 1 indicates that the patient shows no movement in response to stimuli.

The results of the three tests are added up to determine the patient's overall condition. A total score of 3 to 8 indicates a severe head injury, 9 to 12 indicates a moderate head injury, and 13 to 15 indicates a mild head injury.

Imaging tests help in determining the diagnosis and prognosis of a TBI patient. Patients with mild to moderate injuries may receive skull and neck x-rays to check for bone fractures or spinal instability. The patient should remain immobilized in a neck and back restraint until medical personnel are certain that there is no risk of spinal cord injury. For moderate to severe cases, the gold standard imaging test is a computed tomography (CT) scan. The CT scan creates a series of cross-sectional x-ray images of the head and brain and can show bone fractures as well as the presence of hemorrhage, hematomas, contusions, brain tissue swelling, and tumors. Magnetic resonance imaging (MRI) may be used after the initial assessment and treatment of the TBI patient. MRI uses magnetic fields to detect subtle changes in brain tissue content and can show more detail than x-rays or CT. Unfortunately, MRI is not ideal for routine emergency imaging of TBI patients because it is time-consuming and is not available in all hospitals.

Approximately half of severely head-injured patients will need surgery to remove or repair hematomas or contusions. Patients may also need surgery to treat injuries in other parts of the body. These patients usually go to the intensive care unit after surgery.

Sometimes when the brain is injured swelling occurs and fluids accumulate within the brain space. It is normal for bodily injuries to cause swelling and disruptions in fluid balance. Yet when an injury occurs inside the skull-encased brain, there is no place for swollen tissues to expand and no adjoining tissues to absorb excess fluid. This increased pressure is called intracranial pressure (ICP).

Medical personnel measure patients' ICP using a probe or catheter. The instrument is inserted through the skull to the subarachnoid level and is connected to a monitor that registers the patient's ICP. If a patient has high ICP, he or she may undergo a ventriculostomy, a procedure that drains cerebrospinal fluid (CSF) from the brain to bring the pressure down. Drugs that can be used to decrease ICP include mannitol or barbiturates, although the safety and effectiveness of the latter are unknown.

How Does a TBI Affect Consciousness?

A TBI can cause problems with arousal, consciousness, awareness, alertness, and responsiveness. Generally, there are five abnormal states of consciousness that can result from a TBI: stupor, coma, persistent vegetative state, locked-in syndrome, and brain death.

Stupor is a state in which the patient is unresponsive but can be aroused briefly by a strong stimulus, such as sharp pain. Coma is a state in which the patient is totally unconscious, unresponsive, unaware, and unarousable. Patients in a coma do not respond to external stimuli, such as pain or light, and do not have sleep-wake cycles. Coma results from widespread and diffuse trauma to the brain, including the cerebral hemispheres of the upper brain and the lower brain or brainstem. Coma generally is of short duration, lasting a few days to a few weeks. After this time, some patients gradually come out of the coma, some progress to a vegetative state, and others die.

Patients in a vegetative state are unconscious and unaware of their surroundings, but they continue to have a sleep-wake cycle and can have periods of alertness. Unlike coma, where the patient's eyes are closed, patients in a vegetative state often open their eyes and may move, groan, or show reflex responses. A vegetative state can result from diffuse injury to the cerebral hemispheres of the brain without damage to the lower brain and brainstem. Anoxia, or lack of oxygen to the brain, which is a common complication of cardiac arrest, can also bring about a vegetative state.

Many patients emerge from a vegetative state within a few weeks, but those who do not recover within thirty days are said to be in a persistent vegetative state (PVS). The chances of recovery depend on the extent of injury to the brain and the patient's age, with younger patients having a better chance of recovery than older patients. Generally adults have a 50 percent chance and children a 60 percent chance of recovering consciousness from a PVS within the first six months. After a year, the chances that a PVS patient will regain consciousness are very low and most patients who do recover consciousness experience significant disability. The longer a patient is in a PVS, the more severe the resulting disabilities will be. Rehabilitation can contribute to recovery, but many patients never progress to the point of being able to take care of themselves.

Locked-in syndrome is a condition in which a patient is aware and awake, but cannot move or communicate due to complete paralysis of the body.

Unlike PVS, in which the upper portions of the brain are damaged and the lower portions are spared, locked-in syndrome is caused by damage to specific portions of the lower brain and brainstem with no damage to the upper brain. Most locked-in syndrome patients can communicate through movements and blinking of their eyes, which are not affected by the paralysis. Some patients may have the ability to move certain facial muscles as well. The majority of locked-in syndrome patients do not regain motor control, but several devices are available to help patients communicate.

With the development over the last half-century of assistive devices that can artificially maintain blood flow and breathing, the term *brain death* has come into use. Brain death is the lack of measurable brain function due to diffuse damage to the cerebral hemispheres and the brainstem, with loss of any integrated activity among distinct areas of the brain. Brain death is irreversible. Removal of assistive devices will result in immediate cardiac arrest and cessation of breathing.

Advances in imaging and other technologies have led to devices that help differentiate among the variety of unconscious states. For example, an imaging test that shows activity in the brainstem but little or no activity in the upper brain would lead a physician to a diagnosis of vegetative state and exclude diagnoses of brain death and locked-in syndrome. On the other hand, an imaging test that shows activity in the upper brain with little activity in the brainstem would confirm a diagnosis of locked-in syndrome, while invalidating a diagnosis of brain death or vegetative state. The use of CT and MRI is standard in TBI treatment, but other imaging and diagnostic techniques that may be used to confirm a particular diagnosis include cerebral angiography, electroencephalography (EEG), transcranial Doppler ultrasound, and single photon emission computed tomography (SPECT).

What Immediate Post-Injury Complications Can Occur from a TBI?

Sometimes, health complications occur in the period immediately following a TBI. These complications are not types of TBI, but are distinct medical problems that arise as a result of the injury. Although complications are rare, the risk increases with the severity of the trauma. Complications of TBI include immediate seizures, hydrocephalus or post-traumatic ventricular enlargement, CSF leaks, infections, vascular injuries, cranial nerve injuries, pain, bed sores, multiple organ system failure in unconscious patients, and polytrauma (trauma to other parts of the body in addition to the brain).

About 25 percent of patients with brain contusions or hematomas and about 50 percent of patients with penetrating head injuries will develop immediate seizures, seizures that occur within the first twenty-four hours of the injury. These immediate seizures increase the risk of early seizures—defined as seizures occurring within one week after injury—but do not seem to be linked to the development of post-traumatic epilepsy (recurrent seizures occurring more than one week after the initial trauma). Generally, medical professionals use anticonvulsant medications to treat seizures in TBI patients only if the seizures persist.

Hydrocephalus or post-traumatic ventricular enlargement occurs when CSF accumulates in the brain, resulting in dilation of the cerebral ventricles (cavities in the brain filled with CSF) and an increase in ICP. This condition can develop during the acute stage of TBI or may not appear until later. Generally it occurs within the first year of the injury and is characterized by worsening neurological outcome, impaired consciousness, behavioral changes, ataxia (lack of coordination or balance), incontinence, or signs of elevated ICP. The condition may develop as a result of meningitis, subarachnoid hemorrhage, intracranial hematoma, or other injuries. Treatment includes shunting and draining of CSF as well as any other appropriate treatment for the root cause of the condition.

Skull fractures can tear the membranes that cover the brain, leading to CSF leaks. A tear between the dura and the arachnoid membranes, called a CSF fistula, can cause CSF to leak out of the subarachnoid space into the subdural space; this is called a subdural hygroma. CSF can also leak from the nose and the ear. These tears that let CSF out of the brain cavity can also allow air and bacteria into the cavity, possibly causing infections such as meningitis. Pneumocephalus occurs when air enters the intracranial cavity and becomes trapped in the subarachnoid space.

Infections within the intracranial cavity are a dangerous complication of TBI. They may occur outside of the dura, below the dura, below the arachnoid (meningitis), or within the space of the brain itself (abscess). Most of these injuries develop within a few weeks of the initial trauma and result from skull fractures or penetrating injuries. Standard treatment involves antibiotics and sometimes surgery to remove the infected tissue. Meningitis may be especially dangerous, with the potential to spread to the rest of the brain and nervous system.

Any damage to the head or brain usually results in some damage to the vascular system, which provides blood to the cells of the brain. The body's immune system can repair damage to small blood vessels, but damage to larger vessels can result in serious complications. Damage to one of the major arteries leading to the brain can cause a stroke, either through bleeding from the artery (hemorrhagic stroke) or through the formation of a clot at the site of injury, called a thrombus or thrombosis, blocking blood flow to the brain (ischemic stroke). Blood clots also can develop in other parts of the head. Symptoms such as headache, vomiting, seizures, paralysis on one side of the body, and semiconsciousness developing within several days of a head injury may be caused by a blood clot that forms in the tissue of one of the sinuses, or cavities, adjacent to the brain. Thrombotic-ischemic strokes are treated with anticoagulants, while surgery is the preferred treatment for hemorrhagic stroke. Other types of vascular injuries include vasospasm and the formation of aneurysms.

Skull fractures, especially at the base of the skull, can cause cranial nerve injuries that result in compressive cranial neuropathies. All but three of the twelve cranial nerves project out from the brainstem to the head and face. The seventh cranial nerve, called the facial nerve, is the most commonly injured cranial nerve in TBI and damage to it can result in paralysis of facial muscles.

Pain is a common symptom of TBI and can be a significant complication for conscious patients in the period immediately following a TBI. Headache is the most common form of pain experienced by TBI patients, but other forms of pain can also be problematic. Serious complications for patients who are unconscious, in a coma, or in a vegetative state include bed or pressure sores of the skin, recurrent bladder infections, pneumonia or other life-threatening infections, and progressive multiple organ failure.

General Trauma

Most TBI patients have injuries to other parts of the body in addition to the head and brain. Physicians call this polytrauma. These injuries require immediate and specialized care and can complicate treatment of and recovery from the TBI. Other medical complications that may accompany a TBI include pulmonary (lung) dysfunction; cardiovascular (heart) dysfunction from blunt chest trauma; gastrointestinal dysfunction; fluid and hormonal imbalances; and other isolated complications, such as fractures, nerve injuries, deep vein thrombosis, excessive blood clotting, and infections.

Trauma victims often develop hypermetabolism or an increased metabolic rate, which leads to an increase in the amount of heat the body produces. The body redirects into heat the energy needed to keep organ systems functioning, causing muscle wasting and the starvation of other tissues. Complications related to pulmonary dysfunction can include neurogenic pulmonary edema (excess fluid in lung tissue), aspiration pneumonia (pneumonia caused by foreign matter in the lungs), and fat and blood clots in the blood vessels of the lungs.

Fluid and hormonal imbalances can complicate the treatment of hypermetabolism and high ICP. Hormonal problems can result from dysfunction of the pituitary, the thyroid, and other glands throughout the body. Two common hormonal complications of TBI are syndrome of inappropriate secretion of antidiuretic hormone (SIADH) and hypothyroidism.

Blunt trauma to the chest can also cause cardiovascular problems, including damage to blood vessels and internal bleeding, and problems with heart rate and blood flow. Blunt trauma to the abdomen can cause damage to or dysfunction of the stomach, large or small intestines, and pancreas. A serious and common complication of TBI is erosive gastritis, or inflammation and degeneration of stomach tissue. This syndrome can cause bacterial growth in the stomach, increasing the risk of aspiration pneumonia. Standard care of TBI patients includes administration of prophylactic gastric acid inhibitors to prevent the buildup of stomach acids and bacteria.

What Disabilities Can Result from a TBI?

Disabilities resulting from a TBI depend upon the severity of the injury, the location of the injury, and the age and general health of the patient. Some common disabilities include problems with cognition (thinking, memory, and reasoning), sensory processing (sight, hearing, touch, taste, and smell), communication (expression and understanding), and behavior or mental health (depression, anxiety, personality changes, aggression, acting out, and social inappropriateness).

Within days to weeks of the head injury approximately 40 percent of TBI patients develop a host of troubling symptoms collectively called postconcussion syndrome (PCS). A patient need not have suffered a concussion or loss of consciousness to develop the syndrome, and many patients with mild TBI suffer from PCS. Symptoms include headache, dizziness, vertigo (a sensation of spinning around or of objects spinning around the patient), memory problems, trouble concentrating, sleeping problems, restlessness, irritability, apathy, depression, and anxiety. These symptoms may last for a few weeks after the head injury. The syndrome is more prevalent in patients who had psychiatric symptoms, such as depression or anxiety, before the injury. Treatment for PCS may include medicines for pain and psychiatric conditions, and psychotherapy and occupational therapy to develop coping skills.

Cognition is a term used to describe the processes of thinking, reasoning, problem solving, information processing, and memory. Most patients with severe TBI, if they recover consciousness, suffer from cognitive disabilities, including the loss of many higher level mental skills. The most common cognitive impairment among severely head-injured patients is memory loss, characterized by some loss of specific memories and the partial inability to form or store new ones. Some of these patients may experience post-traumatic amnesia (PTA), either anterograde or retrograde. Anterograde PTA is impaired memory of events that happened after the TBI, while retrograde PTA is impaired memory of events that happened before the TBI.

Many patients with mild to moderate head injuries who experience cognitive deficits become easily confused or distracted and have problems with concentration and attention. They also have problems with higher level, so-called executive functions, such as planning, organizing, abstract reasoning, problem solving, and making judgments, which may make it difficult to resume pre-injury work-related activities. Recovery from cognitive deficits is greatest within the first six months after the injury and more gradual after that.

Patients with moderate to severe TBI have more problems with cognitive deficits than patients with mild TBI, but a history of several mild TBIs may have an additive effect, causing cognitive deficits equal to a moderate or severe injury.

Many TBI patients have sensory problems, especially problems with vision. Patients may not be able to register what they are seeing or may be slow to recognize objects. Also, TBI patients often have difficulty with hand-eye coordination. Because of this, TBI patients may be prone to bumping into or dropping objects, or may seem generally unsteady. TBI patients may have difficulty driving a car, working complex machinery, or playing sports. Other sensory deficits may include problems with hearing, smell, taste, or touch. Some TBI patients develop tinnitus, a ringing or roaring in the ears. A person with damage to the part of the brain that processes taste or smell may develop a persistent bitter taste in the mouth or perceive a persistent noxious smell. Damage to the part of the brain that controls the sense of touch may cause a TBI patient to develop persistent skin tingling, itching, or pain. Although rare, these conditions are hard to treat.

Language and communication problems are common disabilities in TBI patients. Some may experience aphasia, defined as difficulty with understanding and producing spoken and written language; others may have difficulty with the more subtle aspects of communication, such as body language and emotional, nonverbal signals.

In nonfluent aphasia, also called Broca's aphasia or motor aphasia, TBI patients often have trouble recalling words and speaking in complete sentences. They may speak in broken phrases and pause frequently. Most patients are aware of these deficits and may become extremely frustrated. Patients with fluent aphasia, also called Wernicke's aphasia or sensory aphasia, display little meaning in their speech, even though they speak in complete sentences and use correct grammar. Instead, they speak in flowing gibberish, drawing out their sentences with nonessential and invented words. Many patients with fluent aphasia are unaware that they make little sense and become angry with others for not understanding them. Patients with global aphasia have extensive damage to the portions of the brain responsible for language and often suffer severe communication disabilities.

TBI patients may have problems with spoken language if the part of the brain that controls speech muscles is damaged. In this disorder, called dysarthria, the patient can think of the appropriate language, but cannot easily speak the words because they are unable to use the muscles needed to form the words and produce the sounds. Speech is often slow, slurred, and garbled. Some may have problems with intonation or inflection, called prosodic dysfunction. An important aspect of speech, inflection conveys emotional meaning and is necessary for certain aspects of language, such as irony.

These language deficits can lead to miscommunication, confusion, and frustration for the patient as well as those interacting with him or her.

Most TBI patients have emotional or behavioral problems that fit under the broad category of psychiatric health. Family members of TBI patients often find that personality changes and behavioral problems are the most difficult disabilities to handle. Psychiatric problems that may surface include depression, apathy, anxiety, irritability, anger, paranoia, confusion, frustration, agitation, insomnia or other sleep problems, and mood swings. Problem behaviors may include aggression and violence, impulsivity, disinhibition, acting out, noncompliance, social inappropriateness, emotional outbursts, childish behavior, impaired self-control, impaired self-awareness, inability to take responsibility or accept criticism, egocentrism, inappropriate sexual activity, and alcohol or drug abuse or addiction. Some patients' personality problems may be so severe that they are diagnosed with borderline personality disorder, a psychiatric condition characterized by many of the problems mentioned previously. Sometimes TBI patients suffer from developmental stagnation, meaning that they fail to mature emotionally, socially, or psychologically after the trauma. This is a serious problem for children and young adults who suffer from a TBI. Attitudes and behaviors that are appropriate for a child or teenager become inappropriate in adulthood. Many TBI patients who show psychiatric or behavioral problems can be helped with medication and psychotherapy.

Are There Other Long-Term Problems Associated with a TBI?

In addition to the immediate post-injury complications discussed previously, other long-term problems can develop after a TBI. These include Parkinson disease and other motor problems, Alzheimer's disease, dementia pugilistica, and post-traumatic dementia.

Alzheimer's disease (AD): AD is a progressive, neurodegenerative disease characterized by dementia, memory loss, and deteriorating cognitive abilities. Recent research suggests an association between head injury in early adulthood and the development of AD later in life; the more severe the head injury, the greater the risk of developing AD. Some evidence indicates that a head injury may interact with other factors to trigger the disease and may hasten the onset of the disease in individuals already at risk. For example, people who have a particular form of the protein apolipoprotein E (apoE4) and suffer a head injury fall into this increased risk category. (ApoE4 is a naturally occurring protein that helps transport cholesterol through the bloodstream.)

Parkinson disease and other motor problems: Movement disorders as a result of TBI are rare but can occur. Parkinson disease may develop years after TBI as a result of damage to the basal ganglia. Symptoms of Parkinson disease include tremor or trembling, rigidity or stiffness, slow movement (bradykinesia), inability to move (akinesia), shuffling walk, and stooped posture. Despite many scientific advances in recent years, Parkinson disease remains a chronic and progressive disorder, meaning that it is incurable and will progress in severity until the end of life. Other movement disorders that may develop after TBI include tremor, ataxia (uncoordinated muscle movements), and myoclonus (shock-like contractions of muscles).

Dementia pugilistica: Also called chronic traumatic encephalopathy, dementia pugilistica primarily affects career boxers. The most common symptoms of the condition are dementia and parkinsonism caused by repetitive blows to the head over a long period of time. Symptoms begin anywhere between six and forty years after the start of a boxing career, with an average onset of about sixteen years.

Post-traumatic dementia: The symptoms of post-traumatic dementia are very similar to those of dementia pugilistica, except that post-traumatic dementia is also characterized by long-term memory problems and is caused by a single, severe TBI that results in a coma.

What Kinds of Rehabilitation Should a TBI Patient Receive?

Rehabilitation is an important part of the recovery process for a TBI patient. During the acute stage, moderately to severely injured patients may receive treatment and care in an intensive care unit of a hospital. Once stable, the patient may be transferred to a subacute unit of the medical center or to an independent rehabilitation hospital. At this point, patients follow many diverse paths toward recovery because there are a wide variety of options for rehabilitation.

In 1998, the NIH held a Consensus Development Conference on Rehabilitation of Persons with Traumatic Brain Injury. The Consensus Development Panel recommended that TBI patients receive an individualized rehabilitation program based upon the patient's strengths and capacities and that rehabilitation services should be modified over time to adapt to the patient's changing needs. (National Institutes of Health Consensus Development Conference Statement, October 26–28, 1998. Rehabilitation of Persons with Traumatic Brain Injury. Bethesda, Maryland, September 1999.) The panel also recommended that moderately to severely injured patients receive rehabilitation treatment that draws on the skills of many specialists. This involves individually tailored treatment programs in the areas of physical therapy, occupational therapy, speech and language therapy, physiatry (physical medicine), psychology and psychiatry, and social support. Medical personnel who provide this care include rehabilitation specialists, such as rehabilitation nurses, psychologists, speech and language pathologists, physical and occupational therapists, physiatrists (physical medicine specialists), social workers, and a team coordinator or administrator.

The overall goal of rehabilitation after a TBI is to improve the patient's ability to function at home and in society. Therapists help the patient adapt to disabilities or change the patient's living space, called environmental modification, to make everyday activities easier.

Some patients may need medication for psychiatric and physical problems resulting from the TBI. Great care must be taken in prescribing medications because TBI patients are more susceptible to side effects and may react adversely to some pharmacological agents. It is important for the family to provide social support for the patient by being involved in the rehabilitation program. Family members may also benefit from psychotherapy.

It is important for TBI patients and their families to select the most appropriate setting for rehabilitation. There are several options, including home-based rehabilitation, hospital outpatient rehabilitation, inpatient rehabilitation centers, comprehensive day programs at rehabilitation centers, supportive living programs, independent living centers, clubhouse programs, school-based programs for children, and others. The TBI patient, the family, and the rehabilitation team members should work together to find the best place for the patient to recover.

How Can TBI Be Prevented?

Unlike most neurological disorders, head injuries can be prevented. The Centers for Disease Control and Prevention (CDC) have issued the following safety tips for reducing the risk of suffering a TBI.

- Wear a seatbelt every time you drive or ride in a car.
- Buckle your child into a child safety seat, booster seat, or seatbelt (depending on the child's age) every time the child rides in a car.
- Wear a helmet and make sure your children wear helmets when
  - riding a bike or motorcycle;
  - playing a contact sport such as football or ice hockey;
  - using in-line skates or riding a skateboard;
  - batting and running bases in baseball or softball;
  - riding a horse;
  - skiing or snowboarding.
- Keep firearms and bullets stored in a locked cabinet when not in use.
- Avoid falls by
  - using a step-stool with a grab bar to reach objects on high shelves;
  - installing handrails on stairways;

- installing window guards to keep young children from falling out of open windows;
- using safety gates at the top and bottom of stairs when young children are around.

- Make sure the surface on your child's playground is made of shock-absorbing material (e.g., hardwood mulch, sand).

What Research Is the NINDS Conducting?

The National Institute of Neurological Disorders and Stroke (NINDS) conducts and supports research to better understand CNS injury and the biological mechanisms underlying damage to the brain, to develop strategies and interventions to limit the primary and secondary brain damage that occurs within days of a head trauma, and to devise therapies to treat brain injury and help in long-term recovery of function.

On a microscopic scale, the brain is made up of billions of cells that interconnect and communicate. The neuron is the main functional cell of the brain and nervous system, consisting of a cell body (soma), a tail or long nerve fiber (axon), and projections of the cell body called dendrites. The axons travel in tracts or clusters throughout the brain, providing extensive interconnections between brain areas.

One of the most pervasive types of injury following even a minor trauma is damage to the nerve cell's axon through shearing; this is referred to as diffuse axonal injury. This damage causes a series of reactions that eventually lead to swelling of the axon and disconnection from the cell body of the neuron. In addition, the part of the neuron that communicates with other neurons degenerates and releases toxic levels of chemical messengers called neurotransmitters into the synapse or space between neurons, damaging neighboring neurons through a secondary neuroexcitatory cascade. Therefore, neurons that were unharmed by the primary trauma suffer damage from this secondary insult. Many of these cells cannot survive the toxicity of the chemical onslaught and initiate programmed cell death, or apoptosis. This process usually takes place within the first twenty-four to forty-eight hours after the initial injury, but can be prolonged.

One area of research that shows promise is the study of the role of calcium ion influx into the damaged neuron as a cause of cell death and general brain tissue swelling. Calcium enters nerve cells through damaged channels in the axon's membrane. The excess calcium inside the cell causes the axon to swell and also activates chemicals, called proteases, that break down proteins. One family of proteases, the calpains, are especially damaging to nerve cells because they break down proteins that maintain the structure of the axon. Excess calcium within the cell is also destructive to the cell's mitochondria, structures that produce the cell's energy. Mitochondria soak up excess calcium until they swell and stop functioning. If enough mitochondria are damaged, the nerve cell degenerates. Calcium influx has other damaging effects: it activates destructive enzymes, such as caspases that damage the DNA in the cell and trigger programmed cell death, and it damages sodium channels in the cell membrane, allowing sodium ions to flood the cell as well. Sodium influx exacerbates swelling of the cell body and axon.

NINDS researchers have shown, in both cell and animal studies, that giving specialized chemicals can reduce cell death caused by calcium ion influx. Other researchers have shown that the use of cyclosporin A, which blocks mitochondrial membrane permeability, protects axons from calcium influx. Another avenue of therapeutic intervention is the use of hypothermia (an induced state of low body temperature) to slow the progression of cell death and axon swelling.

In the healthy brain, the chemical glutamate functions as a neurotransmitter, but an excess amount of glutamate in the brain causes neurons to quickly overload from too much excitation, releasing toxic chemicals. These substances poison the chemical environment of surrounding cells, initiating degeneration and programmed cell death. Studies have shown that a group of enzymes called matrix metalloproteinases contribute to the toxicity by breaking down proteins that maintain the structure and order of the extracellular environment. Other research shows that glutamate reacts with calcium and sodium ion channels on the cell membrane, leading to an influx of calcium and sodium ions into the cell. Investigators are looking for ways to decrease the toxic effects of glutamate and other excitatory neurotransmitters.

The brain attempts to repair itself after a trauma, and is more successful after mild to moderate injury than after severe injury. Scientists have shown that after diffuse axonal injury neurons can spontaneously adapt and recover by sprouting some of the remaining healthy fibers of the neuron into the spaces once occupied by the degenerated axon. These fibers can develop in such a way that the neuron can resume communication with neighboring neurons. This is a very delicate process and can be disrupted by any of a number of factors, such as neuroexcitation, hypoxia (low oxygen levels), and hypotension (low blood flow). Following trauma, excessive neuroexcitation, that is, the electrical activation of nerve cells or fibers, especially disrupts this natural recovery process and can cause sprouting fibers to lose direction and connect with the wrong terminals.

Scientists suspect that these misconnections may contribute to some long-term disabilities, such as pain, spasticity, seizures, and memory problems. NINDS researchers are trying to learn more about the brain's natural recovery process and what factors or triggers control it. They hope that through manipulation of these triggers they can increase repair while decreasing misconnections.

NINDS investigators are also looking at larger, tissue-specific changes within the brain after a TBI. Researchers have shown that trauma to the frontal lobes of the brain can damage specific chemical messenger systems, specifically the dopaminergic system, the collection of neurons in the brain that uses the neurotransmitter dopamine. Dopamine is an important chemical messenger—for example, degeneration of dopamine-producing neurons is the primary cause of Parkinson disease. NINDS researchers are studying how the dopaminergic system responds after a TBI and its relationship to neurodegeneration and Parkinson disease.

The use of stem cells to repair or replace damaged brain tissue is a new and exciting avenue of research. A neural stem cell is a special kind of cell that can multiply and give rise to other more specialized cell types. These cells are found in adult neural tissue and normally develop into several different cell types found within the central nervous system. NINDS researchers are investigating the ability of stem cells to develop into neurotransmitter-producing neurons, specifically dopamine-producing cells. Researchers are also looking at the power of stem cells to develop into oligodendrocytes, a type of brain cell that produces myelin, the fatty sheath that surrounds and insulates axons. One study in mice has shown that bone marrow stem cells can develop into neurons, demonstrating that neural stem cells are not the only type of stem cell that could be beneficial in the treatment of brain and nervous system disorders. At the moment, stem cell research for TBI is in its infancy, but future research may lead to advances for treatment and rehabilitation.

In addition to the basic research described here, NINDS scientists also conduct broader based clinical research involving patients. One area of study focuses on the plasticity of the brain after injury. In the strictest sense, plasticity means the ability to be formed or molded. When speaking of the brain, plasticity means the ability of the brain to adapt to deficits and injury. NINDS researchers are investigating the extent of brain plasticity after injury and developing therapies to enhance plasticity as a means of restoring function.

The plasticity of the brain and the rewiring of neural connections make it possible for one part of the brain to take up the functions of a disabled part. Scientists have long known that the immature brain is generally more plastic than the mature brain, and that the brains of children are better able to adapt and recover from injury than the brains of adults. NINDS researchers are investigating the mechanisms underlying this difference and theorize that children have an overabundance of hard-wired neural networks, many of which naturally decrease through a process called pruning. When an injury destroys an important neural network in children, another less useful neural network that would have eventually died takes over the responsibilities of the damaged network. Some researchers are looking at the role of plasticity in memory, while others are using imaging technologies, such as functional MRI, to map regions of the brain and record evidence of plasticity.

Another important area of research involves the development of improved rehabilitation programs for those who have disabilities from a TBI. The Congressional Children's Health Act of 2000 authorized the NINDS to conduct and support research related to TBI with the goal of designing therapies to restore normal functioning in cognition and behavior.

Clinical Trials Research

The NINDS works to develop treatments that can be given in the first hours after a TBI, hoping that quick action can prevent or reverse much of the brain damage resulting from the injury. A recently completed NINDS-supported clinical trial involved lowering body temperature in TBI patients to 33 degrees Celsius within eight hours of the trauma. Although the investigators found that the treatment did not improve outcome overall, they did learn that patients younger than forty-five years who were admitted to the hospital already in a hypothermic state fared better if they were kept cool than if they were brought to normal body temperature. Other ongoing clinical trials include the use of hypothermia for severe TBI in children, the use of magnesium sulfate to protect nerve cells after TBI, and the effects of lowering ICP and increasing cerebral blood flow.

Section 11.2

Concussion

Reprinted with permission from "Concussion," www.muhealth.org/~neuro medicine/concussion.shtml by D. M. Mueller, M.D., and J. J. Oro, M.D., Division of Neurosurgery, University of Missouri Health Care, Columbia, Missouri. Copyright © 2004 University of Missouri-Columbia.

The brain is composed of soft, delicate structures that lie within the rigid skull. Surrounding the brain is a tough, leathery outer covering called the dura. Within the brain are (cranial) nerves that are responsible for many activities, such as eye opening, facial movements, speech, and hearing. These nerves carry and receive messages that allow the person to think and function normally. There are also centers that control level of consciousness and vital activities, such as breathing. The brain is cushioned by blood and spinal fluid. There is very little extra room within the skull cavity.

An injury to the head causes the brain to bounce against the rigid bone of the skull. This force may cause a tearing or twisting of the structures and blood vessels of the brain, which results in a breakdown of the normal flow of messages within the brain. The damage to the brain generally is found deep within the brain tissue. Because of this damage, the normal function of the brain signals is interrupted.

Concussion Categories

- **Grade 1:** The mild concussion occurs when the person does not lose consciousness (pass out) but may seem dazed.

- **Grade 2:** The slightly more severe form occurs when the person does not lose consciousness but has a period of confusion and does not recall the event.

- **Grade 3:** The classic concussion, which is the most severe form, occurs when the person loses consciousness for a brief period of time and has no memory of the event. Evaluation from a health care provider should be performed as soon as possible after the injury.

A concussion can happen to anyone, at any time. The most common causes of concussion include a blow to the head from a motor vehicle crash, fall, or assault. People at higher risk are those who have difficulty walking and fall often, those who are active in high-impact contact sports, and those who are taking blood thinners, such as Coumadin. Mild head injury, such as concussion, is a frequent cause for hospital admission, with an estimate of more than six hundred thousand cases per year in the United States.

Signs and Symptoms

The signs and symptoms of a concussion include severe headache, dizziness, vomiting, increased size of one pupil, or sudden weakness in an arm or leg. The person may seem restless, agitated, or irritable. Often, the person may have memory loss or seem forgetful. These symptoms may last for several hours to weeks, depending on the seriousness of the injury. Any period of loss of consciousness or amnesia due to the head injury should be evaluated by a health care professional. As the brain tissue swells, the person may feel increasingly drowsy or confused. If the person is difficult to awaken or passes out, medical attention should be sought immediately. This could be a sign of a more severe injury.

Diagnostic Tests

If your health care provider suspects a concussion, the following tests may be ordered.

- **CT scan:** This is a special x-ray image of the brain. The test is performed by having the patient lie on a flat x-ray table that slides into a round, open scanner. The x-ray images are taken as the patient is lying still on the x-ray table. Often, this test involves the injection of a contrast dye to obtain better images of the brain structures (be sure to tell the technician if the person is allergic to contrast dye).

- **MRI (magnetic resonance imaging):** This is a special non-x-ray image of the brain to examine the structures. No x-rays are used in this test. The test is performed by having the patient lie still while in the scanner, as the pictures are very sensitive to any movement. There is a machine-like sound while the pictures are being taken. The space inside the tube is quite snug; therefore be sure to notify the technician if the person has claustrophobia or is uncomfortable in tight places. Because this test is performed with a special high-power magnet, it may not be performed on anyone with a metal implant (i.e. artificial limbs, artificial joints, aneurysm clips, shrapnel, or metal heart valves).

Treatment

The treatment for a concussion is usually to watch the person closely for any change in level of consciousness. The person may need to stay in the hospital for close observation. Surgery is usually not necessary. Headache and dizziness are common, but if the headache persists or becomes severe, it is best to seek medical attention.

Post-concussion syndrome may occur in some people. The syndrome generally consists of a persistent headache, dizziness, irritability, memory changes, and vision changes. The person may seem overly emotional or unable to control his or her emotions. Some people experience unexplained depression. Difficulty with concentration or problems with thinking and planning ahead also are reported. Symptoms may begin weeks or even months after the initial injury. Although the symptoms generally resolve over time, some people need a rehabilitation specialist to oversee a program for recovery.

It is important to keep in mind that recovery from a traumatic brain injury can be very slow. Sometimes several days can go by without seeing any major visible change. This is not unusual, and it is best to ask the health care providers if any changes have occurred. It is also important to try to get enough rest and nutrition while waiting for the patient to recover. It is normal to feel frustrated, overwhelmed, lonely, and worried. Sometimes a friend or support group can help. Before your stress gets out of control, tell someone who can help.

Section 11.3

Coma

Severe Brain Injury and Coma

Severe brain injury occurs when a prolonged unconscious state or coma lasts days, weeks, or months. Severe brain injury is further categorized into subgroups with separate features. These subgroups of Severe Brain Injury are discussed in the following:

- Coma
- Vegetative State
- Persistent Vegetative State
- Minimally Responsive State
- Akinetic Mutism
- Locked-In Syndrome

Coma

When people experience a brain injury, they can become unconscious. When the unconscious state is prolonged, it is termed a "coma." Coma is defined as a state of unconsciousness from which the individual cannot be awakened, in which the individual responds minimally or not at all to stimuli, and initiates no voluntary activities.

- A coma is a continued unconscious state that can occur as part of the natural recovery for a person who has experienced a severe brain injury.

- While in a coma, a person can continue to heal and progress through different states of consciousness.

- Persons who sustain a severe brain injury and experience coma can make significant improvements, but are often left with permanent physical, cognitive, or behavioral impairments.

- A coma can last days, weeks, months, or indefinitely. The length of a coma cannot be accurately predicted or known.

- Physicians may not be able to state how long a person will be in a coma or what the person will be like when he or she comes out of the coma. There is no "treatment" physicians can use to "make" a person "come out of" a coma. Likewise, there is no test physicians can use to "predict" when a person will come out of a coma or what a person's recovery will be like.

- If the person with a brain injury remains in what seems like a comatose state, and there is no clear cut reason for this, it is imperative to get a good evaluation! The evaluation is to differentiate someone who is truly not responding at all to the environment, and someone who is responding in some manner.

Department of Defense and Veteran's Head Injury Program & Brain Injury Association of America (1999).

Appearance

- Persons in a coma may appear to be "asleep" because they cannot be awakened or alerted.

- While in a deep coma, a person may not move at all, even in response to painful stimuli. The person may be unable to produce any voluntary actions or meaningful responses.

- Persons in a coma can show various levels of nonpurposeful movements. The person may respond minimally or not at all to stimuli.

- A person in a coma will not be able to talk to you.

Talk to the person in your regular tone of voice with the assumption that the person can understand what you are saying and discussing while the he or she is nearby. Some people who have emerged from a coma report remembering the conversations of others.

Department of Defense and Veteran's Head Injury Program & Brain Injury Association of America (1999).

Vegetative State (VS)

Vegetative state (VS) describes a severe brain injury in which:

- Arousal is present, but the ability to interact with the environment is not.

- Eye opening can be spontaneous or in response to stimulation
- General responses to pain exist, such as increased heart rate, increased respiration, posturing, or sweating
- Sleep-wakes cycles, respiratory functions, and digestive functions return.

There is no test to specifically diagnose vegetative state; the diagnosis is made only by repetitive neurobehavioral assessments.

Giacino, J. & Zasler, N. (1995). Outcome after severe traumatic brain injury: Coma, the vegetative state, and the minimally responsive state. *Journal of Head Trauma Rehabilitation* 10: 40–56.

Persistent Vegetative State (PVS)

Persistent vegetative state (PVS) is a term used for a vegetative state that has lasted for more than a month.

- The criteria is the same as for vegetative state.

The use of this term is considered controversial because it implies a prognosis.

Giacino, J. & Zasler, N. (1995). Outcome after severe traumatic brain injury: Coma, the vegetative state, and the minimally responsive state. *Journal of Head Trauma Rehabilitation* 10: 40–56.

Minimally Responsive State (MR)

Minimally responsive state (MR) is the term used for a severe traumatic brain injury in which a person is no longer in a coma or a vegetative state. Persons in a minimally responsive state demonstrate:

- Primitive reflexes
- Inconsistent ability to follow simple commands
- An awareness of environmental stimulation

The frequency and the conditions in which a response was made are considered when assessing the meaningfulness or purposefulness of a behavior.

Giacino, J. & Zasler, N. (1995). Outcome after severe traumatic brain injury: Coma, the vegetative state, and the minimally responsive state. *Journal of Head Trauma Rehabilitation* 10: 40–56.

Akinetic Mutism

Akinetic mutism is a neurobehavioral condition that results when the dopaminergic pathways in the brain are damaged. Damage to these pathways results in:

- Minimal amount of body movement
- Little or no spontaneous speech
- Speech that can be elicited (For example, the person can answer a question if asked, but otherwise does not voluntarily start saying anything).
- Eye opening and visual tracking
- Infrequent and incomplete ability to follow commands
- Vigilance and agitation for frontal akinetic mutism

Akinetic mutism is different from the minimally responsive state because the lack of movement and speech with akinetic mutism is not because of neuromuscular disturbance.

Giacino, J. & Zasler, N. (1995). Outcome after severe traumatic brain injury: Coma, the vegetative state, and the minimally responsive state. *Journal of Head Trauma Rehabilitation* 10: 40–56.

Locked-In Syndrome

Locked-in syndrome is a rare neurological condition in which a person cannot physically move any part of the body except the eyes. The person is conscious and able to think.

- Vertical eye movements and eye blinking can be used to communicate with others and operate environmental controls.

Brain Death

Brain death can result from a very severe injury to the brain. When brain death occurs, the brain shows no sign of functioning. The physician performs a specific formal brain death examination.

Treatment in the Intensive Care Unit (ICU)

After receiving emergency medical treatment, persons with severe brain injury and coma may be admitted to a hospital's inpatient intensive care unit. The goals in the intensive care unit include achieving medical stability, medical management, and prevention of medical crisis.

- Medications may be used to decrease brain swelling, treat infections, and prevent seizures. If a person's intracranial pressure is very high or difficult to control, medication may be used to put the person into a medication-induced coma to prevent more swelling.

- Some preventive rehabilitation may be initiated in the intensive care unit such as body positioning, splinting, and range of motion (a therapist moves the person's body limbs).

- Sometimes surgery may be necessary to remove blood clots and pressure.

- To provide life-sustaining medical care, the healthcare staff may have many tubes, wires, and pieces of medical equipment attached to the person with a brain injury.

Possible Medical Equipment in the Intensive Care Unit (ICU)

A ventilator (also called a respirator) is a machine that helps a person breathe.

- A person who has sustained a brain injury may be unable to breathe on his or her own.

- To use a ventilator, a tube is placed through the person's mouth to the breathing passage, (trachea, "windpipe"). This procedure is called intubation.

- Intubation with the use of a ventilator allows a person to breathe and receive oxygen, which is necessary for life.

A tracheotomy (trach) is a tube placed in a person's windpipe to help him or her breathe. A trach may be used if a person has a lot of secretions in the lungs that need to be suctioned, or if he or she is on a ventilator for a long time.

Intravenous lines (IVs) are tubes placed in a person's veins to deliver medications and fluids to the person's body.

Arterial lines are tubes placed in a person's arteries to measure blood pressure.

A Foley catheter is used to collect and monitor a person's urine output.

- A person who has sustained a brain injury may be unable to control bladder functions.

- A rubber tube is inserted into the person's bladder. This allows urine to move from the bladder, through the tube, and to a container at the end of the tube.

A nasogastric tube (NG Tube) is used to deliver medication and nutrients directly to a person's stomach.

- A person who has sustained a brain injury may be unable to swallow.

- A tube is placed through a person's nose or mouth and ran through the swallowing passage (the esophagus), to the stomach.

An EKG machine monitors a person's heart.

- Wires with sticky ends are placed on the body.

An intracranial pressure (ICP) monitor is a device that indicates the amount of pressure in the brain. The device is placed in or on top of the brain through a small hole in the skull.

- As the brain swells, the skull does not also swell; therefore, the brain has limited room to expand in. Swollen brain tissues can compress, causing further injury or death.

- Intracranial pressure is taken to assess a person's condition and to provide information for treatment.

- Intracranial pressure is taken by placing a monitor in or on a person's brain through a small hole in the skull.

A ventricular drain (ventriculostomy) is a small tube placed in the brain that drains cerebral spinal fluid into a drainage bag. It is used as to measure pressure changes and drain fluid from the brain.

A pulse oximeter is a small clamplike device placed on a person's finger, toe, or earlobe. The pulse oximeter measures the amount of oxygen in the bloodstream.

Anti-embolism stockings (TED hose) are worn on the person's legs to help prevent embolisms (blood clots) from forming and to assist in circulation of blood and fluids in the legs. The stockings are long (up to the thighs) and made of tight elastic material.

Sequential compression stockings (Kendalls) are worn on the person's legs to help prevent blood pooling. These are plastic leg wraps operated by a machine to inflate and deflate around the person's legs.

Possible Tests and Assessments

As each person is an individual, the tests and assessments selected by the healthcare professionals may differ from person to person. Possible tests and assessments that may be used are described here.

Arterial Blood Gas (ABG)

- This lab tests measures levels of oxygen and carbon dioxide in the blood to determine breathing efficiency.
- A blood sample from an artery is used for this test.

Electrolytes

- This lab test measures levels of electrolytes (sodium, potassium, chloride, bicarbonate, urea nitrogen, and creatine) in the blood to determine how efficiently the body is managing or producing amounts of electrolytes necessary for bodily functions.
- A blood sample from a vein is used for this test.

EEG (Electroencephalogram)

- An EEG detects electrical brain abnormalities, such as seizures.
- Testing involves placing small metal discs, called electrodes, on a person's scalp.

X-ray

- X-rays are a type of picture taken to check the structural integrity of bones and the lungs.
- X-rays are also used to evaluate the placement of tubes, such as feeding tubes, in the stomach.
- To take an x-ray, a camera is focused on the body area to be examined and a picture is taken.

Angiogram

- An angiogram is a type of picture showing the arteries and veins in the head and neck.

- To take an angiogram, x-ray pictures are taken after dye has been placed in the arteries.

CT or CAT Scan (Computed Tomography Scan)

- CT scans are used to view harm to brain structures, the skull, and facial bones.

- CT scans are a good detector of bleeds, blood clots, swelling, or compression in the brain.

- CT scans take pictures of the brain in layers, so they produce images in the form of slices that make up the brain, like the slices that make up a loaf of bread.

- Because some brain injuries may not show up on the first CT scan, a second CT scan may be taken within the first twenty-four hours. Not all types of brain injuries show up on CT scans.

- To take a CT scan, a camera is focused on the body area to be examined and the pictures are taken.

MRI (Magnetic Resonance Imaging)

- A MRI uses an imaging technique to provide a more detailed view of the brain structure than CT scans.

- A MRI is advantageous for examination of the brain stem and cerebellum structure (deep brain structures), since these views can be limited on a CT scan.

- To take an MRI, the MRI equipment is focused on the body part to be imaged.

PET Scan (Positron Emission Tomography)

- A PET Scan is used to detect brain function and metabolism.

- A PET Scan involves the injection of a radioactive solution, which is detected by imaging equipment to produce a cross-sectional picture of the brain.

SPECT Scan (Single Photon Emitting Computerized Tomography)

- A SPECT scan is a sensitive tool to measure brain function and metabolism.

- Blood flow rates to the brain and cellular tissue are assessed.

- A SPECT scan involves the injection of a radioactive substance intravenously. Imaging equipment picks up the radioactive substance. This information creates a 3-D image of the brain.

Neurological Exam

- A neurological exam is performed through interaction and observation to assist in determining the person's neurological functional ability.

- The healthcare professional may ask the person simple questions, such as "What year is it?" or give simple directions such as "Hold up one finger."

Glasgow Coma Scale (GCS)

- The Glasgow Coma Scale is used to determine the severity of a brain injury. It is often used at the emergency scene or emergency room.

- Motor, verbal, and eye responses are solicited and rated.

- A score of 15 is normal or near normal and a score of 3 indicates the worst possible neurological status.

Rancho Los Amigos Scale

- The Rancho Los Amigos Scale is used to determine a level of cognitive functioning.

- Cognitive abilities are categorized from levels 1 to 10, with level 1 being the lowest based on clinical observations and interactions. The original Rancho Los Amigos Scale, with levels from 1 to 8 may still be in use at some facilities.

- This scale may be used repeatedly to monitor a person's progress throughout recovery and rehabilitation.

Section 11.4

Shaken Baby Syndrome

Several years ago, when a young au pair from Great Britain was charged in the death of the eight-month-old Massachusetts boy in her care, the case received phenomenal media coverage both in the United States and abroad. Lawyers for the prosecution and the defense waged a charged battle throughout the trial, trying to assign the blame for Matthew Eappen's death. But when it was all over, the only thing that was clear was that Matthew's case had become one of the most publicized cases of shaken baby/shaken impact syndrome (SBS).

What Is SBS?

SBS is the leading cause of death in child abuse cases in the United States. The syndrome results from injuries caused by someone vigorously shaking an infant, usually for five to twenty seconds, which causes brain damage. In some cases, the shaking is accompanied by a final impact to the baby's head against a bed, chair, or other surface.

Although SBS is occasionally seen in children up to four years old, the vast majority of incidents occur in infants who are younger than one year old; the average age of victims is between three and eight months. Approximately 60 percent of shaken babies are male, and children of families who live at or below the poverty level are at an increased risk for SBS (and any type of child abuse).

How It Happens

When someone forcefully shakes a baby, the child's head rotates about uncontrollably because infants' neck muscles are not well developed and provide little support for the head. The violent movement pitches the infant's brain back and forth within the skull, rupturing blood vessels and nerves throughout the brain and tearing the brain tissue. The brain strikes the inside of the skull, causing bruising and bleeding to the brain. The damage is even greater when the shaking ends with an impact (hitting a wall or a crib mattress, for example), because the forces of acceleration and deceleration associated with an impact are so strong. After the shaking, swelling in the brain can cause enormous pressure within the skull, compressing blood vessels and increasing overall injury to its delicate structure.

Normal interaction with a child, like bouncing the baby on a knee, will not cause SBS, although it is important never to shake a baby under any circumstances because gentle shaking can rapidly escalate. Pediatrician Allan DeJong, M.D., says, "When you shake your baby hard enough to give them these injuries, you know you've crossed the line. This is something violent."

Diagnosing SBS

To diagnose SBS, doctors look for hemorrhages in the retinas of the eyes (which are extremely rare in any accidental injuries, such as falls), skull fractures, swelling of the brain, subdural hematomas (blood collections pressing on the surface of the brain), rib and long bone (bones in the arms and legs) fractures, and bruises around the head, neck, or chest.

SBS often has irreparable consequences. In the worst cases, the death rate is almost half of all babies involved. Children who survive may suffer partial or total blindness, hearing loss, seizures, developmental delays, impaired intellect, speech and learning difficulties, problems with memory and attention, or paralysis (some particularly traumatic episodes leave children in a coma). Severe mental retardation may also result.

Even in milder cases, where the baby looks normal immediately after the shaking, he may eventually develop one or more of these problems. Sometimes the first sign of a problem isn't noticed until the child enters the school system and exhibits behavioral problems or learning difficulties. By that time, however, it is more difficult to link these problems to a shaking incident from several years before.

Effects of SBS

In any SBS case, the duration and force of the shaking, the number of episodes, and whether impact is involved all affect the severity of the infant's injuries. In the most violent cases, children may arrive at the emergency room unconscious, suffering seizures, or in shock. But in many cases, where the infants don't exhibit such severe symptoms, they may never be brought to medical attention.

In milder cases, the infant may seem lethargic or irritable or perhaps will not be feeding well. Unfortunately, unless a doctor has reason to suspect SBS, these cases are often misdiagnosed as a viral illness or colic. "Their brain may have been scrambled [by the shaking], but not to the point of significant brain injury, yet they could have been a shaken baby," Dr. DeJong notes. Lacking a diagnosis of SBS and subsequent intervention, these children may be shaken again, worsening any brain injury or damage.

Besides lethargy, a baby who has been shaken may experience vomiting, poor sucking or swallowing, decreased appetite, lack of smiling or vocalizing, rigidity, seizures, difficulty breathing, altered consciousness, unequal pupil size, an inability to lift his head, or an inability to focus his eyes or track movement.

What makes SBS so devastating is that it usually involves a total brain injury. Because the infant's brain has little stored information and few developed capacities to make up for the deficit, the brain's adaptive abilities are substantially impaired, says Jane Crowley, PsyD, a pediatric rehabilitation psychologist. For example, a child whose vision is severely impaired will not be able to learn through observation, which decreases his overall ability to learn. The development of language, vision, balance, and motor coordination, all of which occur to varying degrees after birth, are particularly likely to be affected in any child who was a victim of SBS.

Such impairment can require rigorous physical and occupational therapy to help the child acquire skills that would have developed on their own had the brain injury not occurred. Therapists do this by providing a sensory-rich environment, which forces the child to be attentive. Therapists often work one on one with a child, concentrating on building his ability to pay attention. Therapists use sound and other stimuli to increase the child's interest in objects, such as repeatedly squeaking a toy near his ear. As he gets older, a child who was shaken as a baby may require special education and continued therapy to help with language development and daily living skills, such as dressing himself.

Your Child's Development and Education

After your child turns three, it is your school district's responsibility to provide additional special educational services. Before age three, your child can receive speech or physical therapy through the Department of Public Health. Federal law requires that each state provide these services for children who have developmental disabilities as a result of being shaken as babies.

Can SBS Be Prevented?

While the consequences of SBS are terrible, it is important to remember that the syndrome is 100 percent preventable. The perpetrators in SBS cases are almost always parents or caregivers, who shake the baby out of frustration when he is crying inconsolably. It is estimated that males, often in their early twenties, usually either the baby's father or the mother's boyfriend, are the perpetrators in 65 percent to 90 percent of cases. Caregivers who shake babies usually do so out of the stress of dealing with a fussy baby. Sadly, the shaking has the desired effect: although at first the baby cries more out of fear, he eventually stops crying as his brain is damaged.

Finding ways to alleviate the caregiver's stress at these critical moments will significantly reduce the risk to the child. If a baby in your care won't stop crying, try the following:

- make sure the baby's basic needs are met (for example, he isn't hungry and doesn't need to be changed)
- check for signs of illness, like fever or swollen gums
- rock or walk with the baby
- sing or talk to him
- offer the baby a pacifier or a noisy toy
- take him for a ride in his stroller or in his car seat in the car
- swaddle the baby snugly in a blanket
- turn on the stereo, run the vacuum cleaner or the clothes dryer, or run water in the tub (babies like rhythmic noise)
- hold the baby close against your body and breathe calmly and slowly
- call a friend or relative for support or to take care of the baby while you take a break
- if nothing else works, put the baby on his back in his crib, close the door, and check on him in ten minutes

Part Three

Epilepsy and Seizure Disorders

Chapter 12

Epilepsy

Chapter Contents

Section 12.1—Seizures and Epilepsy 246
Section 12.2—Epilepsy: Women's Concerns 274
Section 12.3—Epilepsy in the Elderly 287
Section 12.4—Understanding Vagus Nerve Stimulation 293
Section 12.5—Ketogenic Diet 300

Section 12.1

Seizures and Epilepsy

Reprinted from "Seizures and Epilepsy: Hope through Research," National Institute of Neurological Disorders and Stroke, National Institutes of Health, November 2004.

Few experiences match the drama of a convulsive seizure. A person having a severe seizure may cry out, fall to the floor unconscious, twitch or move uncontrollably, drool, or even lose bladder control. Within minutes the attack is over and the person regains consciousness but is exhausted and dazed. This is the image most people have when they hear the word epilepsy. However, this type of seizure—a generalized tonic-clonic seizure—is only one kind of epilepsy. There are many other kinds, each with a different set of symptoms.

Epilepsy was one of the first brain disorders to be described. It was mentioned in ancient Babylon more than three thousand years ago. The strange behavior caused by some seizures has contributed through the ages to many superstitions and prejudices. The word *epilepsy* is derived from the Greek word for "attack." People once thought that those with epilepsy were being visited by demons or gods. However, in 400 B.C. the early physician Hippocrates suggested that epilepsy was a disorder of the brain—and we now know that he was right.

What is epilepsy?

Epilepsy is a brain disorder in which clusters of nerve cells, or neurons, in the brain sometimes signal abnormally. Neurons normally generate electrochemical impulses that act on other neurons, glands, and muscles to produce human thoughts, feelings, and actions. In epilepsy, the normal pattern of neuronal activity becomes disturbed, causing strange sensations, emotions, and behavior, or sometimes convulsions, muscle spasms, and loss of consciousness. During a seizure, neurons may fire as many as five hundred times a second, much faster than the normal rate of about eighty times a second. In some people, this happens only occasionally; for others it may happen up to hundreds of times a day.

More than two million people in the United States—about one in a hundred—have experienced an unprovoked seizure or been diagnosed with epilepsy. For about 80 percent of those diagnosed with epilepsy, seizures can be controlled with modern medicines and surgical techniques. However, about 20 percent of people with epilepsy will continue to experience seizures even with the best available treatment. Doctors call this situation intractable epilepsy. Having a seizure does not necessarily mean that a person has epilepsy. Only when a person has had two or more seizures is he or she considered to have epilepsy.

Epilepsy is not contagious and is not caused by mental illness or mental retardation. Some people with mental retardation may experience seizures, but seizures do not necessarily mean the person has or will develop mental impairment. Many people with epilepsy have normal or above-average intelligence. Famous people who are known or rumored to have had epilepsy include the Russian writer Dostoyevsky, the philosopher Socrates, the military general Napoleon, and the inventor of dynamite, Alfred Nobel, who established the Nobel Prize. Several Olympic medalists and other athletes also have had epilepsy. Seizures sometimes do cause brain damage, particularly if they are severe. However, most seizures do not seem to have a detrimental effect on the brain. Any changes that do occur are usually subtle, and it is often unclear whether these changes are caused by the seizures themselves or by the underlying problem that caused the seizures.

While epilepsy cannot currently be cured, for some people it does eventually go away. One study found that children with idiopathic epilepsy, or epilepsy with an unknown cause, had a 68 to 92 percent chance of becoming seizure-free by twenty years after their diagnosis. The odds of becoming seizure-free are not as good for adults or for children with severe epilepsy syndromes, but it is nonetheless possible that seizures may decrease or even stop over time. This is more likely if the epilepsy has been well controlled by medication or if the person has had epilepsy surgery.

What causes epilepsy?

Epilepsy is a disorder with many possible causes. Anything that disturbs the normal pattern of neuron activity—from illness to brain damage to abnormal brain development—can lead to seizures.

Epilepsy may develop because of an abnormality in brain wiring, an imbalance of nerve signaling chemicals called neurotransmitters, or some combination of these factors. Researchers believe that some people with epilepsy have an abnormally high level of excitatory neurotransmitters that increase neuronal activity, while others have an abnormally low level of inhibitory neurotransmitters that decrease neuronal activity in the brain. Either situation can result in too much neuronal activity and cause epilepsy. One of the most-studied neurotransmitters that plays a role in epilepsy is GABA, or gamma-aminobutyric acid, which is an inhibitory neurotransmitter. Research on GABA has led to drugs that alter the amount of this neurotransmitter in the brain or change how the brain responds to it. Researchers also are studying excitatory neurotransmitters such as glutamate.

In some cases, the brain's attempts to repair itself after a head injury, stroke, or other problem may inadvertently generate abnormal nerve connections that lead to epilepsy. Abnormalities in brain wiring that occur during brain development also may disturb neuronal activity and lead to epilepsy.

Research has shown that the cell membrane that surrounds each neuron plays an important role in epilepsy. Cell membranes are crucial for a neuron to generate electrical impulses. For this reason, researchers are studying details of the membrane structure, how molecules move in and out of membranes, and how the cell nourishes and repairs the membrane. A disruption in any of these processes may lead to epilepsy. Studies in animals have shown that, because the brain continually adapts to changes in stimuli, a small change in neuronal activity, if repeated, may eventually lead to full-blown epilepsy. Researchers are investigating whether this phenomenon, called kindling, may also occur in humans.

In some cases, epilepsy may result from changes in non-neuronal brain cells called glia. These cells regulate concentrations of chemicals in the brain that can affect neuronal signaling.

About half of all seizures have no known cause. However, in other cases, the seizures are clearly linked to infection, trauma, or other identifiable problems.

Genetic Factors: Research suggests that genetic abnormalities may be some of the most important factors contributing to epilepsy. Some types of epilepsy have been traced to an abnormality in a specific gene. Many other types of epilepsy tend to run in families, which suggests that genes influence epilepsy. Some researchers estimate that more than five hundred genes could play a role in this disorder. However, it is increasingly clear that, for many forms of epilepsy, genetic abnormalities play only a partial role, perhaps by increasing a person's susceptibility to seizures that are triggered by an environmental factor.

Several types of epilepsy have now been linked to defective genes for ion channels, the "gates" that control the flow of ions in and out of cells and regulate neuron signaling. Another gene, which is missing in people with progressive myoclonus epilepsy, codes for a protein called cystatin B. This protein regulates enzymes that break down other proteins. Another gene, which is altered in a severe form of epilepsy called LaFora's disease, has been linked to a gene that helps to break down carbohydrates.

While abnormal genes sometimes cause epilepsy, they also may influence the disorder in subtler ways. For example, one study showed that many people with epilepsy have an abnormally active version of a gene that increases resistance to drugs. This may help explain why anticonvulsant drugs do not work for some people. Genes also may control other aspects of the body's response to medications and each person's susceptibility to seizures, or seizure threshold. Abnormalities in the genes that control neuronal migration—a critical step in brain development—can lead to areas of misplaced or abnormally formed neurons, or dysplasia, in the brain that can cause epilepsy. In some cases, genes may contribute to development of epilepsy even in people with no family history of the disorder. These people may have a newly developed abnormality, or mutation, in an epilepsy-related gene.

Other Disorders: In many cases, epilepsy develops as a result of brain damage from other disorders. For example, brain tumors, alcoholism, and Alzheimer's disease frequently lead to epilepsy because they alter the normal workings of the brain. Strokes, heart attacks, and other conditions that deprive the brain of oxygen also can cause epilepsy in some cases. About 32 percent of all cases of newly developed epilepsy in elderly people appear to be due to cerebrovascular disease, which reduces the supply of oxygen to brain cells. Meningitis, AIDS, viral encephalitis, and other infectious diseases can lead to epilepsy, as can hydrocephalus—a condition in which excess fluid builds up in the brain. Epilepsy also can result from intolerance to wheat gluten (also known as celiac disease), or from a parasitic infection of the brain called neurocysticercosis. Seizures may stop once these disorders are treated successfully. However, the odds of becoming seizure-free after the primary disorder is treated are uncertain and vary depending on the type of disorder, the brain region that is affected, and how much brain damage occurred prior to treatment.

Epilepsy is associated with a variety of developmental and metabolic disorders, including cerebral palsy, neurofibromatosis, pyruvate dependency, tuberous sclerosis, Landau-Kleffner syndrome, and autism. Epilepsy is just one of a set of symptoms commonly found in people with these disorders.

Head Injury: In some cases, head injury can lead to seizures or epilepsy. Safety measures such as wearing seat belts in cars and using helmets when riding a motorcycle or playing competitive sports can protect people from epilepsy and other problems that result from head injury.

Prenatal Injury and Developmental Problems: The developing brain is susceptible to many kinds of injury. Maternal infections, poor nutrition, and oxygen deficiencies are just some of the conditions that may take a toll on the brain of a developing baby. These conditions may lead to cerebral palsy, which often is associated with epilepsy, or they may cause epilepsy that is unrelated to any other disorders. About 20 percent of seizures in children are due to cerebral palsy or other neurological abnormalities. Abnormalities in genes that control development also may contribute to epilepsy. Advanced brain imaging has revealed that some cases of epilepsy that occur with no obvious cause may be associated with areas of dysplasia in the brain that probably develop before birth.

Poisoning: Seizures can result from exposure to lead, carbon monoxide, and many other poisons. They also can result from exposure to street drugs and from overdoses of antidepressants and other medications.

Seizures are often triggered by factors such as lack of sleep, alcohol consumption, stress, or hormonal changes associated with the menstrual cycle. These seizure triggers do not cause epilepsy but can provoke first seizures or cause breakthrough seizures in people who otherwise experience good seizure control with their medication. Sleep deprivation in particular is a universal and powerful trigger of seizures. For this reason, people with epilepsy should make sure to get enough sleep and should try to stay on a regular sleep schedule as much as possible. For some people, light flashing at a certain speed or the flicker of a computer monitor can trigger a seizure; this problem is called photosensitive epilepsy. Smoking cigarettes also can trigger seizures. The nicotine in cigarettes acts on receptors for the excitatory neurotransmitter acetylcholine in the brain, which increases neuronal firing. Seizures are not triggered by sexual activity except in very rare instances.

What are the different kinds of seizures?

Doctors have described more than thirty different types of seizures. Seizures are divided into two major categories—focal seizures and generalized seizures. However, there are many different types of seizures in each of these categories.

Focal Seizures: Focal seizures, also called partial seizures, occur in just one part of the brain. About 60 percent of people with epilepsy have focal seizures. These seizures are frequently described by the area of the brain in which they originate. For example, someone might be diagnosed with focal frontal lobe seizures.

In a simple focal seizure, the person will remain conscious but experience unusual feelings or sensations that can take many forms. The person may experience sudden and unexplainable feelings of joy, anger, sadness, or nausea. He or she also may hear, smell, taste, see, or feel things that are not real.

In a complex focal seizure, the person has a change in or loss of consciousness. His or her consciousness may be altered, producing a dreamlike experience. People having a complex focal seizure may display strange, repetitious behaviors such as blinks, twitches, mouth movements, or even walking in a circle. These repetitious movements are called automatisms. More complicated actions, which may seem purposeful, can also occur involuntarily. Patients may also continue activities they started before the seizure began, such as washing dishes in a repetitive, unproductive fashion. These seizures usually last just a few seconds.

Some people with focal seizures, especially complex focal seizures, may experience auras—unusual sensations that warn of an impending seizure. These auras are actually simple focal seizures in which the person maintains consciousness. The symptoms an individual person has, and the progression of those symptoms, tend to be stereotyped, or similar every time.

The symptoms of focal seizures can easily be confused with other disorders. For instance, the dreamlike perceptions associated with a complex focal seizure may be misdiagnosed as migraine headaches, which also may cause a dreamlike state. The strange behavior and sensations caused by focal seizures also can be mistaken for symptoms of narcolepsy, fainting, or even mental illness. It may take many tests and careful monitoring by an experienced physician to tell the difference between epilepsy and other disorders.

Generalized Seizures: Generalized seizures are a result of abnormal neuronal activity on both sides of the brain. These seizures may cause loss of consciousness, falls, or massive muscle spasms.

There are many kinds of generalized seizures. In absence seizures, the person may appear to be staring into space or have jerking or twitching muscles. These seizures are sometimes referred to as petit mal seizures, which is an older term. Tonic seizures cause stiffening of muscles of the body, generally those in the back, legs, and arms. Clonic seizures cause repeated jerking movements of muscles on both sides of the body. Myoclonic seizures cause jerks or twitches of the upper body, arms, or legs. Atonic seizures cause a loss of normal muscle tone. The affected person will fall down or may drop his or her head involuntarily. Tonic-clonic seizures cause a mixture of symptoms, including stiffening of the body and repeated jerks of the arms or legs as well as loss of consciousness. Tonic-clonic seizures are sometimes referred to by an older term: grand mal seizures.

Not all seizures can be easily defined as either focal or generalized. Some people have seizures that begin as focal seizures but then spread to the entire brain. Other people may have both types of seizures but with no clear pattern.

Society's lack of understanding about the many different types of seizures is one of the biggest problems for people with epilepsy. People who witness a nonconvulsive seizure often find it difficult to understand that behavior that looks deliberate is not under the person's control. In some cases, this has led to the affected person being arrested or admitted to a psychiatric hospital. To combat these problems, people everywhere need to understand the many different types of seizures and how they may appear.

What are the different kinds of epilepsy?

Just as there are many different kinds of seizures, there are many different kinds of epilepsy. Doctors have identified hundreds of different epilepsy syndromes—disorders characterized by a specific set of symptoms that include epilepsy. Some of these syndromes appear to be hereditary. For other syndromes, the cause is unknown. Epilepsy syndromes are frequently described by their symptoms or by where in the brain they originate. People should discuss the implications of their type of epilepsy with their doctors to understand the full range of symptoms, the possible treatments, and the prognosis.

People with absence epilepsy have repeated absence seizures that cause momentary lapses of consciousness. These seizures almost always begin in childhood or adolescence, and they tend to run in families, suggesting that they may be at least partially due to a defective gene or genes. Some people with absence seizures have purposeless movements during their seizures, such as a jerking arm or rapidly blinking eyes. Others have no noticeable symptoms except for brief times when they are "out of it." Immediately after a seizure, the person can resume whatever he or she was doing. However, these seizures may occur so frequently that the person cannot concentrate in school or other situations. Childhood absence epilepsy usually stops when the child reaches puberty. Absence seizures usually have no lasting effect on intelligence or other brain functions.

Temporal lobe epilepsy, or TLE, is the most common epilepsy syndrome with focal seizures. These seizures are often associated with auras. TLE often begins in childhood. Research has shown that repeated temporal lobe seizures can cause a brain structure called the hippocampus to shrink over time. The hippocampus is important for memory and learning. While it may take years of temporal lobe seizures for measurable hippocampal damage to occur, this finding underlines the need to treat TLE early and as effectively as possible.

Neocortical epilepsy is characterized by seizures that originate from the brain's cortex, or outer layer. The seizures can be either focal or generalized. They may include strange sensations, visual hallucinations, emotional changes, muscle spasms, convulsions, and a variety of other symptoms, depending on where in the brain the seizures originate.

There are many other types of epilepsy, each with its own characteristic set of symptoms. Many of these, including Lennox-Gastaut syndrome and Rasmussen's encephalitis, begin in childhood. Children with Lennox-Gastaut syndrome have severe epilepsy with several different types of seizures, including atonic seizures, which cause sudden falls and are also called drop attacks. This severe form of epilepsy can be very difficult to treat effectively. Rasmussen's encephalitis is a progressive type of epilepsy in which half of the brain shows continual inflammation. It sometimes is treated with a radical surgical procedure called hemispherectomy (see the section on Surgery). Some childhood epilepsy syndromes, such as childhood absence epilepsy, tend to go into remission or stop entirely during adolescence, whereas other syndromes such as juvenile myoclonic epilepsy and Lennox-Gastaut syndrome are usually present for life once they develop. Seizure syndromes do not always appear in childhood, however.

Epilepsy syndromes that are easily treated, do not seem to impair cognitive functions or development, and usually stop spontaneously are often described as benign. Benign epilepsy syndromes include benign infantile encephalopathy and benign neonatal convulsions. Other syndromes, such as early myoclonic encephalopathy, include neurological and developmental problems. However, these problems may be caused by underlying neurodegenerative processes rather than by the seizures. Epilepsy syndromes in which the seizures or the person's cognitive abilities get worse over time are called progressive epilepsy.

Several types of epilepsy begin in infancy. The most common type of infantile epilepsy is infantile spasms, clusters of seizures that usually begin before the age of six months. During these seizures the infant may bend and cry out. Anticonvulsant drugs often do not work for infantile spasms, but the seizures can be treated with ACTH (adrenocorticotropic hormone) or prednisone.

When are seizures not epilepsy?

While any seizure is cause for concern, having a seizure does not by itself mean a person has epilepsy. First seizures, febrile seizures, nonepileptic events, and eclampsia are examples of seizures that may not be associated with epilepsy.

First Seizures: Many people have a single seizure at some point in their lives. Often these seizures occur in reaction to anesthesia or a strong drug, but they also may be unprovoked, meaning that they occur without any obvious triggering factor. Unless the person has suffered brain damage or there is a family history of epilepsy or other neurological abnormalities, these single seizures usually are not followed by additional seizures. One recent study that followed patients for an average of eight years found that only 33 percent of people have a second seizure within four years after an initial seizure. People who did not have a second seizure within that time remained seizure-free for the rest of the study. For people who did have a second seizure, the risk of a third seizure was about 73 percent on average by the end of four years.

When someone has experienced a first seizure, the doctor will usually order an electroencephalogram, or EEG, to determine what type of seizure the person may have had and if there are any detectable abnormalities in the person's brain waves. The doctor also may order brain scans to identify abnormalities that may be visible in the brain. These tests may help the doctor decide whether or not to treat the person with antiepileptic drugs. In some cases, drug treatment after the first seizure may help prevent future seizures and epilepsy. However, the drugs also can cause detrimental side effects, so doctors prescribe them only when they feel the benefits outweigh the risks. Evidence suggests that it may be beneficial to begin anticonvulsant medication once a person has had a second seizure, as the chance of future seizures increases significantly after this occurs.

Febrile Seizures: Sometimes a child will have a seizure during the course of an illness with a high fever. These seizures are called febrile seizures (*febrile* is derived from the Latin word for "fever") and can be very alarming to the parents and other caregivers. In the past, doctors usually prescribed a course of anticonvulsant drugs following a febrile seizure in the hope of preventing epilepsy. However, most children who have a febrile seizure do not develop epilepsy, and long-term use of anticonvulsant drugs in children may damage the developing brain or cause other detrimental side effects. Experts at a 1980 consensus conference coordinated by the National Institutes of Health concluded that preventive treatment after a febrile seizure is generally not warranted unless certain other conditions are present: a family history of epilepsy, signs of nervous system impairment prior to the seizure, or a relatively prolonged or complicated seizure. The risk of subsequent nonfebrile seizures is only 2 to 3 percent unless one of these factors is present.

Researchers have now identified several different genes that influence the risk of febrile seizures in certain families. Studying these genes may lead to new understanding of how febrile seizures occur and perhaps point to ways of preventing them.

Nonepileptic Events: Sometimes people appear to have seizures, even though their brains show no seizure activity. This type of phenomenon has various names, including nonepileptic events and pseudoseizures. Both of these terms essentially mean something that looks like a seizure but isn't one. Nonepileptic events that are psychological in origin may be referred to as psychogenic seizures. Psychogenic seizures may indicate dependence, a need for attention, avoidance of stressful situations, or specific psychiatric conditions. Some people with epilepsy have psychogenic seizures in addition to their epileptic seizures. Other people who have psychogenic seizures do not have epilepsy at all. Psychogenic seizures cannot be treated in the same way as epileptic seizures. Instead, they are often treated by mental health specialists.

Other nonepileptic events may be caused by narcolepsy, Tourette syndrome, cardiac arrhythmia, and other medical conditions with symptoms that resemble seizures. Because symptoms of these disorders can look very much like epileptic seizures, they are often mistaken for epilepsy. Distinguishing between true epileptic seizures and nonepileptic events can be very difficult and requires a thorough medical assessment, careful monitoring, and knowledgeable health professionals. Improvements in brain scanning and monitoring technology may improve diagnosis of nonepileptic events in the future.

Eclampsia: Eclampsia is a life-threatening condition that can develop in pregnant women. Its symptoms include sudden elevations of blood pressure and seizures. Pregnant women who develop unexpected seizures should be rushed to a hospital immediately. Eclampsia can be treated in a hospital setting and usually does not result in additional seizures or epilepsy once the pregnancy is over.

How is epilepsy diagnosed?

Doctors have developed a number of different tests to determine whether a person has epilepsy and, if so, what kind of seizures the person has. In some cases, people may have symptoms that look very much like a seizure but in fact are nonepileptic events caused by other disorders. Even doctors may not be able to tell the difference between these disorders and epilepsy without close observation and intensive testing.

EEG Monitoring: An EEG records brain waves detected by electrodes placed on the scalp. This is the most common diagnostic test for epilepsy and can detect abnormalities in the brain's electrical activity. People with epilepsy frequently have changes in their normal pattern of brain waves, even when they are not experiencing a seizure. While this type of test can be very useful in diagnosing epilepsy, it is not foolproof. Some people continue to show normal brain wave patterns even after they have experienced a seizure. In other cases, the unusual brain waves are generated deep in the brain where the EEG is unable to detect them. Many people who do not have epilepsy also show some unusual brain activity on an EEG. Whenever possible, an EEG should be performed within twenty-four hours of a patient's first seizure. Ideally, EEGs should be performed while the patient is sleeping as well as when he or she is awake, because brain activity during sleep is often quite different than at other times.

Video monitoring is often used in conjunction with EEG to determine the nature of a person's seizures. It also can be used in some cases to rule out other disorders such as cardiac arrhythmia or narcolepsy that may look like epilepsy.

Brain Scans: One of the most important ways of diagnosing epilepsy is through the use of brain scans. The most commonly used brain scans include CT (computed tomography), PET (positron emission tomography), and MRI (magnetic resonance imaging). CT and MRI scans reveal the structure of the brain, which can be useful for identifying brain tumors, cysts, and other structural abnormalities. PET and an adapted kind of MRI called functional MRI (fMRI) can be used to monitor the brain's activity and detect abnormalities in how it works. SPECT (single photon emission computed tomography) is a relatively new kind of brain scan that is sometimes used to locate seizure foci in the brain.

In some cases, doctors may use an experimental type of brain scan called a magnetoencephalogram, or MEG. MEG detects the magnetic signals generated by neurons to allow doctors to monitor brain activity at different points in the brain over time, revealing different brain functions. While MEG is similar in concept to EEG, it does not require electrodes and it can detect signals from deeper in the brain than an EEG. Doctors also are experimenting with brain scans called magnetic resonance spectroscopy (MRS) that can detect abnormalities in the brain's biochemical processes, and with near-infrared spectroscopy, a technique that can detect oxygen levels in brain tissue.

Medical History: Taking a detailed medical history, including symptoms and duration of the seizures, is still one of the best methods available to determine if a person has epilepsy and what kind of seizures he or she has. The doctor will ask questions about the seizures and any past illnesses or other symptoms a person may have had. Since people who have suffered a seizure often do not remember what happened, caregivers' accounts of the seizure are vital to this evaluation.

Blood Tests: Doctors often take blood samples for testing, particularly when they are examining a child. These blood samples are often screened for metabolic or genetic disorders that may be associated with the seizures. They also may be used to check for underlying problems such as infections, lead poisoning, anemia, and diabetes that may be causing or triggering the seizures.

Developmental, Neurological, and Behavioral Tests: Doctors often use tests devised to measure motor abilities, behavior, and intellectual capacity as a way to determine how the epilepsy is affecting that person. These tests also can provide clues about what kind of epilepsy the person has.

Can epilepsy be prevented?

Many cases of epilepsy can be prevented by wearing seatbelts and bicycle helmets, putting children in car seats, and other measures that prevent head injury and other trauma. Prescribing medication after first or second seizures or febrile seizures also may help prevent epilepsy in some cases. Good prenatal care, including treatment of high blood pressure and infections during pregnancy, can prevent brain damage in the developing baby that may lead to epilepsy and other neurological problems later. Treating cardiovascular disease, high blood pressure, infections, and other disorders that can affect the brain during adulthood and aging also may prevent many cases of epilepsy. Finally, identifying the genes for many neurological disorders can provide opportunities for genetic screening and prenatal diagnosis that may ultimately prevent many cases of epilepsy.

How can epilepsy be treated?

Accurate diagnosis of the type of epilepsy a person has is crucial for finding an effective treatment. There are many different ways to treat epilepsy. Currently available treatments can control seizures at least some of the time in about 80 percent of people with epilepsy. However, another 20 percent—about six hundred thousand people with epilepsy in the United States—have intractable seizures, and another four hundred thousand feel they get inadequate relief from available treatments. These statistics make it clear that improved treatments are desperately needed.

Doctors who treat epilepsy come from many different fields of medicine. They include neurologists, pediatricians, pediatric neurologists, internists, and family physicians, as well as neurosurgeons and doctors called epileptologists who specialize in treating epilepsy. People who need specialized or intensive care for epilepsy may be treated at large medical centers and neurology clinics at hospitals or by neurologists in private practice. Many epilepsy treatment centers are associated with university hospitals that perform research in addition to providing medical care.

Once epilepsy is diagnosed, it is important to begin treatment as soon as possible. Research suggests that medication and other treatments may be less successful in treating epilepsy once seizures and their consequences become established.

Tailoring the Dosage of Antiepileptic Drugs: When a person starts a new epilepsy drug, it is important to tailor the dosage to achieve the best results. People's bodies react to medications in very different and sometimes unpredictable ways, so it may take some time to find the right drug at the right dose to provide optimal control of seizures while minimizing side effects. A drug that has no effect or very bad side effects at one dose may work very well at another dose. Doctors will usually prescribe a low dose of the new drug initially and monitor blood levels of the drug to determine when the best possible dose has been reached.

Generic versions are available for many antiepileptic drugs. The chemicals in generic drugs are exactly the same as in the brand-name drugs, but they may be absorbed or processed differently in the body because of the way they are prepared. Therefore, patients should always check with their doctors before switching to a generic version of their medication.

Discontinuing Medication: Some doctors will advise people with epilepsy to discontinue their antiepileptic drugs after two years have passed without a seizure. Others feel it is better to wait for four to five years. Discontinuing medication should always be done with a doctor's advice and supervision. It is very important to continue taking epilepsy medication for as long as the doctor prescribes it. People also should ask the doctor or pharmacist ahead of time what they should do if they miss a dose. Discontinuing medication without a doctor's advice is one of the major reasons people who have been seizure-free begin having new seizures. Seizures that result from suddenly stopping medication can be very serious and can lead to status epilepticus. Furthermore, there is some evidence that uncontrolled seizures trigger changes in neurons that can make it more difficult to treat the seizures in the future.

The chance that a person will eventually be able to discontinue medication varies depending on the person's age and his or her type of epilepsy. More than half of children who go into remission with medication can eventually stop their medication without having new seizures. One study showed that 68 percent of adults who had been seizure-free for two years before stopping medication were able to do so without having more seizures, and 75 percent could successfully discontinue medication if they had been seizure-free for three years. However, the odds of successfully stopping medication are not as good for people with a family history of epilepsy, those who need multiple medications, those with focal seizures, and those who continue to have abnormal EEG results while on medication.

Surgery: When seizures cannot be adequately controlled by medications, doctors may recommend that the person be evaluated for surgery. Surgery for epilepsy is performed by teams of doctors at medical centers. To decide if a person may benefit from surgery, doctors consider the type or types of seizures he or she has. They also take into account the brain region involved and how important that region is for everyday behavior. Surgeons usually avoid operating in areas of the brain that are necessary for speech, language, hearing, or other important abilities. Doctors may perform tests such as a Wada test (administration of the drug amobarbital into the carotid artery) to find areas of the brain that control speech and memory. They often monitor the patient intensively prior to surgery in order to pinpoint the exact location in the brain where seizures begin. They also may use implanted electrodes to record brain activity from the surface of the brain. This yields better information than an external EEG.

A 1990 National Institutes of Health consensus conference on surgery for epilepsy concluded that there are three broad categories of epilepsy that can be treated successfully with surgery. These include focal seizures, seizures that begin as focal seizures before spreading to the rest of the brain, and unilateral multifocal epilepsy with infantile hemiplegia (such as Rasmussen's encephalitis). Doctors generally recommend surgery only after patients have tried two or three different medications without success, or if there is an identifiable brain lesion—a damaged or dysfunctional area—believed to cause the seizures.

A study published in 2000 compared surgery to an additional year of treatment with antiepileptic drugs in people with longstanding temporal lobe epilepsy. The results showed that 64 percent of patients receiving surgery became seizure-free, compared to 8 percent of those who continued with medication only. Because of this study and other evidence, the American Academy of Neurology (AAN) now recommends surgery for TLE when antiepileptic drugs are not effective. However, the study and the AAN guidelines do not provide guidance on how long seizures should occur, how severe they should be, or how many drugs should be tried before surgery is considered. A nationwide study is now under way to determine how soon surgery for TLE should be performed.

If a person is considered a good candidate for surgery and has seizures that cannot be controlled with available medication, experts generally agree that surgery should be performed as early as possible. It can be difficult for a person who has had years of seizures to fully re-adapt to a seizure-free life if the surgery is successful. The person may never have had an opportunity to develop independence, and he or she may have had difficulties with school and work that could have been avoided with earlier treatment. Surgery should always be performed with support from rehabilitation specialists and counselors who can help the person deal with the many psychological, social, and employment issues he or she may face.

While surgery can significantly reduce or even halt seizures for some people, it is important to remember that any kind of surgery carries some amount of risk (usually small). Surgery for epilepsy does not always successfully reduce seizures and it can result in cognitive or personality changes, even in people who are excellent candidates for surgery. Patients should ask their surgeon about his or her experience, success rates, and complication rates with the procedure they are considering.

Even when surgery completely ends a person's seizures, it is important to continue taking seizure medication for some time to give the brain time to re-adapt. Doctors generally recommend medication for two years after a successful operation to avoid new seizures.

Surgery to Treat Underlying Conditions: In cases where seizures are caused by a brain tumor, hydrocephalus, or other conditions that can be treated with surgery, doctors may operate to treat these underlying conditions. In many cases, once the underlying condition is successfully treated, a person's seizures will disappear as well.

Surgery to Remove a Seizure Focus: The most common type of surgery for epilepsy is removal of a seizure focus, or small area of the brain where seizures originate. This type of surgery, which doctors may refer to as a lobectomy or lesionectomy, is appropriate only for focal seizures that originate in just one area of the brain. In general, people have a better chance of becoming seizure-free after surgery if they have a small, well-defined seizure focus. Lobectomies have a 55–70 percent success rate when the type of epilepsy and the seizure focus is well defined. The most common type of lobectomy is a temporal lobe resection, which is performed for people with temporal lobe epilepsy. Temporal lobe resection leads to a significant reduction or complete cessation of seizures about 70–90 percent of the time.

Multiple Subpial Transection: When seizures originate in part of the brain that cannot be removed, surgeons may perform a procedure called a multiple subpial transection. In this type of operation, which has been commonly performed since 1989, surgeons make a series of cuts that are designed to prevent seizures from spreading into other parts of the brain while leaving the person's normal abilities intact. About 70 percent of patients who undergo a multiple subpial transection have satisfactory improvement in seizure control.

Corpus Callosotomy: Corpus callosotomy, or severing the network of neural connections between the right and left halves, or hemispheres, of the brain, is done primarily in children with severe seizures that start in one half of the brain and spread to the other side. Corpus callosotomy can end drop attacks and other generalized seizures. However, the procedure does not stop seizures in the side of the brain where they originate, and these focal seizures may even increase after surgery.

Hemispherectomy and Hemispherotomy: These procedures remove half of the brain's cortex, or outer layer. They are used predominantly in children who have seizures that do not respond to medication because of damage that involves only half the brain, as occurs with conditions such as Rasmussen's encephalitis, Sturge-Weber syndrome, and hemimegencephaly. While this type of surgery is very radical and is performed only as a last resort, children often recover very well from the procedure, and their seizures usually cease altogether. With intense rehabilitation, they often recover nearly normal abilities. Since the chance of a full recovery is best in young children, hemispherectomy should be performed as early in a child's life as possible. It is rarely performed in children older than thirteen.

Devices: The vagus nerve stimulator was approved by the U.S. Food and Drug Administration (FDA) in 1997 for use in people with seizures that are not well controlled by medication. The vagus nerve stimulator is a battery-powered device that is surgically implanted under the skin of the chest, much like a pacemaker, and is attached to the vagus nerve in the lower neck. This device delivers short bursts of electrical energy to the brain via the vagus nerve. On average, this stimulation reduces seizures by about 20–40 percent. Patients usually cannot stop taking epilepsy medication because of the stimulator, but they often experience fewer seizures and they may be able to reduce the dose of their medication. Side effects of the vagus nerve stimulator are generally mild but may include hoarseness, ear pain, a sore throat, or nausea. Adjusting the amount of stimulation can usually eliminate most side effects, although the hoarseness typically persists. The batteries in the vagus nerve stimulator need to be replaced about once every five years; this requires a minor operation that can usually be performed as an outpatient procedure.

Several new devices may become available for epilepsy in the future. Researchers are studying whether transcranial magnetic stimulation (TMS), a procedure that uses a strong magnet held outside the head to influence brain activity, may reduce seizures. They also hope to develop implantable devices that can deliver drugs to specific parts of the brain.

Diet: Studies have shown that, in some cases, children may experience fewer seizures if they maintain a strict diet rich in fats and low in carbohydrates. This unusual diet, called the ketogenic diet, causes the body to break down fats instead of carbohydrates to survive. This condition is called ketosis. One study of 150 children whose seizures were poorly controlled by medication found that about one-fourth of the children had a 90 percent or better decrease in seizures with the ketogenic diet, and another half of the group had a 50 percent or better decrease in their seizures. Moreover, some children can discontinue the ketogenic diet after several years and remain seizure-free. The ketogenic diet is not easy to maintain, as it requires strict adherence to an unusual and limited range of foods. Possible side effects include retarded growth due to nutritional deficiency and a buildup of uric acid in the blood, which can lead to kidney stones. People who try the ketogenic diet should seek the guidance of a dietitian to ensure that it does not lead to serious nutritional deficiency.

Researchers are not sure how ketosis inhibits seizures. One study showed that a byproduct of ketosis called beta-hydroxybutyrate (BHB) inhibits seizures in animals. If BHB also works in humans, researchers may eventually be able to develop drugs that mimic the seizure-inhibiting effects of the ketogenic diet.

Other Treatment Strategies: Researchers are studying whether biofeedback—a strategy in which individuals learn to control their own brain waves—may be useful in controlling seizures. However, this type of therapy is controversial and most studies have shown discouraging results. Taking large doses of vitamins generally does not help a person's seizures and may even be harmful in some cases. But a good diet and some vitamin supplements, particularly folic acid, may help reduce some birth defects and medication-related nutritional deficiencies. Use of non-vitamin supplements such as melatonin is controversial and can be risky. One study showed that melatonin may reduce seizures in some children, while another found that the risk of seizures increased measurably with melatonin. Most non-vitamin supplements such as those found in health food stores are not regulated by the FDA, so their true effects and their interactions with other drugs are largely unknown.

How does epilepsy affect daily life?

Most people with epilepsy lead outwardly normal lives. Approximately 80 percent can be significantly helped by modern therapies, and some may go months or years between seizures. However, the condition can and does affect daily life for people with epilepsy, their family, and their friends. People with severe seizures that resist treatment have, on average, a shorter life expectancy and an increased risk of cognitive impairment, particularly if the seizures developed in early childhood. These impairments may be related to the underlying conditions that cause epilepsy or to epilepsy treatment rather than the epilepsy itself.

Behavior and Emotions: It is not uncommon for people with epilepsy, especially children, to develop behavioral and emotional problems. Sometimes these problems are caused by embarrassment or frustration associated with epilepsy. Other problems may result from bullying, teasing, or avoidance in school and other social settings. In children, these problems can be minimized if parents encourage a positive outlook and independence, do not reward negative behavior with unusual amounts of attention, and try to stay attuned to their child's needs and feelings. Families must learn to accept and live with the seizures without blaming or resenting the affected person. Counseling services can help families cope with epilepsy in a positive manner. Epilepsy support groups also can help by providing a way for people with epilepsy and their family members to share their experiences, frustrations, and tips for coping with the disorder.

People with epilepsy have an increased risk of poor self-esteem, depression, and suicide. These problems may be a reaction to a lack of understanding or discomfort about epilepsy that may result in cruelty or avoidance by other people. Many people with epilepsy also live with an ever-present fear that they will have another seizure.

Driving and Recreation: For many people with epilepsy, the risk of seizures restricts their independence, in particular the ability to drive. Most states and the District of Columbia will not issue a driver's license to someone with epilepsy unless the person can document that they have gone a specific amount of time without a seizure (the waiting period varies from a few months to several years). Some states make exceptions for this policy when seizures don't impair consciousness, occur only during sleep, or have long auras or other warning signs that allow the person to avoid driving when a seizure is likely to occur. Studies show that the risk of having a seizure-related accident decreases as the length of time since the last seizure increases. One study found that the risk of having a seizure-related motor vehicle accident is 93 percent less in people who wait at least one year after their last seizure before driving, compared to people who wait for shorter intervals.

The risk of seizures also restricts people's recreational choices. For instance, people with epilepsy should not participate in sports such as skydiving or motor racing where a moment's inattention could lead to injury. Other activities, such as swimming and sailing, should be done only with precautions or supervision. However, jogging, football, and many other sports are reasonably safe for a person with epilepsy. Studies to date have not shown any increase in seizures due to sports, although these studies have not focused on any activity in particular. There is some evidence that regular exercise may even improve seizure control in some people. Sports are often such a positive factor in life that it is best for the person to participate, although the person with epilepsy and the coach or other leader should take appropriate safety precautions. It is important to take steps to avoid potential sports-related problems such as dehydration, overexertion, and hypoglycemia, as these problems can increase the risk of seizures.

Education and Employment: By law, people with epilepsy or other handicaps in the United States cannot be denied employment or access to any educational, recreational, or other activity because of their seizures. However, one survey showed that only about 56 percent of people with epilepsy finish high school and about 15 percent finish college—rates much lower than those for the general population. The same survey found that about 25 percent of working-age people with epilepsy are unemployed. These numbers indicate that significant barriers still exist for people with epilepsy in school and work. Restrictions on driving limit the employment opportunities for many people with epilepsy, and many find it difficult to face the misunderstandings and social pressures they encounter in public situations. Antiepileptic drugs also may cause side effects that interfere with concentration and memory. Children with epilepsy may need extra time to complete schoolwork, and they sometimes may need to have instructions or other information repeated for them. Teachers should be told what to do if a child in their classroom has a seizure, and parents should work with the school system to find reasonable ways to accommodate any special needs their child may have.

Pregnancy and Motherhood: Women with epilepsy are often concerned about whether they can become pregnant and have a healthy child. This is usually possible. While some seizure medications and some types of epilepsy may reduce a person's interest in sexual activity, most people with epilepsy can become pregnant. Moreover, women with epilepsy have a 90 percent or better chance of having a normal, healthy baby, and the risk of birth defects is only about 4 to 6 percent. The risk that children of parents with epilepsy will develop epilepsy themselves is only about 5 percent unless the parent has a clearly hereditary form of the disorder. Parents who are worried that their epilepsy may be hereditary may wish to consult a genetic counselor to determine what the risk might be. Amniocentesis and high-level ultrasound can be performed during pregnancy to ensure that the baby is developing normally, and a procedure called a maternal serum alpha-fetoprotein test can be used for prenatal diagnosis of many conditions if a problem is suspected.

There are several precautions women can take before and during pregnancy to reduce the risks associated with pregnancy and delivery. Women who are thinking about becoming pregnant should talk with their doctors to learn any special risks associated with their epilepsy and the medications they may be taking. Some seizure medications, particularly valproate, trimethadione, and phenytoin, are known to increase the risk of having a child with birth defects such as cleft palate, heart problems, or finger and toe defects. For this reason, a woman's doctor may advise switching to other medications during pregnancy. Whenever possible, a woman should allow her doctor enough time to properly change medications, including phasing in the new medications and checking to determine when blood levels are stabilized, before she tries to become pregnant. Women should also begin prenatal vitamin supplements—especially with folic acid, which may reduce the risk of some birth defects—well before pregnancy. Women who discover that they are pregnant but have not already spoken with their doctor about ways to reduce the risks should do so as soon as possible. However, they should continue taking seizure medication as prescribed until that time to avoid preventable seizures. Seizures during pregnancy can harm the developing baby or lead to miscarriage, particularly if the seizures are severe. Nevertheless, many women who have seizures during pregnancy have normal, healthy babies.

Women with epilepsy sometimes experience a change in their seizure frequency during pregnancy, even if they do not change medications. About 25 to 40 percent of women have an increase in their seizure frequency while they are pregnant, while other women may have fewer seizures during pregnancy. The frequency of seizures during pregnancy may be influenced by a variety of factors, including the woman's increased blood volume during pregnancy, which can dilute the effect of medication. Women should have their blood levels of seizure medications monitored closely during and after pregnancy, and the medication dosage should be adjusted accordingly.

Pregnant women with epilepsy should take prenatal vitamins and get plenty of sleep to avoid seizures caused by sleep deprivation. They also should take vitamin K supplements after thirty-four weeks of pregnancy to reduce the risk of a blood-clotting disorder in infants called neonatal coagulopathy that can result from fetal exposure to epilepsy medications. Finally, they should get good prenatal care, avoid tobacco, caffeine, alcohol, and illegal drugs, and try to avoid stress.

Labor and delivery usually proceed normally for women with epilepsy, although there is a slightly increased risk of hemorrhage, eclampsia, premature labor, and cesarean section. Doctors can administer antiepileptic drugs intravenously and monitor blood levels of anticonvulsant medication during labor to reduce the risk that the labor will trigger a seizure. Babies sometimes have symptoms of withdrawal from the mother's seizure medication after they are born, but these problems wear off in a few weeks or months and usually do not cause serious or long-term effects. A mother's blood levels of anticonvulsant medication should be checked frequently after delivery as medication often needs to be decreased.

Epilepsy medications need not influence a woman's decision about breast-feeding her baby. Only minor amounts of epilepsy medications are secreted in breast milk, usually not enough to harm the baby and much less than the baby was exposed to in the womb. On rare occasions, the baby may become excessively drowsy or feed poorly, and these problems should be closely monitored. However, experts believe the benefits of breast-feeding outweigh the risks except in rare circumstances.

To increase doctors' understanding of how different epilepsy medications affect pregnancy and the chances of having a healthy baby, Massachusetts General Hospital has begun a nationwide registry for women who take antiepileptic drugs while pregnant. Women who enroll in this program are given educational materials on pre-conception planning and perinatal care and are asked to provide information about the health of their children (this information is kept confidential). Women and physicians can contact this registry by calling 1-888-233-2334 or 617-726-1742 (fax: 617-724-8307).

Women with epilepsy should be aware that some epilepsy medications can interfere with the effectiveness of oral contraceptives. Women who wish to use oral contraceptives to prevent pregnancy should discuss this with their doctors, who may be able to prescribe a different kind of antiepileptic medication or suggest other ways of avoiding an unplanned pregnancy.

Are there special risks associated with epilepsy?

Although most people with epilepsy lead full, active lives, they are at special risk for two life-threatening conditions: status epilepticus and sudden unexplained death.

Status Epilepticus: Status epilepticus is a potentially life-threatening condition in which a person either has an abnormally prolonged seizure or does not fully regain consciousness between seizures. Although there is no strict definition for the time at which a seizure turns into status epilepticus, most people agree that any seizure lasting longer than five minutes should, for practical purposes, be treated as though it was status epilepticus.

Status epilepticus affects about 195,000 people each year in the United States and results in about 42,000 deaths. While people with epilepsy are at an increased risk for status epilepticus, about 60 percent of people who develop this condition have no previous seizure history. These cases often result from tumors, trauma, or other problems that affect the brain and may themselves be life-threatening.

While most seizures do not require emergency medical treatment, someone with a prolonged seizure lasting more than five minutes may be in status epilepticus and should be taken to an emergency room immediately. It is important to treat a person with status epilepticus as soon as possible. One study showed that 80 percent of people in status epilepticus who received medication within thirty minutes of seizure onset eventually stopped having seizures, whereas only 40 percent recovered if two hours had passed before they received medication. Doctors in a hospital setting can treat status epilepticus with several different drugs and can undertake emergency life-saving measures, such as administering oxygen, if necessary.

People in status epilepticus do not always have severe convulsive seizures. Instead, they may have repeated or prolonged nonconvulsive seizures. This type of status epilepticus may appear as a sustained episode of confusion or agitation in someone who does not ordinarily have that kind of mental impairment. While this type of episode may not seem as severe as convulsive status epilepticus, it should still be treated as an emergency.

Sudden Unexplained Death: For reasons that are poorly understood, people with epilepsy have an increased risk of dying suddenly for no discernible reason. This condition, called sudden unexplained death, can occur in people without epilepsy, but epilepsy increases the risk about twofold. Researchers are still unsure why sudden unexplained death occurs. One study suggested that use of more than two anticonvulsant drugs may be a risk factor. However, it is not clear whether the use of multiple drugs causes the sudden death, or whether people who use multiple anticonvulsants have a greater risk of death because they have more severe types of epilepsy.

What research is being done on epilepsy?

While research has led to many advances in understanding and treating epilepsy, there are many unanswered questions about how and why seizures develop, how they can best be treated or prevented, and how they influence other brain activity and brain development. Researchers, many of whom are supported by the National Institute of Neurological Disorders and Stroke (NINDS), are studying all of these questions. They also are working to identify and test new drugs and other treatments for epilepsy and to learn how those treatments affect brain activity and development.

The NINDS's Anticonvulsant Screening Program (ASP) studies potential new therapies with the goal of enhancing treatment for patients with epilepsy. Since it began in 1975, more than 390 public-private partnerships have been created. These partnerships have resulted in state-of-the-art evaluations of more than twenty-five thousand compounds for their potential as antiepileptic drugs. This government-sponsored effort has contributed to the development of five drugs that are now approved for use in the United States. It has also aided in the discovery and profiling of six new compounds currently in various stages of clinical development. Besides testing for safer, more efficacious therapies, the program is developing and validating new models that may one day find therapies that intervene in the disease process itself as well as models of resistant or refractory epilepsy.

Scientists continue to study how excitatory and inhibitory neurotransmitters interact with brain cells to control nerve firing. They can apply different chemicals to cultures of neurons in laboratory dishes to study how those chemicals influence neuronal activity. They also are studying how glia and other non-neuronal cells in the brain contribute to seizures. This research may lead to new drugs and other new ways of treating seizures.

Researchers also are working to identify genes that may influence epilepsy in some way. Identifying these genes can reveal the underlying chemical processes that influence epilepsy and point to new ways of preventing or treating this disorder. Researchers also can study rats and mice that have missing or abnormal copies of certain genes to determine how these genes affect normal brain development and resistance to damage from disease and other environmental factors. In the future, researchers may be able to use panels of gene fragments, called "gene chips," to determine each person's genetic makeup. This information may allow doctors to prevent epilepsy or to predict which treatments will be most beneficial.

Doctors are now experimenting with several new types of therapies for epilepsy. In one preliminary clinical trial, doctors have begun transplanting fetal pig neurons that produce GABA into the brains of patients to learn whether the cell transplants can help control seizures. Preliminary research suggests that stem cell transplants also may prove beneficial for treating epilepsy. Research showing that the brain undergoes subtle changes prior to a seizure has led to a prototype device that may be able to predict seizures up to three minutes before they begin. If this device works, it could greatly reduce the risk of injury from seizures by allowing people to move to a safe area before their seizures start. This type of device also may be hooked up to a treatment pump or other device that will automatically deliver an antiepileptic drug or an electric impulse to forestall the seizures.

Researchers are continually improving MRI and other brain scans. Pre-surgical brain imaging can guide doctors to abnormal brain tissue and away from essential parts of the brain. Researchers also are using brain scans such as magnetoencephalograms (MEG) and magnetic resonance spectroscopy (MRS) to identify and study subtle problems in the brain that cannot otherwise be detected. Their findings may lead to a better understanding of epilepsy and how it can be treated.

How can I help research on epilepsy?

There are many ways that people with epilepsy and their families can help with research on this disorder. Pregnant women with epilepsy who are taking antiepileptic drugs can help researchers learn how these drugs affect unborn children by participating in the Antiepileptic Drug Pregnancy Registry, which is maintained by the Genetics and Teratology Unit of Massachusetts General Hospital (see section on Pregnancy and Motherhood). People with epilepsy that may be hereditary can aid research by participating in the Epilepsy Gene Discovery Project, which is supported by the Epilepsy Foundation. This project helps to educate people with epilepsy about new genetic research on the disorder and enlists families with hereditary epilepsy for participation in gene research. People who enroll in this project are asked to create a family tree showing which people in their family have or have had epilepsy. Researchers then examine this information to determine if the epilepsy is in fact hereditary, and they may invite participants to enroll in genetic research studies. In many cases, identifying the gene defect responsible for epilepsy in an individual family leads researchers to new clues about how epilepsy develops. It also can provide opportunities for early diagnosis and genetic screening of individuals in the family.

People with epilepsy can help researchers test new medications, surgical techniques, and other treatments by enrolling in clinical trials. Information on clinical trials can be obtained from the NINDS as well as many private pharmaceutical and biotech companies, universities, and other organizations. A person who wishes to participate in a clinical trial must ask his or her regular physician to refer him or her to the doctor in charge of that trial and to forward all necessary medical records. While experimental therapies may benefit those who participate in clinical trials, patients and their families should remember that all clinical trials also involve some risks. Therapies being tested in clinical trials may not work, and in some cases doctors may not yet be sure that the therapies are safe. Patients should be certain they understand the risks before agreeing to participate in a clinical trial.

Patients and their families also can help epilepsy research by donating their brain to a brain bank after death. Brain banks supply researchers with tissue they can use to study epilepsy and other disorders.

What should you do if you see someone having a seizure?

If you see someone having a seizure with convulsions or loss of consciousness, here's how you can help:

1. Roll the person on his or her side to prevent choking on any fluids or vomit.

2. Cushion the person's head.

3. Loosen any tight clothing around the neck.

4. Keep the person's airway open. If necessary, grip the person's jaw gently and tilt his or her head back.

5. Do not restrict the person from moving unless he or she is in danger.

6. Do not put anything into the person's mouth, not even medicine or liquid. These can cause choking or damage to the person's jaw, tongue, or teeth. Contrary to widespread belief, people cannot swallow their tongues during a seizure or any other time.

7. Remove any sharp or solid objects that the person might hit during the seizure.

8. Note how long the seizure lasts and what symptoms occurred so you can tell a doctor or emergency personnel if necessary.

9. Stay with the person until the seizure ends.

Call 911 if:

- The person is pregnant or has diabetes.
- The seizure happened in water.
- The seizure lasts longer than five minutes.
- The person does not begin breathing again or does not return to consciousness after the seizure stops.
- Another seizure starts before the person regains consciousness.
- The person injures himself or herself during the seizure.
- This is a first seizure or you think it might be. If in doubt, check to see if the person has a medical identification card or jewelry stating that he or she has epilepsy or a seizure disorder.

After the seizure ends, the person will probably be groggy and tired. He or she also may have a headache and be confused or embarrassed. Be patient with the person and try to help him or her find a place to rest if he or she is tired or doesn't feel well. If necessary, offer to call a taxi, a friend, or a relative to help the person get home safely.

If you see someone having a nonconvulsive seizure, remember that the person's behavior is not intentional. The person may wander aimlessly or make alarming or unusual gestures. You can help by following these guidelines:

- Remove any dangerous objects from the area around the person or in his or her path.
- Don't try to stop the person from wandering unless he or she is in danger.
- Don't shake the person or shout.
- Stay with the person until he or she is completely alert.

Many people with epilepsy lead productive and outwardly normal lives. Medical and research advances in the past two decades have led to a better understanding of epilepsy and seizures than ever before. Advanced brain scans and other techniques allow greater accuracy in diagnosing epilepsy and determining when a patient may be helped by surgery. More than twenty different medications and a variety of surgical techniques are now available and provide good control of seizures for most people with epilepsy. Other treatment options include the ketogenic diet and the first implantable device, the vagus nerve stimulator. Research on the underlying causes of epilepsy, including identification of genes for some forms of epilepsy and febrile seizures, has led to a greatly improved understanding of epilepsy that may lead to more effective treatments or even new ways of preventing epilepsy in the future.

Section 12.2

Epilepsy: Women's Concerns

Birth Control

Is there any way to be sure that I don't get pregnant?

All available birth control methods can be used by persons with epilepsy. These include:

- **Barriers:** diaphragms, spermicidal vaginal creams, intrauterine devices (IUDs), and condoms;

- **Timing:** the "rhythm method," where intercourse is avoided during a woman's ovulation period, or withdrawal by the man prior to ejaculation [Editor's note: Regarding these methods of birth control, the U.S. Department of Health and Human Services's Office of Disease Prevention and Health Promotion says "their effectiveness in actual use is lower than that for other methods" ("Chapter 9: Family Planning," *Healthy People 2010*, p.5).];

- **Hormonal contraception:** birth control pills, hormone implants, or hormone injections.

Of these, hormonal contraception is the most reliable method for most women, but it is not 100 percent effective, especially in women with epilepsy. Keep in mind that even in the general population there is always a slight chance of an unwanted pregnancy despite appropriate use of contraceptives.

If you have decided that you never want to have children, you can talk to your doctor about an operation called a tubal ligation. This procedure is the most secure way to ensure that you will never become pregnant. If you are in a monogamous relationship (only one male partner) he can have a similar operation, a vasectomy. This would not protect you from pregnancy with other male partners. These are serious decisions, and you need to think about them carefully before choosing either of these procedures.

How do I know which method is best for me?

You need to work with your gynecologist and your neurologist to choose the birth control method that is most appropriate for you. It is possible that your anti-epileptic drug (AED) may make your hormonal birth control less reliable, resulting in an unwanted pregnancy. You and your physicians may consider different combinations of hormonal birth control and seizure medications to find the one that works best for you.

How will my seizure medication affect my hormonal birth control?

There are complex interactions between the hormones (estrogen and progesterone) contained in birth control pills or devices, and some of the medications used to control seizures. Some of these medications increase the breakdown of contraceptive hormones in the body, making them less effective in preventing pregnancy. The seizure medications that have this effect are often called "liver enzyme-inducing" drugs. They are carbamazepine (Tegretol), phenytoin (Dilantin), phenobarbital (Luminal), primidone (Mysoline), and topiramate (Topamax). Valproate (Depakote and Epival) does not increase breakdown of hormones, and may even increase hormonal levels, which may require an adjustment in the dose of your birth control. Gabapentin (Neurontin) and lamotrigine (Lamictal) have no effect on this system and do not interfere with the effectiveness of hormonal birth control.

Are there special concerns about "the pill" for women with epilepsy?

Yes, there are. The popular "mini pill" has a relatively small amount of estrogen (less than 35 micrograms). That's not enough to protect women with epilepsy from becoming pregnant, because many of the commonly prescribed seizure medications reduce the amount of time that hormones are in your bloodstream. You may need contraceptive pills with higher doses of estrogen, and even then, there is a risk of unexpected pregnancy. It is a good idea to use barrier methods (a diaphragm, spermicidal cream, or a condom) in addition to the contraceptive pill, if you are taking one of the seizure medications that speed up the breakdown of the hormones in birth control pills.

Are there problems with other forms of hormonal birth control?

Hormonal implants, like levonorgestrel (Norplant), which is placed under the skin, may not provide effective birth control protection if you are taking certain epilepsy drugs. The medications that cause the most problems with Norplant are the "liver enzyme-inducing" seizure medications such as carbamazepine (Tegretol), phenytoin (Dilantin), phenobarbital (Luminal), primidone (Mysoline), and topiramate (Topamax). These anti-epileptic drugs increase the rate of breakdown of birth control hormones.

Medroxyprogesterone (Depo-Provera) is a hormonal injection used for birth control and it may need to be given more frequently in women with epilepsy taking medications such as those mentioned previously. If you are using one of these forms of birth control, and you take one of the liver enzyme-inducing medications, it is a good idea to use a second barrier method of contraception in addition, such as a diaphragm, a spermicidal cream, or a condom.

Are there any warning signals if my contraception is not working?

Bleeding in the middle of your cycle while you're on hormonal contraception could be a sign that you are ovulating and may become pregnant. If bleeding occurs, ask your doctor to help you select an additional form of contraception such as a diaphragm, spermicidal vaginal cream, or a condom. It is important for you to know that hormonal contraception can fail without mid-cycle bleeding.

Does it matter that my periods aren't regular?

Yes, because it may make hormonal birth control and timing methods more complicated. Usually, irregular menstrual cycles mean that hormones are out of balance in some way. It is important for your gynecologist and your neurologist to know if your periods are irregular so that they can help you choose the best method of contraception. It may be necessary to consult with an endocrinologist, a doctor who specializes in diagnosing and treating hormonal problems.

Will my seizure pattern change if I use hormonal birth control?

Current research does not indicate changes in seizure frequency when women with epilepsy use hormonal birth control, but individual reports suggest they may change. Some women have reported more seizures, some have reported less. If you notice a change in your seizure pattern when you use hormonal birth control, contact your physician.

Pregnancy

Can women with epilepsy have healthy babies?

Yes. In the past, women with epilepsy were discouraged from having children, and, in some cases, were sterilized against their will to prevent pregnancy. Yet public understanding of epilepsy has grown, and the medical community has useful information to share with women who happen to have seizures and want to consider pregnancy. Over 90 percent of women with epilepsy who choose to become pregnant have healthy babies. However, there may be special concerns for women with epilepsy to consider.

Do women with epilepsy have problems getting pregnant?

Overall, women with epilepsy have fewer children than other women. This may be partly personal choice, but research has indicated that women with epilepsy have a higher rate of menstrual cycle irregularities and other gynecological problems that may interfere with fertility. It is important that you talk with your gynecologist/obstetrician and your neurologist before getting pregnant, if possible. Your epilepsy can affect the pregnancy, and pregnancy can change your seizure pattern and how your body uses anti-epileptic drugs (AEDs). There is a slight risk that epilepsy or your seizure medication may have adverse effects on your baby. There are important prenatal vitamins containing folic acid that should be taken prior to getting pregnant, as some of the potential problems with your baby occur in the first few weeks of pregnancy, often before you realize you are pregnant. Check with your doctor about the exact dose of the folic acid supplement. You and your physicians can plan together about medication changes, and other factors that can make your pregnancy as safe as possible for you and your baby.

How can pregnancy affect my seizures?

Up to one-third of women with epilepsy who become pregnant will have increased seizures during their pregnancy despite continued use of antiepileptic medication. During pregnancy, concentrations of seizure medication in your bloodstream may change or decrease, putting you at greater risk for seizures.

Your physician may need to check blood levels of your medication more frequently, and may need to adjust your dose.

The weeks right after delivery are another time when your hormones and your body chemistry may change, affecting levels of your seizure medication. Extra lab work may be necessary.

Is it true that medication taken for seizures may affect my child?

Women with epilepsy do have a greater risk of having a baby with certain kinds of birth defects. The rate is 4–6 percent for women with epilepsy, compared with a rate of 2–3 percent in the general population. We do not understand all the reasons for this difference. Some of the malformations may be caused by your seizure medication, or by your epilepsy, and for some we have no good explanation. Some may be due to inherited traits within a specific family, and genetic counseling may be helpful to you in assessing your risk. It is important to remember that even with the increased rate of certain kinds of birth defects, women with epilepsy who become pregnant have a better than 90 percent chance of having a healthy baby.

Should I stop my anti-epileptic medication before I get pregnant?

This is a complicated decision. Pregnancy without anti-epileptic medication might lessen some of the possible risks to the baby. If a woman has been seizure-free for many years, it may be possible for her and the physician to slowly discontinue medication before she attempts to become pregnant. Remember, you should never stop your seizure medication without the advice and supervision of your doctor.

However, the danger of seizures to both the mother and the child is a serious one. Seizures can result in falls, or cause oxygen deficiency for the baby. They can increase the risk of miscarriage or stillbirths. For most women with epilepsy, staying on medications poses less risk to their own health and the health of their babies than discontinuing medication and the subsequent risk of having uncontrolled seizures.

In most cases, a single medication at the lowest possible dose that provides seizure control is the best option.

Are there other problems to consider besides my epilepsy?

Yes, women with epilepsy are more likely to have morning sickness and vaginal bleeding during pregnancy. There is an increased risk for premature labor and delivery. Sometimes labor does not progress normally, and more women with epilepsy need to have cesarean sections to deliver their babies than other women.

There is a small risk that your baby will develop a bleeding problem in the first twenty-four hours after birth. Women with epilepsy are often given oral vitamin K supplements during the last month of pregnancy to lessen the chances of this happening to their babies.

I'm taking birth control pills now. What if I get pregnant without meaning to?

If you have doubts about your birth control method, talk to your physician or nurse about alternatives.

Contact your physician immediately about an unplanned pregnancy. For any woman, the early weeks of pregnancy pose the greatest risk of possible birth defects. Since the risk for women with epilepsy is even higher, it is important to have early prenatal care. Your physician can talk to you about tests that may detect some types of early malformations, and refer you for genetic counseling if necessary.

Parenting Concerns

I am pregnant. How can I keep my child safe and healthy?

Epilepsy affects people in different ways. Some parents will need to make several changes in their lives to provide a safe environment for the baby. Others will need to make very few changes. It is helpful to think about your personal seizure pattern and the specific risks or problems that you might have. Then choose lifestyle adaptations that will provide solutions for you. Every prospective parent has to think through issues like these. There may be additional factors for people with epilepsy to consider.

During pregnancy and after delivery, the best thing you can do for your baby is to take good care of yourself. Get enough sleep, eat well, exercise regularly, and take your prescribed seizure medication. Keep in close contact with your neurologist and your gynecologist/obstetrician, and talk with them about necessary adjustments in your lifestyle.

Do I need to be concerned about my seizure pattern?

It depends on your seizure type, and the frequency of your seizures. It may be helpful to ask yourself, "Do I fall with my seizures? Do I lose consciousness? Do I get a warning?" Some women with epilepsy may have changes in their seizures while they are pregnant. During pregnancy, concentrations of your anti-epileptic drug (AED) may change or decrease, putting you at greater risk for seizures. After delivery, medication levels in your bloodstream tend to rise, increasing the possibility of side effects. These factors may make it necessary for your physician to check medication blood levels more frequently in the first few months after delivery.

I want to breast-feed my baby. Will that be safe?

For most women with epilepsy, breast-feeding is a safe option. All seizure medications will be found in small amounts in breast milk, but this usually does not affect the baby. Some women who are taking phenobarbital (Luminol) or primidone (Mysoline) may notice that their babies are too sleepy or irritable. If this is a significant problem, ask your physician or the pediatrician about supplemental bottle feedings. Breast-feeding may create more demands on you, particularly at night, with loss of sleep. Explore all your options including bottle-feeding, or a combination of breast and bottle, to find what works best for you.

Can I manage alone?

The birth of a baby is a monumental event for any woman! It changes your life, and the first few weeks can seem overwhelming. Every mother has disturbed sleep, extra work, and hormonal changes—and for a woman with epilepsy these factors can increase the risk of seizures. So it makes sense to include other family members or friends in the care of your baby. That will give you a chance to rest. The best way to take care of your baby is to take good care of yourself.

I often fall during my seizures. What if I have a seizure while I'm feeding my baby?

Feed your baby in a comfortable chair, or on your bed with good back support. Or feed the baby while seated on a pad on the floor. Keep the baby next to your bed at night, and feed him or her in bed with you. If you are using a bottle, have a family member help you— one of you can hold the baby and the other can fix the bottle. If you are alone, don't carry the baby to the kitchen—leave your baby in the crib while you prepare the bottle and bring it back. When your baby is older, always strap him or her into a high chair or infant seat for feedings.

What is the best way to diaper my baby?

The safest way to dress or diaper a newborn is to sit on the floor with a pad. A changing table is not as safe, but if you use one, be sure to strap your baby on securely. Keep diapers and infant care supplies on every level of the house to limit stair climbing.

How can I safely give my baby a bath?

If you are using a tub, it makes sense to have another person with you when you bathe your baby. When you're alone, give sponge baths on the floor, with a separate bowl of water.

I want to have my baby with me, but I often have seizures. What should I do?

Use an "umbrella stroller" in the house, instead of carrying your baby. Keep toys and baby supplies in different areas of the house so they are there when you need them. Use a playpen or other enclosed area to provide a safe place for your baby to sleep and play when you are caring for him or her by yourself.

Are there household chores that might be dangerous?

Yes. Avoid holding your baby while you are cooking. If you have frequent seizures, use a microwave when you're alone. Delay ironing or other potentially dangerous activities until another person is there.

Once my baby starts to walk, how can I keep him or her safe if I have a seizure?

There are many childcare books that give parents advice about "child-proofing" a home. It helps to get down on the floor and look at the world like your toddler does. Added factors you need to consider are what happens when you have a seizure, and how often you have seizures. Think about what might happen if you were confused or lost consciousness, even briefly.

Keep outside doors locked, and close inside doors to rooms where your toddler could hurt him- or herself (kitchen or bathroom) if you lose consciousness during a seizure. Use a safety gate across stairs, cover electrical outlets, and get childproof latches for drawers and cabinets (especially ones where you store medication, sharp objects, or other dangerous substances). Consider an enclosed play area, in the house and outside, where your child can be safe if you have a seizure while you are alone with him or her. When your child is ready to be toilet-trained, try a child-size "potty chair," not a booster seat on the toilet. Whenever your child is in the bathroom, be sure the toilet is covered and cabinets and drawers are locked.

How can I keep my toddler from walking away if I have a seizure?

If you have seizures that make you confused or unaware, consider using a stroller, a child safety harness, or a wrist bungee cord to keep your child nearby, both at home and when you are outside. This may reduce the risk of your child wandering away if you have a seizure and no one else is there.

How should I tell my child about my epilepsy?

Explain your condition in simple words that your child can understand. Let him or her know that between seizures you are healthy and normal. As your child gets older, it may help everyone feel more secure to have "seizure drills"—to practice seizure first aid and how to call for help. If your child is fearful about seizures, talk about it and answer questions honestly. Ask your physician or nurse for more information.

Sexual Relationships

What makes a person want to have sex?

Sexual relationships are a normal part of healthy living. Three things lead to sexual activity: first there is desire—wanting to have sex with a partner. When that feeling is strong, there is arousal—the physical feeling that you "need" to have sex. Finally, there is orgasm—the height of physical pleasure during intercourse. These processes depend on many reflexes that are coordinated by the nervous system, and involve hormones, nerves, and blood vessels.

How often should a person have sex?

The desire for sex varies widely in the general population and in people with epilepsy. A person who does not think about sex or want to have sex one to three times a month probably has unusually low sexual desire. But remember, this is a very personal matter, and if you are satisfied with your level of sexual activity, you have no problem.

Could my epilepsy cause problems when I'm sexually active?

We do not yet fully understand all the complex causes for sexual problems, especially how they may be related to epilepsy. For example, some people have a low level of sexual desire; others have difficulty becoming sexually aroused; or intercourse can be painful for some women. It is not unusual for people to have problems with sexual performance at times, and people with epilepsy are no exception. However, people with complex partial seizures, particularly when the seizures start in the temporal lobe, seem to have more sexual problems, such as the ones listed here.

I would like to have a close relationship with another person, but I'm afraid to have sex. Is that unusual?

No. Low self-esteem or cosmetic effects from medication may make women and men with epilepsy feel sexually unattractive. Those feelings can lead to a lack of sexual desire and arousal. Acceptance of yourself and your epilepsy are important in developing an intimate relationship with another person. Perhaps you are afraid you might have a seizure during intercourse. Seizures often involve the same areas of the brain that are important to maintaining healthy sexual function, and some of the sensations felt during lovemaking can be similar to those experienced during auras or simple partial seizures.

I don't like sex because it hurts. What can I do?

Many women with epilepsy say that intercourse is painful for them. This is especially common in people who have temporal lobe epilepsy. Painful intercourse can be caused by dryness of the vagina or painful vaginal spasms during intercourse. Ask your physician about creams or gels for lubricating the vagina to ease the discomfort of intercourse. Gynecologists can do gradual dilations of the vaginal opening for women who have severe problems with pain and spasm.

Do men with epilepsy have sexual problems too?

Yes, almost a third of all men with epilepsy have difficulty achieving and maintaining an erection. Specialists called urologists offer help to men with sexual problems, including some medications that ease problems with erection.

Can seizures have anything to do with how I feel about sex?

Yes, they may. When seizures are under control, people seem to have improved sexual desire and performance. Any of the anti-epileptic drugs (AEDs) can possibly cause sexual difficulties. However, this reaction to one medication does not mean you will have the same experience with another. Talk with your doctor about trying another anti-convulsant medication for your seizures if you suspect this is a part of your sexual problem.

Hormones play an important role in sexual function and some people with epilepsy have alterations in normal hormone levels. Both seizures and epilepsy medicine can interfere with the way your body uses hormones, resulting in sexual problems. You may need referral to an endocrine specialist to sort out the complex interactions between hormones, seizures, and medications.

I am embarrassed to talk to my doctor about sex. What can I do?

It may be difficult, but it is very important to talk to your doctor about sexual difficulties. In addition to epilepsy, there are other causes for sexual dysfunction that can be diagnosed and treated (medical conditions like diabetes, thyroid disorders, or high blood pressure). Your physician may ask questions about religious beliefs, uncomfortable experiences in your past related to sex, any stress or recent illness, and details of your sexual relationships. These are private, personal issues, but it is important to share the information openly, to help your doctor understand your problems and provide the appropriate help in solving them.

I've heard about sex therapy. Would that help?

Talking about your sexual difficulties with a trained therapist can be very helpful. Sometimes, anxiety or depression is causing problems with sex. It is often important to bring your partner for couples therapy. Some people need information about sexual feelings and activities and suggestions for making their relationship more pleasurable.

Menopause and Epilepsy

In general, we need more information to determine how seizures are affected by the changes in women's bodies during and after menopause. Currently, little is known about how physical changes associated with this stage of life cause increases or decreases in seizures or what precise relationship exists, if any. There are, however, a few indicators that may aid in prediction and there are some studies that measure how commonly women experience onset, exacerbation, or diminishment of seizures during this time.

Menopause

Although it has been suggested that women with epilepsy experience menopause earlier than on average, the relationship has not been established. Many women report that their seizure frequency reduces or does not change during and after menopause. A minority of women with epilepsy report that their seizures increase during menopause. The reasons for these changes are not clear.

Everything has been reported to happen during menopause:

- no change in seizures
- a recurrence of previously well controlled seizures
- a worsening of seizures
- the first-time appearance of seizures
- improvement of seizures

Most studies show that hormones influence seizures in women. Therefore, menopause has been associated with changes in seizures in many individual women. Menopause may be an unrecognized factor for some new-onset seizures. More research is needed for this life-stage and its relationship to seizure disorders.

There have been documented patterns of seizure changes in women during menopause. Some suggest that women with epilepsy who are menopausal should be considered in two separate groups:

- perimenopausal (the early stages of menopause), and
- postmenopausal (having had no periods for years)

Studies show that seizures are less likely to improve noticeably if:

- seizures begin early in your life
- seizures have never been well controlled
- you have tonic-clonic, or complex partial seizures
- you are early in your menopausal stage. This is for hormonal reasons. There may be altered estrogen: progesterone ratios at the beginning of menopause. When a woman moves into the perimenopausal period, there may be an exacerbation of seizures. When you reach menopause itself (at least one year of not having periods), the seizures may improve, because estrogen production may be extremely low or undetectable.

Anecdotal reports suggest seizures that are most likely to improve are:

- seizures that occur later in life, prior to menopause (therefore in a catamenial pattern);
- seizures that have been well controlled throughout life.

Osteoporosis

Antiepileptic drugs are a risk factor for developing osteoporosis. Women with epilepsy who are taking antiepileptic drugs should ask their health care practitioners about this risk and should take preventative measures. These might involve changes in diet, the use of vitamins, and exercise programs. If you are taking antiepileptic drugs, you should be evaluated for osteoporosis as you mature.

Section 12.3

Epilepsy in the Elderly

In the twentieth century, we witnessed a dramatic increase in the incidence of senior epilepsy, especially in people eighty-five years and older. Until recently, epilepsy was believed to be predominantly a childhood disorder. Research now shows that the incidence of epilepsy in people age seventy-five and over is higher than in the first ten years of life. In fact, statistics have illustrated that approximately 7 percent of seniors have epilepsy.

Due to the large "baby boomer" generation, there will be an anticipated increase in the number of senior citizens in the near future. For this reason, epilepsy occurrence and diagnosis in seniors is an issue that must not be ignored. Being diagnosed with epilepsy at any age takes getting used to. Seniors diagnosed with epilepsy have unique and sometimes shattered expectations for themselves, as many were raised to believe that epilepsy is something to be kept quiet.

People with seizure disorders often find themselves having to lead a different lifestyle than the one they have grown used to over the years. Metabolism changes with age, which means that treatments will affect different people in different ways. As a result of the changes, everyone who loves and cares for a senior with epilepsy will find their lives affected by the disorder.

With patience and the willingness to learn about epilepsy in seniors, we can look beyond ignorance and mistreatment. This section of the chapter will explore current issues concerning seniors today, and offer suggestions for an improved quality of life.

Causes and Diagnosis

How Does One Recognize the Signs of Epilepsy?

Acute and chronic states of confusion, dizziness, and amnesia ordinarily appear in a large number of seniors, but they are also common symptoms of a seizure disorder. The actual causes of epilepsy in seniors are unknown in almost half of the cases.

There are a number of reasons why a person develops epilepsy. Seizures experienced by seniors may be either an ongoing challenge or the return of a seizure disorder that was in remission.

At any age, epilepsy may be caused by:

- infections in the brain and central nervous system (encephalitis or meningitis)
- multiple drug therapy
- severe brain injury from accidents or other head trauma
- certain genetic conditions

Causes of Epilepsy Related to Aging

- **Nervous System:** The nervous system changes as people grow older, making seniors more susceptible to abnormal electric discharges in the brain (seizures).

- **Stroke:** This is the most frequent cause of epilepsy in seniors. Arteries narrow or clog with age, which results in deprivation of blood and oxygen in some parts of the brain. Sometimes bleeding occurs in the brain. This can also result in damage that causes seizures.

- **Heart Attacks:** Oxygen carried to the brain can be cut off temporarily, resulting in damage that can produce seizures.

- **Disease:** Alzheimer's and other brain diseases alter the internal structure of the brain and therefore may be likely to induce seizure activity. Other diseases, such as complications of kidney disease, liver disease, alcoholism, and diabetes, increase the likelihood of seizures in seniors.

- **Brain Tumors:** Any kind of tumor may cause seizures. Sometimes, the removal of a tumor stops seizures.

- **Surgery:** Scars left from an operation may cause seizures later in life.

Preventative Measures: Healthy Tips for People over Sixty

- Maintain a good level of blood pressure to reduce the chance of stroke.

- Eat a diet low in fat, sugar, and salt to reduce the chance of heart problems.

- Use canes and walkers when necessary to avoid accidental falls.

- Be cautious if drinking alcoholic beverages.

- If you smoke, consider quitting.

- Use a microwave oven instead of a stove or kettle for cooking and for heating water.

- Lower the temperature of the water heater to prevent scalds.

- Ensure that a television is in good working order. To reduce contrast, always have a light on in the room, situated above and behind you. Watch television at a distance of at least 3 meters [10 feet], at a 45° angle.

- If you drive, make sure that your eyesight and reflexes are sufficient.

- Discuss the medications you are taking with your doctor regularly.

- Wear a MedicAlert™ or similar bracelet.

- Ask for help. It may be difficult. Counseling is a great idea to help you to identify your needs and risks, and to advocate for yourself.

- Inform your neighbors of your epilepsy, outlining the type(s) of seizures you experience and what they can do to assist you, should the need arise.

Medications for Seniors with Epilepsy

Seniors may take several medications, both prescription and non-prescription, at one time. The distribution of any drug in the body changes with age as the body fat content increases and muscle mass decreases. As a result, the absorption, distribution, metabolism, and excretion of medications are all affected. This is why checking the level of medication in your blood regularly becomes important as you grow older.

Everybody reacts differently to medicine; some people are more sensitive to the effects of a drug than others. Consequently, antiepileptic drugs (AEDs) have different effects on everyone. You may find that your AED has reduced the frequency and severity of your seizures, or perhaps it has stopped seizure activity completely.

Choosing an Antiepileptic Drug

Choosing the right medication takes time and a willingness to be open and honest with your doctor. You and your health care provider must have a common understanding of your general health and the nature of every medication you are presently taking. Some drugs should not be taken simultaneously. This means that your doctor will have to know your entire medical history in order to prescribe the right medication for you.

Communication with your family and caregivers is most important. Your partner, adult children, and caregivers should understand the goals of your treatment, the possible side effects of your AEDs, and your monitoring strategies. Communicating clearly will eliminate confusion and feelings of helplessness when you need support.

Everyone's AED dosage may be different, depending on the severity of their seizures, the other drugs they are taking, and allergies. If you are not completely honest about your medical history, the dosage prescribed may be wrong and could be a dangerous amount. With the wrong prescription, you may experience symptoms of sedation or hyperactivity, a disruption in vision and balance, and states of confusion, among other side effects.

It is always a good idea to carry a list with you of the medications you are presently taking.

Stopping Medication

Do not stop taking your medication without consulting your doctor first.

Abruptly stopping an AED may cause serious rebound seizures and can even be life threatening. If you are experiencing problems with your AED, talk to your neurologist about it. You may consider other treatment options together.

Compliance: Remembering Your Medication

Multiple medications can be overwhelming, especially when they must be taken at scheduled times every day. Sometimes it is easy to forget the last time you took your medication or when the next dosage should be taken. To avoid missing dosages or double dosing, try using memory aids. Your family and friends can assist you.

Suggestions for Memory Aids

- Use divided, labeled pill containers. If you cannot find one that suits your needs, label it yourself.

- Wear a wristwatch with an alarm set to sound when you should take your next dose.

- Try to make a routine: if you need to take a pill when you wake up in the morning, always bring one to the breakfast table with you.

- Post a schedule of what medications you should take and when to take them.

- Let friends and relatives know medication times and where the medication is stored.

- Schedule more frequent visits to your doctor as a motivator to stick with your drug regimen.

- If these strategies fail, consult your physician. It may be possible to switch to another AED with a simpler dosing regimen.

Sometimes medication is not taken properly for reasons other than memory.

- Many seniors find it difficult to read small print, as is always found on the label of a pill container. If this keeps you from reading the instructions to take your medication, ask your doctor and pharmacist if it is possible to use large print on the label.

- To avoid confusion, ask for the prescriptions to be fully and clearly labeled. Usually, a pamphlet or information about the drug is given to a patient. Make sure you are given the information you need to know.

- If you have arthritis, ask for a container with a cap that is easy to open.

Financial constraints sometimes force seniors to withhold food as well as their medication. People on low or fixed incomes who have small pensions often try to make their medication last longer by taking fewer pills than they are supposed to.

If you are suffering from this problem, tell someone. Your doctor may be able to suggest something. Perhaps you qualify for certain government pensions you do not know about. Either way, your medication must be taken as directed in order to stop the seizure activity.

Risks in Taking Multiple Medications

On average, seniors take approximately seven drugs a day. As you grow older, taking multiple medications becomes more of a risk. This need not be a problem, though: careful planning on your doctor's part will result in proper treatment. Agreeing to take proper care with your medications on your part should yield better health.

Factors when Taking Multiple Medications

• **Physical/Physiological Changes:** With age, the liver becomes less efficient at breaking down drugs and the kidneys may be less efficient at excreting waste. This can result in drug accumulation in the body. Other physiological changes may affect sleep (medications may make a person need to sleep more), sexuality (some AEDs affect sexual function), and overall nutritional (appetite alters with medications, as well as with age) and metabolic patterns.

• **Drug Interactions:** Other medications can increase the likelihood of drug interaction. As the body ages, changes occur in the immune system and in the ratio of body fat. As well, the brain and the nervous system become more sensitive to drugs. These factors increase the likelihood of adverse drug reactions.

• **Compliance:** Some seniors may not be able to take proper care of their medications. Misuse may result from misinformation about the drug or vague instructions about its use. A declining memory and intellect due to aging also contribute to the misuse of antiepileptic drugs. Some seniors may not be able to remember whether they have already taken their medication at the proper time, bringing the risk of double dosage. Furthermore, if a senior is taking multiple medications in addition to AEDs, which is very common, general confusion and temporary memory loss may arise, especially if one of the drugs taken is sedative.

Section 12.4

Understanding Vagus Nerve Stimulation

Seizures are caused by electrical events in the brain that occur when there is a brief disturbance in the way the brain's electrical system works. Vagal nerve stimulation (VNS) is a surgical treatment that reduces the frequency and duration of seizures in certain patients diagnosed with epilepsy. VNS was first introduced experimentally in 1988. By the mid 1990s, the safety and efficacy of VNS was firmly established through numerous clinical trials across North America and Europe.

VNS uses regular pulses of electrical energy to prevent or interrupt the electrical disturbances in the brain, thus decreasing the frequency and duration of seizures. The vagus nerve originates in the brainstem (where the brain becomes the spinal cord) and travels through the neck into the chest and abdomen. It is one of the longest nerves in the human body, and it affects a large number of bodily functions including speech, swallowing, heart rate, and digestion. Every person has two vagal nerves, one for each side of the body. VNS therapy involves the left vagus nerve, and the stimulation is applied to the nerve as it passes through the middle of the neck or "mid-cervical" region.

The electrical signals to the vagus nerve come from a thin, round pulse generator—a battery—about the size of a pocket watch. The device is usually implanted under the skin on the upper left side of the chest. A flexible, insulated plastic tube containing electrodes runs under the skin from the little generator and connects to the left vagus nerve on the left side of the neck.

VNS has been found effective in controlling some epilepsies when anti-epileptic drugs have been inadequate, their side effects intolerable, or neurosurgery has not been an option. In some cases, VNS has also been effective in stopping seizures.

VNS is currently approved in more than twenty countries.

How Does Vagal Nerve Stimulation Control Seizures?

The exact mechanism by which VNS prevents or inhibits seizure formation is currently unknown. However, what is known is that VNS works by interfering with the electrical activity of the brain. Epileptic seizures are associated with highly synchronized, characteristic patterns of brain wave activity. The vagus nerve disrupts these synchronized brain wave patterns by providing a sudden stimulation to the vagal nerve, which carries the impulse from the neck back up to the brain. Therefore, with every stimulation from the pulse generator, epileptic electrical activity may be interrupted, thus preventing a seizure before it occurs. This would explain why manually activating the pulse generator (with a hand-held magnet) at the onset of an aura is often effective at preventing progression to a seizure.

VNS Surgery

Implanting the VNS battery in a patient and connecting it to the vagus nerve takes approximately an hour. The procedure is usually done under general anesthesia, and can be done on an inpatient or outpatient basis. Two incisions are required, one in the neck to gain access to the vagal nerve, and one below the collarbone in the chest wall or armpit. A 5–6 cm incision is made below the collarbone where the pulse generator is inserted into a pocket of fat between the surface of the skin and the ribs of the chest wall. After the pulse generator is in place, the surgeon threads a plastic tube containing the electrodes from the neck to the generator in the chest. Then, the surgeon gently wraps the flexible ends of silicone-coated electrodes around the vagus nerve.

Programming the Device

The device is programmed to begin stimulation at one to two weeks after surgery. Programming is performed with the aid of a computer and a "programming wand." The wand is held above the chest directly over the pulse generator (the procedure is completely noninvasive). Doctors program the device to deliver pulses of electrical stimulation automatically, twenty-four hours a day. The device can be reprogrammed as many times as necessary. It is important to note that the system is not designed to provide constant stimulation, but rather to generate a series of short, repeated electrical impulses. The device usually gives the patient a stimulation for about thirty seconds on and five minutes off, but settings may vary. This occurs automatically throughout the day during both wake and sleep. The device continues the cycle until the neurologist reprograms it or until the battery runs out, usually in about six years. In addition, the patient can manually trigger a stimulus at any time, or turn the device off altogether, by holding a hand-held magnet over the pulse generator. When the battery runs out, another surgical procedure is required, which involves the chest only.

Monitoring Treatment

After the surgery, the doctor schedules a series of follow-up visits. At first, a person with a new VNS implant may see the doctor every two weeks. Later, if everything is going well, the doctor may schedule the visits every two to six months, or as needed.

The manufacturer of the device recommends that people being treated with VNS visit their doctors at least every six months throughout the life of the device.

Also, people who have the VNS implant should let their doctor know if at any time the device becomes uncomfortable, if the stimulation seems to be coming on too often, if it seems to have stopped altogether, or if they have any concerns about its operation or effects.

Some people worry that their body may reject the VNS device; however, rejection is not a problem because the device is made of titanium. Titanium is a material that is widely used for pacemakers and does not trigger an immune response. If the device has to be removed, it is usually because it is not effective or, in about 1 percent of cases, it is due to malfunction or infection.

How Well Does VNS Work?

The efficacy of VNS varies widely from patient to patient. It is hard to know in advance how someone with epilepsy will respond to the VNS therapy. In some people with epilepsy, their seizures are eliminated completely, but in others the device may have no effect.

Studies have shown that one-third of VNS patients will experience a major improvement in seizure control (i.e., greater than 50 percent reduction in seizure frequency), one-third will experience a moderate improvement in seizure control, and one-third will continue to have seizures as before the device was implanted.

Please remember that improvement may not happen overnight; it usually takes time. Several months may go by before there is any change, followed by a slow but steady improvement.

Safety and Side Effects

The VNS implant has not yet been officially approved for use in children less than twelve years old, pregnant women, or the elderly (more than sixty years of age).

The most common side effects associated with the VNS implant are hoarseness, breathlessness, voice change, coughing, and sore throat. These side effects occur only when the stimulator is "on." Most of the side effects usually become less noticeable with time. In addition, smoking has been shown to worsen the hoarseness, sore throat, and inflammation. As well, patients with chronic obstructive pulmonary disease may have an increased risk of shortness of breath.

Other less common side effects reported in clinical trials include: lack of coordination of voluntary muscles, difficulty swallowing, aspiration (inhaling fluid into the lungs), insomnia, indigestion, infection, inflammation of the throat, twitching, nausea, vomiting, pain, and prickling or decreased skin sensation.

There are also side effects associated with the surgery itself. These are rare, and include: blood clots, damage to nerves or blood vessels in the neck, facial paralysis, foreign body reaction to the implant, scarring or infection at the incision site, fever, muscle pain, and ringing in the ears.

Furthermore, after the device is implanted, any trauma to the chest or neck may result in damage to the pulse generator or disconnection of the leads. This can damage the vagus nerve or inactivate the device, resulting in increased seizure frequency.

The mode of action of VNS is still unknown. It is, therefore, difficult to determine which medications (if any) might cause adverse reactions for VNS patients.

Summary Chart of the Major Advantages and Disadvantages of VNS

Table 12.1 is a brief summary of the major benefits and concerns associated with vagal nerve stimulation. Please note that important issues of safety and risk associated with the surgery itself are not included in the table, and should be discussed with your physician. No two patients are the same, and actual benefits and side effects experienced will vary greatly from patient to patient.

Table 12.1. Major Advantages and Disadvantages of VNS (*continued on next page*)

Advantages	Disadvantages
A potentially effective therapy for the treatment of partial seizures (with or without generalization) or generalized seizures.	Surgical procedure required (involves a general anesthesia and overnight stay at the hospital).
Nonpharmacological option for patients with intractable or inoperable seizures.	Contraindicated in patients after a bilateral or left cervical vagotomy, or in patients with cardiac conduction defects.
May generally reduce frequency or duration of seizures, and shorten the length of the post-ictal period.	Two-thirds of patients will experience light or no reduction in frequency or duration of seizures.
May eliminate the need for antiepileptic medications (AEDs), or reduce the required dose.	Most patients still require AEDs for optimal control of seizures (all AEDs continue for at least three months following implantation).
Improvement is both short-term (months) and long-term (years).	Long term commitment may be required to see improvement.
The device maintains its constant stimulation cycle without any effort or assistance from the patient.	Stimulation pulses are often notice able, and may lead to hoarseness of voice, breathlessness, or swallowing difficulties.
For patients who experience auras, seizures may be averted at onset by use of the hand-held magnet.	The magnet may have no effect.
The magnet may be used to stop stimulation momentarily (i.e., to prevent hoarseness while singing) or to inactivate the device continuously (i.e., if patient experiences stimulation-induced pain or discomfort).	Continuous or frequent magnet use will use up the battery and could potentially cause damage to the left vagus nerve.
The pulse generator is not affected by microwave ovens, power lines, metal detectors, or cellular phones.	The pulse generator is adversely affected by MRI, therapeutic radiation, external defibrillation, strong magnets, and hair clippers. The unit may interfere with transistor radios, hearing aids, cardiac pacemakers, and defibrillators.

Table 12.1. Major Advantages and Disadvantages of VNS (*continued from previous page*)

Advantages	Disadvantages
A special "magnet guard" will be provided for the hand-held horseshoe magnet.	The magnet may damage televisions, computer disks, and credit cards, and should be kept away from these items at all times.
An irregular stimulation will alert the patient that the battery is approaching exhaustion.	The pulse generator will require surgical replacement when the battery runs out, at significant cost to the patient.
The intensity of the stimulation can be individualized to the needs and tolerance of each patient.	Programming of the device will require several follow-up appointments, and should be performed by only a qualified, experienced physician.

Source: The above summary chart of the major advantages and disadvantages of VNS was compiled by Epilepsy Kingston & Area, Ontario, Canada, and is reproduced with permission.

What Will the VNS Implant Cost?

The implant device alone costs $14,000 (Canadian). It is important to note that the implant has to be replaced when the batteries run out, and the replacement is as expensive as the original implant. The full implant including the entire surgical procedure and hospital stay costs approximately $29,000 (Canadian). [Information provided by Irene Elliot at the Hospital for Sick Children in Toronto, Ontario, Canada.]

Using the Magnet

The magnet involved in the VNS treatment allows the patient some control over the device and how it works. The special, thin blocked magnet is attached to a strap. It can be worn on the wrist like a watch, or clipped to a belt like a pager. Although the VNS system delivers stimulation automatically in regular pulses all the time, the magnet can be used to deliver extra electronic stimulation in between cycles. The patient does this by passing the magnet over the area of the chest where the VNS device is implanted.

Tips on Handling the Magnet

- Don't place or store the magnet near credit cards, televisions, computers, computer disks, microwave ovens, or other magnets. Keep it at least ten inches away from these items.

- Do not drop the magnet. It can break if it falls on a hard surface.

- Carry the magnet with you. If your seizures stop or are shorter when the extra stimulation is turned on, show family members or caregivers how to use the magnet when you have a seizure.

- Ask your doctor about how much and for how long you can safely use the magnet to activate the device.

Who Is Using VNS?

The VNS system was approved for people with partial onset seizures—seizures that begin in one part of the brain. VNS is intended for people whose seizures do not respond to medications and who are either not good candidates for brain surgery or don't want to have brain surgery. People who are considering VNS must not have any other medical conditions that might be affected by the device. For example, VNS should not be used in people who have had certain throat operations or disorders affecting the throat.

Currently, about ten thousand people have received the VNS system, including about 33 percent under the age of eighteen. A registry system that tracks about five thousand people living with VNS includes about 60 percent with partial seizures; 15 percent with Lennox Gastaut Syndrome (mixed seizures); and 25 percent with generalized seizures.

Section 12.5

Ketogenic Diet

The ketogenic diet is a special high-fat, low-carbohydrate diet that helps to control seizures in some people with epilepsy. It is prescribed by a physician. It is not the same as other popular low-carbohydrate diets, such as the Atkins diet.

The name *ketogenic* means that it produces ketones in the body (keto = ketone, genic = producing). Ketones are formed when the body uses fat for its source of energy. Usually the body usually uses carbohydrates (such as sugar, bread, pasta) for its fuel, but because the ketogenic diet is very low in carbohydrates, fats become the primary fuel instead. Ketones are not dangerous. They can be detected in the urine.

Who will it help?

Doctors usually recommend the ketogenic diet for children whose seizures have not responded to several different seizure medicines. It is particularly recommended for children with the Lennox-Gastaut syndrome.

Doctors seldom recommend the ketogenic diet for adults. When it has been tried with adults, it doesn't seem to work nearly as well. The reasons for this difference are unclear.

What is it like?

The typical ketogenic diet, called the "long-chain triglyceride diet," provides 3 to 4 grams of fat for every 1 gram of carbohydrate and protein. The dietitian recommends a daily diet that contains 75 to 100 calories for every kilogram (2.2 pounds) of body weight and 1 to 2 grams of protein for every kilogram of body weight. If this sounds complicated, it is! That's why parents need a dietitian's help.

The kinds of foods that provide fat for the ketogenic diet are butter, cream, mayonnaise, and peanut butter. Because the amount of carbohydrate and protein in the diet have to be restricted, it is very important that the meals be prepared carefully. No other sources of carbohydrates can be eaten. (Even toothpaste might have some sugar in it!) For this reason, the ketogenic diet is supervised by a dietitian. The parents and the child become very familiar with what can and cannot be eaten.

What happens first?

Typically the diet is started in the hospital. The child usually begins by fasting (except for water) under close medical supervision for thirty-eight hours (twenty-four hours for infants). For instance, the child might go into the hospital on Monday, start fasting at 6 p.m., and continue to have only water until 8 a.m. on Wednesday. Then the child's urine is tested to see if it shows ketones. If ketones are found, the diet is then begun. The child stays in the hospital for another two to three days for close monitoring. During this time, the parents are taught more about the diet.

Does it work?

Several studies have shown that the ketogenic diet does reduce or prevent seizures in many children whose seizures could not be controlled by medications. Over half of the children who go on the diet have at least a 50 percent reduction in the number of their seizures. Some children even become seizure-free.

Children who are on the ketogenic diet continue to take seizure medicines. Some are able to take smaller doses or fewer medicines than before they started the diet, however.

It is not clear how the diet works, though doctors have some theories. What is clear is that it must be followed precisely. If the person goes off the diet for even one meal, it loses its good effect. So it is very important to stick with the diet as prescribed. It can be especially hard to follow the diet 100 percent if there are other children at home who are on a normal diet. Small children who have free access to the refrigerator are tempted by "forbidden" foods. Parents need to work as closely as possible with a dietitian.

Are there any side effects?

A person starting the ketogenic diet may feel sluggish for a few days after the diet is started. This can continue if the patient takes phenobarbital or benzodiazepines.

Other side effects that might occur if the person stays on the diet for a long time are:

- thinning of bone
- kidney stones
- abnormal liver function
- hair thinning
- high cholesterol levels in the blood
- dehydration
- constipation
- changes in behavior
- slowed growth

Because the diet does not provide all the vitamins and minerals found in a balanced diet, the dietitian will recommend vitamin and mineral supplements. The most important of these are calcium and vitamin D (to prevent thinning of the bones), iron, and folic acid.

To avoid complications, the seizure medicines Topamax (topiramate) and Diamox (acetazolamide) must be stopped before the diet is started.

How is the patient monitored over time?

Early on, the doctor will usually see the child every month. Blood tests are performed to make sure there are no medical problems. The height, weight, and head size are measured to see if growth has slowed down. As the child gains weight, the diet must be adjusted by the dietitian.

Can the diet ever be stopped?

If seizures have been well controlled for some time, the doctor might suggest going off the diet. Usually, the patient is gradually taken off the diet over several months or even longer. Just as happens if seizure medicines are stopped suddenly, seizures may become much worse if the ketogenic diet is stopped all at once. Children usually continue to take seizure medicines after they go off the diet.

Chapter 13

Nonepileptic Seizures

Psychogenic Seizures

What are they?

Events that look like seizures but are not due to epilepsy are called "nonepileptic seizures." A common type is described as psychogenic, which means beginning in the mind. Psychogenic seizures are caused by subconscious mental activity, not abnormal electrical activity in the brain. Doctors consider most of them psychological in nature, but not purposely produced. Usually the person is not aware that the spells are not "epileptic." The term "pseudoseizures" has also been used (mostly in the past) to refer to these events.

Are they common?

Psychogenic nonepileptic seizures are common. About 20 percent of the patients referred to comprehensive epilepsy centers for study with video-EEG are found to have nonepileptic seizures. About one in six of these patients either also has epileptic seizures or has had them, however. These people need different treatment for each disorder. Psychogenic nonepileptic seizures have been more widely recognized

"Psychogenic Seizures" is reprinted with permission from http://www.epilepsy.com, the public education website of The Epilepsy Project. © 2004. All rights reserved. "Febrile Seizures" is reprinted from "Febrile Seizures Fact Sheet," National Institute of Neurological Disorders and Stroke, National Institutes of Health, NIH Publication Number 95-3930, updated November 2004.

during the past several decades. They are most often seen in adolescents and young adults, but they also can occur in children and the elderly. They are three times more common in females.

What do they look like?

The seizures most often imitate complex partial or tonic-clonic (grand mal) seizures. Family members report episodes in which the patient stiffens and jerks. Doctors rarely witness the actual event, so they are drawn toward the diagnosis of epilepsy. Often years can be spent trying to treat the spells as epileptic seizures without success.

How are they recognized?

Doctors have identified certain kinds of movements and other patterns that seem to be more common in psychogenic nonepileptic seizures than in seizures caused by epilepsy. Some of these patterns do occur occasionally in epileptic seizures, however, so having one of them does not necessarily mean that the seizure was nonepileptic. Video-EEG monitoring is the most effective way of diagnosing nonepileptic seizures. The doctor may take steps to provoke a seizure and then ask a family member or friend of the patient to confirm that the event was the same as the usual kind.

Can they be treated?

Psychogenic nonepileptic seizures do not necessarily indicate that the person has a serious psychiatric disorder. The problem does need to be addressed, and many patients need treatment. Sometimes the episodes stop when the person learns that they are psychological. Some people have depression or anxiety disorders that can be helped by medication. Counseling for a limited time is often helpful. The person needs to accept the diagnosis (at least as a possibility) and follow through with therapy.

Febrile Seizures

What are febrile seizures?

Febrile seizures are convulsions brought on by a fever in infants or small children. During a febrile seizure, a child often loses consciousness and shakes, moving limbs on both sides of the body. Less commonly, the child becomes rigid or has twitches in only a portion of the body, such as an arm or a leg, or on the right or the left side only. Most febrile seizures last a minute or two, although some can be as brief as a few seconds while others last for more than fifteen minutes.

The majority of children with febrile seizures have rectal temperatures greater than 102 degrees F. Most febrile seizures occur during the first day of a child's fever. Children prone to febrile seizures are not considered to have epilepsy, since epilepsy is characterized by recurrent seizures that are not triggered by fever.

How common are febrile seizures?

Approximately one in every twenty-five children will have at least one febrile seizure, and more than one-third of these children will have additional febrile seizures before they outgrow the tendency to have them. Febrile seizures usually occur in children between the ages of six months and five years and are particularly common in toddlers. Children rarely develop their first febrile seizure before the age of six months or after three years of age. The older a child is when the first febrile seizure occurs, the less likely that child is to have more.

What makes a child prone to recurrent febrile seizures?

A few factors appear to boost a child's risk of having recurrent febrile seizures, including young age (less than fifteen months) during the first seizure, frequent fevers, and having immediate family members with a history of febrile seizures. If the seizure occurs soon after a fever has begun or when the temperature is relatively low, the risk of recurrence is higher. A long initial febrile seizure does not substantially boost the risk of recurrent febrile seizures, either brief or long.

Are febrile seizures harmful?

Although they can be frightening to parents, the vast majority of febrile seizures are harmless. During a seizure, there is a small chance that the child may be injured by falling or may choke from food or saliva in the mouth. Using proper first aid for seizures can help avoid these hazards (see section entitled "What should be done for a child having a febrile seizure?").

There is no evidence that febrile seizures cause brain damage. Large studies have found that children with febrile seizures have normal school achievement and perform as well on intellectual tests as their siblings who don't have seizures. Even in the rare instances of very prolonged seizures (more than one hour), most children recover completely.

Between 95 and 98 percent of children who have experienced febrile seizures do not go on to develop epilepsy. However, although the absolute risk remains very small, certain children who have febrile seizures face an increased risk of developing epilepsy. These children include those who have febrile seizures that are lengthy, that affect only part of the body, or that recur within twenty-four hours, and children with cerebral palsy, delayed development, or other neurological abnormalities. Among children who don't have any of these risk factors, only one in one hundred develops epilepsy after a febrile seizure.

What should be done for a child having a febrile seizure?

Parents should stay calm and carefully observe the child. To prevent accidental injury, the child should be placed on a protected surface such as the floor or ground. The child should not be held or restrained during a convulsion. To prevent choking, the child should be placed on his or her side or stomach. When possible, the parent should gently remove all objects in the child's mouth. The parent should never place anything in the child's mouth during a convulsion. Objects placed in the mouth can be broken and obstruct the child's airway. If the seizure lasts longer than ten minutes, the child should be taken immediately to the nearest medical facility for further treatment. Once the seizure has ended, the child should be taken to his or her doctor to check for the source of the fever. This is especially urgent if the child shows symptoms of stiff neck, extreme lethargy, or abundant vomiting.

How are febrile seizures diagnosed and treated?

Before diagnosing febrile seizures in infants and children, doctors sometimes perform tests to be sure that seizures are not caused by something other than simply the fever itself. For example, if a doctor suspects the child has meningitis (an infection of the membranes surrounding the brain), a spinal tap may be needed to check for signs of the infection in the cerebrospinal fluid (fluid that bathes the brain and spinal cord). If there have been severe diarrhea or vomiting, dehydration could be responsible for seizures. Also, doctors often perform other tests such as examining the blood and urine to pinpoint the cause of the child's fever.

A child who has a febrile seizure usually doesn't need to be hospitalized. If the seizure is prolonged or is accompanied by a serious infection, or if the source of the infection cannot be determined, a doctor may recommend that the child be hospitalized for observation.

How are febrile seizures prevented?

If a child has a fever most parents will use fever-lowering drugs such as acetaminophen or ibuprofen to make the child more comfortable, although there are no studies that prove that this will reduce the risk of a seizure. One preventive measure would be to try to reduce the number of febrile illnesses, although this is often not a practical possibility.

Prolonged daily use of oral anticonvulsants, such as phenobarbital or valproate, to prevent febrile seizures is usually not recommended because of their potential for side effects and questionable effectiveness for preventing such seizures.

Children especially prone to febrile seizures may be treated with the drug diazepam, orally or rectally, whenever they have a fever. The majority of children with febrile seizures do not need to be treated with medication, but in some cases a doctor may decide that medicine given only while the child has a fever may be the best alternative. This medication may lower the risk of having another febrile seizure. It is usually well tolerated, although it occasionally can cause drowsiness, a lack of coordination, or hyperactivity. Children vary widely in their susceptibility to such side effects.

What research is being done on febrile seizures?

The National Institute of Neurological Disorders and Stroke (NINDS), a part of the National Institutes of Health (NIH), sponsors research on febrile seizures in medical centers throughout the country. NINDS-supported scientists are exploring what environmental and genetic risk factors make children susceptible to febrile seizures. Some studies suggest that women who smoke or drink alcohol during their pregnancies are more likely to have children with febrile seizures, but more research needs to be done before this link can be clearly established. Scientists are also working to pinpoint factors that can help predict which children are likely to have recurrent or long-lasting febrile seizures.

Investigators continue to monitor the long-term impact that febrile seizures might have on intelligence, behavior, school achievement, and the development of epilepsy. For example, scientists conducting studies in animals are assessing the effects of seizures and anticonvulsant drugs on brain development.

Investigators also continue to explore which drugs can effectively treat or prevent febrile seizures and to check for side effects of these medicines.

Chapter 14

First Aid for Seizures

First Aid Information

Tonic Clonic Seizure (Grand Mal)

Convulsive seizures where the body stiffens (tonic phase) followed by general muscle jerking (clonic phase).
Do:

- Remain calm
- Stay with person
- Time seizure
- Protect from harm
- Place something soft under head
- Loosen tight neckwear
- Roll onto side
  - after jerking stops, or
  - immediately if vomited
- Maintain privacy and dignity
- Observe and reassure until recovered

Do not:

- Put anything in the person's mouth
- Restrain
- Move person unless in danger
- Apply CPR/EAR

In the unlikely event resuscitation is necessary, commence once jerking stops.

If seizure occurs while seated in a wheelchair, car, or stroller, support the person's head and leave safely strapped in seat until seizure is finished. If there is food, water, or vomit in the person's mouth, remove him or her from seat and roll onto side immediately.

Complex Partial Seizure (Focal)

Nonconvulsive seizure with outward signs of confusion, unresponsiveness, or inappropriate behavior.

- Remain calm
- Stay with person
- Time the seizure
- Gently guide to avoid harm
- Reassure until recovered
- Do not restrain unless in danger

Absence Seizure (Petit Mal)

Mostly affects children. Nonconvulsive with brief blank periods with loss of awareness. Can be mistaken for daydreaming.

- Remain calm
- Reassure
- Repeat missed information

When to Call For Help

Call an ambulance if :

- You are in any doubt
- You arrive after the seizure has started
- Injury has occurred

- Food or water is in mouth during seizure
- The seizure occurs in water
- The seizure lasts longer than normal for that person
- The jerking lasts longer than five minutes
- Another seizure follows quickly
- A complex partial seizure lasts longer than fifteen minutes
- The person has breathing difficulties after the jerking stops
- The person has diabetes
- The woman is pregnant and having a tonic clonic seizure
- It is the first known seizure

Seizures in Water

For many people, the scariest aspect of epilepsy is not knowing when or where a seizure will occur. In certain situations, a loss of consciousness is especially dangerous and emergency care must go beyond the routine procedures. A seizure in water is one of these life-threatening situations.

Here are steps to follow if someone is having a seizure in water:

- Support the person in the water with the head tilted so the face and head stay above the surface.
- Remove the person from the water as quickly as possible.
- Check to see whether the person is breathing. If not, begin CPR immediately.
- Call an ambulance. Even if the person appears to be fully recovered, he or she should have a full medical checkup. Inhaling water can cause lung or heart damage.

Seizures in Airplanes

If a person is having a major seizure in a crowded plane miles above the earth, the rules for first aid are different.

Here are some tips:

- Clear space by folding up seat arms. Ask a flight attendant to find new seats for the other passengers in the row.
- Lie the person down across the seats with the head and body turned on one side. Make sure that the airway is clear and breathing is not obstructed.

- Arrange pillows or blankets to prevent the person's head from hitting unpadded areas.

- When the seizure stops, help the person into a resting position in a single reclining seat.

- If the seizure continues for more than about five minutes or is immediately followed by another one, tell the flight attendant that the person may be experiencing a medical emergency and may need emergency care.

Part Four

Degenerative
Neurological Disorders

Chapter 15

Amyotrophic Lateral Sclerosis (ALS)

Chapter Contents

Section 15.1—ALS: An Overview 316
Section 15.2—Recent Research on ALS 325

Section 15.1

ALS: An Overview

Excerpted from "Amyotrophic Lateral Sclerosis Fact Sheet," National Institute of Neurological Disorders and Stroke, National Institutes of Health, NIH Publication No. 00-916, updated November 2004.

What is amyotrophic lateral sclerosis?

Amyotrophic lateral sclerosis (ALS), sometimes called Lou Gehrig's disease, is a rapidly progressive, invariably fatal neurological disease that attacks the nerve cells (neurons) responsible for controlling voluntary muscles. The disease belongs to a group of disorders known as motor neuron diseases, which are characterized by the gradual degeneration and death of motor neurons.

Motor neurons are nerve cells located in the brain, brainstem, and spinal cord that serve as controlling units and vital communication links between the nervous system and the voluntary muscles of the body. Messages from motor neurons in the brain (called upper motor neurons) are transmitted to motor neurons in the spinal cord (called lower motor neurons) and from them to particular muscles. In ALS, both the upper motor neurons and the lower motor neurons degenerate or die, ceasing to send messages to muscles. Unable to function, the muscles gradually weaken, waste away (atrophy), and twitch (fasciculations). Eventually, the ability of the brain to start and control voluntary movement is lost.

ALS causes weakness with a wide range of disabilities (see section titled "What are the symptoms?"). Eventually, all muscles under voluntary control are affected, and patients lose their strength and the ability to move their arms, legs, and body. When muscles in the diaphragm and chest wall fail, patients lose the ability to breathe without ventilatory support. Most people with ALS die from respiratory failure, usually within three to five years from the onset of symptoms. However, about 10 percent of ALS patients survive for ten or more years.

Because ALS affects only motor neurons, the disease does not impair a person's mind, personality, intelligence, or memory. Nor does it affect a person's ability to see, smell, taste, hear, or recognize touch.

Patients usually maintain control of eye muscles and bladder and bowel functions.

Who gets ALS?

As many as twenty thousand Americans have ALS, and an estimated five thousand people in the United States are diagnosed with the disease each year. ALS is one of the most common neuromuscular diseases worldwide, and people of all races and ethnic backgrounds are affected. ALS most commonly strikes people between forty and sixty years of age, but younger and older people also can develop the disease. Men are affected more often than women.

In 90 to 95 percent of all ALS cases, the disease occurs apparently at random with no clearly associated risk factors. Patients do not have a family history of the disease, and their family members are not considered to be at increased risk for developing ALS.

About 5 to 10 percent of all ALS cases are inherited. The familial form of ALS usually results from a pattern of inheritance that requires only one parent to carry the gene responsible for the disease. About 20 percent of all familial cases result from a specific genetic defect that leads to mutation of the enzyme known as superoxide dismutase 1 (SOD1). Research on this mutation is providing clues about the possible causes of motor neuron death in ALS. Not all familial ALS cases are due to the SOD1 mutation, therefore other unidentified genetic causes clearly exist.

What are the symptoms?

The onset of ALS may be so subtle that the symptoms are frequently overlooked. The earliest symptoms may include twitching, cramping, or stiffness of muscles; muscle weakness affecting an arm or a leg; slurred and nasal speech; or difficulty chewing or swallowing. These general complaints then develop into more obvious weakness or atrophy that may cause a physician to suspect ALS.

The parts of the body affected by early symptoms of ALS depend on which muscles in the body are damaged first. In some cases, symptoms initially affect one of the legs, and patients experience awkwardness when walking or running or they notice that they are tripping or stumbling more often. Some patients first see the effects of the disease on a hand or arm as they experience difficulty with simple tasks requiring manual dexterity such as buttoning a shirt, writing, or turning a key in a lock. Other patients notice speech problems.

317

Regardless of the part of the body first affected by the disease, muscle weakness and atrophy spread to other parts of the body as the disease progresses. Patients have increasing problems with moving, swallowing (dysphagia), and speaking or forming words (dysarthria). Symptoms of upper motor neuron involvement include tight and stiff muscles (spasticity) and exaggerated reflexes (hyperreflexia) including an overactive gag reflex. An abnormal reflex commonly called Babinski's sign (the large toe extends upward as the sole of the foot is stimulated in a certain way) also indicates upper motor neuron damage. Symptoms of lower motor neuron degeneration include muscle weakness and atrophy, muscle cramps, and fleeting twitches of muscles that can be seen under the skin (fasciculations).

To be diagnosed with ALS, patients must have signs and symptoms of both upper and lower motor neuron damage that cannot be attributed to other causes.

Although the sequence of emerging symptoms and the rate of disease progression vary from person to person, eventually patients will not be able to stand or walk, get in or out of bed on their own, or use their hands and arms. Difficulty swallowing and chewing impair the patient's ability to eat normally and increase the risk of choking. Maintaining weight will then become a problem. Because the disease usually does not affect cognitive abilities, patients are aware of their progressive loss of function and may become anxious and depressed. Health care professionals need to explain the course of the disease and describe available treatment options so that patients can make informed decisions in advance. In later stages of the disease, patients have difficulty breathing as the muscles of the respiratory system weaken. Patients eventually lose the ability to breathe on their own and must depend on ventilatory support for survival. Patients also face an increased risk of pneumonia during later stages of ALS.

How is ALS diagnosed?

No one test can provide a definitive diagnosis of ALS, although the presence of upper and lower motor neuron signs in a single limb is strongly suggestive. Instead, the diagnosis of ALS is primarily based on the symptoms and signs the physician observes in the patient and a series of tests to rule out other diseases. Physicians obtain the patient's full medical history and usually conduct a neurologic examination at regular intervals to assess whether symptoms such as muscle weakness, atrophy of muscles, hyperreflexia, and spasticity are getting progressively worse.

Because symptoms of ALS can be similar to those of a wide variety of other, more treatable diseases or disorders, appropriate tests must be conducted to exclude the possibility of other conditions. One of these tests is electromyography (EMG), a special recording technique that detects electrical activity in muscles. Certain EMG findings can support the diagnosis of ALS. Another common test measures nerve conduction velocity (NCV). Specific abnormalities in the NCV results may suggest, for example, that the patient has a form of peripheral neuropathy (damage to peripheral nerves) or myopathy (muscle disease) rather than ALS. The physician may order magnetic resonance imaging (MRI), a noninvasive procedure that uses a magnetic field and radio waves to take detailed images of the brain and spinal cord. Although these MRI scans are often normal in patients with ALS, they can reveal evidence of other problems that may be causing the symptoms, such as a spinal cord tumor, a herniated disk in the neck, syringomyelia, or cervical spondylosis.

Based on the patient's symptoms and findings from the examination and from these tests, the physician may order tests on blood and urine samples to eliminate the possibility of other diseases as well as routine laboratory tests. In some cases, for example, if a physician suspects that the patient may have a myopathy rather than ALS, a muscle biopsy may be performed.

Infectious diseases such as human immunodeficiency virus (HIV), human T-cell leukemia virus (HTLV), and Lyme disease can in some cases cause ALS-like symptoms. Neurological disorders such as multiple sclerosis, post-polio syndrome, multifocal motor neuropathy, and spinal muscular atrophy also can mimic certain facets of the disease and should be considered by physicians attempting to make a diagnosis.

Because of the prognosis carried by this diagnosis and the variety of diseases or disorders that can resemble ALS in the early stages of the disease, patients may wish to obtain a second neurological opinion.

What causes ALS?

The cause of ALS is not known, and scientists do not yet know why ALS strikes some people and not others. An important step toward answering that question came in 1993 when scientists supported by the National Institute of Neurological Disorders and Stroke (NINDS) discovered that mutations in the gene that produces the SOD1 enzyme were associated with some cases of familial ALS. This enzyme is a powerful antioxidant that protects the body from damage caused by free radicals. Free radicals are highly reactive molecules produced by cells during normal metabolism. If not neutralized, free radicals can accumulate and cause random damage to the DNA and proteins within cells. Although it is not yet clear how the SOD1 gene mutation leads to motor neuron degeneration, researchers have theorized that an accumulation of free radicals may result from the faulty functioning of this gene. In support of this, animal studies have shown that motor neuron degeneration and deficits in motor function accompany the presence of the SOD1 mutation.

Studies also have focused on the role of glutamate in motor neuron degeneration. Glutamate is one of the chemical messengers or neurotransmitters in the brain. Scientists have found that, compared to healthy people, ALS patients have higher levels of glutamate in the serum and spinal fluid. Laboratory studies have demonstrated that neurons begin to die off when they are exposed over long periods to excessive amounts of glutamate. Now, scientists are trying to understand what mechanisms lead to a buildup of unneeded glutamate in the spinal fluid and how this imbalance could contribute to the development of ALS.

Autoimmune responses—which occur when the body's immune system attacks normal cells—have been suggested as one possible cause for motor neuron degeneration in ALS. Some scientists theorize that antibodies may directly or indirectly impair the function of motor neurons, interfering with the transmission of signals between the brain and muscles.

In searching for the cause of ALS, researchers have also studied environmental factors such as exposure to toxic or infectious agents. Other research has examined the possible role of dietary deficiency or trauma. However, as of yet, there is insufficient evidence to implicate these factors as causes of ALS.

Future research may show that many factors, including a genetic predisposition, are involved in the development of ALS.

How is ALS treated?

No cure has yet been found for ALS. However, the Food and Drug Administration (FDA) has approved the first drug treatment for the disease—riluzole (Rilutek). Riluzole is believed to reduce damage to motor neurons by decreasing the release of glutamate. Clinical trials with ALS patients showed that riluzole prolongs survival by several months, mainly in those with difficulty swallowing. The drug also extends the time before a patient needs ventilation support. Riluzole does not reverse the damage already done to motor neurons, and patients taking the drug must be monitored for liver damage and other possible side effects. However, this first disease-specific therapy offers hope that the progression of ALS may one day be slowed by new medications or combinations of drugs.

Other treatments for ALS are designed to relieve symptoms and improve the quality of life for patients. This supportive care is best provided by multidisciplinary teams of health care professionals such as physicians; pharmacists; physical, occupational, and speech therapists; nutritionists; social workers; and home care and hospice nurses. Working with patients and caregivers, these teams can design an individualized plan of medical and physical therapy and provide special equipment aimed at keeping patients as mobile and comfortable as possible.

Physicians can prescribe medications to help reduce fatigue, ease muscle cramps, control spasticity, and reduce excess saliva and phlegm. Drugs also are available to help patients with pain, depression, sleep disturbances, and constipation. Pharmacists can give advice on the proper use of medications and monitor a patient's prescriptions to avoid risks of drug interactions.

Physical therapy and special equipment can enhance patients' independence and safety throughout the course of ALS. Gentle, low-impact aerobic exercise such as walking, swimming, and stationary bicycling can strengthen unaffected muscles, improve cardiovascular health, and help patients fight fatigue and depression. Range of motion and stretching exercises can help prevent painful spasticity and shortening (contracture) of muscles. Physical therapists can recommend exercises that provide these benefits without overworking muscles. Occupational therapists can suggest devices such as ramps, braces, walkers, and wheelchairs that help patients conserve energy and remain mobile.

ALS patients who have difficulty speaking may benefit from working with a speech therapist. These health professionals can teach patients adaptive strategies such as techniques to help them speak louder and more clearly. As ALS progresses, speech therapists can help patients develop ways for responding to yes-or-no questions with their eyes or by other nonverbal means and can recommend aids such as speech synthesizers and computer-based communication systems. These methods and devices help patients communicate when they can no longer speak or produce vocal sounds.

Patients and caregivers can learn from speech therapists and nutritionists how to plan and prepare numerous small meals throughout the day that provide enough calories, fiber, and fluid and how to avoid foods that are difficult to swallow. Patients may begin using suction devices to remove excess fluids or saliva and prevent choking. When patients can no longer get enough nourishment from eating, doctors may advise inserting a feeding tube into the stomach. The use of a feeding tube also reduces the risk of choking and pneumonia that can result from inhaling liquids into the lungs. The tube is not painful and does not prevent patients from eating food orally if they wish.

When the muscles that assist in breathing weaken, use of nocturnal ventilatory assistance (intermittent positive pressure ventilation [IPPV] or bilevel positive airway pressure [BIPAP]) may be used to aid breathing during sleep. Such devices artificially inflate the patient's lungs from various external sources that are applied directly to the face or body. When muscles are no longer able to maintain oxygen and carbon dioxide levels, these devices may be used full time.

Patients may eventually consider forms of mechanical ventilation (respirators) in which a machine inflates and deflates the lungs. To be effective, this may require a tube that passes from the nose or mouth to the windpipe (trachea) and for long-term use, an operation such as a tracheostomy, in which a plastic breathing tube is inserted directly in the patient's windpipe through an opening in the neck. Patients and their families should consider several factors when deciding whether and when to use one of these options. Ventilation devices differ in their effect on the patient's quality of life and in cost. Although ventilation support can ease problems with breathing and prolong survival, it does not affect the progression of ALS. Patients need to be fully informed about these considerations and the long-term effects of life without movement before they make decisions about ventilation support.

Social workers and home care and hospice nurses help patients, families, and caregivers with the medical, emotional, and financial challenges of coping with ALS, particularly during the final stages of the disease. Social workers provide support such as assistance in obtaining financial aid, arranging durable power of attorney, preparing a living will, and finding support groups for patients and caregivers. Home care nurses are available not only to provide medical care but also to teach caregivers about tasks such as maintaining respirators, giving tube feedings, and moving patients to avoid painful skin problems and contractures. Home hospice nurses work in consultation with physicians to ensure proper medication, pain control, and other care affecting the quality of life of patients who wish to remain at home.

The home hospice team can also counsel patients and caregivers about end-of-life issues.

What research is being done?

The National Institute of Neurological Disorders and Stroke, part of the National Institutes of Health, is the federal government's leading supporter of biomedical research on ALS. The goals of this research are to find the cause or causes of ALS, understand the mechanisms involved in the progression of the disease, and develop effective treatment.

Scientists are seeking to understand the mechanisms that trigger selective motor neurons to degenerate in ALS and to find effective approaches to halt the processes leading to cell death. This work includes studies in animals to identify the means by which SOD1 mutations lead to the destruction of neurons. The excessive accumulation of free radicals, which has been implicated in a number of neurodegenerative diseases including ALS, is also being closely studied. In addition, researchers are examining how the loss of neurotrophic factors may be involved in ALS. Neurotrophic factors are chemicals found in the brain and spinal cord that play a vital role in the development, specification, maintenance, and protection of neurons. Studying how these factors may be lost and how such a loss may contribute to motor neuron degeneration may lead to a greater understanding of ALS and the development of neuroprotective strategies. By exploring these and other possible factors, researchers hope to find the cause or causes of motor neuron degeneration in ALS and develop therapies to slow the progression of the disease.

Researchers are also conducting investigations to increase their understanding of the role of programmed cell death or apoptosis in ALS. In normal physiological processes, apoptosis acts as a means to rid the body of cells that are no longer needed by prompting the cells to commit "cell suicide." The critical balance between necessary cell death and the maintenance of essential cells is thought to be controlled by trophic factors. In addition to ALS, apoptosis is pervasive in other chronic neurodegenerative conditions such as Parkinson disease and Alzheimer's disease and is thought to be a major cause of the secondary brain damage seen after stroke and trauma. Discovering what triggers apoptosis may eventually lead to therapeutic interventions for ALS and other neurological diseases.

Scientists have not yet identified a reliable biological marker for ALS—a biochemical abnormality shared by all patients with the disease.

Once such a biomarker is discovered and tests are developed to detect the marker in patients, allowing early detection and diagnosis of ALS, physicians will have a valuable tool to help them follow the effects of new therapies and monitor disease progression.

NINDS-supported researchers are studying families with ALS who lack the SOD1 mutation to locate additional genes that cause the disease. Identification of additional ALS genes will allow genetic testing useful for diagnostic confirmation of ALS and prenatal screening for the disease. This work with familial ALS could lead to a greater understanding of sporadic ALS as well. Because familial ALS is virtually indistinguishable from sporadic ALS clinically, some researchers believe that familial ALS genes may also be involved in the manifestations of the more common sporadic form of ALS. Scientists also hope to identify genetic risk factors that predispose people to sporadic ALS.

Potential therapies for ALS are being investigated in animal models. Some of this work involves experimental treatments with normal SOD1 and other antioxidants. In addition, neurotrophic factors are being studied for their potential to protect motor neurons from pathological degeneration. Investigators are optimistic that these and other basic research studies will eventually lead to treatments for ALS.

Section 15.2

Recent Research on ALS

This section includes the following press releases from the National Institute of Neurological Disorders and Stroke: "Minocycline Delays Onset and Slows Progression of ALS in Mice," May 2, 2002; "Doubling Up: Researchers Combine a Common Dietary Supplement with an Antibiotic to Treat Lou Gehrig's Disease," January 31, 2003; "Misbehaving Molecules: 3-Dimensional Pictures of ALS Mutant Proteins Support Two Major Theories about How the Disease Is Caused," May 18, 2003; and "Senataxin Gene Linked to Juvenile-Onset ALS," June 23, 2004.

Minocycline Delays Onset and Slows Progression of ALS in Mice

The antibiotic minocycline delays onset and slows progression of symptoms in a mouse model for amyotrophic lateral sclerosis (ALS), a new study shows. The study also revealed that the drug may work by blocking release of a molecule that triggers cell death. The findings may lead to new ways of treating ALS or other neurodegenerative disorders.

ALS, also called Lou Gehrig's disease, is a progressive and fatal neurological disease that attacks the nerve cells responsible for controlling movement. More than five thousand people in the United States are diagnosed with ALS each year. Most patients die within three to five years after symptoms begin.

Previous studies have shown that minocycline protects neurons from dying in animal models for a variety of disorders, including Huntington disease, Parkinson disease, stroke, and traumatic brain injury, and it is currently being tested in human clinical trials of Huntington disease. However, until now researchers did not know how the drug prevented cell death. The new study shows that minocycline prevents release of a mitochondrial protein called cytochrome c into the body of the cell. Mitochondria are tiny rod-shaped compartments within cells that break down food and produce energy. Release of cytochrome c activates an enzyme that enables cells to commit suicide and is a common feature of many neurological disorders. The study was funded in part by the National Institute of Neurological

Disorders and Stroke (NINDS) and appears in the May 2, 2002, issue of *Nature*.

Researchers led by Robert M. Friedlander, M.D., of Brigham and Women's Hospital in Boston, injected minocycline into mice with mutations, or abnormalities, in the gene for an enzyme called superoxide dismutase-1 (SOD1). Another group of mice received saline (saltwater) injections. SOD1 mutations are found in about 20 percent of patients with familial ALS; mice with these mutations develop nerve damage and neurological symptoms that resemble the human disease. The researchers found that minocycline delayed the onset of movement problems in the mouse model by an average of several weeks. The minocycline-treated mice also lived slightly longer than the saline-treated mice.

The researchers also tested the effects of minocycline on neurons in culture and on isolated mitochondria. These studies indicate that minocycline inhibited cell death by preventing release of cytochrome c. Minocycline also significantly inhibited release of cytochrome c in the SOD1 mice. A previous report had shown that release of cytochrome c in spinal cords of these mice correlates with progression of the disease.

The effect of minocycline on survival in the SOD1 mice is roughly equivalent to that of riluzole, the only drug currently approved by the Food and Drug Administration (FDA) to treat ALS, says Dr. Friedlander. In humans, riluzole extends survival by approximately three months. However, the new study shows that minocycline works in a very different way than riluzole, which inhibits release of the neurotransmitter glutamate. This suggests that a combination of riluzole and minocycline may be more effective than either drug alone, Dr. Friedlander says. The researchers plan to test combinations of minocycline and other drugs in animals to see if they can identify a drug combination, or "cocktail," that would be a safe, powerful therapy for ALS.

Minocycline is the first nontoxic drug with a proven human safety record that has been shown to inhibit cytochrome c release, says Dr. Friedlander. It also crosses the blood-brain barrier and is effective when taken orally, which makes it a good candidate for human clinical trials. Knowing how minocycline works also will help researchers design and test similar drugs that may be more effective against ALS and other neurological diseases.

Reference

Zhu S, Stavrovskaya IG, Drozda M, Kim BYS, Ona V, Li M, Sarang S, Liu AS, Hartley DM, Wu DC, Gullans S, Ferrante RJ, Przedborski S,

Kristal BS, Friedlander RM. "Minocycline inhibits cytochrome c release and delays progression of amyotrophic lateral sclerosis in mice." *Nature,* May 2, 2002, Vol. 417, No. 6884, pp. 74–78.

Doubling Up: Researchers Combine a Common Dietary Supplement with an Antibiotic to Treat Lou Gehrig's Disease

A new study shows that combining the supplement creatine and the antibiotic minocycline significantly slows disease progression and prolongs survival in a mouse model of amyotrophic lateral sclerosis (ALS), or Lou Gehrig's disease. The combined treatment was significantly more effective than either compound administered alone. Both creatine and minocycline have previously been shown to improve outcomes in a mouse model of this disabling neurological disease, but this study is the first to test a combination of the two.

"Given that these two compounds each work in ALS mouse models, we thought combining them might have an even stronger effect on symptoms and disease progression," says lead author Robert Friedlander, M.D., M.A., associate professor of neurosurgery at Brigham and Women's Hospital and Harvard Medical School in Boston. "Our results show that this kind of cocktail approach might be a new potential strategy for treating ALS." The study was funded in part by the DHHS's National Institute of Neurological Disorders and Stroke (NINDS) and appears in the February 2003 issue of *Annals of Neurology*.[1]

ALS is a progressive and fatal neurological disease affecting nerve cells that control movement. More than five thousand Americans are diagnosed with ALS each year, and most patients die within three to five years after symptoms begin.

Creatine is an amino acid that is found naturally in meats and fish, and is also marketed as a dietary supplement. In 1999, researchers showed that creatine was better at prolonging survival in a mouse model for ALS than the prescription drug riluzole, which is already used to treat people with ALS. Diets supplemented with creatine extended the lives of ALS mice by about 18 percent compared to unsupplemented diets, while riluzole extended survival in mice by about 9 percent.

Researchers do not know how creatine works to slow the progression of ALS in mice, but Dr. Friedlander says there are several different hypotheses. "We are working very hard to understand the mechanism of creatine in mice with ALS," he says, adding that the most widely accepted hypothesis is that creatine may improve neurons' energy supply, making them more resistant to degeneration.

Minocycline is an antibiotic that has been used for about thirty years to treat a variety of infections, as well as acne and rheumatoid arthritis. In May 2002, Dr. Friedlander and colleagues published a study demonstrating neuroprotective effects of minocycline in an ALS mouse model.[2] Previous studies have also shown that minocycline protects neurons from dying in animal models of Huntington disease, Parkinson disease, stroke, traumatic brain injury, and a variety of other disorders.

Minocycline has at least two possible mechanisms of action for treating ALS. Recent studies have shown that problems in mitochondria—tiny rod-shaped compartments within cells that break down food and produce energy—lead to the death of nerve cells controlling movement in ALS mice. Dr. Friedlander and colleagues recently published findings demonstrating that minocycline makes the mitochondria more resistant to changes that may trigger cell death. ALS also causes certain immune cells in the brain, called microglia, to release toxic compounds, Dr. Friedlander says. Minocycline appears to block this reactivity of microglia.

In the new study, Dr. Friedlander and colleagues studied mice with a mutation in the human SOD1 gene, which is found in about 20 percent of patients with familial ALS. Mice with this mutation develop nerve damage and neurological symptoms that mimic those of ALS in humans.

The researchers fed one group of ten mice a diet supplemented with 2 percent creatine beginning at three weeks of age. Once the mice reached four weeks of age, the researchers also gave them injections of minocycline once daily until they died or were too sick to be tested further. For comparison, three other groups of mice received a creatine-supplemented diet plus saline (saltwater) injections, minocycline injections alone, or saline injections alone.

The researchers assessed each mouse's motor strength and coordination on a weekly basis, starting at ten weeks, by observing its ability to remain standing on a rod rotating at five and fifteen revolutions per minute (rpm) for up to seven minutes. Disease onset was defined as the first day a mouse could not remain on the rod for seven minutes at fifteen rpm.

The minocycline injections and creatine supplements delayed disease onset to 113 and 111 days, respectively, compared with 94 days in the untreated group. The two drugs delayed mortality to 142 and 141 days, respectively, compared to 126 days in the control group—a 13 and 12 percent improvement in survival. However, mice in the minocycline-creatine combination group did significantly better than mice receiving either creatine or minocycline alone. They did not show disease onset until 122 days and they survived for an average of 157 days—a 25 percent improvement in survival compared to untreated mice.

Dr. Friedlander says that this particular combination is especially promising because the mechanisms of action of the two compounds are different. "To block a disease pathway, you want to target different steps within the pathway. Although we don't fully understand the mechanism of creatine-mediated neuroprotection, we do know that it is not the same as the minocycline mechanism."

Researchers are currently testing the safety and efficacy of both creatine and minocycline in clinical trials for ALS. So far, there have been no significant negative side effects for either compound, although extremely high doses of creatine can cause kidney problems, says Dr. Friedlander. Both compounds also cross the blood-brain barrier and are effective when taken orally, making them good candidates for human clinical trials.

Before human trials of minocycline plus creatine can be conducted, researchers need to do further studies to better understand the disease process of ALS and to understand the mechanism, safety, and appropriate doses of the combination treatment. Researchers are also working to develop new drug combinations for treating ALS in animal models.

References

1. Zhang W, Narayanan M, Friedlander RM. "Additive Neuroprotective Effects of Minocycline with Creatine in a Transgenic Mouse Model of ALS," *Annals of Neurology,* February 2003, Vol. 53, Issue 2, pp. 267–70.

2. Zhu S, Stavrovskaya IG, Drozda M, Kim BYS, Ona V, Li M, Sarang S, Liu AS, Hartley DM, Wu DC, Gullans S, Ferrante RJ, Przedborski S, Kristal BS, Friedlander RM. "Minocycline inhibits cytochrome c release and delays progression of amyotrophic lateral sclerosis in mice." *Nature,* May 2, 2002, Vol. 417, No. 6884, pp. 74–78.

Misbehaving Molecules: 3-Dimensional Pictures of ALS Mutant Proteins Support Two Major Theories about How the Disease Is Caused

A new study reveals for the first time how gene mutations lead to the inherited form of amyotrophic lateral sclerosis (ALS), or Lou

Gehrig's disease. The study suggests that the two most prominent theories of how familial ALS (FALS) and other related diseases develop are both right in part.

"No one has ever demonstrated at the molecular level how ALS mutations might lead to disease," says study author John Hart, Ph.D., director of the University of Texas Health Science Center X-ray Crystallographic Core Laboratory in San Antonio. "Using a technique commonly used in structural biology, we could see the intimate details of how toxic familial ALS proteins interact. And we found out that the proteins are interacting in a way they shouldn't be." The study was funded by the National Institute of Neurological Disorders and Stroke and appears in the June 2003 issue of *Nature Structural Biology*.[1]

ALS is a progressive, fatal neurological disease that usually strikes in mid-life. It causes muscle weakness, leads to paralysis, and usually ends in death within two to five years of diagnosis. Affecting as many as twenty thousand Americans, ALS occurs when specific nerve cells in the brain and spinal cord that control voluntary movement gradually degenerate.

About 10 percent of ALS cases are familial ALS. Only one parent needs to have FALS to pass it on to his or her children, although men are about one-and-a-half times more likely to develop the disease than women. Studies that reveal how FALS develops may give researchers new clues about the other 90 percent of ALS cases—known as sporadic ALS—and other neurodegenerative diseases, such as Alzheimer's, Parkinson, and Huntington diseases.

Scientists studying FALS patients have identified more than ninety mutations in the gene that directs the production of the protein copper-zinc superoxide dismutase (SOD1). In FALS, proteins accumulate in a way they shouldn't to form large protein complexes. Scientists believe these complexes interfere with nerve cell transport, cellular waste management, and other cellular activities that prevent cell death. Similar large protein complexes have been implicated in other neurodegenerative diseases.

Using a three-dimensional imaging technique called x-ray crystallography, Dr. Hart and his colleagues compared the interactions among proteins in the FALS mutant protein complexes to interactions among normal proteins.

Normally, proteins protect themselves from sticking to one another by covering their edges with loop-shaped ends. The researchers found that in the mutant proteins, the loops were in the wrong position. This loss of protection appears to lead to the toxic accumulation of proteins in FALS. The finding reveals a new mechanism for researchers to exploit in their efforts to find ways to prevent or treat neurodegenerative diseases.

For years scientists have speculated about the disease mechanisms in ALS. Researchers initially thought that the FALS mutation in SOD1 led to a decrease in SOD1 activity and subsequent oxidative damage to cells. But a recent study disproved the idea, showing that mice completely lacking SOD1 lived to adulthood without developing movement disorders. Mice with the human FALS-SOD1 mutation, however, became paralyzed despite normal SOD1 levels.

Scientists now have two primary theories for why the mere presence of the mutant SOD1 protein seems to cause FALS without interfering with SOD1 activity.

The new oxidative damage theory holds that mutant SOD1 proteins produce chemicals called oxidants that damage and kill cells. In a nutshell, the SOD1 protein needs to bind to a reactive metal in order to form loops to protect its edges. The oxidants, however, often damage the mutant SOD1 protein itself, interfering with metal binding and leaving the protein unprotected.

The aggregation theory, on the other hand, maintains that mutant SOD1 proteins fold improperly, causing them to stick together and form large toxic protein complexes. Researchers believe that those protein complexes interfere specifically with transport machinery within the nerve cells that control voluntary movement.

A recently substantiated addition to the aggregation theory, suggested by studies in Parkinson and Alzheimer's diseases, is that pore-like precursors of the protein aggregates—not the aggregates themselves—may be killing the nerve cells. In this study, Dr. Hart and Dr. Samar Hasnain saw those helical, pore-like precursors using x-ray crystallography, providing striking evidence implicating the aggregation theory in ALS.

"Our study provides a model for how protein aggregation in FALS occurs," says Dr. Hart. "But it also suggests that deadly oxidative chemistry can lead to metal loss which in turn can lead to aggregation. These are very exciting findings, because we have 3-D pictures that support two separate hypotheses."

These findings offer a unique contribution to the enormous effort to understand not only the causes of, but also the possible ways to treat or prevent FALS and other neurodegenerative disorders.

"If we can understand what is going on at the molecular level, we may eventually be able to develop a drug to prevent the defect that leads to disease," says study co-author Jennifer Stine Elam, a graduate student in Dr. Hart's laboratory.

References

1. Stine Elam J, Taylor AB, Strange R, Antonyuk S, Doucette PA, Rodriguez JA, Hasnain SS, Hayward LJ, Selverstone Valentine J, Yeates TO, Hart PJ. "Amyloid-like filaments and water-filled nanotubes formed by SOD1 mutants linked to familial ALS." *Nature Structural Biology*, June 2003; online May 19, 2003.

Senataxin Gene Linked to Juvenile-Onset ALS

Researchers funded in part by the National Institute of Neurological Disorders and Stroke (NINDS) have identified the gene that causes a rare juvenile-onset form of amyotrophic lateral sclerosis (ALS). The discovery of the Senataxin gene, on chromosome 9q34, may provide clues to the mechanisms of related brain disorders. The study appears in the June 2004 issue of the *American Journal of Human Genetics*.[1]

ALS is a progressive disorder that destroys motor neurons, the cells that control voluntary muscle activity such as speaking, walking, and writing. Affected muscles gradually weaken and waste away, and patients eventually are unable to move voluntarily. About 10 percent of all cases of ALS are inherited.

Mutations in the Senataxin gene cause ALS4, a juvenile-onset form that usually begins before age twenty-five. These mutations likely lead to a protein that has harmful cellular effects. Unlike classical ALS, which is a fatal disease, ALS4 causes weakness that is slowly progressive, and affected individuals typically have a normal life span. Sensation in ALS4 is not altered.

A team of researchers led by Phillip F. Chance, M.D, a professor of pediatrics and neurology at the University of Washington, Seattle, studied four unrelated families (from the United States, Belgium, Austria, and England), each of whom had multiple family members affected by a childhood- or adolescent-onset, slowly progressive motor neuron disorder with minimal or no sensory nerve impairment. Electrophysiological studies and autopsies confirmed the diagnosis of a chronic motor nerve disorder that initially affected distal muscles (those farthest away from the center of the body). Further analysis revealed an alteration in the DNA sequence of the Senataxin gene on chromosome 9 in the U.S. family. The scientists then studied DNA samples from the other three families, and similar mutations were found in two additional families.

Although the exact function of the Senataxin gene is unknown, scientists believe that the mutated protein may disrupt normal mechanisms through which cells rid themselves of defective RNA transcripts.

"The abnormal Senataxin protein in ALS4 may impair the capacity of neurons to produce error-free mature messenger RNA, leading to neuronal degeneration," said Dr. Chance. "Given the precedence for RNA processing defects in other forms of motor neuron disease, it is hoped this discovery will bring additional insight into motor neuron degeneration."

"We are excited to find the cause of ALS4," said Kenneth H. Fischbeck, M.D., scientific team member and chief of the NINDS Neurogenetics Branch. "Each discovery of a gene responsible for motor neuron disease brings us closer to new therapies and hopefully ways to prevent the onset and progression of ALS."

The findings may provide insight into the mechanisms of other forms of ALS and motor neuron diseases in general, since many of these disorders have overlapping features. The same gene is mutated in a rare form of ataxia, a disorder that is unrelated to motor neuron disease.

Classical ALS (also known as Lou Gehrig's disease) typically strikes people between forty and sixty years of age, and most patients die within three to five years of symptom onset. Intellect, memory, and personality are not affected in most cases.

Reference

1. Chen Y, Bennett CL, Huynh HM, Blair IP, Puls I, Irobi J, Dierick I, Abel A, Kennerson ML, Rabin BA, Nicholson GA, Auer-Grumbach M, Wagner K, De Jonghe P, Griffin JW, Fischbeck KH, Timmerman V, Cornblath DR, Chance PF. "DNA/RNA helicase gene mutations in a form of juvenile Amyotrophic Lateral Sclerosis (ALS4)." *American Journal of Human Genetics*, Vol. 74, No. 6, pp. 1128–35.

Chapter 16

Dementias:
Hope through Research

Introduction

A woman in her early fifties was admitted to a hospital because of increasingly odd behavior. Her family reported that she had been showing memory problems and strong feelings of jealousy. She also had become disoriented at home and was hiding objects. During a doctor's examination, the woman was unable to remember her husband's name, the year, or how long she had been at the hospital. She could read but did not seem to understand what she read, and she stressed the words in an unusual way. She sometimes became agitated and seemed to have hallucinations and irrational fears.

This woman, known as Auguste D., was the first person reported to have the disease now known as Alzheimer's disease (AD) after Alois Alzheimer, the German doctor who first described it. After Auguste D. died in 1906, doctors examined her brain and found that it appeared shrunken and contained several unusual features, including strange clumps of protein called plaques and tangled fibers inside the nerve cells. Memory impairments and other symptoms of dementia, which means "deprived of mind," had been described in older adults since ancient times. However, because Auguste D. began to show symptoms at a relatively early age, doctors did not think her disease could be related to what was then called "senile

Excerpted from "The Dementias: Hope through Research," National Institute of Neurological Disorders and Stroke, National Institutes of Health, NIH Publication Number 04-2252, updated November 2004.

dementia. "The word senile is derived from a Latin term that means, roughly, "old age."

It is now clear that AD is a major cause of dementia in elderly people as well as in relatively young adults. Furthermore, we know that it is only one of many disorders that can lead to dementia. The U.S. Congress Office of Technology Assessment estimates that as many as 6.8 million Americans have dementia, and at least 1.8 million of those are severely affected. Studies in some communities have found that almost half of all people age eighty-five and older have some form of dementia. Although it is common in very elderly individuals, dementia is not a normal part of the aging process. Many people live into their nineties and even hundreds without any symptoms of dementia.

Besides senile dementia, other terms often used to describe dementia include senility and organic brain syndrome. Senility and senile dementia are outdated terms that reflect the formerly widespread belief that dementia was a normal part of aging. Organic brain syndrome is a general term that refers to physical disorders (not psychiatric in origin) that impair mental functions.

Research in the last thirty years has led to a greatly improved understanding of what dementia is, who gets it, and how it develops and affects the brain. This work is beginning to pay off with better diagnostic techniques, improved treatments, and even potential ways of preventing these diseases.

What Is Dementia?

Dementia is not a specific disease. It is a descriptive term for a collection of symptoms that can be caused by a number of disorders that affect the brain. People with dementia have significantly impaired intellectual functioning that interferes with normal activities and relationships. They also lose their ability to solve problems and maintain emotional control, and they may experience personality changes and behavioral problems, such as agitation, delusions, and hallucinations. While memory loss is a common symptom of dementia, memory loss by itself does not mean that a person has dementia. Doctors diagnose dementia only if two or more brain functions—such as memory, language skills, perception, or cognitive skills including reasoning and judgment—are significantly impaired without loss of consciousness.

There are many disorders that can cause dementia. Some, such as AD, lead to a progressive loss of mental functions. Yet other types of dementia can be halted or reversed with appropriate treatment.

With AD and many other types of dementia, disease processes cause many nerve cells to stop functioning, lose connections with other neurons, and die. In contrast, normal aging does not result in the loss of large numbers of neurons in the brain.

What Are the Different Kinds of Dementia?

Dementing disorders can be classified many different ways. These classification schemes attempt to group disorders that have particular features in common, such as whether they are progressive or what parts of the brain are affected. Some frequently used classifications include the following:

- **Cortical dementia:** dementia where the brain damage primarily affects the brain's cortex, or outer layer. Cortical dementias tend to cause problems with memory, language, thinking, and social behavior.

- **Subcortical dementia:** dementia that affects parts of the brain below the cortex. Subcortical dementia tends to cause changes in emotions and movement in addition to problems with memory.

- **Progressive dementia:** dementia that gets worse over time, gradually interfering with more and more cognitive abilities.

- **Primary dementia:** dementia such as AD that does not result from any other disease.

- **Secondary dementia:** dementia that occurs as a result of a physical disease or injury.

Some types of dementia fit into more than one of these classifications. For example, AD is considered both a progressive and a cortical dementia.

Alzheimer's Disease

Alzheimer's disease is the most common cause of dementia in people aged sixty-five and older. Experts believe that up to four million people in the United States are currently living with the disease: one in ten people over the age of sixty-five and nearly half of those over eighty-five have AD. At least 360,000 Americans are diagnosed with AD each year and about 50,000 are reported to die from it.

In most people, symptoms of AD appear after age sixty. However, there are some early-onset forms of the disease, usually linked to a specific gene defect, which may appear as early as age thirty. AD usually causes a gradual decline in cognitive abilities, usually during a span of seven to ten years. Nearly all brain functions, including memory, movement, language, judgment, behavior, and abstract thinking, are eventually affected.

AD is characterized by two abnormalities in the brain: amyloid plaques and neurofibrillary tangles. Amyloid plaques, which are found in the tissue between the nerve cells, are unusual clumps of a protein called beta amyloid along with degenerating bits of neurons and other cells.

Neurofibrillary tangles are bundles of twisted filaments found within neurons. These tangles are largely made up of a protein called tau. In healthy neurons, the tau protein helps the functioning of microtubules, which are part of the cell's structural support and deliver substances throughout the nerve cell. However, in AD, tau is changed in a way that causes it to twist into pairs of helical filaments that collect into tangles. When this happens, the microtubules cannot function correctly and they disintegrate. This collapse of the neuron's transport system may impair communication between nerve cells and cause them to die.

Researchers do not know if amyloid plaques and neurofibrillary tangles are harmful or if they are merely side effects of the disease process that damages neurons and leads to the symptoms of AD. They do know that plaques and tangles usually increase in the brain as AD progresses.

In the early stages of AD, patients may experience memory impairment, lapses of judgment, and subtle changes in personality. As the disorder progresses, memory and language problems worsen and patients begin to have difficulty performing activities of daily living, such as balancing a checkbook or remembering to take medications. They also may have visuospatial problems, such as difficulty navigating an unfamiliar route. They may become disoriented about places and times, may suffer delusions (such as the idea that someone is stealing from them or that their spouse is being unfaithful), and may become short-tempered and hostile. During the late stages of the disease, patients begin to lose the ability to control motor functions. They may have difficulty swallowing and lose bowel and bladder control. They eventually lose the ability to recognize family members and to speak. As AD progresses, it begins to affect the person's emotions and behavior. Most people with AD eventually develop symptoms such as aggression, agitation, depression, sleeplessness, or delusions.

On average, patients with AD live for eight to ten years after they are diagnosed. However, some people live as long as twenty years.

Patients with AD often die of aspiration pneumonia because they lose the ability to swallow late in the course of the disease.

Vascular Dementia

Vascular dementia is the second most common cause of dementia, after AD. It accounts for up to 20 percent of all dementias and is caused by brain damage from cerebrovascular or cardiovascular problems—usually strokes. It also may result from genetic diseases, endocarditis (infection of a heart valve), or amyloid angiopathy (a process in which amyloid protein builds up in the brain's blood vessels, sometimes causing hemorrhagic or "bleeding" strokes). In many cases, it may coexist with AD. The incidence of vascular dementia increases with advancing age and is similar in men and women.

Symptoms of vascular dementia often begin suddenly, frequently after a stroke. Patients may have a history of high blood pressure, vascular disease, or previous strokes or heart attacks. Vascular dementia may or may not get worse with time, depending on whether the person has additional strokes. In some cases, symptoms may get better with time. When the disease does get worse, it often progresses in a stepwise manner, with sudden changes in ability. Vascular dementia with brain damage to the mid-brain regions, however, may cause a gradual, progressive cognitive impairment that may look much like AD. Unlike people with AD, people with vascular dementia often maintain their personality and normal levels of emotional responsiveness until the later stages of the disease.

People with vascular dementia frequently wander at night and often have other problems commonly found in people who have had a stroke, including depression and incontinence.

There are several types of vascular dementia, which vary slightly in their causes and symptoms. One type, called multi-infarct dementia (MID), is caused by numerous small strokes in the brain. MID typically includes multiple damaged areas, called infarcts, along with extensive lesions in the white matter, or nerve fibers, of the brain.

Because the infarcts in MID affect isolated areas of the brain, the symptoms are often limited to one side of the body or they may affect just one or a few specific functions, such as language. Neurologists call these "local" or "focal" symptoms, as opposed to the "global" symptoms seen in AD, which affect many functions and are not restricted to one side of the body.

Although not all strokes cause dementia, in some cases a single stroke can damage the brain enough to cause dementia. This condition is called single-infarct dementia. Dementia is more common when the stroke takes place on the left side (hemisphere) of the brain or when it involves the hippocampus, a brain structure important for memory.

Another type of vascular dementia is called Binswanger's disease. This rare form of dementia is characterized by damage to small blood vessels in the white matter of the brain (white matter is found in the inner layers of the brain and contains many nerve fibers coated with a whitish, fatty substance called myelin). Binswanger's disease leads to brain lesions, loss of memory, disordered cognition, and mood changes. Patients with this disease often show signs of abnormal blood pressure, stroke, blood abnormalities, disease of the large blood vessels in the neck, or disease of the heart valves. Other prominent features include urinary incontinence, difficulty walking, clumsiness, slowness, lack of facial expression, and speech difficulty. These symptoms, which usually begin after the age of sixty, are not always present in all patients and may sometimes appear only temporarily. Treatment of Binswanger's disease is symptomatic, and may include the use of medications to control high blood pressure, depression, heart arrhythmias, and low blood pressure. The disorder often includes episodes of partial recovery.

Another type of vascular dementia is linked to a rare hereditary disorder called CADASIL, which stands for cerebral autosomal dominant arteriopathy with subcortical infarct and leukoencephalopathy. CADASIL is linked to abnormalities of a specific gene, Notch3, which is located on chromosome 19. This condition causes multi-infarct dementia as well as stroke, migraine with aura, and mood disorders. The first symptoms usually appear in people who are in their twenties, thirties, or forties, and affected individuals often die by age sixty-five. Researchers believe most people with CADASIL go undiagnosed, and the actual prevalence of the disease is not yet known.

Other causes of vascular dementia include vasculitis, an inflammation of the blood vessel system; profound hypotension (low blood pressure); and lesions caused by brain hemorrhage. The autoimmune disease lupus erythematosus and the inflammatory disease temporal arteritis can also damage blood vessels in a way that leads to vascular dementia.

Lewy Body Dementia

Lewy body dementia (LBD) is one of the most common types of progressive dementia. LBD usually occurs sporadically, in people with no known family history of the disease. However, rare familial cases have occasionally been reported.

In LBD, cells die in the brain's cortex, or outer layer, and in a part of the mid-brain called the substantia nigra. Many of the remaining nerve cells in the substantia nigra contain abnormal structures called Lewy bodies that are the hallmark of the disease. Lewy bodies may also appear in the brain's cortex, or outer layer. Lewy bodies contain a protein called alpha-synuclein that has been linked to Parkinson disease and several other disorders. Researchers, who sometimes refer to these disorders collectively as "synucleinopathies," do not yet know why this protein accumulates inside nerve cells in LBD.

The symptoms of LBD overlap with AD in many ways, and may include memory impairment, poor judgment, and confusion. However, LBD typically also includes visual hallucinations, parkinsonian symptoms such as a shuffling gait and flexed posture, and day-to-day fluctuations in the severity of symptoms. Patients with LBD live an average of seven years after symptoms begin.

There is no cure for LBD, and treatments are aimed at controlling the parkinsonian and psychiatric symptoms of the disorder. Patients sometimes respond dramatically to treatment with antiparkinsonian drugs or cholinesterase inhibitors, such as those used for AD. Some studies indicate that neuroleptic drugs, such as clozapine and olanzapine, also can reduce the psychiatric symptoms of this disease. Yet neuroleptic drugs may cause severe adverse reactions, so other therapies should be tried first and patients using these drugs should be closely monitored.

Lewy bodies are often found in the brains of people with Parkinson and AD. These findings suggest that either LBD is related to these other causes of dementia or that the diseases sometimes coexist in the same person.

Frontotemporal Dementia

Frontotemporal dementia (FTD), sometimes called frontal lobe dementia, describes a group of diseases characterized by degeneration of nerve cells—especially those in the frontal and temporal lobes of the brain. Unlike AD, FTD usually does not include formation of amyloid plaques. In many people with FTD, there is an abnormal form of tau protein in the brain, which accumulates into neurofibrillary tangles. This disrupts normal cell activities and may cause the cells to die.

Experts believe FTD accounts for 2 to 10 percent of all cases of dementia. Symptoms of FTD usually appear between the ages of forty and sixty-five. In many cases, people with FTD have a family history of dementia, suggesting that there is a strong genetic factor in the disease. The duration of FTD varies, with some patients declining rapidly over two to three years and others showing only minimal changes for many years. People with FTD live with the disease for an average of five to ten years after diagnosis.

Because structures found in the frontal and temporal lobes of the brain control judgment and social behavior, people with FTD often have problems maintaining normal interactions and following social conventions. They may steal or exhibit impolite and socially inappropriate behavior, and they may neglect their normal responsibilities. Other common symptoms include loss of speech and language, compulsive or repetitive behavior, increased appetite, and motor problems such as stiffness and balance problems. Memory loss also may occur, although it typically appears late in the disease.

In one type of FTD called Pick's disease, certain nerve cells become abnormal and swollen before they die. These swollen, or ballooned, neurons are one hallmark of the disease. The brains of people with Pick's disease also have abnormal structures called Pick bodies, composed largely of the protein tau, inside the neurons. The cause of Pick's disease is unknown, but it runs in some families and thus it is probably due at least in part to a faulty gene or genes. The disease usually begins after age fifty and causes changes in personality and behavior that gradually worsen over time. The symptoms of Pick's disease are very similar to those of AD, and may include inappropriate social behavior, loss of mental flexibility, language problems, and difficulty with thinking and concentration. There is currently no way to slow the progressive degeneration found in Pick's disease. However, medication may be helpful in reducing aggression and other behavioral problems, and in treating depression.

In some cases, familial FTD is linked to a mutation in the tau gene. This disorder, called frontotemporal dementia with parkinsonism linked to chromosome 17 (FTDP-17), is much like other types of FTD but often includes psychiatric symptoms such as delusions and hallucinations.

Primary progressive aphasia (PPA) is a type of FTD that may begin in people as early as their forties. "Aphasia" is a general term used to refer to deficits in language functions, such as speaking, understanding what others are saying, and naming common objects. In PPA one or more of these functions can become impaired. Symptoms often begin gradually and progress slowly over a period of years. As the disease progresses, memory and attention may also be impaired and patients may show personality and behavior changes. Many, but not all, people with PPA eventually develop symptoms of dementia.

HIV-Associated Dementia

HIV-associated dementia (HAD) results from infection with the human immunodeficiency virus (HIV) that causes AIDS. HAD can cause widespread destruction of the brain's white matter. This leads to a type of dementia that generally includes impaired memory, apathy, social withdrawal, and difficulty concentrating. People with HAD often develop movement problems as well. There is no specific treatment for HAD, but AIDS drugs can delay onset of the disease and may help to reduce symptoms.

Huntington Disease

Huntington disease (HD) is a hereditary disorder caused by a faulty gene for a protein called huntingtin. The children of people with the disorder have a 50 percent chance of inheriting it. The disease causes degeneration in many regions of the brain and spinal cord. Symptoms of HD usually begin when patients are in their thirties or forties, and the average life expectancy after diagnosis is about fifteen years.

Cognitive symptoms of HD typically begin with mild personality changes, such as irritability, anxiety, and depression, and progress to severe dementia. Many patients also show psychotic behavior. HD causes chorea—involuntary jerky, arrhythmic movements of the body—as well as muscle weakness, clumsiness, and gait disturbances.

Dementia Pugilistica

Dementia pugilistica, also called chronic traumatic encephalopathy or Boxer's syndrome, is caused by head trauma, such as that experienced by people who have been punched many times in the head during boxing. The most common symptoms of the condition are dementia and parkinsonism, which can appear many years after the trauma ends. Affected individuals may also develop poor coordination and slurred speech. A single traumatic brain injury may also lead to a disorder called post-traumatic dementia (PTD). PTD is much like dementia pugilistica but usually also includes long-term memory problems. Other symptoms vary depending on which part of the brain was damaged by the injury.

Corticobasal Degeneration

Corticobasal degeneration (CBD) is a progressive disorder characterized by nerve cell loss and atrophy of multiple areas of the brain.

343

Brain cells from people with CBD often have abnormal accumulations of the protein tau. CBD usually progresses gradually over the course of six to eight years. Initial symptoms, which typically begin at or around age sixty, may first appear on one side of the body but eventually will affect both sides. Some of the symptoms, such as poor coordination and rigidity, are similar to those found in Parkinson disease. Other symptoms may include memory loss, dementia, visual-spatial problems, apraxia (loss of the ability to make familiar, purposeful movements), hesitant and halting speech, myoclonus (involuntary muscular jerks), and dysphagia (difficulty swallowing). Death is often caused by pneumonia or other secondary problems such as sepsis (severe infection of the blood) or pulmonary embolism (a blood clot in the lungs).

There are no specific treatments available for CBD. Drugs such as clonazepam may help with myoclonus, however, and occupational, physical, and speech therapy can help in managing the disabilities associated with this disease. The symptoms of the disease often do not respond to Parkinson medications or other drugs.

Creutzfeldt-Jakob Disease

Creutzfeldt-Jakob disease (CJD) is a rare, degenerative, fatal brain disorder that affects about one in every million people per year worldwide. Symptoms usually begin after age sixty, and most patients die within one year. Many researchers believe CJD results from an abnormal form of a protein called a prion. Most cases of CJD occur sporadically—that is, in people who have no known risk factors for the disease. However, about 5 to 10 percent of cases of CJD in the United States are hereditary, caused by a mutation in the gene for the prion protein. In rare cases, CJD can also be acquired through exposure to diseased brain or nervous system tissue, usually through certain medical procedures. There is no evidence that CJD is contagious through the air or through casual contact with a CJD patient.

Patients with CJD may initially experience problems with muscular coordination; personality changes, including impaired memory, judgment, and thinking; and impaired vision. Other symptoms may include insomnia and depression. As the illness progresses, mental impairment becomes severe. Patients often develop myoclonus and they may go blind. They eventually lose the ability to move and speak, and go into a coma. Pneumonia and other infections often occur in these patients and can lead to death.

CJD belongs to a family of human and animal diseases known as the transmissible spongiform encephalopathies (TSEs). Spongiform refers to the characteristic appearance of infected brains, which become filled with holes until they resemble sponges when viewed under a microscope. CJD is the most common of the known human TSEs. Others include fatal familial insomnia and Gerstmann-Straussler-Scheinker disease.

In recent years, a new type of CJD, called variant CJD (vCJD), has been found in Great Britain and several other European countries. The initial symptoms of vCJD are different from those of classic CJD, and the disorder typically occurs in younger patients. Research suggests that vCJD may result from human consumption of beef from cattle with a TSE disease called bovine spongiform encephalopathy (BSE), also known as "mad cow disease."

Other Dementias

Other rare hereditary dementias include Gerstmann-Straussler-Scheinker (GSS) disease, fatal familial insomnia, familial British dementia, and familial Danish dementia. Symptoms of GSS typically include ataxia and progressive dementia that begins when people are between fifty and sixty years old. The disease may last for several years before patients eventually die. Fatal familial insomnia causes degeneration of a brain region called the thalamus, which is partially responsible for controlling sleep. It causes a progressive insomnia that eventually leads to a complete inability to sleep. Other symptoms may include poor reflexes, dementia, hallucinations, and eventually coma. It can be fatal within seven to thirteen months after symptoms begin but may last longer. Familial British dementia and familial Danish dementia have been linked to two different defects in a gene found on chromosome 13. The symptoms of both diseases include progressive dementia, paralysis, and loss of balance.

Secondary Dementias

Dementia may occur in patients who have other disorders that primarily affect movement or other functions. These cases are often referred to as secondary dementias. The relationship between these disorders and the primary dementias is not always clear. For instance, people with advanced Parkinson disease, which is primarily a movement disorder, sometimes develop symptoms of dementia. Many Parkinson patients also have amyloid plaques and neurofibrillary tangles like those found in AD. The two diseases may be linked in a yet-unknown way, or they may simply coexist in some people. People with

Parkinson and associated dementia sometimes show signs of Lewy body dementia or progressive supranuclear palsy at autopsy, suggesting that these diseases may also overlap with Parkinson or that Parkinson is sometimes misdiagnosed.

Other disorders that may include symptoms of dementia include multiple sclerosis; presenile dementia with motor neuron disease, also called ALS dementia; olivopontocerebellar atrophy (OPCA); Wilson's disease; and normal pressure hydrocephalus (NPH).

Dementias in Children

While it is usually found in adults, dementia can also occur in children. For example, infections and poisoning can lead to dementia in people of any age. In addition, some disorders unique to children can cause dementia.

Niemann-Pick Disease

Niemann-Pick disease is a group of inherited disorders that affect metabolism and are caused by specific genetic mutations. Patients with Niemann-Pick disease cannot properly metabolize cholesterol and other lipids. Consequently, excessive amounts of cholesterol accumulate in the liver and spleen and excessive amounts of other lipids accumulate in the brain. Symptoms may include dementia, confusion, and problems with learning and memory. These diseases usually begin in young school-age children but may also appear during the teen years or early adulthood.

Batten Disease

Batten disease is a fatal, hereditary disorder of the nervous system that begins in childhood. Symptoms are linked to a buildup of substances called lipopigments in the body's tissues. The early symptoms include personality and behavior changes, slow learning, clumsiness, or stumbling. Over time, affected children suffer mental impairment, seizures, and progressive loss of sight and motor skills. Eventually, children with Batten disease develop dementia and become blind and bedridden. The disease is often fatal by the late teens or twenties.

Lafora Body Disease

Lafora body disease is a rare genetic disease that causes seizures, rapidly progressive dementia, and movement problems. These problems usually begin in late childhood or the early teens. Children with Lafora body disease have microscopic structures called Lafora bodies in the brain, skin, liver, and muscles. Most affected children die within two to ten years after the onset of symptoms.

A number of other childhood-onset disorders can include symptoms of dementia. Among these are mitochondrial myopathies, Rasmussen's encephalitis, mucopolysaccharidosis III (Sanfilippo syndrome), neuro-degeneration with brain iron accumulation, and leukodystrophies such as Alexander disease, Schilder's disease, and metachromatic leu-kodystrophy.

What Other Conditions Can Cause Dementia?

Doctors have identified many other conditions that can cause de-mentia or dementia-like symptoms. Many of these conditions are re-versible with appropriate treatment.

- **Reactions to medications:** Medications can sometimes lead to reactions or side effects that mimic dementia. These dementia-like effects can occur in reaction to just one drug or they can re-sult from drug interactions. They may have a rapid onset or they may develop slowly over time.

- **Metabolic problems and endocrine abnormalities:** Thy-roid problems can lead to apathy, depression, or dementia. Hy-poglycemia, a condition in which there is not enough sugar in the bloodstream, can cause confusion or personality changes. Too little or too much sodium or calcium can also trigger mental changes. Some people have an impaired ability to absorb vita-min B_{12}, which creates a condition called pernicious anemia that can cause personality changes, irritability, or depression. Tests can determine if any of these problems are present.

- **Nutritional deficiencies:** Deficiencies of thiamine (vitamin B_1) frequently result from chronic alcoholism and can seriously impair mental abilities, in particular memories of recent events. Severe deficiency of vitamin B_6 can cause a neurological illness called pellagra that may include dementia. Deficiencies of vita-min B_{12} also have been linked to dementia in some cases. Dehy-dration can also cause mental impairment that can resemble dementia.

- **Infections:** Many infections can cause neurological symptoms, including confusion or delirium, due to fever or other side effects of the body's fight to overcome the infection. Meningitis and encephalitis, which are infections of the brain or the membrane that covers it, can cause confusion, sudden severe dementia, withdrawal from social interaction, impaired judgment, or memory loss. Untreated syphilis also can damage the nervous system and cause dementia. In rare cases, Lyme disease can cause memory or thinking difficulties. People in the advanced stages of AIDS also may develop a form of dementia. People with compromised immune systems, such as those with leukemia and AIDS, may also develop an infection called progressive multifocal leukoencephalopathy (PML). PML is caused by a common human polyomavirus, JC virus, and leads to damage or destruction of the myelin sheath that covers nerve cells. PML can lead to confusion, difficulty with thinking or speaking, and other mental problems.

- **Subdural hematomas:** Subdural hematomas, or bleeding between the brain's surface and its outer covering (the dura), can cause dementia-like symptoms and changes in mental function.

- **Poisoning:** Exposure to lead, other heavy metals, or other poisonous substances can lead to symptoms of dementia. These symptoms may or may not resolve after treatment, depending on how badly the brain is damaged. People who have abused substances such as alcohol and recreational drugs sometimes display signs of dementia even after the substance abuse has ended. This condition is known as substance-induced persisting dementia.

- **Brain tumors:** In rare cases, people with brain tumors may develop dementia because of damage to their brains. Symptoms may include changes in personality, psychotic episodes, or problems with speech, language, thinking, and memory.

- **Anoxia:** Anoxia and a related term, hypoxia, are often used interchangeably to describe a state in which there is a diminished supply of oxygen to an organ's tissues. Anoxia may be caused by many different problems, including heart attack, heart surgery, severe asthma, smoke or carbon monoxide inhalation, high-altitude exposure, strangulation, or an overdose of anesthesia. In severe cases of anoxia the patient may be in a stupor or a coma for periods ranging from hours to days, weeks, or months. Recovery depends on the severity of the oxygen deprivation. As recovery proceeds, a variety of psychological and neurological abnormalities, such as dementia or psychosis, may occur. The person also may experience confusion, personality changes, hallucinations, or memory loss.

- **Heart and lung problems:** The brain requires a high level of oxygen in order to carry out its normal functions. Therefore, problems such as chronic lung disease or heart problems that prevent the brain from receiving adequate oxygen can starve brain cells and lead to the symptoms of dementia.

What Conditions Are Not Dementia?

- **Age-related cognitive decline:** As people age, they usually experience slower information processing and mild memory impairment. In addition, their brains frequently decrease in volume and some nerve cells, or neurons, are lost. These changes, called age-related cognitive decline, are normal and are not considered signs of dementia.

- **Mild cognitive impairment:** Some people develop cognitive and memory problems that are not severe enough to be diagnosed as dementia but are more pronounced than the cognitive changes associated with normal aging. This condition is called mild cognitive impairment. Although many patients with this condition later develop dementia, some do not. Many researchers are studying mild cognitive impairment to find ways to treat it or prevent it from progressing to dementia.

- **Depression:** People with depression are frequently passive or unresponsive, and they may appear slow, confused, or forgetful. Other emotional problems can also cause symptoms that sometimes mimic dementia.

- **Delirium:** Delirium is characterized by confusion and rapidly altering mental states. The person may also be disoriented, drowsy, or incoherent, and may exhibit personality changes. Delirium is usually caused by a treatable physical or psychiatric illness, such as poisoning or infections. Patients with delirium often, though not always, make a full recovery after their underlying illness is treated.

What Causes Dementia?

All forms of dementia result from the death of nerve cells or the loss of communication among these cells. The human brain is a very complex and intricate machine and many factors can interfere with its functioning. Researchers have uncovered many of these factors, but they have not yet been able to fit these puzzle pieces together in order to form a complete picture of how dementias develop.

Many types of dementia, including AD, Lewy body dementia, Parkinson's dementia, and Pick's disease, are characterized by abnormal structures called inclusions in the brain. Because these inclusions, which contain abnormal proteins, are so common in people with dementia, researchers suspect that they play a role in the development of symptoms. However, that role is unknown, and in some cases the inclusions may simply be a side effect of the disease process that leads to the dementia.

Genes clearly play a role in the development of some kinds of dementia. However, in AD and many other disorders, the dementia usually cannot be tied to a single abnormal gene. Instead, these forms of dementia appear to result from a complex interaction of genes, lifestyle factors, and other environmental influences.

Researchers have identified several genes that influence susceptibility to AD. Mutations in three of the known genes for AD—genes that control the production of proteins such as amyloid precursor protein (APP), presenilin 1, and presenilin 2—are linked to early-onset forms of the disease.

Variations in another gene, called apolipoprotein E (apoE), have been linked to an increased risk of late-onset AD. The apoE gene does not cause the disease by itself, but one version of the gene, called apoE epsilon4 (apoE E4), appears to increase the risk of AD. People with two copies of the apoE E4 gene have about ten times the risk of developing AD compared to people without apoE E4. This gene variant seems to encourage amyloid deposition in the brain. One study also found that this gene is associated with shorter survival in men with AD. In contrast, another version of the apoE gene, called apoE E2, appears to protect against AD.

Studies have suggested that mutations in another gene, called CYP46, may contribute to an increased risk of developing late-onset sporadic AD. This gene normally produces a protein that helps the brain metabolize cholesterol.

Scientists are trying to determine how beta amyloid influences the development of AD. A number of studies indicate that the buildup of this protein initiates a complex chain of events that culminates in dementia. One study found that beta amyloid buildup in the brain triggers cells called microglia, which act like janitors that mop up potentially harmful substances in the brain, to release a potent neurotoxin called peroxynitrite. This may contribute to nerve cell death in AD. Another study found that beta amyloid causes a protein called p35 to be split into two proteins. One of the resulting proteins triggers changes in the tau protein that lead to formation of neurofibrillary tangles. A third study found that beta amyloid activates cell-death enzymes called caspases that alter the tau protein in a way that causes it to form tangles. Researchers believe these tangles may contribute to the neuron death in AD.

Vascular dementia can be caused by cerebrovascular disease or any other condition that prevents normal blood flow to the brain. Without a normal supply of blood, brain cells cannot obtain the oxygen they need to work correctly, and they often become so deprived that they die.

The causes of other types of dementias vary. Some, such as CJD and GSS, have been tied to abnormal forms of specific proteins. Others, including Huntington disease and FTDP-17, have been linked to defects in a single gene. Post-traumatic dementia is directly related to brain cell death after injury. HIV-associated dementia is clearly tied to infection by the HIV virus, although the exact way the virus causes damage is not yet certain. For other dementias, such as corticobasal degeneration and most types of frontotemporal dementia, the underlying causes have not yet been identified.

What Are the Risk Factors for Dementia?

Researchers have identified several risk factors that affect the likelihood of developing one or more kinds of dementia. Some of these factors are modifiable, while others are not.

- **Age:** The risk of AD, vascular dementia, and several other dementias goes up significantly with advancing age.

- **Genetics and family history:** As described previously, researchers have discovered a number of genes that increase the risk of developing AD. Although people with a family history of AD are generally considered to be at heightened risk of developing the disease themselves, many people with a family history never develop the disease, and many without a family history of the disease do get it. In most cases, it is still impossible to predict a specific person's risk of the disorder based on family history alone. Some families with CJD, GSS, or fatal familial insomnia have mutations in the prion protein gene, although these disorders can also occur in people without the

351

gene mutation. Individuals with these mutations are at significantly higher risk of developing these forms of dementia. Abnormal genes are also clearly implicated as risk factors in Huntington disease, FTDP-17, and several other kinds of dementia.

- **Smoking and alcohol use:** Several recent studies have found that smoking significantly increases the risk of mental decline and dementia. People who smoke have a higher risk of atherosclerosis and other types of vascular disease, which may be the underlying causes for the increased dementia risk. Studies also have found that drinking large amounts of alcohol appears to increase the risk of dementia. However, other studies have suggested that people who drink moderately have a lower risk of dementia than either those who drink heavily or those who completely abstain from drinking.

- **Atherosclerosis:** Atherosclerosis is the buildup of plaque—deposits of fatty substances, cholesterol, and other matter—in the inner lining of an artery. Atherosclerosis is a significant risk factor for vascular dementia, because it interferes with the delivery of blood to the brain and can lead to stroke. Studies have also found a possible link between atherosclerosis and AD.

- **Cholesterol:** High levels of low-density lipoprotein (LDL), the so-called bad form of cholesterol, appear to significantly increase a person's risk of developing vascular dementia. Some research has also linked high cholesterol to an increased risk of AD.

- **Plasma homocysteine:** Research has shown that a higher-than-average blood level of homocysteine—a type of amino acid—is a strong risk factor for the development of AD and vascular dementia.

- **Diabetes:** Diabetes is a risk factor for both AD and vascular dementia. It is also a known risk factor for atherosclerosis and stroke, both of which contribute to vascular dementia.

- **Mild cognitive impairment:** While not all people with mild cognitive impairment develop dementia, people with this condition do have a significantly increased risk of dementia compared to the rest of the population. One study found that approximately 40 percent of people over age sixty-five who were diagnosed with mild cognitive impairment developed dementia within three years.

- **Down syndrome:** Studies have found that most people with
  Down syndrome develop characteristic AD plaques and neurofibrillary tangles by the time they reach middle age. Many,
  but not all, of these individuals also develop symptoms of dementia.

How Is Dementia Diagnosed?

Doctors employ a number of strategies to diagnose dementia. It is
important that they rule out any treatable conditions, such as depression, normal pressure hydrocephalus, or vitamin B_{12} deficiency, which
can cause similar symptoms.

Early, accurate diagnosis of dementia is important for patients and
their families because it allows early treatment of symptoms. For
people with AD or other progressive dementias, early diagnosis may
allow them to plan for the future while they can still help to make
decisions. These people also may benefit from drug treatment.

The "gold standard" for diagnosing dementia, autopsy, does not help
the patient or caregivers. Therefore, doctors have devised a number
of techniques to help identify dementia with reasonable accuracy
while the patient is still alive.

Patient History

Doctors often begin their examination of a patient suspected of
having dementia by asking questions about the patient's history. For
example, they may ask how and when symptoms developed and about
the patient's overall medical condition. They also may try to evaluate the patient's emotional state, although patients with dementia
often may be unaware of or in denial about how their disease is affecting them. Family members also may deny the existence of the disease because they do not want to accept the diagnosis and because,
at least in the beginning, AD and other forms of dementia can resemble normal aging. Therefore additional steps are necessary to confirm or rule out a diagnosis of dementia.

Physical Examination

A physical examination can help rule out treatable causes of dementia and identify signs of stroke or other disorders that can contribute to dementia. It can also identify signs of other illnesses, such
as heart disease or kidney failure, that can overlap with dementia. If

a patient is taking medications that may be causing or contributing to his or her symptoms, the doctor may suggest stopping or replacing some medications to see if the symptoms go away.

Neurological Evaluations

Doctors will perform a neurological examination, looking at balance, sensory function, reflexes, and other functions, to identify signs of conditions—for example movement disorders or stroke—that may affect the patient's diagnosis or are treatable with drugs.

Cognitive and Neuropsychological Tests

Doctors use tests that measure memory, language skills, math skills, and other abilities related to mental functioning to help them diagnose a patient's condition accurately. For example, people with AD often show changes in so-called executive functions (such as problem-solving), memory, and the ability to perform once-automatic tasks.

Doctors often use a test called the Mini-Mental State Examination (MMSE) to assess cognitive skills in people with suspected dementia. This test examines orientation, memory, and attention, as well as the ability to name objects, follow verbal and written commands, write a sentence spontaneously, and copy a complex shape. Doctors also use a variety of other tests and rating scales to identify specific types of cognitive problems and abilities.

Brain Scans

Doctors may use brain scans to identify strokes, tumors, or other problems that can cause dementia. Also, cortical atrophy—degeneration of the brain's cortex (outer layer)—is common in many forms of dementia and may be visible on a brain scan. The brain's cortex normally appears very wrinkled, with ridges of tissue (called gyri) separated by "valleys" called sulci. In individuals with cortical atrophy, the progressive loss of neurons causes the ridges to become thinner and the sulci to grow wider. As brain cells die, the ventricles (or fluid-filled cavities in the middle of the brain) expand to fill the available space, becoming much larger than normal. Brain scans also can identify changes in the brain's structure and function that suggest AD.

The most common types of brain scans are computed tomographic (CT) scans and magnetic resonance imaging (MRI). Doctors frequently request a CT scan of the brain when they are examining a patient with suspected dementia. These scans, which use x-rays to detect brain structures, can show evidence of brain atrophy, strokes and transient ischemic attacks (TIAs), changes to the blood vessels, and other problems such as hydrocephalus and subdural hematomas. MRI scans use magnetic fields and focused radio waves to detect hydrogen atoms in tissues within the body. They can detect the same problems as CT scans but they are better for identifying certain conditions, such as brain atrophy and damage from small TIAs.

Doctors also may use electroencephalograms (EEGs) in people with suspected dementia. In an EEG, electrodes are placed on the scalp over several parts of the brain in order to detect and record patterns of electrical activity and check for abnormalities. This electrical activity can indicate cognitive dysfunction in part or all of the brain. Many patients with moderately severe to severe AD have abnormal EEGs. An EEG may also be used to detect seizures, which occur in about 10 percent of AD patients as well as in many other disorders. EEGs also can help diagnose CJD.

Several other types of brain scans allow researchers to watch the brain as it functions. These scans, called functional brain imaging, are not often used as diagnostic tools, but they are important in research and they may ultimately help identify people with dementia earlier than is currently possible. Functional brain scans include functional MRI (fMRI), single photon-emission computed tomography (SPECT), positron emission tomography (PET), and magnetoencephalography (MEG). fMRI uses radio waves and a strong magnetic field to measure the metabolic changes that take place in active parts of the brain. SPECT shows the distribution of blood in the brain, which generally increases with brain activity. PET scans can detect changes in glucose metabolism, oxygen metabolism, and blood flow, all of which can reveal abnormalities of brain function. MEG shows the electromagnetic fields produced by the brain's neuronal activity.

Laboratory Tests

Doctors may use a variety of laboratory tests to help diagnose dementia and rule out other conditions, such as kidney failure, that can contribute to symptoms. A partial list of these tests includes a complete blood count, blood glucose test, urinalysis, drug and alcohol tests (toxicology screen), cerebrospinal fluid analysis (to rule out specific infections that can affect the brain), and analysis of thyroid and thyroid-stimulating hormone levels. A doctor will order only the tests that he or she feels are necessary and likely to improve the accuracy of a diagnosis.

Psychiatric Evaluation

A psychiatric evaluation may be obtained to determine if depression or another psychiatric disorder may be causing or contributing to a person's symptoms.

Presymptomatic Testing

Testing people before symptoms begin to determine if they will develop dementia is not possible in most cases. However, in disorders such as Huntington where a known gene defect is clearly linked to the risk of the disease, a genetic test can help identify people who are likely to develop the disease. Since this type of genetic information can be devastating, people should carefully consider whether they want to undergo such testing.

Researchers are examining whether a series of simple cognitive tests, such as matching words with pictures, can predict who will develop dementia. One study suggested that a combination of a verbal learning test and an odor-identification test can help identify AD before symptoms become obvious. Other studies are looking at whether memory tests and brain scans can be useful indicators of future dementia.

Is There Any Treatment?

While treatments to reverse or halt disease progression are not available for most of the dementias, patients can benefit to some extent from treatment with available medications and other measures, such as cognitive training.

Drugs to specifically treat AD and some other progressive dementias are now available and are prescribed for many patients. Although these drugs do not halt the disease or reverse existing brain damage, they can improve symptoms and slow the progression of the disease. This may improve the patient's quality of life, ease the burden on caregivers, and delay admission to a nursing home. Many researchers are also examining whether these drugs may be useful for treating other types of dementia.

Many people with dementia, particularly those in the early stages, may benefit from practicing tasks designed to improve performance in specific aspects of cognitive functioning. For example, people can sometimes be taught to use memory aids, such as mnemonics, computerized recall devices, or note taking.

Behavior modification—rewarding appropriate or positive behavior and ignoring inappropriate behavior—also may help control unacceptable or dangerous behaviors.

Alzheimer's Disease

Most of the drugs currently approved by the U.S. Food and Drug Administration for AD fall into a category called cholinesterase inhibitors. These drugs slow the breakdown of the neurotransmitter acetylcholine, which is reduced in the brains of people with AD. Acetylcholine is important for the formation of memories and it is used in the hippocampus and the cerebral cortex, two brain regions that are affected by AD. There are currently four cholinesterase inhibitors approved for use in the United States: tacrine (Cognex), donepezil (Aricept), rivastigmine (Exelon), and galantamine (Reminyl). These drugs temporarily improve or stabilize memory and thinking skills in some individuals. Many studies have shown that cholinesterase inhibitors help to slow the decline in mental functions associated with AD, and that they can help reduce behavioral problems and improve the ability to perform everyday tasks. However, none of these drugs can stop or reverse the course of AD.

A fifth drug, memantine (Namenda), was recently approved for use in the United States. Unlike other drugs for AD, which affect acetylcholine levels, memantine works by regulating the activity of a neurotransmitter called glutamate that plays a role in learning and memory. Glutamate activity is often disrupted in AD. Because this drug works differently from cholinesterase inhibitors, combining memantine with other AD drugs may be more effective than any single therapy. One controlled clinical trial found that patients receiving donepezil plus memantine had better cognition and other functions than patients receiving donepezil alone.

Doctors may also prescribe other drugs, such as anticonvulsants, antipsychotics, sedatives, and antidepressants, to treat seizures, depression, agitation, sleep disorders, and other specific problems that can be associated with dementia.

Vascular Dementia

There is no standard drug treatment for vascular dementia, although some of the symptoms, such as depression, can be treated. Most other treatments aim to reduce the risk factors for further brain damage. However, some studies have found that cholinesterase inhibitors, such as galantamine and other AD drugs, can improve cognitive function and behavioral symptoms in patients with early vascular dementia.

The progression of vascular dementia can often be slowed significantly or halted if the underlying vascular risk factors for the disease are treated. To prevent strokes and TIAs, doctors may prescribe medicines to control high blood pressure, high cholesterol, heart disease, and diabetes. Doctors also sometimes prescribe aspirin, warfarin, or other drugs to prevent clots from forming in small blood vessels. When patients have blockages in blood vessels, doctors may recommend surgical procedures, such as carotid endarterectomy, stenting, or angioplasty, to restore the normal blood supply. Medications to relieve restlessness or depression or to help patients sleep better may also be prescribed.

Other Dementias

Some studies have suggested that cholinesterase inhibitors, such as donepezil (Aricept), can reduce behavioral symptoms in some patients with Parkinson's dementia.

At present, no medications are approved specifically to treat or prevent FTD and most other types of progressive dementia. However, sedatives, antidepressants, and other medications may be useful in treating specific symptoms and behavioral problems associated with these diseases.

Scientists continue to search for specific treatments to help people with Lewy body dementia. Current treatment is symptomatic, often involving the use of medication to control the parkinsonian and psychiatric symptoms. Although antiparkinsonian medication may help reduce tremor and loss of muscle movement, it may worsen symptoms such as hallucinations and delusions. Also, drugs prescribed for psychiatric symptoms may make the movement problems worse. In general, newer antipsychotic medications are more successful than older drugs such as haloperidol. Several studies have suggested that cholinesterase inhibitors may be able to improve cognitive function and behavioral symptoms in patients with Lewy body disease.

There is no known treatment that can cure or control CJD. Current treatment is aimed at alleviating symptoms and making the patient as comfortable as possible. Opiate drugs can help relieve pain, and the drugs clonazepam and sodium valproate may help relieve myoclonus. During later stages of the disease, treatment focuses on supportive care, such as administering intravenous fluids and changing the person's position frequently to prevent bedsores.

Can Dementia Be Prevented?

Research has revealed a number of factors that may be able to prevent or delay the onset of dementia in some people. For example, studies have shown that people who maintain tight control over their glucose levels tend to score better on tests of cognitive function than those with poorly controlled diabetes. Several studies also have suggested that people who engage in intellectually stimulating activities, such as social interactions, chess, crossword puzzles, and playing a musical instrument, significantly lower their risk of developing AD and other forms of dementia. Scientists believe mental activities may stimulate the brain in a way that increases the person's "cognitive reserve"—the ability to cope with or compensate for the pathologic changes associated with dementia.

Researchers are studying other steps people can take that may help prevent AD in some cases. So far, none of these factors has been definitively proven to make a difference in the risk of developing the disease. Moreover, most of the studies addressed only AD, and the results may or may not apply to other forms of dementia. Nevertheless, scientists are encouraged by the results of these early studies and many believe it will eventually become possible to prevent some forms of dementia. Possible preventive actions include:

- **Lowering homocysteine:** In one study, elevated blood levels of the amino acid homocysteine were associated with a 2.9 times greater risk of AD and a 4.9 times greater risk of vascular dementia. A preliminary study has shown that high doses of three B vitamins that help lower homocysteine levels—folic acid, B_{12}, and B_6—appear to slow the progression of AD. Researchers are now conducting a multi-center clinical trial to test this effect in a larger group of patients.

- **Lowering cholesterol levels:** Research has suggested that people with high cholesterol levels have an increased risk of developing AD. Cholesterol is involved in formation of amyloid plaques in the brain. Mutations in a gene called CYP46 and the apoE E4 gene variant, both of which have been linked to an increased risk of AD, are also involved in cholesterol metabolism. Several studies have also found that the use of drugs called statins, which lower cholesterol levels, is associated with a lower likelihood of cognitive impairment.

- **Lowering blood pressure:** Several studies have shown that antihypertensive medicine reduces the odds of cognitive impairment in elderly people with high blood pressure. One large European study found a 55 percent lower risk of dementia in people over sixty who received drug treatment for hypertension. These people had a reduced risk of both AD and vascular dementia.

- **Exercise:** Regular exercise stimulates production of chemicals called growth factors that help neurons survive and adapt to new situations. These gains may help to delay the onset of dementia symptoms. Exercise also may reduce the risk of brain damage from atherosclerosis.

- **Education:** Researchers have found evidence that formal education may help protect people against the effects of AD. In one study, researchers found that people with more years of formal education had relatively less mental decline than people with less schooling, regardless of the number of amyloid plaques and neurofibrillary tangles each person had in his or her brain. The researchers think education may cause the brain to develop robust nerve cell networks that can help compensate for the cell damage caused by AD.

- **Controlling inflammation:** Many studies have suggested that inflammation may contribute to AD. Moreover, autopsies of people who died with AD have shown widespread inflammation in the brain that appeared to be caused by the accumulation of beta amyloid. Another study found that men with high levels of C-reactive protein, a general marker of inflammation, had a significantly increased risk of AD and other kinds of dementia.

- **Nonsteroidal anti-inflammatory drugs (NSAIDs):** Research indicates that long-term use of NSAIDs—ibuprofen, naproxen, and similar drugs—may prevent or delay the onset of AD. Researchers are not sure how these drugs may protect against the disease, but some or all of the effect may be due to reduced inflammation. A 2003 study showed that these drugs also bind to amyloid plaques and may help to dissolve them and prevent formation of new plaques.

The risk of vascular dementia is strongly correlated with risk factors for stroke, including high blood pressure, diabetes, elevated cholesterol levels, and smoking. This type of dementia may be prevented in many cases by changing lifestyle factors, such as excessive weight and high blood pressure, which are associated with an increased risk of cerebrovascular disease. One European study found that treating isolated systolic hypertension (high blood pressure in which only the systolic or top number is high) in people age sixty and older reduced the risk of dementia by 50 percent. These studies strongly suggest that effective use of current treatments can prevent many future cases of vascular dementia.

What Kind of Care Does a Person with Dementia Need?

People with moderate and advanced dementia typically need round-the-clock care and supervision to prevent them from harming themselves or others. They also may need assistance with daily activities such as eating, bathing, and dressing. Meeting these needs takes patience, understanding, and careful thought by the person's caregivers.

A typical home environment can present many dangers and obstacles to a person with dementia, but simple changes can overcome many of these problems. For example, sharp knives, dangerous chemicals, tools, and other hazards should be removed or locked away. Other safety measures include installing bed and bathroom safety rails, removing locks from bedroom and bathroom doors, and lowering the hot water temperature to 120°F (48.9°C) or less to reduce the risk of accidental scalding. People with dementia also should wear some form of identification at all times in case they wander away or become lost. Caregivers can help prevent unsupervised wandering by adding locks or alarms to outside doors.

People with dementia often develop behavior problems because of frustration with specific situations. Understanding and modifying or preventing the situations that trigger these behaviors may help to make life more pleasant for the person with dementia as well as his or her caregivers. For instance, the person may be confused or frustrated by the level of activity or noise in the surrounding environment. Reducing unnecessary activity and noise (such as limiting the number of visitors and turning off the television when it's not in use) may make it easier for the person to understand requests and perform simple tasks. Confusion also may be reduced by simplifying home decorations, removing clutter, keeping familiar objects nearby, and following a predictable routine throughout the day. Calendars and clocks also may help patients orient themselves.

People with dementia should be encouraged to continue their normal leisure activities as long as they are safe and do not cause frustration. Activities such as crafts, games, and music can provide important mental stimulation and improve mood. Some studies have suggested that participating in exercise and intellectually stimulating activities may slow the decline of cognitive function in some people.

Many studies have found that driving is unsafe for people with dementia. They often get lost and they may have problems remembering or following rules of the road. They also may have difficulty processing information quickly and dealing with unexpected circumstances. Even a second of confusion while driving can lead to an accident. Driving with impaired cognitive functions can also endanger others. Some experts have suggested that regular screening for changes in cognition might help to reduce the number of driving accidents among elderly people, and some states now require that doctors report people with AD to their state motor vehicle department. However, in many cases, it is up to the person's family and friends to ensure that the person does not drive.

The emotional and physical burden of caring for someone with dementia can be overwhelming. Support groups can often help caregivers deal with these demands and they can also offer helpful information about the disease and its treatment. It is important that caregivers occasionally have time off from round-the-clock nursing demands. Some communities provide respite facilities or adult day care centers that will care for dementia patients for a period of time, giving the primary caregivers a break. Eventually, many patients with dementia require the services of a full-time nursing home.

What Research Is Being Done?

Current research focuses on many different aspects of dementia. This research promises to improve the lives of people affected by the dementias and may eventually lead to ways of preventing or curing these disorders.

Causes and Prevention

Research on the causes of AD and other dementias includes studies of genetic factors, neurotransmitters, inflammation, factors that influence programmed cell death in the brain, and the roles of tau, beta amyloid, and the associated neurofibrillary tangles and plaques in AD. Some other researchers are trying to determine the possible roles of cholesterol metabolism, oxidative stress (chemical reactions that can damage proteins, DNA, and lipids inside cells), and microglia in the development of AD. Scientists also are investigating the role of aging-related proteins such as the enzyme telomerase.

Since many dementias and other neurodegenerative diseases have been linked to abnormal clumps of proteins in cells, researchers are trying to learn how these clumps develop, how they affect cells, and how the clumping can be prevented.

Some studies are examining whether changes in white matter—nerve fibers lined with myelin—may play a role in the onset of AD. Myelin may erode in AD patients before other changes occur. This may be due to a problem with oligodendrocytes, the cells that produce myelin.

Researchers are searching for additional genes that may contribute to AD, and they have identified a number of gene regions that may be involved. Some researchers suggest that people will eventually be screened for a number of genes that contribute to AD and that they will be able to receive treatments that specifically address their individual genetic risks. However, such individualized screening and treatment is still years away.

Insulin resistance is common in people with AD, but it is not clear whether the insulin resistance contributes to the development of the disease or if it is merely a side effect.

Several studies have found a reduced risk of dementia in people who take cholesterol-lowering drugs called statins. However, it is not yet clear if the apparent effect is due to the drugs or to other factors.

One clinical trial is testing estrogen to see if it can help prevent AD. Early studies of estrogen looked promising. However, a clinical study of several thousand postmenopausal women aged sixty-five or older found that combination therapy with estrogen and progestin substantially increased the risk of AD. The study is continuing to examine whether taking estrogen alone may decrease the risk of AD.

A 2003 study found that people with HIV-associated dementia have different levels of activity for more than thirty different proteins, compared to people who have HIV but no signs of dementia. The study suggests a possible way to screen HIV patients for the first signs of cognitive impairment, and it may lead to ways of intervening to prevent this form of dementia.

Diagnosis

Improving early diagnosis of AD and other types of dementia is important not only for patients and families, but also for researchers who seek to better understand the causes of dementing diseases and find ways to reverse or halt them at early stages. Improved diagnosis can also reduce the risk that people will receive inappropriate treatments.

Some researchers are investigating whether three-dimensional computer models of PET and MRI images can identify brain changes typical of early AD, before any symptoms appear. This research may lead to ways of preventing the symptoms of the disease.

One study found that levels of beta amyloid and tau in spinal fluid can be used to diagnose AD with a sensitivity of 92 percent. If other studies confirm the validity of this test, it may allow doctors to identify people who are beginning to develop the disorder before they start to show symptoms. This would allow treatment at very early stages of the disorder, and may help in testing new treatments to prevent or delay symptoms of the disease. Other researchers have identified factors in the skin and blood of AD patients that are different from those in healthy people. They are trying to determine if these factors can be used to diagnose the disease.

Treatment

Researchers are continually working to develop new drugs for AD and other types of dementia. Many researchers believe a vaccine that reduces the number of amyloid plaques in the brain might ultimately prove to be the most effective treatment for AD. In 2001, researchers began one clinical trial of a vaccine called AN-1792. The study was halted after a number of people developed inflammation of the brain and spinal cord. Despite these problems, one patient appeared to have reduced numbers of amyloid plaques in the brain. Other patients showed little or no cognitive decline during the course of the study, suggesting that the vaccine may slow or halt the disease. Researchers are now trying to find safer and more effective vaccines for AD.

Researchers are also investigating possible methods of gene therapy for AD. In one case, researchers used cells genetically engineered to produce nerve growth factor and transplanted them into monkeys' forebrains. The transplanted cells boosted the amount of nerve growth factors in the brain and seemed to prevent degeneration of acetylcholine-producing neurons in the animals. This suggests that gene therapy might help to reduce or delay symptoms of the disease. Researchers are now testing a similar therapy in a small number of patients. Other researchers have experimented with gene therapy that adds a gene called neprilysin in a mouse model that produces human beta amyloid. They found that increasing the level of neprilysin greatly reduced the amount of beta amyloid in the mice and halted the amyloid-related brain degeneration. They are now trying to determine whether neprilysin gene therapy can improve cognition in mice.

A clinical trial called the Vitamins to Slow Alzheimer's Disease (VITAL) study is testing whether high doses of three common B vitamins—folic acid, B_{12}, and B_6—can reduce homocysteine levels and slow the rate of cognitive decline in AD.

Since many studies have found evidence of brain inflammation in AD, some researchers have proposed that drugs that control inflammation, such as NSAIDs, might prevent the disease or slow its progression. Studies in mice have suggested that these drugs can limit production of amyloid plaques in the brain. Clinical trials are now studying whether NSAIDs and related drugs can slow or prevent development of AD in humans.

Other clinical trials for AD are investigating whether antipsychotic drugs are useful in treating symptoms of AD, whether use of a shunt to increase the flow of cerebrospinal fluid and improve clearance of potential neurotoxins can halt or slow progression of the disease, and whether insulin-sensitizing drugs may be useful in treating AD.

Some researchers are investigating the effects of two drugs, pentoxifylline and propentofylline, to treat vascular dementia. Pentoxifylline improves blood flow, while propentofylline appears to interfere with some of the processes that cause cell death in the brain.

One study is testing the safety and effectiveness of donepezil (Aricept) for treating mild dementia in patients with Parkinson dementia, while another is investigating whether skin patches with the drug selegiline can improve mental function in patients with cognitive problems related to HIV.

How Can I Help Research?

People with dementia and others who wish to help research on dementing disorders may be able to do so by participating in clinical studies designed to learn more about the disorders or to test potential new therapies. Information about many such studies is available free of charge from the federal government's database of clinical trials, clinicaltrials.gov (http://clinicaltrials.gov).

Information about clinical trials specific to AD is available from the Alzheimer's Disease Clinical Trials Database (www.alzheimers .org/trials), a joint project of the U.S. Food and Drug Administration and the National Institute on Aging (NIA) that is maintained by the NIA's Alzheimer's Disease Education and Referral Center.

Another important way that people can help dementia research is by arranging to donate their brains to brain and tissue banks after they die. Tissue from these banks is made available to qualified researchers so that they can continue their studies of how these diseases develop and how they affect the brain.

Chapter 17

Huntington Disease

Chapter Contents

Section 17.1—Understanding Huntington Disease 368
Section 17.2—Recent Research on Huntington Disease 387

Section 17.1

Understanding Huntington Disease

Excerpted from "Huntington's Disease: Hope through Research," National Institute of Neurological Disorders and Stroke, National Institutes of Health, NIH Publication No. 98-49, updated November 2004.

In 1872, the American physician George Huntington wrote about an illness that he called "an heirloom from generations away back in the dim past." He was not the first to describe the disorder, which has been traced back to the Middle Ages at least. One of its earliest names was chorea, which, as in "choreography," is the Greek word for dance. The term chorea describes how people affected with the disorder writhe, twist, and turn in a constant, uncontrollable dance-like motion. Later, other descriptive names evolved. "Hereditary chorea" emphasizes how the disease is passed from parent to child. "Chronic progressive chorea" stresses how symptoms of the disease worsen over time. Today, physicians commonly use the simple term Huntington disease (HD) to describe this highly complex disorder that causes untold suffering for thousands of families.

In the United States alone, about 30,000 people have HD; estimates of its prevalence are about 1 in every 10,000 persons. At least 150,000 others have a 50 percent risk of developing the disease, and thousands more of their relatives live with the possibility that they, too, might develop HD.

Until recently, scientists understood very little about HD and could only watch as the disease continued to pass from generation to generation. Families saw the disease destroy their loved ones' ability to feel, think, and move. In the last several years, scientists working with support from the National Institute of Neurological Disorders and Stroke (NINDS) have made several breakthroughs in the area of HD research. With these advances, our understanding of the disease continues to improve.

This chapter presents information about HD, and about current research progress, to health professionals, scientists, caregivers, and, most important, to those already too familiar with the disorder: the many families who are affected by HD.

What causes Huntington disease (HD)?

HD results from genetically programmed degeneration of nerve cells, called neurons, in certain areas of the brain. This degeneration causes uncontrolled movements, loss of intellectual faculties, and emotional disturbance. Specifically affected are cells of the basal ganglia, structures deep within the brain that have many important functions, including coordinating movement. Within the basal ganglia, HD especially targets neurons of the striatum, particularly those in the caudate nuclei and the pallidum. Also affected is the brain's outer surface, or cortex, which controls thought, perception, and memory.

How is HD inherited?

HD is found in every country of the world. It is a familial disease, passed from parent to child through a mutation or misspelling in the normal gene.

A single abnormal gene, the basic biological unit of heredity, produces HD. Genes are composed of deoxyribonucleic acid (DNA), a molecule shaped like a spiral ladder. Each rung of this ladder is composed of two paired chemicals called bases. There are four types of bases—adenine, thymine, cytosine, and guanine—each abbreviated by the first letter of its name: A, T, C, and G. Certain bases always "pair" together, and different combinations of base pairs join to form coded messages. A gene is a long string of this DNA in various combinations of A, T, C, and G. These unique combinations determine the gene's function, much like letters join together to form words. Each person has about thirty thousand genes—a billion base pairs of DNA or bits of information repeated in the nuclei of human cells—which determine individual characteristics or traits.

Genes are arranged in precise locations along twenty-three rod-like pairs of chromosomes. One chromosome from each pair comes from an individual's mother, the other from the father. Each half of a chromosome pair is similar to the other, except for one pair, which determines the sex of the individual. This pair has two X chromosomes in females and one X and one Y chromosome in males. The gene that produces HD lies on chromosome 4, one of the twenty-two non-sex-linked, or "autosomal," pairs of chromosomes, placing men and women at equal risk of acquiring the disease.

The impact of a gene depends partly on whether it is dominant or recessive. If a gene is dominant, then only one of the paired chromosomes is required to produce its called-for effect. If the gene is recessive, both parents must provide chromosomal copies for the trait to be present. HD is called an autosomal dominant disorder because only one copy of the defective gene, inherited from one parent, is necessary to produce the disease.

The genetic defect responsible for HD is a small sequence of DNA on chromosome 4 in which several base pairs are repeated many, many times. The normal gene has three DNA bases, composed of the sequence CAG. In people with HD, the sequence abnormally repeats itself dozens of times. Over time—and with each successive generation—the number of CAG repeats may expand further.

Each parent has two copies of every chromosome but gives only one copy to each child. Each child of an HD parent has a 50-50 chance of inheriting the HD gene. If a child does not inherit the HD gene, he or she will not develop the disease and cannot pass it to subsequent generations. A person who inherits the HD gene, and survives long enough, will sooner or later develop the disease. In some families, all the children may inherit the HD gene; in others, none do. Whether one child inherits the gene has no bearing on whether others will or will not share the same fate.

A small number of cases of HD are sporadic, that is, they occur even though there is no family history of the disorder. These cases are thought to be caused by a new genetic mutation—an alteration in the gene that occurs during sperm development and that brings the number of CAG repeats into the range that causes disease.

What are the major effects of the disease?

Early signs of the disease vary greatly from person to person. A common observation is that the earlier the symptoms appear, the faster the disease progresses.

Family members may first notice that the individual experiences mood swings or becomes uncharacteristically irritable, apathetic, passive, depressed, or angry. These symptoms may lessen as the disease progresses or, in some individuals, may continue and include hostile outbursts or deep bouts of depression.

HD may affect the individual's judgment, memory, and other cognitive functions. Early signs might include having trouble driving, learning new things, remembering a fact, answering a question, or making a decision. Some may even display changes in handwriting. As the disease progresses, concentration on intellectual tasks becomes increasingly difficult.

In some individuals, the disease may begin with uncontrolled movements in the fingers, feet, face, or trunk. These movements—which are signs of chorea—often intensify when the person is anxious. HD can also begin with mild clumsiness or problems with balance. Some people develop choreic movements later, after the disease has progressed. They may stumble or appear uncoordinated. Chorea often creates serious problems with walking, increasing the likelihood of falls.

The disease can reach the point where speech is slurred and vital functions, such as swallowing, eating, speaking, and especially walking, continue to decline. Some individuals cannot recognize other family members. Many, however, remain aware of their environment and are able to express emotions.

Some physicians have employed a recently developed Unified HD Rating Scale, or UHDRS, to assess the clinical features, stages, and course of HD. In general, the duration of the illness ranges from ten to thirty years. The most common causes of death are infection (most often pneumonia), injuries related to a fall, or other complications.

At what age does HD appear?

The rate of disease progression and the age at onset vary from person to person. Adult-onset HD, with its disabling, uncontrolled movements, most often begins in middle age. There are, however, other variations of HD distinguished not just by age at onset but by a distinct array of symptoms. For example, some persons develop the disease as adults, but without chorea. They may appear rigid and move very little, or not at all, a condition called akinesia.

Some individuals develop symptoms of HD when they are very young—before age twenty. The terms "early-onset" or "juvenile" HD are often used to describe HD that appears in a young person. A common sign of HD in a younger individual is a rapid decline in school performance. Symptoms can also include subtle changes in handwriting and slight problems with movement, such as slowness, rigidity, tremor, and rapid muscular twitching, called myoclonus. Several of these symptoms are similar to those seen in Parkinson's disease, and they differ from the chorea seen in individuals who develop the disease as adults. These young individuals are said to have "akinetic-rigid" HD or the Westphal variant of HD. People with juvenile HD may also have seizures and mental disabilities. The earlier the onset, the faster the disease seems to progress. The disease progresses most rapidly in individuals with juvenile or early-onset HD, and death often follows within ten years.

Individuals with juvenile HD usually inherit the disease from their fathers. These individuals also tend to have the largest number of CAG repeats. The reason for this may be found in the process of sperm production. Unlike eggs, sperm are produced in the millions. Because DNA is copied millions of times during this process, there is an increased possibility for genetic mistakes to occur. To verify the link between the number of CAG repeats in the HD gene and the age at onset of symptoms, scientists studied a boy who developed HD symptoms at the age of two, one of the youngest and most severe cases ever recorded. They found that he had the largest number of CAG repeats of anyone studied so far—nearly one hundred. The boy's case was central to the identification of the HD gene and at the same time helped confirm that juveniles with HD have the longest segments of CAG repeats, the only proven correlation between repeat length and age at onset.

A few individuals develop HD after age fifty-five. Diagnosis in these people can be very difficult. The symptoms of HD may be masked by other health problems, or the person may not display the severity of symptoms seen in individuals with HD of earlier onset. These individuals may also show symptoms of depression rather than anger or irritability, or they may retain sharp control over their intellectual functions, such as memory, reasoning, and problem solving.

There is also a related disorder called senile chorea. Some elderly individuals display the symptoms of HD, especially choreic movements, but do not become demented, have a normal gene, and lack a family history of the disorder. Some scientists believe that a different gene mutation may account for this small number of cases, but this has not been proven.

How is HD diagnosed?

The great American folk singer and composer Woody Guthrie died on October 3, 1967, after suffering from HD for thirteen years. He had been misdiagnosed, considered an alcoholic, and shuttled in and out of mental institutions and hospitals for years before being properly diagnosed. His case, sadly, is not extraordinary, although the diagnosis can be made easily by experienced neurologists.

A neurologist will interview the individual intensively to obtain the medical history and rule out other conditions. A tool used by physicians to diagnose HD is to take the family history, sometimes called a pedigree or genealogy. It is extremely important for family members to be candid and truthful with a doctor who is taking a family history.

The doctor will also ask about recent intellectual or emotional problems, which may be indications of HD, and will test the person's hearing, eye movements, strength, coordination, involuntary movements (chorea), sensation, reflexes, balance, movement, and mental status, and will probably order a number of laboratory tests as well.

People with HD commonly have impairments in the way the eye follows or fixes on a moving target. Abnormalities of eye movements vary from person to person and differ, depending on the stage and duration of the illness.

The discovery of the HD gene in 1993 resulted in a direct genetic test to make or confirm a diagnosis of HD in an individual who is exhibiting HD-like symptoms. Using a blood sample, the genetic test analyzes DNA for the HD mutation by counting the number of repeats in the HD gene region. Individuals who do not have HD usually have twenty-eight or fewer CAG repeats. Individuals with HD usually have forty or more repeats. A small percentage of individuals, however, have a number of repeats that fall within a borderline region (see Table 17.1).

Table 17.1. Diagnosis of Huntington Disease

No. of CAG repeats	Outcome
less than or equal to 28	Normal range; individual will not develop HD
29–34	Individual will not develop HD but the next generation is at risk
35–39	Some, but not all, individuals in this range will develop HD; next generation is also at risk
greater than or equal to 40	Individual will develop HD

The physician may ask the individual to undergo a brain imaging test. Computed tomography (CT) and magnetic resonance imaging (MRI) provide excellent images of brain structures with little if any discomfort. Those with HD may show shrinkage of some parts of the brain—particularly two areas known as the caudate nuclei and putamen—and enlargement of fluid-filled cavities within the brain called ventricles. These changes do not definitely indicate HD, however, because they can also occur in other disorders. In addition, a person can have early symptoms of HD and still have a normal CT scan. When used in conjunction with a family history and record of clinical symptoms, however, CT can be an important diagnostic tool.

Another technology for brain imaging includes positron emission tomography (PET), which is important in HD research efforts but is not often needed for diagnosis.

What is presymptomatic testing?

Presymptomatic testing is used for people who have a family history of HD but have no symptoms themselves. If either parent had HD, the person's chance would be 50-50. In the past, no laboratory test could positively identify people carrying the HD gene—or those fated to develop HD—before the onset of symptoms. That situation changed in 1983, when a team of scientists supported by the NINDS located the first genetic marker for HD—the initial step in developing a laboratory test for the disease.

A marker is a piece of DNA that lies near a gene and is usually inherited with it. Discovery of the first HD marker allowed scientists to locate the HD gene on chromosome 4. The marker discovery quickly led to the development of a presymptomatic test for some individuals, but this test required blood or tissue samples from both affected and unaffected family members in order to identify markers unique to that particular family. For this reason, adopted individuals, orphans, and people who had few living family members were unable to use the test.

Discovery of the HD gene has led to a less expensive, scientifically simpler, and far more accurate presymptomatic test that is applicable to the majority of at-risk people. The new test uses CAG repeat length to detect the presence of the HD mutation in blood. This is discussed further in the next section.

There are many complicating factors that reflect the complexity of diagnosing HD. In a small number of individuals with HD—1 to 3 percent—no family history of HD can be found. Some individuals may not be aware of their genetic legacy, or a family member may conceal a genetic disorder from fear of social stigma. A parent may not want to worry children, scare them, or deter them from marrying. In other cases, a family member may die of another cause before he or she begins to show signs of HD. Sometimes, the cause of death for a relative may not be known, or the family is not aware of a relative's death. Adopted children may not know their genetic heritage, or early symptoms in an individual may be too slight to attract attention.

How is the presymptomatic test conducted?

An individual who wishes to be tested should contact the nearest testing center. (A list of such centers can be obtained from the Huntington Disease Society of America at 1-800-345-HDSA.) The testing process should include several components. Most testing programs include a neurological examination, pretest counseling, and follow-up. The purpose of the neurological examination is to determine whether or not the person requesting testing is showing any clinical symptoms of HD. It is important to remember that if an individual is showing even slight symptoms of HD, he or she risks being diagnosed with the disease during the neurological examination, even before the genetic test. During pretest counseling, the individual will learn about HD, about his or her own level of risk, and about the testing procedure. The person will be told about the test's limitations, the accuracy of the test, and possible outcomes. He or she can then weigh the risks and benefits of testing and may even decide at that time against pursuing further testing.

If a person decides to be tested, a team of highly trained specialists will be involved, which may include neurologists, genetic counselors, social workers, psychiatrists, and psychologists. This team of professionals helps the at-risk person decide if testing is the right thing to do and carefully prepares the person for a negative, positive, or inconclusive test result.

Individuals who decide to continue the testing process should be accompanied to counseling sessions by a spouse, a friend, or a relative who is not at risk. Other interested family members may participate in the counseling sessions if the individual being tested so desires.

The genetic testing itself involves donating a small sample of blood that is screened in the laboratory for the presence or absence of the HD mutation. Testing may require a sample of DNA from a closely related affected relative, preferably a parent, for the purpose of confirming the diagnosis of HD in the family. This is especially important if the family history for HD is unclear or unusual in some way.

Results of the test should be given only in person and only to the individual being tested. Test results are confidential. Regardless of test results, follow-up is recommended.

In order to protect the interests of minors, including confidentiality, testing is not recommended for those under the age of eighteen unless there is a compelling medical reason (for example, the child is exhibiting symptoms).

Testing of a fetus (prenatal testing) presents special challenges and risks; in fact some centers do not perform genetic testing on fetuses.

Because a positive test result using direct genetic testing means the at-risk parent is also a gene carrier, at-risk individuals who are considering a pregnancy are advised to seek genetic counseling prior to conception.

Some at-risk parents may wish to know the risk to their fetus but not their own. In this situation, parents may opt for prenatal testing using linked DNA markers rather than direct gene testing. In this case, testing does not look for the HD gene itself but instead indicates whether or not the fetus has inherited a chromosome 4 from the affected grandparent or from the unaffected grandparent on the side of the family with HD. If the test shows that the fetus has inherited a chromosome 4 from the affected grandparent, the parents then learn that the fetus's risk is the same as that of the parent (50-50), but they learn nothing new about the parent's risk. If the test shows that the fetus has inherited a chromosome 4 from the unaffected grandparent, the risk to the fetus is very low (less than 1 percent) in most cases.

Another option open to parents is in vitro fertilization with preimplantation screening. In this procedure, embryos are screened to determine which ones carry the HD mutation. Embryos determined not to have the HD gene mutation are then implanted in the woman's uterus.

In terms of emotional and practical consequences, not only for the individual taking the test but for his or her entire family, testing is enormously complex and has been surrounded by considerable controversy. For example, people with a positive test result may risk losing health and life insurance, suffer loss of employment, and other liabilities. People undergoing testing may wish to cover the cost themselves, since coverage by an insurer may lead to loss of health insurance in the event of a positive result, although this may change in the future.

With the participation of health professionals and people from families with HD, scientists have developed testing guidelines. All individuals seeking a genetic test should obtain a copy of these guidelines, which should be available at their testing center. It is strongly recommend that individuals avoid testing that does not adhere to these guidelines.

How does a person decide whether to be tested?

The anxiety that comes from living with a 50 percent risk for HD can be overwhelming. How does a young person make important choices about long-term education, marriage, and children? How do older parents of adult children cope with their fears about children and grandchildren? How do people come to terms with the ambiguity and uncertainty of living at risk?

Some individuals choose to undergo the test out of a desire for greater certainty about their genetic status. They believe the test will enable them to make more informed decisions about the future. Others choose not to take the test. They are able to make peace with the uncertainty of being at risk, preferring to forgo the emotional consequences of a positive result, as well as possible losses of insurance and employment. There is no right or wrong decision, as each choice is highly individual. The guidelines for genetic testing for HD, discussed in the previous section, were developed to help people with this life-changing choice.

Whatever the results of genetic testing, the at-risk individual and family members can expect powerful and complex emotional responses. The health and happiness of spouses, brothers and sisters, children, parents, and grandparents are affected by a positive test result, as are an individual's friends, work associates, neighbors, and others. Because receiving test results may prove to be devastating, testing guidelines call for continued counseling even after the test is complete and the results are known.

Is there a treatment for HD?

Physicians may prescribe a number of medications to help control emotional and movement problems associated with HD. It is important to remember, however, that while medicines may help keep these clinical symptoms under control, there is no treatment to stop or reverse the course of the disease.

Antipsychotic drugs, such as haloperidol, or other drugs, such as clonazepam, may help to alleviate choreic movements and may also be used to help control hallucinations, delusions, and violent outbursts. Antipsychotic drugs, however, are not prescribed for another form of muscle contraction associated with HD, called dystonia, and may in fact worsen the condition, causing stiffness and rigidity. These medications may also have severe side effects, including sedation, and for that reason should be used in the lowest possible doses.

For depression, physicians may prescribe fluoxetine, sertraline, nortriptyline, or other compounds. Tranquilizers can help control anxiety and lithium may be prescribed to combat pathological excitement and severe mood swings. Medications may also be needed to treat the severe obsessive-compulsive rituals of some individuals with HD.

Most drugs used to treat the symptoms of HD have side effects such as fatigue, restlessness, or hyperexcitability. Sometimes it may be difficult to tell if a particular symptom, such as apathy or incontinence, is a sign of the disease or a reaction to medication.

What kind of care does the individual with HD need?

Although a psychologist or psychiatrist, a genetic counselor, and other specialists may be needed at different stages of the illness, usually the first step in diagnosis and in finding treatment is to see a neurologist. While the family doctor may be able to diagnose HD, and may continue to monitor the individual's status, it is better to consult with a neurologist about management of the varied symptoms.

Problems may arise when individuals try to express complex thoughts in words they can no longer pronounce intelligibly. It can be helpful to repeat words back to the person with HD so that he or she knows that some thoughts are understood. Sometimes people mistakenly assume that if individuals do not talk, they also do not understand. Never isolate individuals by not talking, and try to keep their environment as normal as possible. Speech therapy may improve the individual's ability to communicate.

It is extremely important for the person with HD to maintain physical fitness as much as his or her condition and the course of the disease allows. Individuals who exercise and keep active tend to do better than those who do not. A daily regimen of exercise can help the person feel better physically and mentally. Although their coordination may be poor, individuals should continue walking, with assistance if necessary. Those who want to walk independently should be allowed to do so as long as possible, and careful attention should be given to keeping their environment free of hard, sharp objects. This will help ensure maximal independence while minimizing the risk of injury from a fall. Individuals can also wear special padding during walks to help protect against injury from falls. Some people have found that small weights around the ankles can help stability. Wearing sturdy shoes that fit well can help too, especially shoes without laces that can be slipped on or off easily.

Impaired coordination may make it difficult for people with HD to feed themselves and to swallow. As the disease progresses, persons with HD may even choke. In helping individuals to eat, caregivers should allow plenty of time for meals. Food can be cut into small pieces, softened, or pureed to ease swallowing and prevent choking. While some foods may require the addition of thickeners, other foods may need to be thinned. Dairy products, in particular, tend to increase the secretion of mucus, which in turn increases the risk of choking. Some individuals may benefit from swallowing therapy, which is especially helpful if started before serious problems arise. Suction cups for plates, special tableware designed for people with disabilities, and plastic cups with tops can help prevent spilling. The individual's physician can offer additional advice about diet and about how to handle swallowing difficulties or gastrointestinal problems that might arise, such as incontinence or constipation.

Caregivers should pay attention to proper nutrition so that the individual with HD takes in enough calories to maintain his or her body weight. Sometimes people with HD, who may burn as many as five thousand calories a day without gaining weight, require five meals a day to take in the necessary number of calories. Physicians may recommend vitamins or other nutritional supplements. In a long-term care institution, staff will need to assist with meals in order to ensure that the individual's special caloric and nutritional requirements are met. Some individuals and their families choose to use a feeding tube; others choose not to.

Individuals with HD are at special risk for dehydration and therefore require large quantities of fluids, especially during hot weather. Bendable straws can make drinking easier for the person. In some cases, water may have to be thickened with commercial additives to give it the consistency of syrup or honey.

What community resources are available?

Individuals and families affected by HD can take steps to ensure that they receive the best advice and care possible. Physicians and state and local health service agencies can provide information on community resources and family support groups that may exist. Possible types of help include:

- **Legal and social aid:** HD affects a person's capacity to reason, make judgments, and handle responsibilities. Individuals may need help with legal affairs. Wills and other important documents should be drawn up early to avoid legal problems when the person with HD may no longer be able to represent his or her own interests. Family members should also seek out assistance if they face discrimination regarding insurance, employment, or other matters.

- **Home care services:** Caring for a person with HD at home
  can be exhausting, but part-time assistance with household
  chores or physical care of the individual can ease this burden.
  Domestic help, meal programs, nursing assistance, occupational
  therapy, or other home services may be available from federal,
  state, or local health service agencies.

- **Recreation and work centers:** Many people with HD are
  eager and able to participate in activities outside the home.
  Therapeutic work and recreation centers give individuals an
  opportunity to pursue hobbies and interests and to meet new
  people. Participation in these programs, including occupational,
  music, and recreational therapy, can reduce the person's dependence on family members and provides home caregivers with a
  temporary, much-needed break.

- **Group housing:** A few communities have group housing facilities that are supervised by a resident attendant and that provide meals, housekeeping services, social activities, and local
  transportation services for residents. These living arrangements
  are particularly suited to the needs of individuals who are alone
  and who, although still independent and capable, risk injury
  when they undertake routine chores like cooking and cleaning.

- **Institutional care:** The individual's physical and emotional demands on the family may eventually become overwhelming. While
  many families may prefer to keep relatives with HD at home
  whenever possible, a long-term care facility may prove to be best.
  To hospitalize or place a family member in a care facility is a difficult decision; professional counseling can help families with this.

Finding the proper facility can itself prove difficult. Organizations
such as the Huntington's Disease Society of America may be able to
refer the family to facilities that have met standards set for the care
of individuals with HD. Very few of these exist, however, and even
fewer have experience with individuals with juvenile or early-onset
HD who require special care because of their age and symptoms.

What research is being done?

Although HD attracted considerable attention from scientists in
the early twentieth century, there was little sustained research on the
disease until the late 1960s, when the Committee to Combat Huntington's Disease and the Huntington's Chorea Foundation, later called

the Hereditary Disease Foundation, first began to fund research and to campaign for federal funding. In 1977, Congress established the Commission for the Control of Huntington's Disease and Its Consequences, which made a series of important recommendations. Since then, Congress has provided consistent support for federal research, primarily through the National Institute of Neurological Disorders and Stroke, the government's lead agency for biomedical research on disorders of the brain and nervous system. The effort to combat HD proceeds along the following lines of inquiry, each providing important information about the disease:

- **Basic neurobiology:** Now that the HD gene has been located, investigators in the field of neurobiology—which encompasses the anatomy, physiology, and biochemistry of the nervous system—are continuing to study the HD gene with an eye toward understanding how it causes disease in the human body.

- **Clinical research:** Neurologists, psychologists, psychiatrists, and other investigators are improving our understanding of the symptoms and progression of the disease in patients while attempting to develop new therapeutics.

- **Imaging:** Scientific investigations using PET and other technologies are enabling scientists to see what the defective gene does to various structures in the brain and how it affects the body's chemistry and metabolism.

- **Animal models:** Laboratory animals, such as mice, are being bred in the hope of duplicating the clinical features of HD and can soon be expected to help scientists learn more about the symptoms and progression of the disease.

- **Fetal tissue research:** Investigators are implanting fetal tissue in rodents and nonhuman primates with the hope that success in this area will lead to understanding, restoring, or replacing functions typically lost by neuronal degeneration in individuals with HD.

These areas of research are slowly converging and, in the process, are yielding important clues about the gene's relentless destruction of mind and body. The NINDS supports much of this exciting work.

Molecular Genetics: For ten years, scientists focused on a segment of chromosome 4 and, in 1993, finally isolated the HD gene. The process of isolating the responsible gene—motivated by the desire to find a cure—was more difficult than anticipated. Scientists now believe that identifying the location of the HD gene is the first step on the road to a cure.

Finding the HD gene involved an intense molecular genetics research effort with cooperating investigators from around the globe. In early 1993, the collaborating scientists announced they had isolated the unstable triplet repeat DNA sequence that has the HD gene. Investigators relied on the NINDS-supported Research Roster for Huntington's Disease, based at Indiana University in Indianapolis, to accomplish this work. First started in 1979, the roster contains data on many American families with HD, provides statistical and demographic data to scientists, and serves as a liaison between investigators and specific families. It provided the DNA from many families affected by HD to investigators involved in the search for the gene and was an important component in the identification of HD markers.

For several years, NINDS-supported investigators involved in the search for the HD gene made yearly visits to the largest known kindred with HD—fourteen thousand individuals—who live on Lake Maracaibo in Venezuela. The continuing trips enable scientists to study inheritance patterns of several interrelated families.

The HD Gene and Its Product: Although scientists know that certain brain cells die in HD, the cause of their death is still unknown. Recessive diseases are usually thought to result from a gene that fails to produce adequate amounts of a substance essential to normal function. This is known as a loss-of-function gene. Some dominantly inherited disorders, such as HD, are thought to involve a gene that actively interferes with the normal function of the cell. This is known as a gain-of-function gene.

How does the defective HD gene cause harm? The HD gene encodes a protein—which has been named huntingtin—the function of which is as yet unknown. The repeated CAG sequence in the gene causes an abnormal form of huntingtin to be made, in which the amino acid glutamine is repeated. It is the presence of this abnormal form, and not the absence of the normal form, that causes harm in HD. This explains why the disease is dominant and why two copies of the defective gene—one from both the mother and the father—do not cause a more serious case than inheritance from only one parent. With the HD gene isolated, NINDS-supported investigators are now turning their attention toward discovering the normal function of huntingtin and how the altered form causes harm. Scientists hope to reproduce, study, and correct these changes in animal models of the disease.

Huntingtin is found everywhere in the body but only outside the cell's nucleus. Mice called "knockout mice" are bred in the laboratory to produce no huntingtin; they fail to develop past a very early embryo stage and quickly die. Huntingtin, scientists now know, is necessary for life. Investigators hope to learn why the abnormal version of the protein damages only certain parts of the brain. One theory is that cells in these parts of the brain may be supersensitive to this abnormal protein.

Cell Death in HD: Although the precise cause of cell death in HD is not yet known, scientists are paying close attention to the process of genetically programmed cell death that occurs deep within the brains of individuals with HD. This process involves a complex series of interlinked events leading to cellular suicide. Related areas of investigation include:

- **Excitotoxicity:** Overstimulation of cells by natural chemicals found in the brain.

- **Defective energy metabolism:** A defect in the power plant of the cell, called mitochondria, where energy is produced.

- **Oxidative stress:** Normal metabolic activity in the brain that produces toxic compounds called free radicals.

- **Trophic factors:** Natural chemical substances found in the human body that may protect against cell death.

Several HD studies are aimed at understanding losses of nerve cells and receptors in HD. Neurons in the striatum are classified both by their size (large, medium, or small) and appearance (spiny or aspiny). Each type of neuron contains combinations of neurotransmitters. Scientists know that the destructive process of HD affects different subsets of neurons to varying degrees. The hallmark of HD, they are learning, is selective degeneration of medium-sized spiny neurons in the striatum. NINDS-supported studies also suggest that losses of certain types of neurons and receptors are responsible for different symptoms and stages of HD.

What do these changes look like? In spiny neurons, investigators have observed two types of changes, each affecting the nerve cells' dendrites. Dendrites, found on every nerve cell, extend out from the cell body and are responsible for receiving messages from other nerve cells. In the intermediate stages of HD, dendrites grow out of control. New, incomplete branches form and other branches become contorted.

In advanced, severe stages of HD, degenerative changes cause sections of dendrites to swell, break off, or disappear altogether. Investigators believe that these alterations may be an attempt by the cell to rebuild nerve cell contacts lost early in the disease. As the new dendrites establish connections, however, they may in fact contribute to nerve cell death. Such studies give compelling, visible evidence of the progressive nature of HD and suggest that new experimental therapies must consider the state of cellular degeneration. Scientists do not yet know exactly how these changes affect subsets of nerve cells outside the striatum.

Animal Models of HD: As more is learned about cellular degeneration in HD, investigators hope to reproduce these changes in animal models and to find a way to correct or halt the process of nerve cell death. Such models serve the scientific community in general by providing a means to test the safety of new classes of drugs in nonhuman primates. NINDS-supported scientists are currently working to develop both nonhuman primate and mouse models to investigate nerve degeneration in HD and to study the effects of excitotoxicity on nerve cells in the brain.

Investigators are working to build genetic models of HD using transgenic mice. To do this, scientists transfer the altered human HD gene into mouse embryos so that the animals will develop the anatomical and biological characteristics of HD. This genetic model of mouse HD will enable in-depth study of the disease and testing of new therapeutic compounds.

Another idea is to insert into mice a section of DNA containing CAG repeats in the abnormal, disease gene range. This mouse equivalent of HD could allow scientists to explore the basis of CAG instability and its role in the disease process.

Fetal Tissue Research: A relatively new field in biomedical research involves the use of brain tissue grafts to study, and potentially treat, neurodegenerative disorders. In this technique, tissue that has degenerated is replaced with implants of fresh, fetal tissue, taken at the very early stages of development. Investigators are interested in applying brain tissue implants to HD research. Extensive animal studies will be required to learn if this technique could be of value in patients with HD.

Clinical Studies: Scientists are pursuing clinical studies that may one day lead to the development of new drugs or other treatments to halt the disease's progression. Examples of NINDS-supported investigations, using both asymptomatic and symptomatic individuals, include:

- **Genetic studies on age of onset, inheritance patterns, and markers found within families:** These studies may shed additional light on how HD is passed from generation to generation.

- **Studies of cognition, intelligence, and movement:** Studies of abnormal eye movements, both horizontal and vertical, and tests of patients' skills in a number of learning, memory, neuropsychological, and motor tasks may serve to identify when the various symptoms of HD appear and to characterize their range and severity.

- **Clinical trials of drugs:** Testing of various drugs may lead to new treatments and at the same time improve our understanding of the disease process in HD. Classes of drugs being tested include those that control symptoms, slow the rate of progression of HD, and block effects of excitotoxins, and those that might correct or replace other metabolic defects contributing to the development and progression of HD.

Imaging: NINDS-supported scientists are using positron emission tomography (PET) to learn how the gene affects the chemical systems of the body. PET visualizes metabolic or chemical abnormalities in the body, and investigators hope to ascertain if PET scans can reveal any abnormalities that signal HD. Investigators conducting HD research are also using PET to characterize neurons that have died and chemicals that are depleted in parts of the brain affected by HD.

Like PET, a form of magnetic resonance imaging (MRI) called functional MRI can measure increases or decreases in certain brain chemicals thought to play a key role in HD. Functional MRI studies are also helping investigators understand how HD kills neurons in different regions of the brain.

Imaging technologies allow investigators to view changes in the volume and structures of the brain and to pinpoint when these changes occur in HD. Scientists know that in brains affected by HD, the basal ganglia, cortex, and ventricles all show atrophy or other alterations.

How can I help?

In order to conduct HD research, investigators require samples of tissue or blood from families with HD. Access to individuals with HD and their families may be difficult, however, because families with HD are often scattered across the country or around the world. A research project may need individuals of a particular age or gender or from a certain geographic area. Some scientists need only statistical data while others may require a sample of blood, urine, or skin from family members. All of these factors complicate the task of finding volunteers. NINDS-supported efforts bring together families with HD, voluntary health agencies, and scientists in an effort to advance science and speed a cure.

The NINDS-sponsored HD Research Roster at the Indiana University Medical Center in Indianapolis, which was discussed earlier, makes research possible by matching scientists with patient and family volunteers. The first DNA bank was established through the roster. Although the gene has already been located, DNA from individuals who have HD is still of great interest to investigators. Of continuing interest are twins, unaffected individuals who have affected offspring, and individuals with two defective HD genes, one from each parent—a very rare occurrence. Participation in the roster and in specific research projects is voluntary and confidential. For more information about the roster and DNA bank, contact the Indiana University Medical Center, Department of Medical and Molecular Genetics at 317-274-5744 (call collect).

The NINDS supports two national brain specimen banks. These banks supply research scientists around the world with nervous system tissue from patients with neurological and psychiatric disorders. They need tissue from patients with HD so that scientists can study and understand the disorder. Those who may be interested in donating will find more information at http://www.loni.ucla.edu/~nnrsb/ NNRSB or www.brainbank.mclean.org.

Section 17.2

Recent Research on Huntington Disease

This section includes the following press releases from the National Institute of Neurological Disorders and Stroke: "Trial Drugs for Huntington's Disease Inconclusive in Slowing Disease" (August 13, 2001) and "Scientists Identify Potential New Treatment for Huntington's Disease" (February 27, 2002).

Trial Drugs for Huntington Disease Inconclusive in Slowing Disease

A large-scale clinical trial that tested the ability of the investigational drugs remacemide and Coenzyme Q10 to slow the progression of Huntington disease showed that neither drug resulted in any significant improvement for the patients. Although after one year of treatment the disease seemed to progress more slowly in patients treated with Coenzyme Q10, the investigators say that overall the results are inconclusive as to whether there is real benefit from this drug. The study is published in the August 14, 2001, issue of *Neurology*.

"The Coenzyme Q10 and Remacemide Evaluation in Huntington's Disease," or CARE-HD trial, was conducted for thirty months by the Huntington Study Group at twenty-three sites in the United States and Canada. The trial included 347 people in the early stages of the disease. It was funded by the National Institute of Neurological Disorders and Stroke (NINDS), and is the largest study to investigate treatments for Huntington disease.

Remacemide is a new investigational drug that blocks a neurotransmitter in the brain (the NMDA glutamate receptor) that has long been suspected of contributing to the death of brain cells in Huntington disease. Coenzyme Q10 is a substance that occurs naturally in the body and plays a role in the function of mitochondria, the energy factories of human cells. It is also an antioxidant, meaning that it can neutralize potentially injurious oxygen-containing chemicals called free radicals, which may play a role in the nerve cell death that occurs in Huntington disease. Coenzyme Q10 is sold as a nutritional supplement in pharmacies and health food stores.

Participants in the randomized, double-blind CARE-HD study were assigned to one of four treatments: 25 percent received remacemide, 25 percent received Coenzyme Q10, 25 percent received the combination of Coenzyme Q10 and remacemide, and 25 percent received placebo (no active medication). Each participant was followed with standardized tests for neurological and neuropsychological function.

To determine the effectiveness of the study drugs, investigators looked for a reduction in the patients' functional decline as measured by the Total Functional Capacity scale (TFC). A score of 13 represents a normal degree of function and a score of 0 represents a severely disabled state. CARE-HD participants had a mean TFC score of approximately 10.

The investigators reported the following results:

- The condition of patients in the placebo group worsened by 2.7 units on the TFC scale over the thirty months of the trial.

- The condition of patients who were treated with remacemide also worsened by 2.7 points on the TFC scale over the course of the study, showing that the drug had no appreciable effect on functional decline. In the remacemide-treated group, however, there was a trend toward improvement in the degree of the patients' chorea. Although this effect was not considered statistically significant, it was seen during the patients' first visit after treatment began, suggesting that the drug may decrease chorea. Remacemide was well tolerated overall, although there was an increase in some side effects, primarily lightheadedness, dizziness, and nausea.

- Patients who were treated with Coenzyme Q10 also failed to show a statistically significant decrease in TFC decline over the duration of the thirty-month trial. However, after the first year, the condition of the study participants treated with Coenzyme Q10 worsened at a slower rate, with approximately 13 percent less decline on the TFC scale compared to those not receiving Coenzyme Q10. A similar trend toward a decrease in functional decline was seen in two other scales that measure functional capacity. In addition, on two cognitive scales there was a slower decline in the group receiving Coenzyme Q10. On no measure was Coenzyme Q10 associated with a worsening of the disease, and there were no apparent side effects, with the exception of gastrointestinal upset.

The CARE-HD investigators, the Huntington's Disease Society of America, the Huntington's Disease Society of Canada, and the Hereditary Disease Foundation, who jointly cooperated on the study, all agree that the data are inconclusive about whether there is clear benefit of Coenzyme Q10 on functional decline. The statistical analysis of the CARE-HD data indicates that the apparent benefit attributed to Coenzyme Q10 could have occurred by chance. The investigators and the cooperating groups urge patients with Huntington disease to discuss the pros and cons of changing their therapy with their physicians.

"Despite the fact that the results of this trial are inconclusive, the study does provide the hope that an agent many someday be found which will slow the progression of Huntington disease and other neurodegenerative disorders, " said Eugene J. Oliver, Ph.D., program director at the NINDS.

Because Coenzyme Q10 is an unregulated dietary supplement, formulations may differ. The authors point out that there were no adverse effects (outside of gastrointestinal upset) with Coenzyme Q10, but given the lack of definite evidence that any benefit will result, the cost of taking the drug over years may be significant. In addition, the results of the CARE-HD study cannot be applied to persons at risk for Huntington disease or those whose are in later disease stages.

"CARE-HD is important because it is the first study to show a hopeful trend toward slowing of disease with a particular therapy and gives us some good clues to work with in future studies," said Walter J. Koroshetz, M.D., of Massachusetts General Hospital in Boston, and a co-principal investigator of the study. "We hope that further research will build on the CARE-HD trial and lead to an effective treatment that significantly slows progression of Huntington disease and eventually to a cure for these patients," said Dr. Koroshetz. "The real heroes of this study were the participants with HD and their families," he added.

Huntington disease is an inherited disorder affecting thirty thousand Americans. It is caused by a single genetic mutation identified in 1993. People who inherit the defective gene from one of their parents develop degeneration of specific brain regions. Symptoms usually begin in early to mid-adulthood, but children are occasionally affected. Signs of the illness include involuntary movements called chorea, as well as motor and cognitive difficulties. It is a progressive disease that leads to death fifteen to twenty years after diagnosis.

Additional support for this study was provided by Astra Zeneca, the makers of remacemide, and by Vitaline Corporation, which supplied the Coenzyme Q10.

NINDS is a component of the National Institutes of Health in Bethesda, Maryland, and is the nation's primary supporter of biomedical research on the brain and nervous system.

Reference

"A Randomized, Placebo-Controlled Trial of Coenzyme Q10 and Remacemide in Huntington's Disease (CARE-HD)," Huntington Study Group, *Neurology*, August 14, 2001, 57:397.

Scientists Identify Potential New Treatment for Huntington Disease

A drug called cystamine alleviates tremors and prolongs life in mice with the gene mutation for Huntington disease (HD), a new study shows. The drug appears to work by increasing the activity of proteins that protect nerve cells, or neurons, from degeneration. The study suggests that a similar treatment may one day be useful in humans with HD and related disorders.

Previous studies have identified several other drugs with potential for treating HD. However, cystamine appears to work differently than those drugs, and it may add to the benefits of other therapies if it is used in combination with them, says senior author Lawrence Steinman, M.D., of Stanford University in California. The study was supported by the National Institute of Neurological Disorders and Stroke (NINDS) and the Hereditary Disease Foundation. It appears in the February 2002 issue of *Nature Medicine*.

In HD, a defective gene produces an abnormal form of a protein named huntingtin. This abnormal protein triggers a process that kills neurons in a brain region called the corpus striatum and leads to the symptoms of the disorder. The abnormal protein aggregates, or clumps together, inside many kinds of neurons. Some researchers believe these clumps contribute to the problems seen in HD, although it is not yet clear if this is the case. Previous studies have found that cystamine inactivates an enzyme called transglutaminase that helps create the clumps of huntingtin protein.

In the study, lead scientist Marcela Karpuj, Ph.D., and colleagues injected cystamine into mice with an abnormal huntingtin gene. The mice that received the drug had fewer tremors and other abnormal movements and less weight loss than the untreated mice. They also lived about 20 percent longer. However, cystamine did not reduce the number of huntingtin clumps found in the brain.

Using gene chips, which can analyze the activity of many different genes at once, the researchers identified two genes that had increased activity in the mice treated with cystamine, as well as in brain tissue collected during autopsies of HD patients. A third, related gene had increased activity in HD patients but not in mice. Previous studies have shown that the proteins produced by these genes protect brain cells from damage. The presence of these proteins in brains of HD patients who were not treated with cystamine may result from a natural attempt at recovery that ultimately failed, the researchers say.

Cystamine may be able to stop huntingtin clumps from forming, even though it does not destroy clumps that are already there, says Dr. Steinman. If so, treatment earlier in the disease process may be able to prevent the clumps entirely. In addition, the protective proteins that increase with cystamine treatment may be able to disarm errant huntingtin proteins before they cause damage. For example, a recent study showed that the abnormal huntingtin protein interferes with another protein called CBP that is crucial for cell survival.

While these findings may lead to a new way of treating HD, they also may be relevant to other disorders, such as the spinocerebellar ataxias and spinobulbar muscular atrophy (SBMA), which have the same type of gene defect and the same kind of protein clumps as HD. The protective proteins identified in this study have also been found in several of these related diseases.

Cystamine is closely related to another drug called cysteamine that is approved to treat a kidney disease called cystinosis in humans. Researchers at Massachusetts General Hospital in Boston are now planning a clinical study of cysteamine for Huntington disease. In addition, several other substances, including the antibiotic minocycline and the dietary supplement creatine, are currently being tested in clinical trials for Huntington disease.

Reference

Karpuj MV, Becher MW, Springer JE, Chabas D, Youssef S, Pedotti R, Mitchell D, Steinman L. "Prolonged survival and decreased abnormal movements in transgenic model of Huntington's disease, with administration of the transglutaminase inhibitor cystamine." *Nature Medicine*, February 2002, vol. 8, no. 2, pp. 143–49.

Chapter 18

Multiple Sclerosis (MS)

Chapter Contents

Section 18.1—MS: An Overview 394
Section 18.2—MS Treatment: Some Safety Issues 415
Section 18.3—MS and Cooling 420
Section 18.4—New Research on MS 426

Section 18.1

MS: An Overview

Excerpted from "Multiple Sclerosis: Hope through Research," National Institute of Neurological Disorders and Stroke, National Institutes of Health, updated November 2004.

Although multiple sclerosis (MS) was first diagnosed in 1849, the earliest known description of a person with possible MS dates from fourteenth-century Holland. An unpredictable disease of the central nervous system, MS can range from relatively benign to somewhat disabling to devastating as communication between the brain and other parts of the body is disrupted.

The vast majority of patients are mildly affected, but in the worst cases MS can render a person unable to write, speak, or walk. A physician can diagnose MS in some patients soon after the onset of the illness. In others, however, physicians may not be able to readily identify the cause of the symptoms, leading to years of uncertainty and multiple diagnoses punctuated by baffling symptoms that mysteriously wax and wane.

Once a diagnosis is made with confidence, patients must consider a profusion of information—and misinformation—associated with this complex disease. This chapter is designed to convey the latest information on the diagnosis, course, and possible treatment of MS, as well as highlights of current research. Although a book cannot substitute for the advice and expertise of a physician, it can provide patients and their families with information to understand MS better so that they can actively participate in their care and treatment.

What is multiple sclerosis?

During an MS attack, inflammation occurs in areas of the white matter of the central nervous system in random patches called plaques. This process is followed by destruction of myelin, the fatty covering that insulates nerve cell fibers in the brain and spinal cord. Myelin facilitates the smooth, high-speed transmission of electrochemical messages between the brain, the spinal cord, and the rest of the body; when it is damaged, neurological transmission of messages may be slowed or blocked completely, leading to diminished or lost function. The name "multiple sclerosis" signifies both the number (multiple) and condition (sclerosis, from the Greek term for scarring or hardening) of the demyelinated areas in the central nervous system.

How many people have MS?

No one knows exactly how many people have MS. It is believed that, currently, there are approximately 250,000 to 350,000 people in the United States with MS diagnosed by a physician. This estimate suggests that approximately 200 new cases are diagnosed each week.

Who gets MS?

Most people experience their first symptoms of MS between the ages of twenty and forty, but a diagnosis is often delayed. This is due to both the transitory nature of the disease and the lack of a specific diagnostic test—specific symptoms and changes in the brain must develop before the diagnosis is confirmed.

Although scientists have documented cases of MS in young children and elderly adults, symptoms rarely begin before age fifteen or after age sixty. Whites are more than twice as likely as other races to develop MS. In general, women are affected at almost twice the rate of men; however, among patients who develop the symptoms of MS at a later age, the gender ratio is more balanced.

MS is five times more prevalent in temperate climates—such as those found in the northern United States, Canada, and Europe—than in tropical regions. Furthermore, the age of fifteen seems to be significant in terms of risk for developing the disease: some studies indicate that a person moving from a high-risk (temperate) to a low-risk (tropical) area before the age of fifteen tends to adopt the risk (in this case, low) of the new area and vice versa. Other studies suggest that people moving after age fifteen maintain the risk of the area where they grew up.

These findings indicate a strong role for an environmental factor in the cause of MS. It is possible that, at the time of or immediately following puberty, patients acquire an infection with a long latency period. Or, conversely, people in some areas may come in contact with an unknown protective agent during the time before puberty. Other studies suggest that the unknown geographic or climatic element may actually be simply a matter of genetic predilection and reflect racial and ethnic susceptibility factors.

Periodically, scientists receive reports of MS "clusters." The most famous of these MS "epidemics" took place in the Faeroe Islands north of Scotland in the years following the arrival of British troops during World War II. Despite intense study of this and other clusters, no direct environmental factor has been identified. Nor has any definitive evidence been found to link daily stress to MS attacks, although there is evidence that the risk of worsening is greater after acute viral illnesses.

How much does MS cost America?

MS is a lifelong chronic disease diagnosed primarily in young adults who have a virtually normal life expectancy. Consequently, the economic, social, and medical costs associated with the disease are significant. Estimates place the annual cost of MS in the United States in the billions of dollars.

What causes MS?

Scientists have learned a great deal about MS in recent years; still, its cause remains elusive. Many investigators believe MS to be an autoimmune disease—one in which the body, through its immune system, launches a defensive attack against its own tissues. In the case of MS, it is the nerve-insulating myelin that comes under assault. Such assaults may be linked to an unknown environmental trigger, perhaps a virus.

The Immune System: To understand what is happening when a person has MS, it is first necessary to know a little about how the healthy immune system works. The immune system—a complex network of specialized cells and organs—defends the body against attacks by "foreign" invaders such as bacteria, viruses, fungi, and parasites. It does this by seeking out and destroying the interlopers as they enter the body. Substances capable of triggering an immune response are called antigens.

The immune system displays both enormous diversity and extraordinary specificity. It can recognize millions of distinctive foreign molecules and produce its own molecules and cells to match up with and counteract each of them. In order to have room for enough cells to match the millions of possible foreign invaders, the immune system stores just a few cells for each specific antigen. When an antigen appears, those few specifically matched cells are stimulated to multiply into a full-scale army. Later, to prevent this army from overexpanding, powerful mechanisms to suppress the immune response come into play.

T cells, so named because they are processed in the thymus, appear to play a particularly important role in MS. They travel widely and continuously throughout the body, patrolling for foreign invaders. In order to recognize and respond to each specific antigen, each T cell's surface carries special receptor molecules for particular antigens.

T cells contribute to the body's defenses in two major ways. Regulatory T cells help orchestrate the elaborate immune system. For instance, they assist other cells to make antibodies, proteins programmed to match one specific antigen much as a key matches a lock. Antibodies typically interact with circulating antigens, such as bacteria, but are unable to penetrate living cells. Chief among the regulatory T cells are those known as helper (or inducer) cells. Helper T cells are essential for activating the body's defenses against foreign substances. Yet another subset of regulatory T cells acts to turn off, or suppress, various immune system cells when their job is done.

Killer T cells, on the other hand, directly attack diseased or damaged body cells by binding to them and bombarding them with lethal chemicals called cytokines. Since T cells can attack cells directly, they must be able to discriminate between "self" cells (those of the body) and "nonself" cells (foreign invaders). To enable the immune system to distinguish the self, each body cell carries identifying molecules on its surface. T cells likely to react against the self are usually eliminated before leaving the thymus; the remaining T cells recognize the molecular markers and coexist peaceably with body tissues in a state of self-tolerance.

In autoimmune diseases such as MS, the détente between the immune system and the body is disrupted when the immune system seems to wrongly identify self as nonself and declares war on the part of the body (myelin) it no longer recognizes. Through intensive research efforts, scientists are unraveling the complex secrets of the malfunctioning immune system of patients with MS.

Components of myelin such as myelin basic protein have been the focus of much research because, when injected into laboratory animals, they can precipitate experimental allergic encephalomyelitis (EAE), a chronic relapsing brain and spinal cord disease that resembles MS. The injected myelin probably stimulates the immune system to produce anti-myelin T cells that attack the animal's own myelin.

Investigators are also looking for abnormalities or malfunctions in the blood-brain barrier, a protective membrane that controls the passage of substances from the blood into the central nervous system. It is possible that, in MS, components of the immune system get through the barrier and cause nervous system damage.

Scientists have studied a number of infectious agents (such as viruses) that have been suspected of causing MS, but have been unable to implicate any one particular agent. Viral infections are usually accompanied by inflammation and the production of gamma interferon, a naturally occurring body chemical that has been shown to worsen the clinical course of MS. It is possible that the immune response to viral infections may itself precipitate an MS attack. There seems to be little doubt that something in the environment is involved in triggering MS.

Genetics: In addition, increasing scientific evidence suggests that genetics may play a role in determining a person's susceptibility to MS. Some populations, such as Gypsies, Eskimos, and Bantus, never get MS. Native Indians of North and South America, the Japanese, and other Asian peoples have very low incidence rates. It is unclear whether this is due mostly to genetic or environmental factors.

In the population at large, the chance of developing MS is less than a tenth of one percent. However, if one person in a family has MS, that person's first-degree relatives—parents, children, and siblings—have a 1 to 3 percent chance of getting the disease.

For identical twins, the likelihood that the second twin may develop MS if the first twin does is about 30 percent; for fraternal twins (who do not inherit identical gene pools), the likelihood is closer to that for non-twin siblings, or about 4 percent. The fact that the rate for identical twins both developing MS is significantly less than 100 percent suggests that the disease is not entirely genetically controlled. Some (but definitely not all) of this effect may be due to shared exposure to something in the environment, or to the fact that some people with MS lesions remain essentially asymptomatic throughout their lives.

Further indications that more than one gene is involved in MS susceptibility come from studies of families in which more than one member has MS. Several research teams found that people with MS inherit certain regions on individual genes more frequently than people without MS. Of particular interest is the human leukocyte antigen (HLA) or major histocompatibility complex region on chromosome 6. HLAs are genetically determined proteins that influence the immune system.

The HLA patterns of MS patients tend to be different from those of people without the disease. Investigations in northern Europe and America have detected three HLAs that are more prevalent in people with MS than in the general population. Studies of American MS patients have shown that people with MS also tend to exhibit these HLAs in combination—that is, they have more than one of the three HLAs—more frequently than the rest of the population. Furthermore, there is evidence that different combinations of the HLAs may correspond to variations in disease severity and progression.

Studies of families with multiple cases of MS and research comparing genetic regions of humans to those of mice with EAE suggest that another area related to MS susceptibility may be located on chromosome 5. Other regions on chromosomes 2, 3, 7, 11, 17, 19, and X have also been identified as possibly containing genes involved in the development of MS.

These studies strengthen the theory that MS is the result of a number of factors rather than a single gene or other agent. Development of MS is likely to be influenced by the interactions of a number of genes, each of which (individually) has only a modest effect. Additional studies are needed to specifically pinpoint which genes are involved, determine their function, and learn how each gene's interactions with other genes and with the environment make an individual susceptible to MS. In addition to leading to better ways to diagnose MS, such studies should yield clues to the underlying causes of MS and, eventually, to better treatments or a way to prevent the disease.

What is the course of MS?

Each case of MS displays one of several patterns of presentation and subsequent course. Most commonly, MS first manifests itself as a series of attacks followed by complete or partial remissions as symptoms mysteriously lessen, only to return later after a period of stability. This is called relapsing-remitting (RR) MS. Primary-progressive (PP) MS is characterized by a gradual clinical decline with no distinct remissions, although there may be temporary plateaus or minor relief from symptoms. Secondary-progressive (SP) MS begins with a relapsing-remitting course followed by a later primary-progressive course. Rarely, patients may have a progressive-relapsing (PR) course in which the disease takes a progressive path punctuated by acute attacks. PP, SP, and PR are sometimes lumped together and called chronic progressive MS.

In addition, 20 percent of the MS population has a benign form of the disease in which symptoms show little or no progression after the initial attack; these patients remain fully functional. A few patients experience malignant MS, defined as a swift and relentless decline resulting in significant disability or even death shortly after disease onset. However, MS is very rarely fatal and most people with MS have a fairly normal life expectancy.

Studies throughout the world are causing investigators to redefine the natural course of the disease. These studies use a technique called magnetic resonance imaging (MRI) to visualize the evolution of MS lesions in the white matter of the brain. Bright spots on a T2 MRI scan indicate the presence of lesions, but do not provide information about when they developed.

Because investigators speculate that the breakdown of the blood-brain barrier is the first step in the development of MS lesions, it is important to distinguish new lesions from old. To do this, physicians give patients injections of gadolinium, a chemical contrast agent that normally does not cross the blood-brain barrier, before performing a scan. On this type of scan, called T1, the appearance of bright areas indicates periods of recent disease activity (when gadolinium is able to cross the barrier). The ability to estimate the age of lesions through MRI has allowed investigators to show that, in some patients, lesions occur frequently throughout the course of the disease even when no symptoms are present.

Can life events affect the course of MS?

While there is no good evidence that daily stress or trauma affects the course of MS, there is data on the influence of pregnancy. Since MS generally strikes during childbearing years, a common concern among women with the disease is whether or not to have a baby. Studies on the subject have shown that MS has no adverse effects on the course of pregnancy, labor, or delivery; in fact, symptoms often stabilize or remit during pregnancy. This temporary improvement is thought to relate to changes in a woman's immune system that allow her body to carry a baby: because every fetus has genetic material from the father as well as the mother, the mother's body should identify the growing fetus as foreign tissue and try to reject it in much the same way the body seeks to reject a transplanted organ. To prevent this from happening, a natural process takes place to suppress the mother's immune system in the uterus during pregnancy.

However, women with MS who are considering pregnancy need to be aware that certain drugs used to treat MS should be avoided during pregnancy and while breast feeding. These drugs can cause birth defects and can be passed to the fetus via blood and to an infant via breast milk. Among them are prednisone, corticotropin, azathioprine, cyclophosphamide, diazepam, phenytoin, carbamazepine, and baclofen.

Unfortunately, between 20 and 40 percent of women with MS do have a relapse in the three months following delivery. However, there is no evidence that pregnancy and childbirth affect the overall course of the disease one way or the other. Also, while MS is not in itself a reason to avoid pregnancy and poses no significant risks to the fetus, physical limitations can make child care more difficult. It is therefore important that MS patients planning families discuss these issues with both their partner and physician.

What are the symptoms of MS?

Symptoms of MS may be mild or severe, of long duration or short, and may appear in various combinations, depending on the area of the nervous system affected. Complete or partial remission of symptoms, especially in the early stages of the disease, occurs in approximately 70 percent of MS patients.

The initial symptom of MS is often blurred or double vision, red-green color distortion, or even blindness in one eye. Inexplicably, visual problems tend to clear up in the later stages of MS. Inflammatory problems of the optic nerve may be diagnosed as retrobulbar or optic neuritis. Fifty-five percent of MS patients will have an attack of optic neuritis at some time or other and it will be the first symptom of MS in approximately 15 percent. This has led to general recognition of optic neuritis as an early sign of MS, especially if tests also reveal abnormalities in the patient's spinal fluid.

Most MS patients experience muscle weakness in their extremities and difficulty with coordination and balance at some time during the course of the disease. These symptoms may be severe enough to impair walking or even standing. In the worst cases, MS can produce partial or complete paralysis. Spasticity—the involuntary increased tone of muscles leading to stiffness and spasms—is common, as is fatigue. Fatigue may be triggered by physical exertion and improve with rest, or it may take the form of a constant and persistent tiredness.

Most people with MS also exhibit paresthesias, transitory abnormal sensory feelings such as numbness, prickling, or "pins and needles" sensations; uncommonly, some may also experience pain. Loss of sensation sometimes occurs. Speech impediments, tremors, and dizziness are other frequent complaints. Occasionally, people with MS have hearing loss.

Approximately half of all people with MS experience cognitive impairments such as difficulties with concentration, attention, memory, and poor judgment, but such symptoms are usually mild and are frequently overlooked. In fact, they are often detectable only through comprehensive testing. Patients themselves may be unaware of their cognitive loss; it is often a family member or friend who first notices a deficit. Such impairments are usually mild, rarely disabling, and intellectual and language abilities are generally spared.

Cognitive symptoms occur when lesions develop in brain areas responsible for information processing. These deficits tend to become more apparent as the information to be processed becomes more complex. Fatigue may also add to processing difficulties. Scientists do not yet know whether altered cognition in MS reflects problems with information acquisition, retrieval, or a combination of both. Types of memory problems may differ depending on the individual's disease course (relapsing-remitting, primary-progressive, etc.), but there does not appear to be any direct correlation between duration of illness and severity of cognitive dysfunction.

Depression, which is unrelated to cognitive problems, is another common feature of MS. In addition, about 10 percent of patients suffer from more severe psychotic disorders such as manic-depression and paranoia. Five percent may experience episodes of inappropriate euphoria and despair—unrelated to the patient's actual emotional state—known as "laughing/weeping syndrome." This syndrome is thought to be due to demyelination in the brainstem, the area of the brain that controls facial expression and emotions, and is usually seen only in severe cases.

As the disease progresses, sexual dysfunction may become a problem. Bowel and bladder control may also be lost.

In about 60 percent of MS patients, heat—whether generated by temperatures outside the body or by exercise—may cause temporary worsening of many MS symptoms. In these cases, eradicating the heat eliminates the problem. Some temperature-sensitive patients find that a cold bath may temporarily relieve their symptoms. For the same reason, swimming is often a good exercise choice for people with MS.

The erratic symptoms of MS can affect the entire family as patients may become unable to work at the same time they are facing high medical bills and additional expenses for housekeeping assistance and modifications to homes and vehicles. The emotional drain on both patient and family is immeasurable. Support groups and counseling may help MS patients, their families, and friends find ways to cope with the many problems the disease can cause.

Possible symptoms of multiple sclerosis:

- Muscle weakness
- Spasticity
- Impairment of pain, temperature, touch senses
- Pain (moderate to severe)
- Ataxia
- Tremor
- Speech disturbances
- Vision disturbances
- Vertigo
- Bladder dysfunction
- Bowel dysfunction
- Sexual dysfunction
- Depression
- Euphoria
- Cognitive abnormalities
- Fatigue

How is MS diagnosed?

There is no single test that unequivocally detects MS. When faced with a patient whose symptoms, neurological exam results, and medical history suggest MS, physicians use a variety of tools to rule out other possible disorders and perform a series of laboratory tests that, if positive, confirm the diagnosis.

Imaging technologies such as MRI can help locate central nervous system lesions resulting from myelin loss. MRI is painless, noninvasive, and does not expose the body to radiation. It is often used in conjunction with the contrast agent gadolinium, which helps distinguish new plaques from old. However, since these lesions can also occur in several other neurological disorders, they are not absolute evidence of MS.

Several new MRI techniques may help quantify and characterize MS lesions that are too subtle to be detected using conventional MRI scans. While standard MRI provides an anatomical picture of lesions, magnetic resonance spectroscopy (MRS) yields information about the brain's biochemistry; specifically, it can measure the brain chemical N-acetyl aspartate. Decreased levels of this chemical can indicate nerve damage.

Magnetization transfer imaging (MTI) is able to detect white matter abnormalities before lesions can be seen on standard MRI scans by calculating the amount of "free" water in tissues. Demyelinated tissues and damaged nerves show increased levels of free" (versus "bound") water particles.

Diffusion-tensor magnetic resonance imaging (DT-MRI or DTI) measures the random motion of water molecules. Individual water molecules are constantly in motion, colliding with each other at extremely high speeds. This causes them to spread out, or diffuse. DT-MRI maps this diffusion to produce intricate, three-dimensional images indicating the size and location of demyelinated areas of the brain. Changes in this process can then be measured and correlated with disease progression.

Functional MRI (fMRI) uses radio waves and a strong magnetic field to measure the correlation between physical changes in the brain (such as blood flow) and mental functioning during the performance of cognitive tasks.

In addition to helping scientists and physicians better understand how MS develops—an important first step in devising new treatments—these approaches offer earlier diagnosis and enhance efforts to monitor disease progression and the effects of treatment.

Other tests that may be used to diagnosis MS include visual evoked potential (VEP) tests and studies of cerebrospinal fluid (the colorless liquid that circulates through the brain and spinal cord). VEP tests measure the speed of the brain's response to visual stimuli. VEP can sometimes detect lesions that the scanners miss and is particularly useful when abnormalities seen on MRI do not meet the specific criteria for MS. Auditory and sensory evoked potentials have also been used in the past, but are no longer believed to contribute significantly to the diagnosis of MS. Like imaging technologies, VEP is helpful but not conclusive because it cannot identify the cause of lesions.

Examination of cerebrospinal fluid can show cellular and chemical abnormalities often associated with MS. These abnormalities include increased numbers of white blood cells and higher-than-average amounts of protein, especially myelin basic protein and an antibody called immunoglobulin G. Physicians can use several different laboratory techniques to separate and graph the various proteins in MS patients' cerebrospinal fluid. This process often identifies the presence of a characteristic pattern called oligoclonal bands.

While it can still be difficult for the physician to differentiate between an MS attack and symptoms that can follow a viral infection or even an immunization, our growing understanding of disease mechanisms and the expanded use of MRI is enabling physicians to diagnose MS with far more confidence than ever before. Today, most patients who undergo a diagnostic evaluation for MS will be classified as either having MS or not having MS, although there are still cases where a person may have the clinical symptoms of MS but not meet all the criteria to confirm a diagnosis of MS. In these cases, a diagnosis of "possible MS" is used.

A number of other diseases may produce symptoms similar to those seen in MS. Other conditions with an intermittent course and MS-like lesions of the brain's white matter include polyarteritis, lupus erythematosus, syringomyelia, tropical spastic paraparesis, some cancers, and certain tumors that compress the brainstem or spinal cord. Progressive multifocal leukoencephalopathy can mimic the acute stage of an MS attack. Physicians will also need to rule out stroke, neurosyphilis, spinocerebellar ataxias, pernicious anemia, diabetes, Sjögren disease, and vitamin B_{12} deficiency. Acute transverse myelitis may signal the first attack of MS, or it may indicate other problems such as infection with the Epstein-Barr or herpes simplex B viruses. Recent reports suggest that the neurological problems associated with Lyme disease may present a clinical picture much like MS.

Investigators are continuing their search for a definitive test for MS. Until one is developed, however, evidence of both multiple attacks and central nervous system lesions must be found before a diagnosis of MS is given.

Can MS be treated?

There is as yet no cure for MS. Many patients do well with no therapy at all, especially since many medications have serious side effects and some carry significant risks. Naturally occurring or spontaneous remissions make it difficult to determine therapeutic effects of experimental treatments; however, the emerging evidence that MRIs can chart the development of lesions is already helping scientists evaluate new therapies.

In the past, the principal medications physicians used to treat MS were steroids possessing anti-inflammatory properties; these include adrenocorticotropic hormone (better known as ACTH), prednisone, prednisolone, methylprednisolone, betamethasone, and dexamethasone. Studies suggest that intravenous methylprednisolone may be superior to the more traditional intravenous ACTH for patients experiencing acute relapses; no strong evidence exists to support the use of these drugs to treat progressive forms of MS. Also, there is some indication that steroids may be more appropriate for people with movement, rather than sensory, symptoms.

While steroids do not affect the course of MS over time, they can reduce the duration and severity of attacks in some patients. The mechanism behind this effect is not known; one study suggests the medications work by restoring the effectiveness of the blood-brain barrier. Because steroids can produce numerous adverse side effects (acne, weight gain, seizures, psychosis), they are not recommended for long-term use.

One of the most promising MS research areas involves naturally occurring antiviral proteins known as interferons. Three forms of beta interferon (Avonex, Betaseron, and Rebif) have now been approved by the Food and Drug Administration for treatment of relapsing-remitting MS. Beta interferon has been shown to reduce the number of exacerbations and may slow the progression of physical disability. When attacks do occur, they tend to be shorter and less severe. In addition, MRI scans suggest that beta interferon can decrease myelin destruction.

Investigators speculate that the effects of beta interferon may be due to the drug's ability to correct an MS-related deficiency of certain white blood cells that suppress the immune system or its ability to inhibit gamma interferon, a substance believed to be involved in MS attacks. Alpha interferon is also being studied as a possible treatment for MS. Common side effects of interferons include fever, chills, sweating, muscle aches, fatigue, depression, and injection site reactions.

Scientists continue their extensive efforts to create new and better therapies for MS. Goals of therapy are threefold: to improve recovery from attacks, to prevent or lessen the number of relapses, and to halt disease progression. Some therapies currently under investigation are discussed in the following.

Immunotherapy: As evidence of immune system involvement in the development of MS has grown, trials of various new treatments to alter or suppress immune response are being conducted. These therapies are, at this time, still considered experimental.

Results of recent clinical trials have shown that immunosuppressive agents and techniques can positively (if temporarily) affect the course of MS; however, toxic side effects often preclude their widespread use. In addition, generalized immunosuppression leaves the patient open to a variety of viral, bacterial, and fungal infections.

Over the years, MS investigators have studied a number of immunosuppressant treatments. One such treatment, Novantrone (mitoxantrone), was approved by the FDA for the treatment of advanced or chronic MS. Other therapies being studied are cyclosporine (Sandimmune), cyclophosphamide (Cytoxan), methotrexate, azathioprine (Imuran), and total lymphoid irradiation (a process whereby the MS patient's lymph nodes are irradiated with x-rays in small doses over a few weeks to destroy lymphoid tissue, which is actively involved in tissue destruction in autoimmune diseases). Inconclusive or contradictory results of these trials, combined with the therapies' potentially dangerous side effects, dictate that further research is necessary to determine what, if any, role they should play in the management of MS. Studies are also being conducted with the immune system modulating drug cladribine (Leustatin).

Two other experimental treatments—one involving the use of monoclonal antibodies and the other involving plasma exchange, or plasmapheresis—may have fewer dangerous side effects. Monoclonal antibodies are identical, laboratory-produced antibodies that are highly specific for a single antigen. They are injected into the patient in the hope that they will alter the patient's immune response. Plasmapheresis is a procedure in which blood is removed from the patient, and the plasma is separated from other blood substances, which may contain antibodies and other immunologically active products. These other blood substances are discarded and the plasma is then transfused back into the patient. Because their worth as treatments for MS has not yet been proven, these experimental treatments remain at the stage of clinical testing.

Bone marrow transplantation (a procedure in which bone marrow from a healthy donor is infused into patients who have undergone drug or radiation therapy to suppress their immune system so they will not reject the donated marrow) and injections of venom from honey bees are also being studied. Each of these therapies carries the risk of potentially severe side effects.

Therapy to Improve Nerve Impulse Conduction: Because the transmission of electrochemical messages between the brain and body is disrupted in MS, medications to improve the conduction of nerve impulses are being investigated. Since demyelinated nerves show abnormalities of potassium activity, scientists are studying drugs that block the channels through which potassium moves, thereby restoring conduction of the nerve impulse. In several small experimental trials, derivatives of a drug called aminopyridine temporarily improved vision, coordination, and strength when given to MS patients who suffered from both visual symptoms and heightened sensitivity to temperature. Possible side effects of these therapies include paresthesias (tingling sensations), dizziness, and seizures.

Therapies Targeting an Antigen: Trials of a synthetic form of myelin basic protein, called copolymer I (Copaxone), were successful, leading the FDA to approve the agent for the treatment of relapsing-remitting MS. Copolymer I, unlike so many drugs tested for the treatment of MS, has few side effects, and studies indicate that the agent can reduce the relapse rate by almost one-third. In addition, patients given copolymer I are more likely to show neurologic improvement than those given a placebo.

Investigators are also looking at the possibility of developing an MS vaccine. Myelin-attacking T cells were removed, inactivated, and injected back into animals with experimental allergic encephalomyelitis (EAE). This procedure results in destruction of the immune system cells that were attacking myelin basic protein. In a couple of small trials scientists have tested a similar vaccine in humans. The product was well tolerated and had no side effects, but the studies were too small to establish efficacy. Patients with progressive forms of MS did not appear to benefit, although relapsing-remitting patients showed some neurologic improvement and had fewer relapses and reduced numbers of lesions in one study. Unfortunately, the benefits did not last beyond two years.

A similar approach, known as peptide therapy, is based on evidence that the body can mount an immune response against the T cells that destroy myelin, but this response is not strong enough to overcome the disease. To induce this response, the investigator scans the myelin-attacking T cells for the myelin-recognizing receptors on the cells' surface. A fragment, or peptide, of those receptors is then injected into the body. The immune system "sees" the injected peptide as a foreign invader and launches an attack on any myelin-destroying T cells that carry the peptide. The injection of portions of T cell receptors may heighten the immune system reaction against the errant T cells much the same way a booster shot heightens immunity to tetanus. Or, peptide therapy may jam the errant cells' receptors, preventing the cells from attacking myelin.

Despite these promising early results, there are some major obstacles to developing vaccine and peptide therapies. Individual patients'

T cells vary so much that it may not be possible to develop a standard vaccine or peptide therapy beneficial to all, or even most, MS patients. At this time, each treatment involves extracting cells from each individual patient, purifying the cells, and then growing them in culture before inactivating and chemically altering them. This makes the production of quantities sufficient for therapy extremely time consuming, labor intensive, and expensive. Further studies are necessary to determine whether universal inoculations can be developed to induce suppression of MS patients' overactive immune systems.

Protein antigen feeding is similar to peptide therapy, but is a potentially simpler means to the same end. Whenever we eat, the digestive system breaks each food or substance into its primary "non-antigenic" building blocks, thereby averting a potentially harmful immune attack. So, strange as it may seem, antigens that trigger an immune response when they are injected can encourage immune system tolerance when taken orally. Furthermore, this reaction is directed solely at the specific antigen being fed; wholesale immunosuppression, which can leave the body open to a variety of infections, does not occur. Studies have shown that when rodents with EAE are fed myelin protein antigens, they experience fewer relapses. Data from a small, preliminary trial of antigen feeding in humans found limited suggestion of improvement, but the results were not statistically significant. A multicenter trial is being conducted to determine whether protein antigen feeding is effective.

Cytokines: As our growing insight into the workings of the immune system gives us new knowledge about the function of cytokines, the powerful chemicals produced by T cells, the possibility of using them to manipulate the immune system becomes more attractive. Scientists are studying a variety of substances that may block harmful cytokines, such as those involved in inflammation, or that encourage the production of protective cytokines.

A drug that has been tested as a depression treatment, rolipram, has been shown to reduce levels of several destructive cytokines in animal models of MS. Its potential as a therapy for MS is not known at this time, but side effects seem modest. Protein antigen feeding, discussed above, may release transforming growth factor beta (TGF), a protective cytokine that inhibits or regulates the activity of certain immune cells. Preliminary tests indicate that it may reduce the number of immune cells commonly found in MS patients' spinal fluid. Side effects include anemia and altered kidney function.

Interleukin 4 (IL-4) is able to diminish demyelination and improve the clinical course of mice with EAE, apparently by influencing developing T cells to become protective rather than harmful. This also appears to be true of a group of chemicals called retinoids. When fed to rodents with EAE, retinoids increase levels of TGF and IL-4, which encourage protective T cells, while decreasing numbers of harmful T cells. This results in improvement of the animals' clinical symptoms.

Remyelination: Some studies focus on strategies to reverse the damage to myelin and oligodendrocytes (the cells that make and maintain myelin in the central nervous system), both of which are destroyed during MS attacks. Scientists now know that oligodendrocytes may proliferate and form new myelin after an attack. Therefore, there is a great deal of interest in agents that may stimulate this reaction. To learn more about the process, investigators are looking at how drugs used in MS trials affect remyelination. Studies of animal models indicate that monoclonal antibodies and two immunosuppressant drugs, cyclophosphamide and azathioprine, may accelerate remyelination, while steroids may inhibit it. The ability of intravenous immunoglobulin (IVIg) to restore visual acuity and muscle strength is also being investigated.

Diet: Over the years, many people have tried to implicate diet as a cause of or treatment for MS. Some physicians have advocated a diet low in saturated fats; others have suggested increasing the patient's intake of linoleic acid, a polyunsaturated fat, via supplements of sunflower seed, safflower, or evening primrose oils. Other proposed dietary "remedies" include megavitamin therapy, including increased intake of vitamins B_{12} or C; various liquid diets; and sucrose-, tobacco-, or gluten-free diets. To date, clinical studies have not been able to confirm benefits from dietary changes; in the absence of any evidence that diet therapy is effective, patients are best advised to eat a balanced, wholesome diet.

Unproven Therapies: MS is a disease with a natural tendency to remit spontaneously, and for which there is no universally effective treatment and no known cause. These factors open the door for an array of unsubstantiated claims of cures. At one time or another, many ineffective and even potentially dangerous therapies have been promoted as treatments for MS. A partial list of these "therapies" includes: injections of snake venom, electrical stimulation of the spinal cord's dorsal column, removal of the thymus gland, breathing pressurized (hyperbaric) oxygen in a special chamber, injections of beef heart and hog pancreas extracts, intravenous or oral calcium orotate (calcium EAP), hysterectomy, removal of dental fillings containing silver or mercury amalgams, and surgical implantation of pig brain into the patient's abdomen. None of these treatments is an effective therapy for MS or any of its symptoms.

Are any MS symptoms treatable?

While some scientists look for therapies that will affect the overall course of the disease, others are searching for new and better medications to control the symptoms of MS without triggering intolerable side effects.

Many people with MS have problems with spasticity, a condition that primarily affects the lower limbs. Spasticity can occur either as a sustained stiffness caused by increased muscle tone or as spasms that come and go, especially at night. It is usually treated with muscle relaxants and tranquilizers. Baclofen (Lioresal), the most commonly prescribed medication for this symptom, may be taken orally or, in severe cases, injected into the spinal cord. Tizanidine (Zanaflex), used for years in Europe and now approved in the United States, appears to function similarly to baclofen. Diazepam (Valium), clonazepam (Klonopin), and dantrolene (Dantrium) can also reduce spasticity. Although its beneficial effect is temporary, physical therapy may also be useful and can help prevent the irreversible shortening of muscles known as contractures. Surgery to reduce spasticity is rarely appropriate in MS.

Weakness and ataxia (incoordination) are also characteristic of MS. When weakness is a problem, some spasticity can actually be beneficial by lending support to weak limbs. In such cases, medication levels that alleviate spasticity completely may be inappropriate. Physical therapy and exercise can also help preserve remaining function, and patients may find that various aids—such as foot braces, canes, and walkers—can help them remain independent and mobile. Occasionally, physicians can provide temporary relief from weakness, spasms, and pain by injecting a drug called phenol into the spinal cord, muscles, or nerves in the arms or legs. Further research is needed to find or develop effective treatments for MS-related weakness and ataxia.

Although improvement of optic symptoms usually occurs even without treatment, a short course of treatment with intravenous methylprednisolone (Solu-Medrol) followed by treatment with oral steroids is sometimes used. A trial of oral prednisone in patients with visual problems suggests that this steroid is not only ineffective in speeding recovery but may also increase patients' risk for future MS attacks. Curiously, prednisone injected directly into the veins—at ten times the oral dose—did seem to produce short-term recovery. Because of the link between optic neuritis and MS, the study's investigators believe these findings may hold true for the treatment of MS as well. A follow-up study of optic neuritis patients will address this and other questions.

Fatigue, especially in the legs, is a common symptom of MS and may be both physical and psychological. Avoiding excessive activity and heat are probably the most important measures patients can take to counter physiological fatigue. If psychological aspects of fatigue such as depression or apathy are evident, antidepressant medications may help. Other drugs that may reduce fatigue in some, but not all, patients include amantadine (Symmetrel), pemoline (Cylert), and the still-experimental drug aminopyridine.

People with MS may experience several types of pain. Muscle and back pain can be helped by aspirin or acetaminophen and physical therapy to correct faulty posture and strengthen and stretch muscles. The sharp, stabbing facial pain known as trigeminal neuralgia is commonly treated with carbamazepine or other anticonvulsant drugs or, occasionally, surgery. Intense tingling and burning sensations are harder to treat. Some people get relief with antidepressant drugs; others may respond to electrical stimulation of the nerves in the affected area. In some cases, the physician may recommend codeine.

As the disease progresses, some patients develop bladder malfunctions. Urinary problems are often the result of infections that can be treated with antibiotics. The physician may recommend that patients take vitamin C supplements or drink cranberry juice, as these measures acidify urine and may reduce the risk of further infections. Several medications are also available. The most common bladder problems encountered by MS patients are urinary frequency, urgency, or incontinence. A small number of patients, however, retain large amounts of urine. In these patients, catheterization may be necessary. In this procedure, a catheter or drainage tube is temporarily inserted (by the patient or a caretaker) into the urethra several times a day to drain urine from the bladder. Surgery may be indicated in severe, intractable cases. Scientists have developed a "bladder pacemaker" that has helped people with urinary incontinence in preliminary trials. The pacemaker, which is surgically implanted, is controlled by a hand-held unit that allows the patient to electrically stimulate the nerves that control bladder function.

MS patients with urinary problems may be reluctant to drink enough fluids, leading to constipation. Drinking more water and adding fiber to the diet usually alleviates this condition. Sexual dysfunction may also occur, especially in patients with urinary problems. Men may experience occasional failure to attain an erection. Penile implants, injection of the drug papaverine, and electrostimulation are techniques used to resolve the problem. Women may experience insufficient lubrication or have difficulty reaching orgasm; in these cases, vaginal gels and vibrating devices may be helpful. Counseling is also beneficial, especially in the absence of urinary problems, since psychological factors can also cause these symptoms. For instance, depression can intensify symptoms of fatigue, pain, and sexual dysfunction. In addition to counseling, the physician may prescribe antidepressant or antianxiety medications. Amitriptyline is used to treat laughing/weeping syndrome.

Tremors are often resistant to therapy, but can sometimes be treated with drugs or, in extreme cases, surgery. Investigators are currently examining a number of experimental treatments for tremor.

Table 18.1. Drugs Used to Treat Symptoms of Multiple Sclerosis

Symptom	Drug
Spasticity	Baclofen (Lioresal) Tizanidine (Zanaflex) Diazepam (Valium) Clonazepam (Klonopin) Dantrolene (Dantrium)
Optic neuritis	Methylprednisolone (Solu-Medrol) Oral steroids
Fatigue	Antidepressants Amantadine (Symmetrel) Pemoline (Cylert)
Pain	Aspirin or acetaminophen Antidepressants Codeine
Trigeminal neuralgia	Carbamazepine, other anticonvulsant
Sexual dysfunction	Papaverine injections (in men)

What recent advances have been made in MS research?

Many advances, on several fronts, have been made in the war against MS. Each advance interacts with the others, adding greater depth and meaning to each new discovery. Four areas, in particular, stand out.

Over the last decade, our knowledge about how the immune system works has grown at an amazing rate. Major gains have been made in recognizing and defining the role of this system in the development of MS lesions, giving scientists the ability to devise ways to alter the immune response. Such work is expected to yield a variety of new potential therapies that may ameliorate MS without harmful side effects.

New tools such as MRI have redefined the natural history of MS and are proving invaluable in monitoring disease activity. Scientists are now able to visualize and follow the development of MS lesions in the brain and spinal cord using MRI; this ability is a tremendous aid in the assessment of new therapies and can speed the process of evaluating new treatments.

Other tools have been developed that make the painstaking work of teasing out the disease's genetic secrets possible. Such studies have strengthened scientists' conviction that MS is a disease with many genetic components, none of which is dominant. Immune system–related genetic factors that predispose an individual to the development of MS have been identified, and may lead to new ways to treat or prevent the disease.

In fact, a treatment that may actually slow the course of the disease has been found and a growing number of therapies are now available that effectively treat some MS symptoms. In addition, there are a number of treatments under investigation that may curtail attacks or improve function of demyelinated nerve fibers. Over a dozen clinical trials testing potential therapies are under way, and additional new treatments are being devised and tested in animal models.

What research remains to be done?

The role of genetic risk factors, and how they can be modified, must be more clearly defined. Environmental triggers, such as viruses or toxins, need to be investigated further. The specific cellular and subcellular targets of immune attack in the brain and spinal cord, and the subsets of T cells involved in that attack, need to be identified. Knowledge of these aspects of the disease will enable scientists to develop new methods for halting—or reversing and repairing—the destruction of myelin that causes the symptoms of MS.

What is the outlook for people with MS?

The 1990s—proclaimed the "Decade of the Brain" in 1989 by President Bush and Congress—have seen an unparalleled explosion of knowledge about neurological disorders. New technologies are forcing even complex diseases like MS to yield up their secrets. These burgeoning opportunities in the field of neurological research have prompted the National Advisory Neurological Disorders and Stroke Council to suggest that an effective treatment for and the cause of MS may be found during the Decade of the Brain. The former has already been achieved; scientists continue to diligently search for the latter. Their dedication is the best hope for a cure, or, better yet, a way to prevent MS altogether.

Section 18.2

MS Treatment: Some Safety Issues

Reprinted from Aguilar, M., "Multiple Sclerosis Treatment: Some Safety Issues to Keep in Mind," *Neurology* 2004 February 24; 62 (4): E8–E9. © 2004 American Academy of Neurology. Reprinted by permission of Lippincott Williams and Willkins.

Interferon Drugs and the Treatment of Multiple Sclerosis

The treatment of multiple sclerosis (MS) has been revolutionized by the discovery of interferons. The interferons are man-made molecules that mimic the action of interferon molecules that are made by the body. The interferons are part of the immune system, which works to clear invaders from the body. The name "interferon" comes from "interference," because they interfere with the growth of viruses.

In MS, part of the immune system reacts against myelin. Myelin is a cover that surrounds the nerves in the brain and allows them to carry impulses through the brain more efficiently. We believe treatment with interferons decreases the number of attacks on myelin.

How Are Interferon Drugs Made?

The interferon drugs are produced by bacteria (*Escherichia coli*) in the laboratory. All the interferon drugs have been shown to cause liver damage in some people. We detect this damage by measuring liver function tests in the blood. The interferon drugs are not only used for the treatment of MS. These medications have been used also for the treatment of hepatitis, myeloma, leukemia, and other diseases.

How Many Interferon Drugs Are There?

There are three interferon drugs available for the treatment of MS: interferon B1a (Avonex), interferon B1b (Betaseron), and interferon B1a (Rebif). All of the interferon drugs must be injected. None are available to take by mouth. The interferon drugs have different doses and routes of injection. Betaseron is injected every other day subcutaneously (under the skin). Rebif is injected three times per week subcutaneously. Avonex is injected once a week intramuscularly (into a muscle).

Interferon Drugs Can Affect the Liver

In the February 24, 2004, issue of *Neurology*, Tremlett and colleagues reviewed the liver function tests of 835 patients with MS who were using one of the three available interferon drugs. The investigators reviewed medical records for patients aged eighteen to sixty years who had had two or more attacks of MS during the two years prior to entering the study. Liver function tests were checked before treatment with interferon drugs and at three, six, and twelve months after treatment was started. After the first year of interferon treatment, liver function tests were checked every year. Patients who had been on interferon treatment in the past or who had any other medical problems that could cause liver abnormalities were not included in the study.

Overall, nearly one third (36 percent) of the patients treated with interferon drugs developed abnormal liver function tests. All of the three interferon drugs caused some abnormality in liver function tests. Avonex caused slightly fewer problems than Betaseron and Rebif. Most patients had minimal abnormalities (33 to 38 percent), 4 to 7 percent had mild to moderate abnormalities, and only 1 to 2 percent had severe abnormalities on the liver function tests. The "highest risk" period for developing liver abnormalities seemed to be in the first twelve months after beginning treatment.

Risk Factors for Liver Problems in Patients Taking Interferon Drugs

Men seemed to be at higher risk than women for developing liver function abnormalities. Other factors, such as obesity, alcohol use, and other medications (i.e., acetaminophen) used simultaneously, also increased the risk of developing liver function abnormalities. The medical significance of a slight abnormality in liver function tests is unknown.

What Have We Learned from This Study?

In conclusion, MS patients must be aware of the risk of developing liver abnormalities while on interferon therapy. It could be harmful to the liver if patients taking interferon therapy use alcohol, become obese, or take other medications that can also be harmful to the liver. Liver function tests should be checked periodically during interferon therapy, especially during the first year of treatment.

What Is MS?

MS is a disabling neurologic disorder of young adults, affecting at least three hundred thousand Americans. The average age at diagnosis is thirty, typically starting between the ages of fifteen and fifty. Women are affected at least twice as often as men. It is more common in persons of northern European heritage and those living furthest from the equator.

MS involves inflammation within the central nervous system (the brain and spinal cord), followed by the loss of the protective myelin sheaths that surround nerve fibers. When the myelin is damaged, nerve impulses are not quickly and efficiently transmitted. Besides damage to the myelin sheaths, it is now recognized that the nerve fibers, called axons, also are damaged in MS to varying extent. Lesions (called plaques) develop in the brain and spinal cord and can cause the symptoms of MS listed in the following.

What Are the Symptoms?

There are several types of MS. Most people with MS begin with relapsing-remitting disease. This means that the symptoms come and go, often leaving the person feeling nearly normal until another relapse, or MS attack, occurs. Symptoms associated with relapses usually develop over a period of days. The problems can last for a matter of days or weeks and then go away, sometimes even without any treatment. New attacks occur at irregular intervals, usually one attack every one to two years. Common symptoms include the following:

- Vision loss
- Numbness or tingling
- Weakness or fatigue
- Unsteadiness in walking
- Double vision
- Heat intolerance
- Partial or complete paralysis
- Electric shock sensations when bending the neck

About 50 percent of patients with relapsing-remitting MS develop a progressive form of MS, called secondary progressive MS, in which there is continual worsening. In this phase of the disease, patients may continue to have relapses or may stop having them altogether. About 15 percent of patients have progressive worsening from the beginning of their MS and do not experience relapses of MS. This form of MS is called primary progressive MS.

How Is MS Diagnosed?

The diagnosis of MS is based on a history of multiple attacks over time of neurologic lesions that affect different parts of the central nervous system. A neurologist will order tests that will help confirm the diagnosis. Usually a magnetic resonance imaging (MRI) scan of the brain (and possibly the spinal cord) is ordered to find evidence of abnormal areas. Lumbar puncture (spinal tap) is also helpful to detect specific problems with the cerebrospinal fluid.

What Causes MS?

The cause of MS is unknown. There is strong evidence that MS is immune mediated. This means that the person's own immune system attacks the central nervous system (an autoimmune disease).

What Are the Treatments?

Currently, there is no prevention or cure for MS. However, this is a promising time for people with MS, as several new medications that affect the underlying disease process have been approved or are awaiting approval by the U.S. Food and Drug Administration (FDA). You should ask your neurologist about the best treatment options for you. Current treatments are divided into three categories:

1. Medications that treat the symptoms of MS. These include medications to treat depression, decrease muscle stiffness, reduce fatigue, control bladder symptoms, reduce pain, and address sexual dysfunction.

2. Medications that modify attacks when they occur. These are primarily corticosteroids (a synthesized adrenal hormone) that can shorten an attack.

3. Medications that modify disease activity. These are taken on a regular basis to help reduce the frequency of attacks and the long-term damage to brain caused by MS. FDA-approved disease-modifying therapies for treating MS include recombinant beta-interferons (Avonex, Betaseron, and Rebif), glatiramer acetate (Copaxone), and an immunosuppressant/chemotherapy drug, mitoxantrone (Novantrone).

Section 18.3

MS and Cooling

Introduction: Multiple Sclerosis

Multiple Sclerosis (MS) is the most commonly diagnosed neurological disorder among young adults. MS is characterized by a disruption of nerve impulses traveling from the brain or spinal cord to other parts of the body, along the nerves of the central nervous system (CNS). Researchers believe that once a person acquires MS, his or her immune system malfunctions and damages or destroys the protective layer, known as myelin, in the brain and spinal cord. Myelin can be thought of as the insulation around the body's circuitry. Nerve fibers, called axons, may become damaged as well.

When myelin or axons are damaged, nerve impulses "short-circuit" before they can complete their journey. The resulting variety of symptoms may include difficulties with vision, numbness, fatigue, balance, spasticity, bladder and bowel function, cognition, and depression, among others. Many individuals with MS may experience only a few, while others may experience a number of symptoms. For most, these symptoms are temporary, particularly for the first several years following diagnosis.

Cooling and Multiple Sclerosis

Studies have shown that nerves with damaged myelin are sensitive to changes in temperatures.[1] Researchers note that a rise in temperature may cause a failure in the effective transmission of signals from the brain to the body (nerve conduction), and a reduction in temperature may allow more signals to be transmitted across the damaged nerve.

The idea of cooling individuals with MS to alleviate symptoms is not a new one. Several research programs were conducted during the 1950s using cool baths.[2] These studies and many unconfirmed personal accounts seemed to substantiate the theory that cooling the body may provide temporary symptom relief for people with MS. Unfortunately, cooling practices such as taking cold baths several times a day and sitting close to air-conditioning are often uncomfortable, impractical, and dangerous, due to the body's defense mechanisms of shivering and vasoconstriction. The answer to these problems is found in the technology developed for eliminating the physical stress of extreme heat and cold for astronauts in space.

Space Technology Refines Cooling

The National Aeronautics and Space Administration (NASA) developed space suits to protect astronauts from the hazards of space. A space suit, however, will also trap heat inside the suit. To stabilize an astronaut's body temperature, space suits are equipped with an undergarment containing a network of small tubes held against the body. A chilled liquid is pumped through these tubes, removing the body's heat by heat transfer between the skin and the tubes. These garments are known as liquid-cooled garments (LCGs), but are often referred to as "cool suits." Cool suits are now used in a variety of industrial and military applications.

Known for their expertise with LCGs, NASA scientists continued to refine and adapt this technology for the advancement of biomedical research. These advancements include cooling systems for cancer patients undergoing chemotherapy, children who suffer from HED (hypohidrotic ectodermal dysplasia; insufficient sweat glands), and those diagnosed with MS.

How to Use Active Cool Suits

The first step to safe cooling is to establish a baseline temperature. This is an average of temperatures over at least seven days. This is important because a maximum cooling of two degrees Fahrenheit from a person's baseline is generally considered safe. A one-degree Fahrenheit drop in a person's temperature, however, has been found to be sufficient for effective active-cooling therapy.

The next step is to choose a room with a stable and moderate room temperature (70 to 75 degrees Fahrenheit). Room temperature plays a vital role in effective cooling. If the room is too cool, the body will

421

react against the cooling. If the room is too warm, the cooling suit will be ineffective.

Active suits are always started at room temperature and then the temperature is slowly reduced during the first fifteen minutes. Most in-home cooling sessions are conducted for one hour. They may be repeated with or without exercise (as recommended by one's physician) up to three times per day, waiting at least two hours between each session. These units can also be used with a battery pack, enabling individuals who are heat intolerant to once again enjoy the outdoors.

Cooling therapy, when used correctly, may help reduce some symptoms of MS, including problems with fatigue, vision, spasticity, motor function, and cognition. As with any therapy, not all people receive the same benefit or any benefit at all. Cooling therapy should be viewed as an adjunct to disease-modifying drugs, not as an alternative, and should be done only with the approval of a medical professional.

How Passive Cooling Can Help

"Passive" cooling refers to cooling with no "active" cooling mechanism, such as a separate pump. Passive cooling can be accomplished through a simple transfer of heat by wearing a garment containing a cooling source.

Evaporation garments include bandanas, skullcaps, and vests. These garments are usually soaked in water, rung out, and occasionally chilled in the refrigerator. As the water in the garments evaporates, they provide limited relief from heat, depending on climate conditions. These garments are less effective in areas with high humidity.

Most passive-cooling garments work by placing ice or gel packs into pockets of a vest. This type of system can provide immediate and simple relief from the heat. These vests allow many people with MS to enjoy outside activities that would otherwise be intolerable.

Studies have shown that an immediate loss of cognitive and physical function can occur due to an increase in either internal (through exercise) or external (room or outside) temperature. Passive cooling can significantly reduce the impact of these factors by providing a simple cooling mechanism. Passive cooling cannot be viewed as a symptomatic therapy, but can be seen as a valuable preventative tool to help reduce the impact of heat in people with MS.

Endnotes

1. Davis F. A. and Jacobson S., Altered thermal sensitivity in injured and demyelinated nerve, *Journal Neurosurg Psychiat,*

1971, 34, pp. 551–61; Davis F. A., Axonal conduction studies based on some considerations of temperature effects in multiple sclerosis, *Electroencephalog Clin Neurophysiol*, 1970, 28, pp. 281–86; McDonald W. I. and Sears T. A., Effect of a demyelinating lesion on conduction in the central nervous system studied in single nerve fibers, *Journal Physio.* (Lond), 1970, 207, pp. 53–54P.

2. Watson C.W., Effect of lowering of body temperature on the symptoms and signs of multiple sclerosis, *New Eng. Journal Med*, 1951, 261, pp. 1253–59; Boynton, B.L., Garramone P.M., and Buca J.T., Observations on the effects of cool baths for patients with multiple sclerosis, *Phys Ther Rev*, 1959, 39, pp. 297–99.

List of Suggested Reference Works Regarding Neurohypothermia as a Symptomatic Therapy for MS

Please Note: This is not an inclusive listing, merely the editor's choice.

Basic Cooling Theory

Boynton B.L., Garramone P.M., and Buca J., Cool baths as adjunct treatment in patients with multiple sclerosis, *Quart Bull (Northwest Univ M School)*, 1959, 33, p. 6.

Boynton B.L., Garramone P.M., and Buca J.T., Observations on the effects of cool baths for patients with multiple sclerosis, *Phys Ther Rev*, 1959, 39, pp. 297–99.

Davis F.A. and Jacobson S., Altered thermal sensitivity in injured and demyelinated nerve. *Journal Neuro Psychiat*, 1971, 34, pp. 551–61.

Davis F.A., Axonal conduction studies based on some considerations of temperature effects in multiple sclerosis, *Electroencephalog Clin Neurophysiol*, 1970, 28, pp. 281–86.

Harbison J.W., Calabrese V.P., and Edlich R.F., A fatal case of sun exposure in multiple sclerosis patient, *Journal of Emergency Medicine*, 1989, 7, pp. 465–67.

McDonald W.I. and Sears T.A., Effect of a demyelinating lesion on conduction in the central nervous system studied in single nerve fibers, *Journal Physiol* (Lond.), 1970, 207, pp. 53–54P.

Nelson D.A., Jeffreys W.H., and McDowell F., Effects of induced hyperthermia on some neurological diseases, *Arch Neurol Psychiatry*, 1958, 79, pp. 31–39.

Schauf, C.L., Pencek T.L., Davis F.A., and Rooney M.W., Physiological basis for neuroelectric blocking activity in multiple sclerosis, *Neurology*, 1981, 31, pp. 1338–41.

Watson C.W., Effect of lowering of body temperature on the symptoms and signs of multiple sclerosis, *New Eng Journal Med*, 1951, 261, pp. 1253–59.

Cooling Therapy in MS

Bassett S. and Lake B., Use of cold applications in the management of spasticity, *Phys Therapy Rev*, 1958, 38 (5), pp. 333–34.

Beenakker E.A.C., Oparina T.I., Hartgring A., Teelken A., Arutjunyan A.V., and De Keyser J., Cooling Garment Treatment in MS: Clinical Improvement and Decrease in Leukocyte Nitric Oxide (NO) Production, *Neurology*, 2001, 57, pp. 892–94.

Capello E., Gardella M., Leandri M., et al, Lowering body temperature with a cooling suit as symptomatic treatment for thermosensitive multiple sclerosis patients, *Ital Journal Neuro Sci*, Nov. 16, 1995, 8, pp. 533–39.

Kinnman J., Anderson U.A., and Kinnman Y., Temporary improvement of motor function in patient with multiple sclerosis after treatment with a cooling suit, *Journal Neuro Rehab*, 1997, 11, pp. 109–14.

Kinnman J., Anderson U.A., Anderson A., Wetterquist L., and Kinnman Y., Cooling Suit for Multiple Sclerosis: Functional Improvement in Daily Living, *Scand Journal Rehab Med*, 2000, 33, pp. 20–24.

Kraft G. and Alquist A., Effect of microclimate cooling on physical function in multiple sclerosis, *Cooling and Multiple Sclerosis*, 1997, 1, pp. 6–9.

Ku Y.E., Montgomery L.D., and Webbon B.W., Hemodynamic and thermal responses to head and neck cooling in men and women, *Am Journal Phys Med Rehabil*, 1996, 75, pp. 443–50.

Ku Y.E., Montgomery L.D., and Lee H., et al, Physiologic and functional responses of MS patients to body cooling, *Am. Journal Phys Med Rehabil*, 2000, 13, 8994–9115.

Montgomery L.D., Montgomery R.W., and Ku Y.E., Enhancement of cognitive processing by multiple sclerosis patients using liquid cooling technology: a case study, Submitted in 1998 for publication to *Am. Journal Phys Med Rehabil.*

Nelson D.A. and McDowell F., The effects of induced hyperthermia on patients with multiple sclerosis, *J Neurol Neurosurg Psychiatry*, 1959, 79, pp. 31–39.

Pellegrino R.G., Roberts A.J., and Harper-Bennie J., The use of in-home portable conductive cooling units from the study to evaluate the chronic effects of conductive cooling in multiple sclerosis patients, *Cooling and Multiple Sclerosis*, 1997, 1, pp. 9–10.

Schauf C.L. and Davis F.A., Impulse conduction in multiple sclerosis: a theoretical basis for modification by temperature and pharmacological agents, *Journal Neurol Neurosurg Psychiatry*, 1974, 37, pp. 152–61.

Schwid S.R., Petrie M.D., Murray R., Leitch J., Bowen J., Alquist A., Pellegrino R.G., Milan M.D., Roberts A., Harper-Bennie J.E., Guisado R., Luna B., Montgomery L., Lamparter R., Ku Y.T., Lee H., Goldwater D., Cutter G., Webbon B., A Randomized Controlled Study of the Acute and Chronic Effects of Cooling Therapy for MS, *Neurology*, 2003, 60, pp. 1955–60.

Section 18.4

New Research on MS

This section includes the following press releases from the National Institute of Neurological Disorders and Stroke: "Brain Produces New Cells
in Multiple Sclerosis" (February 26, 2002); "Old Drug, New Use: New
Research Shows Common Cholesterol-Lowering Drug Reduces Multiple
Sclerosis Symptoms in Mice" (January 6, 2003); and "Small Trial Shows
Daclizumab Add-On Therapy Improves Multiple Sclerosis Outcome" (May
24, 2004).

Brain Produces New Cells in Multiple Sclerosis

The brain produces new cells to repair the damage from multiple
sclerosis (MS) for years after symptoms of the disorder appear, according to a recent study. However, in most cases the cells are unable to
complete the repairs. These findings suggest that an unknown factor
limits the repair process and may lead to new ways of treating this
disorder.

"The brain is making a serious attempt to repair the damage," says
Bruce D. Trapp, Ph.D., of the Cleveland Clinic Foundation in Ohio,
who led the study. The findings are consistent with those of other recent studies showing that the adult brain has the capacity to replace
cells, he adds. The study was supported by the National Institute of
Neurological Disorders and Stroke (NINDS) and appears in the January 17, 2002, issue of the *New England Journal of Medicine*.

In patients with multiple sclerosis, brain inflammation in random
patches, or lesions, leads to destruction of myelin, the fatty covering
that insulates nerve cell fibers called axons in the brain and spinal
cord and aids in transmission of signals to other neurons. This inflammation causes the myelin to deteriorate and leads to the symptoms
of MS. Previous studies have shown that some brain lesions are repaired during the early years of multiple sclerosis. However, many
other lesions are not repaired.

In the study, Dr. Trapp and colleagues examined brain tissue obtained during autopsies of ten patients with MS to see if new myelin-
producing cells, called oligodendrocytes, were being produced in the
chronic MS lesions. They found that most of the lesions contained

newly produced oligodendrocytes. The percentage of lesions from each brain that had these new cells decreased as the duration of the disease increased, but the decline was not related to the type of MS the patients had or to their ages at death. The new oligodendrocytes extended "arms" that produced myelin-related proteins and grew around the damaged axons as if they were trying to repair the myelin. However, in most cases the axons were not repaired.

One of the central questions in MS research is how to promote myelin repair. Many researchers have concentrated on increasing the number of oligodendrocytes through stem cell transplantation or other means. However, this study suggests that problems with the axons or with the tissue that surrounds them may prevent remyelination. Many of the axons that were not remyelinated looked abnormal, whereas remyelinated axons appeared healthy. This suggests that therapies that prevent axon degeneration or help oligodendrocytes complete the repair process in other ways may be necessary. More research is needed to identify drugs that may be useful for this purpose, says Dr. Trapp. While the study shows that the brain's attempts to repair itself decrease over time, new cells were produced even in patients who had had MS for as long as fifteen years, implying that there is a long window of opportunity for treatment.

Researchers must now determine how long the new oligodendrocytes survive in the brain and whether the brain can produce enough of them to repair all the damage from MS, says Dr. Trapp. If the brain produces enough new cells on its own, then transplantation of additional cells may not be necessary. Research using brain scanning or other techniques may help to identify patients who are most likely to benefit from these therapies.

Reference

Chang A, Tourtellotte WW, Rudick R, Trapp BD. "Premyelinating oligodendrocytes in chronic lesions of multiple sclerosis." *New England Journal of Medicine*, Vol. 346, No. 3, January 17, 2002, pp. 165–73.

Old Drug, New Use: New Research Shows Common Cholesterol-Lowering Drug Reduces Multiple Sclerosis Symptoms in Mice

A new study shows that a widely prescribed cholesterol-lowering drug dramatically reduces symptoms of multiple sclerosis (MS) in mice. Results of the study suggest that statins, which are commonly used to prevent heart attack and stroke, could be a possible new treatment for MS and other autoimmune disorders. The study was funded in part by the National Institute of Neurological Disorders and Stroke (NINDS) and appears in the November 7, 2002, issue of *Nature*.[1]

"These are very provocative results, because we've shown that statins can regulate the immune system response in an animal model for multiple sclerosis," says Scott Zamvil, M.D., Ph.D., assistant professor of neurology at the University of California at San Francisco and senior author of the study.

In the study, a daily dose of atorvastatin (brand name Lipitor), given for several weeks, reduced inflammation in the central nervous system and reversed some emerging paralysis in mice with a disease closely resembling MS, a disabling immune disorder affecting about 2.5 million people worldwide.

If the drug proves effective in human trials, statins, which can be taken in pill form, would offer an attractive alternative or complement to existing therapies for MS. Currently approved treatments are given by injection, often have serious side effects, and are only partly effective, Dr. Zamvil says.

"We don't know if or how well statins would work in reducing symptoms of MS in humans, but we do know that they are well tolerated when given orally," says Dr. Zamvil. Still, there are some risks. Statins can cause liver damage in a small percentage of patients, and they carry a small risk of serious muscle damage.

Scientists believe MS develops when the body's immune cells led by so-called helper T cells attack myelin, the fatty insulating sheath surrounding nerve cells. The damage to myelin and the underlying neurons in both the brain and spinal cord leads to impaired cell communication and progressive physical disability.

MS symptoms include fatigue, vision problems, numbness, impaired balance, and paralysis. There are currently no treatments that can stop the disease, although a few treatments do slow its progression.

Atorvastatin appears to help the body produce protective molecules that fight inflammation and inhibit the production of toxic molecules, the researchers say. Previous studies in test tubes have also shown neuroprotective effects, suggesting that the drug might be used to treat such neurodegenerative diseases as Alzheimer's. "In the very near future we may have a variety of new uses for statins," Dr. Zamvil says.

Because statins have a different mechanism of action than current treatments, they may be able to work in tandem with other MS treatments. Since MS is a multistage disease, statins might be used along with approved treatments—Copaxone or beta interferons—to treat the early, inflammatory stage of the disease and possibly to delay later stages, Dr. Zamvil says. Another drug, Novantrone, is approved to treat symptoms related to later-stage neuron loss, he says.

The mouse findings support the results of a test-tube study of human blood samples published in the October 8, 2002, issue of *Neurology*,[2] which compared the effectiveness of three statin drugs to interferon beta proteins at reducing inflammation in human tissue samples. Dr. Zamvil says that because the two studies use different methods they are difficult to compare, but they both clearly show an anti-inflammatory effect of statins.

"Our study is a new stimulus for examining how statins might help patients in the early stages of MS and many other autoimmune diseases," says Dr. Zamvil. "But we'll have to wait for clinical trial results to see whether we can apply what we've learned to patients."

The researchers say their next step is to test the effectiveness of atorvastatin in patients with early stage MS.

References

1. Youssef S, Stuve O, Patarroyo JC, Ruiz PJ, Radosevich JL, Hur EM, Bravo M, Mitchell DJ, Sobel RA, Steinman L, Zamvil SS. "The HMG-CoA reductase inhibitor, atorvastatin, promotes a Th2 bias and reverses paralysis in central nervous system autoimmune disease." *Nature*, November 7, 2002; vol. 420, pp. 78–84.

2. Neuhaus O, Strasser-Fuchs S, Fazekas F, Kieseier BC, Niederweiser G, Hartung HP, Archelos JJ. "Statins as immunomodulators: Comparison with interferon-Beta1b in MS." *Neurology*, October 8, 2002; vol. 59, pp. 990–97.

Small Trial Shows Daclizumab Add-On Therapy Improves Multiple Sclerosis Outcome

A small clinical trial of patients with multiple sclerosis (MS) who did not respond to interferon alone found that adding the human antibody Daclizumab improved patient outcome. Patients who received the combined therapy had a 78 percent reduction in new brain lesions and a 70 percent reduction in total lesions, along with other significant clinical improvements. The trial was led by investigators at the National Institute of Neurological Disorders and Stroke (NINDS), a component of the National Institutes of Health. Findings will appear in the Early Edition of the *Proceedings of the National Academy of Sciences* the week of May 24–28, 2004.[1]

MS is a chronic disease marked by inflammation in the central nervous system and development of lesions in the brain. Messages from the brain to the body are interrupted as nerve fibers begin to lose their protective coating of myelin, resulting in muscle weakness, problems with vision and coordination, pain, and, in some patients, cognitive impairments. Approximately 250,000 to 350,000 people in the United States suffer from MS and about two hundred new cases are diagnosed by physicians each week. There is no cure for the disorder.

NINDS investigator Roland Martin, M.D., and colleagues studied eleven patients with either relapsing-remitting[2] or secondary progressive[3] MS. Each patient was treated with beta interferon—a naturally occurring antiviral protein commonly used to treat MS. Patients also received seven treatments of Daclizumab (a genetically engineered human antibody that blocks the interleukin-2 receptor on immune cells) administered intravenously at two-week, and later, four-week intervals.

Ten patients showed a dramatic reduction in both the severity and number of brain lesions as demonstrated by magnetic resonance imaging. The decrease in new lesions, as well as the total decrease in lesions, occurred gradually over a two-month span. Improvement was also seen on a neurological rating scale and in a test of hand function. The clinical improvement was unexpected in such a small trial, since a larger number of patients is usually required to show clinical effects. One patient with extremely high inflammation activity responded initially to Daclizumab but, as disease activity returned, was given higher doses of the antibody and was excluded from final analysis.

"There is great interest now in new approaches and new therapies for a disorder about which we know too little and have only moderately effective therapies," said Dr. Martin. "The combined therapy was well tolerated by all patients, with side effects that were either mild or clearly not caused by Daclizumab." He said the therapy limits the activity of T-cells that attack the myelin coating around the nerves, without shutting down the entire immune system.

"While these results are preliminary, this discovery offers hope for thousands of patients with certain forms of MS. Findings like this are helping us to better understand how this disease affects the immune system, which offers hope for all MS patients," said Story C. Landis, Ph.D., NINDS director.

Further studies are needed to confirm the extent of the clinical benefit of Daclizumab on typical MS patients and whether Daclizumab is similarly effective as a stand-alone therapy.

The study was a collaboration between the NINDS and its sister agency, the National Cancer Institute (NCI). Thomas Waldmann, M.D., chief of the metabolism branch for NCI's Center for Cancer Research, developed the antibody used in the trial.

Daclizumab (trade name Zenapax®) received FDA approval in 1997 for use in kidney transplantation.

The NINDS is a component of the National Institutes of Health within the Department of Health and Human Services and is the nation's primary supporter of biomedical research on the brain and nervous system.

References

1. Bielekova B, Richert N, Howard T, Blevins G, Markovic-Plese S, McCartin J, Wirfel J, Ohayon J, Waldmann TA, McFarland HF, and Martin R. "Humanized Anti-CD25 (Daclizumab) Inhibits Disease Activity in Multiple Sclerosis Patients Failing to Respond to Interferon-beta." *Proceedings of the National Academy of Sciences*, Vol. 101, Issue 23, pp. 8705–8.

2. A course of MS in which some patients experience a series of attacks followed by complete or partial remission of symptoms that return after a period of stability.

3. MS that may begin with a relapsing-remitting course, followed by gradual clinical decline with no distinct remissions.

Chapter 19

Parkinson Disease

Chapter Contents

Section 19.1—Parkinson Disease: An Overview 434
Section 19.2—Recent Research on Parkinson Disease 443

Section 19.1

Parkinson Disease: An Overview

What Is Parkinson Disease?

Parkinson disease belongs to a group of conditions called movement disorders. It is both chronic, meaning it persists over a long period of time, and progressive, meaning its symptoms grow worse over time.

Parkinson disease occurs when a group of cells, in an area of the brain called the substantia nigra, that produce a chemical called dopamine begin to malfunction and eventually die. Dopamine is a neurotransmitter, or chemical messenger, that transports signals to the parts of the brain that control movement initiation and coordination. When Parkinson disease occurs, for unexplained reasons, these cells begin to die at a faster rate and the amount of dopamine produced in the brain decreases. The four primary symptoms are:

- tremor of the hands, arms, legs, jaw, and face;
- rigidity or stiffness of the limbs and trunk;
- bradykinesia or slowness of movement; and
- postural instability or impaired balance and coordination.

As many as one million Americans suffer from Parkinson disease. While approximately 15 percent of Parkinson patients are diagnosed before the age of forty, incidence increases with age. The cause is unknown, and although there is presently no cure, there are many treatment options such as medication and surgery to manage the symptoms.

Common Symptoms

The symptoms vary from patient to patient and not everyone is affected by all of them. In some people, the disease progresses quickly;

in others it does not. The following are the most common primary symptoms of Parkinson disease.

- **Tremor:** In the early stages of the disease, about 70 percent of people experience a slight tremor in the hand or foot on one side of the body, or less commonly in the jaw or face. It appears as a "beating" or oscillating movement and is regular (four to six beats per second). Because tremor usually appears when the muscles are relaxed, it is called "resting tremor." This means that the affected body part trembles when it is at rest and not doing work and often subsides with action. The tremor often spreads to the other side of the body as the disease progresses, but remains most apparent on the original side of occurrence.

- **Rigidity:** Rigidity or increased muscle tone means stiffness or inflexibility of the muscles. Normally muscles contract when they move, and then relax when they are at rest. In rigidity, the muscle tone of an affected limb is stiff. Rigidity can result in a decreased range of motion. For example a patient may not swing his or her arms when walking. Rigidity can also cause pain and cramps at the muscle site.

- **Bradykinesia:** Bradykinesia is a slowing of voluntary movement. In addition to slow movements, a person with bradykinesia will likely also have incompleteness of movement, difficulty in initiating movements, and arrests of ongoing movement. Patients may begin to walk with short, shuffling steps (festination), which, combined with other symptoms such as loss of balance, increases the incidence of falls. They may also experience difficulty making turns or abrupt movements. They may go through periods of "freezing," which is when the patient is stuck and finds it difficult to stop or start walking. Bradykinesia and rigidity can occur in the facial muscles, causing a "mask-like" expression with little or no movement of the face. The slowness and incompleteness of movement can also affect speaking and swallowing.

There are many secondary symptoms of Parkinson disease. These include stooped posture, a tendency to lean forward or backward, and speech problems, such as softness of voice or slurred speech caused by lack of muscle control. Non-motor symptoms also impact the life of a person with Parkinson. A survey published in October 2003, "The Impact of Parkinson's Disease on Quality of Life," revealed that two of the top three most disabling symptoms for people with Parkinson are non-motor symptoms, including loss of energy and pain.

The following is a list of secondary symptoms of Parkinson disease:

- Speech changes
- Loss of facial expression
- Micrographia (small, cramped handwriting)
- Difficulty swallowing
- Drooling
- Pain
- Dementia or confusion
- Sleep disturbances
- Constipation
- Skin problems
- Depression
- Fear or anxiety
- Memory difficulties and slowed thinking
- Sexual dysfunction
- Urinary problems
- Fatigue and aching
- Loss of energy

What Causes Parkinson?

Why an individual develops Parkinson disease remains undetermined. The causes likely include both genetic and environmental factors. A variety of mechanisms that are believed to cause accelerated cell death have also been suggested, including oxidative stress, excitotoxicity and mitochondrial dysfunction. These are described in the following.

- **Genetics:** About 15 to 25 percent of Parkinson patients report having a relative with Parkinson. Researchers have found a defective gene in some rare families, with a high incidence of Parkinson disease. These rare cases have an inherited form of Parkinson disease. Scientists have discovered several "Parkinson genes" and there is conclusive evidence that genetics play a role in at least some patients. There appears to be a two- to threefold increased risk of PD in first-degree relatives compared to matched control populations. However, the majority of cases of PD still appear to be sporadic.

- **Environmental Factors:** Some scientists have suggested that Parkinson disease may occur when a toxin selectively destroys dopaminergic neurons. Scientists have known for a number of years of several toxins that can cause Parkinson-like symptoms, such as MPTP. Several studies have suggested a link between rural living, herbicide use, and exposure to pesticides as possible factors that may contribute to a person's developing Parkinson. Some people with Parkinson recall a time when they were exposed to chemicals, and believe this exposure may be a possible cause. Scientists are continuing to pursue these clues to establish more concrete linkages.

While the debate concerning environmental factors and genetics as causative factors in PD continues, there has been extensive investigation of the mechanisms involved in the cell death process. A number of cell death concepts have been put forward, including oxidative stress, mitochondrial dysfunction, and excitotoxicity.

- **Oxidative damage:** This theory suggests that free radicals— unstable molecules whose toxic effects are believed to be caused by oxidation—may contribute to cell death, thereby leading to Parkinson disease. Oxidation is thought to cause damage to tissues, including neurons. In addition, antioxidant defenses appear to be markedly reduced in PD brains. In particular, reduced levels of glutathione (an acid that plays a role in the detoxification of harmful compounds) have been discovered. The cause of the deficiency and the potential role that antioxidants like glutathione play in the development of PD remain unresolved.

- **Mitochondrial dysfunction:** The mitochondria are small bodies within cells that produce energy. They can be described as the "powerhouse" of the cell. Scientific findings indicate a reduction in the function of mitochondria, and this may play a role in PD.

- **Excitotoxicity:** This occurs when selected neurotransmitters in the brain get out of balance leading to cell death. This mechanism has been documented in Parkinson, and scientists believe that glutamate excitotoxicity is the main culprit within this mechanism. Finding a way to correct this imbalance may be neuroprotective.

Most experts in the field share the opinion that Parkinson disease is caused by a combination of genetic and environmental factors, and other contributing mechanisms of cell death.

Medications for Parkinson Disease

There are several symptomatic treatments for people with Parkinson, including medication, surgery, and physical therapy. The degree of success of each treatment varies among individuals, as does the length of time the treatment option remains effective.

Levodopa is a dopamine precursor, a substance that is converted into dopamine by an enzyme in the brain. The use of levodopa was a breakthrough in the treatment of PD. Unfortunately, patients experienced debilitating side effects, including severe nausea and vomiting. With increased dosing and prolonged use of levodopa, patients experienced other side effects, including dyskinesias (spontaneous, involuntary movements) and "on-off" periods when the medication would suddenly start or stop working.

Check with a doctor before taking any of the following to avoid possible interactions: antacids, anti-seizure drugs, anti-hypertensives, anti-depressants, and high-protein food.

Combining Levodopa with Carbidopa (Sinemet) represented a significant improvement in the treatment of Parkinson disease. The addition of carbidopa prevents levodopa from being metabolized in the gut, liver, and other tissues, and allows more of it to get to the brain. Therefore, a smaller dose of levodopa is needed to treat symptoms. In addition, the severe nausea and vomiting often associated with levodopa treatment was greatly reduced.

Consult a doctor before taking any medications to avoid possible interactions. In particular, antacids, anti-seizure drugs, anti-hypertensives, anti-depressants, and high-protein food may adversely affect the function of Levodopa and carbidopa.

Stalevo (carbidopa, levodopa, and entacapone) is a new (September 2003) combination tablet for patients who experience signs and symptoms of end-of-dose "wearing-off." The tablet combines carbidopa and levodopa (the most widely used agent for PD), with entacapone. While carbidopa reduces the side effects of levodopa, entacapone extends the time levodopa is active in the brain (up to 10 percent longer). The same drugs that interact with carbidopa, levodopa, and entacapone interact with Stalevo.

Symmetrel (amantadine hydrochloride) is thought to work in PD because it has several actions. It activates the release of dopamine from storage sites and possibly blocks the re-uptake of dopamine into nerve terminals. It also has a glutamate receptor blocking activity. Its dopaminergic actions result in its usefulness in reducing dyskinesia induced by levodopa. It is thus called an indirect-acting dopamine agonist, and is widely used as an early monotherapy (treatment of a condition by means of a single drug), with the more powerful Sinemet added when needed. Unfortunately, its benefit in more advanced PD is often short-lived, with patients reporting a fall-off effect.

Symmetrel may interact with Cogentin (benztropine), Disipal (orphenadrine), Sinemet (levodopa), Artane (trihexyphenidyl), amphetamines, and alcohol.

Anticholinergics (trihexyphenidyl, benztropine mesylate, procyclidine, etc.) do not act directly on the dopaminergic system. Instead they act to decrease the activity of another neurotransmitter, acetylcholine. There is a complex interaction between levels of acetylcholine in the brain and levels of dopamine. Many clinicians find that if an agonist or levodopa does not relieve tremor, then the addition of an anticholinergic drug is often effective. Adverse effects include blurred vision, dry mouth, and urinary retention. These drugs may be contraindicated in older patients since they can cause confusion and hallucination.

Check with a doctor before using anticholinergics with antihistamines, Haldol, Thorazine, Symmetrel, Clozaril, and alcohol.

Selegiline or deprenyl (Eldepryl) has been shown to delay the need for Sinemet when prescribed in the earliest stage of PD, and has also been approved for use in later stages to boost the effects of Sinemet. Eldepryl may interact with anti-depressants, narcotic painkillers, and decongestants. Check with a doctor before taking any new medications.

Dopamine agonists are drugs that activate dopamine receptors directly, and can be taken alone or in combination with Sinemet. Agonists available in the United States include bromocriptine (Parlodel), pergolide (Permax), pramipexole (Mirapex), and ropinirole (Requip).

Consult a doctor before taking any of the following to avoid possible interactions: alcohol, anti-psychotics, medications that lower blood pressure, Navane (thiothixene), Taractan (chlorprothixene), Haldol (haloperidol), Reglan (metoclopramide), phenothiazines, thioxanthenes, cimetidine, butyrophenones, Cipro, and benzodiazepines.

COMT [catecholamine-O-methyltransferase] inhibitors such as tolcapone (Tasmar) and entacapone (Comtan) represent a different class of Parkinson medications. These drugs must be taken with levodopa. They prolong the duration of symptom relief by blocking the action of an enzyme that breaks down levodopa.

Side Effects from Medications

Like the symptoms of PD themselves, the side effects caused by Parkinson medications vary from patient to patient. They may include dry mouth, nausea, dizziness, confusion, hallucinations, drowsiness, insomnia, and other unwelcome symptoms. Some patients experience no side effects from a drug, while others may have to discontinue its use because of them.

Surgical Treatment for Parkinson Disease

Surgery is an option for patients to explore after they have had experience with medications and are no longer satisfied with the results. A patient should discuss surgery thoroughly with his or her neurologist before making any decision.

Two older, and somewhat outdated, lesioning procedures that provide relief from Parkinson symptoms are pallidotomy and thalamotomy. Pallidotomy can alleviate rigidity and bradykinesia symptoms, and thalamotomy helps to control tremors. Doctors rarely perform either procedure because both permanently destroy parts of the brain and have serious side effects. The damage could make it impossible to perform surgeries that may become available in the future, such as brain tissue transplants.

Deep brain stimulation (DBS), a safer and more effective surgery, has replaced these methods. It is a preferred surgical option because it has the same, if not better, results than pallidotomy and thalamotomy. DBS also leaves open the possibility of other therapies, should they become available in the future. As with any surgical procedure, there are risks and side effects. The main benefit of DBS surgery is to reduce motor fluctuations such as the ups and downs caused by a decreasing effectiveness of Sinemet.

The electrode is usually placed on one side of the brain. The DBS electrode implanted in the left side of the brain will control the symptoms on the right side of the body and vice versa. In some cases, patients will need to have stimulators on both sides of the brain.

During surgery, a device is implanted to provide an electrical impulse to a part of the brain involved in motor function. This is often the subthalamic nucleus, in a deep part of the brain called the thalamus.

During the procedure, electrodes are inserted into the targeted brain region using MRI and neurophysiological mapping to ensure that they are implanted in the right place. The electrodes are connected to wires that lead to an impulse generator or IPG (similar to a pacemaker) that is placed under the collarbone and beneath the skin. Patients have a controller, which allows them to verify whether the DBS is on or off. They can use this device to check the battery and to turn the device on or off. An IPG battery lasts for about three to five years and is relatively easy to replace under local anesthesia.

Patients considering one or another surgical procedure should discuss the options first with their movement disorder specialists and then with their families or caregivers.

The Role of the Patient

Treating Parkinson disease is not exclusively the doctor's job; there is much the individual can do to stay as well as possible for as long as possible. Regular exercise, being part of a support group, maintaining a healthy diet, or taking part in a clinical trial are just some of the things you might consider.

Exercise

For people with Parkinson, regular exercise or physical therapy are essential for maintaining and improving mobility, flexibility, balance, and a range of motion, and for warding off many of the secondary symptoms mentioned previously. Exercise is as important as medication for the management of PD.

Support Groups

For many people, these groups play an important role in the emotional well-being of patients and families. They provide a caring environment for asking questions about PD, for laughing and crying and sharing stories and getting advice from other sufferers, and for forging friendships with people who understand each other's problems.

Diet

There is no specific diet to prevent or slow PD but there are several suggestions to help manage the disease. A vegetable-rich diet may aid digestion and prevent constipation. Parkinson patients should also take a balanced approach to protein intake because protein inhibits the absorption of levodopa in the gut. Avoiding high-protein meals when taking levodopa helps prevent this potential problem. However, a patient should not make dietary changes without discussing this first with his or her doctor. Parkinson disease nutrition author Kathrynne Holden offers several books, including *Eat Well, Stay Well* and *Cook Well, Stay Well,* that provide beneficial eating and cooking tips.

A Healthy Patient/Doctor Relationship

A neurologist can most effectively help a patient manage his or her PD if the neurologist and the patient have a good working relationship. Doctors need the patient to be honest, forthright, and inquisitive in order to give the best medical attention possible. Patients should also require that a doctor treat them in the same honest, open manner, engaging them in dialogue about the patient's experiences. Doctors can provide a wealth of information and suggestions for improving quality of life.

Physical, Speech, and Occupational Therapy

These therapies can help Parkinson patients control their symptoms and make daily life easier. Physical therapy may increase muscle strength and flexibility and decrease the incidence of falls. Speech therapy is available to increase voice volume and assist with word pronunciation. The Lee Silverman technique is a special speech therapy that can be very beneficial to people with PD.

Occupational therapy affords patients alternative methods of doing tasks that they can no longer perform with ease. These options may give patients a stronger sense of control when living with Parkinson disease, which seems to take control from them. The patient should ask a physician for recommendations if he or she does not provide them. These therapies may or may not be covered by insurance.

Clinical Trials

Getting involved in a clinical trial may be a way for a patient to feel empowered and help researchers understand more about Parkinson disease in order to improve treatment options for this disorder. Increased clinical trial participation will result in a better understanding of the disease and will also help treatments that are in the research and developmental phases reach patients more quickly. A patient should understand what the trial entails and be educated about the patient's responsibilities and obligations.

Section 19.2

Recent Research on Parkinson Disease

This section contains the following press releases from the National Institute of Neurological Disorders and Stroke: "Researchers Find Genetic
Links for Late-Onset Parkinson's Disease" (December 19, 2001); "Parkinsonian Symptoms Decrease in Rats Given Stem Cell Transplants" (January 9, 2002); "Study Finds Widespread Sympathetic Nerve Damage in
Parkinson's Disease" (April 22, 2002); "Embryonic Mouse Stem Cells Reduce Symptoms in Model for Parkinson's Disease" (June 20, 2002); "Study
Suggests Coenzyme Q10 Slows Functional Decline in Parkinson's Disease"
(October 14, 2002); "New Findings about Parkinson's Disease: Coffee and
Hormones Don't Mix" (April 17, 2003); and "Yeast Model Yields Insight
into Parkinson's Disease" (December 4, 2003).

Researchers Find Genetic Links for Late-Onset Parkinson Disease

Recent studies provide strong evidence that genetic factors influence susceptibility to the common, late-onset form of Parkinson disease (PD). The findings improve scientists' understanding of how PD
develops and may lead to new treatments or even ways of preventing
the disease.

Until 1996, few people believed there was a genetic component to
PD. The prevailing evidence suggested that environmental factors
were largely or entirely to blame. Since then, studies have identified a
clear genetic basis for two forms of PD that affect people younger than
fifty: one that affects a few families from Europe and another called
autosomal recessive juvenile parkinsonism (ARJP) that affects some
families in Japan. The first disorder is linked to a mutation in the gene
for a protein called alpha-synuclein, and the second is linked to mutations in the gene for a protein called parkin. However, the role of genetics in the common, late-onset form of PD has remained controversial. In
fact, several studies of twins have suggested that genes do not influence
this form of PD. The new studies challenge that earlier work and suggest that multiple genes play a role in susceptibility to the disease.

One of the recent studies,[1] led by Margaret A. Pericak-Vance, Ph.D.,
of the Center for Human Genetics at Duke University Medical Center

in Durham, North Carolina, and funded by the National Institute of Neurological Disorders and Stroke (NINDS), looked for a relationship between specific genetic markers and PD in 870 people from 174 families in which more than one person had been diagnosed with the disorder. They found evidence that five distinct regions, on chromosomes 5, 6, 8, 9, and 17, were associated with susceptibility to PD. The chromosome 6 region contains the parkin gene, which was previously associated only with early-onset PD. The familial link to chromosome 9 was found primarily in patients who do not respond to levodopa (a common treatment for PD) and the marker is located near a gene that is altered in another disorder called idiopathic torsion dystonia. This suggests that there may be a relationship between PD and dystonia. The strongest genetic association in families with late-onset PD was on chromosome 17, near the gene for a protein called tau. Tau is a component of neurofibrillary tangles, a specific brain abnormality found in other neurodegenerative diseases, including Alzheimer's disease, frontotemporal dementia with parkinsonism (FTDP), and progressive supranuclear palsy (PSP). Because people with PD do not have neurofibrillary tangles, researchers did not previously suspect tau as a factor in the disease. However, tau is important to normal cell function and it is possible that even minor abnormalities in how it works may lead to cell death, the researchers say.

A second NINDS-funded study,[2] led by Jeffrey M. Vance of Duke University, looked at specific variations within the tau gene and found evidence that three of the variations were linked to increased susceptibility for late-onset PD. A third study,[3] conducted by scientists at deCODE genetics, Inc., of Reykjavik, Iceland, looked at fifty-one Icelandic families with late-onset PD and linked the disease in these families to a region on chromosome 1.

Previous studies have suggested that other genes, including ubiquitin carboxy-terminal hydrolase (UCH-L1) and genes on chromosomes X, 1, 2, and 4, influence susceptibility to PD in some families. It also is possible that additional, still-unidentified genes may play a role in specific populations, the researchers say.

Knowledge of the genes that influence PD is potentially useful in a number of ways. For example, testing people for specific genes may help to identify subtypes of PD and lead to a better understanding of how to treat different groups of patients. "We could be talking about Parkinson's diseases—not just one disease," says William K. Scott, Ph.D., of Duke. Certain drugs and other treatments may be more or less effective in people with specific subtypes of PD.

The researchers stress that the genes linked to the late-onset form of PD are susceptibility genes—they do not cause the disorder all by themselves. Environmental factors probably interact with these genetic variations in ways that cause the disorder in some people.

While it is still unclear how the different genes may interact with the environment to cause PD, each identified factor represents an important piece in the puzzle, the researchers say. Parkinson disease is a complex disease, and each genetic factor could have many effects and interactions with other genes that may influence the development and symptoms of the disorder. "We've got the outside of the puzzle—now we need to fill in the middle," says Dr. Pericak-Vance. Researchers think the various genes and environmental factors that influence PD may all affect a single pathway, or series of biochemical interactions, that leads to the disease. Understanding the steps of the pathway should help researchers develop strategies to interrupt the process and lead to new treatments or even ways to prevent the devastating disease.

References

1. Scott WK, Nance MA, Watts RL, et. al. "Complete genomic screen in Parkinson disease: evidence for multiple genes." *Journal of the American Medical Association* 2001 Nov 14; 286(18): 2239–44.

2. Martin ER, Scott WK, Nance MA, et. al. "Association of single-nucleotide polymorphisms of the tau gene with late-onset Parkinson disease." *Journal of the American Medical Association* 2001 Nov 14; 286(18): 2245–50.

3. Hicks A, Petursson H, Jonsson T, et. al. "A susceptibility gene for late-onset idiopathic Parkinson's disease successfully mapped." *American Journal of Human Genetics* Oct 2001, 69, Abstract 123: 200 (Supplement).

Parkinsonian Symptoms Decrease in Rats Given Stem Cell Transplants

A new study shows that mouse embryonic stem cells transplanted into rats with brain damage resembling Parkinson disease spontaneously acquire many of the features of dopamine-producing neurons. Animals that received the transplants showed a gradual reduction in their parkinsonian symptoms, and brain scans revealed evidence that the transplanted cells integrated with the surrounding area and began to produce dopamine. The findings raise the possibility that embryonic stem cell transplants may one day be useful in treating Parkinson disease and other brain disorders.

Many of the symptoms of Parkinson disease result from the loss of neurons that produce dopamine, a nerve-signaling chemical. Previous studies have shown that embryonic stem cells can take on the characteristics of dopamine-producing neurons in culture. However, this is the first study to show that undifferentiated (unspecialized) embryonic stem cells transplanted into the brains of an animal model for Parkinson disease can develop into dopamine-producing cells with no special pretreatment to control their fate. The study was carried out by Dr. Ole Isacson of McLean Hospital and Harvard Medical School in Belmont, Massachusetts, and colleagues. It appears in the January 8, 2002, early edition of the *Proceedings of the National Academy of Sciences* and was supported by the National Institute of Neurological Disorders and Stroke (NINDS).

While the results of this study are intriguing, they also reveal the need for additional research. The transplanted cells did not survive in six of the twenty-five rats treated, and five of the animals developed tumors near the site of the transplants within the first nine weeks. These complications illustrate the importance of learning how to control the differentiation and proliferation of stem cells before planning similar therapies in humans. Researchers still need to learn how the stem cells develop into dopamine-producing cells and identify genes and chemical signals that control this process. This information should help researchers learn to control the cells in ways that improve their effectiveness and reduce the risk of tumors and other side effects.

Reference

Bjorklund LM, Sanchez-Pernaute R, and Chung S, et. al. "Embryonic stem cells develop into functional dopaminergic neurons after transplantation in a Parkinson rat model." *Proceedings of the National Academy of Sciences*, January 8, 2002, early edition.

Study Finds Widespread Sympathetic Nerve Damage in Parkinson Disease

For years, researchers have known that the symptoms of Parkinson disease (PD) result from damage to a specific region of the brain. A new study shows that the disease also causes widespread damage to the sympathetic nervous system, which controls blood pressure, pulse rate, perspiration, and many other automatic responses to stress. The findings help explain the blood pressure regulation problems commonly found in PD and may lead to new treatments for the disease.

Physicians have long known that patients with PD often have incontinence and other symptoms of autonomic nervous system function, and previous studies have found evidence of sympathetic nerve damage in PD patients' hearts. The sympathetic nervous system is one component of the autonomic nervous system. However, this study is the first to show that the disease affects sympathetic nerve endings in the thyroid gland and the kidney, says David S. Goldstein, M.D., Ph.D., of the National Institute of Neurological Disorders and Stroke in Bethesda, Maryland, who led the study. It also shows that this damage is unrelated to treatment with the most commonly used PD drug, levodopa. The study appears in the April 23, 2002, issue of *Neurology*.

Many people with PD develop a problem called orthostatic hypotension (OH), in which blood pressure falls suddenly when a person stands up. This condition can lead to dizziness, lightheadedness, and fainting. OH increases the risk of falls and other types of accidents, which can be disabling or even life-threatening. Patients with PD frequently have other symptoms of sympathetic nervous system failure, including intolerance to heat or cold and sexual dysfunction. However, the underlying cause of these problems has been unclear.

In the study, the researchers examined eighteen patients with PD and OH, twenty-three patients with PD only, and sixteen normal volunteers. The participants were given positron emission tomography (PET) scans of the heart, kidney, and several other organs using a chemical (fluorodopamine) that highlights sympathetic nerve endings. The researchers also measured levels of the sympathetic nerve signaling chemical norepinephrine in the blood coming from the heart and studied blood pressure responses to the Valsalva maneuver, a common test of sympathetic nervous system function in which patients blow into a tube against a resistance. The Valsalva maneuver causes a temporary decrease in the amount of blood pumped by the heart. People with a fully functioning sympathetic nervous system are able to compensate for the decrease in blood output by the heart because the brain responds by signaling the sympathetic nervous system to constrict the blood vessels. If the sympathetic nervous system is damaged, however, the blood vessels do not constrict and blood pressure progressively decreases.

The researchers found that all of the patients with PD and OH had abnormal blood pressure responses to the Valsalva maneuver and significant loss of sympathetic nerve endings in the left side of the heart. About 75 percent of the patients without OH also had lost sympathetic nerve endings in one or more areas of the heart, and six of the patients without OH had an abnormal Valsalva response. The abnormal blood pressure response to the Valsalva maneuver and loss of fluorodopamine-derived radioactivity in the heart were not seen in any age-matched normal volunteers. These findings suggest that most PD patients have at least some loss of sympathetic nerves, even if they do not develop OH, says Dr. Goldstein. In the patients who have OH, the loss of sympathetic nerves seems more widespread in the body.

The study also found that patients with PD had fewer sympathetic nerve endings in the thyroid and kidneys than the normal volunteers. PET scans of the PD patients showed normal numbers of nerve endings in the liver, spleen, and several other organs. However, patients with both PD and OH had lower norepinephrine levels in their blood than patients with PD alone, suggesting that they had a widespread loss of sympathetic nerve endings.

For years, neurologists have believed that OH in PD was due to treatment with the drug levodopa. However, several of the patients in this study who had OH had never taken levodopa, and blood levels of levodopa were the same in patients with and without OH. This shows that the development of OH is unrelated to treatment with levodopa, although it is possible that the levodopa may cause the blood vessel walls to dilate, making the OH worse, Dr. Goldstein says. Since significant loss of sympathetic nerve endings in the heart was found in all the patients with OH, the study suggests that OH in PD is due to the loss of these nerve endings.

"One implication of this finding is that if we can understand what causes the sympathetic nerve loss, we may be able to identify the cause of the entire disease," says Dr. Goldstein. Since norepinephrine and dopamine are part of the same family of chemicals, called catecholamines, the findings suggest that whatever causes the loss of dopamine-producing nerve fibers in the brain also causes the loss of sympathetic nerve endings in other parts of the body. The pattern of sympathetic nerve fiber loss in the heart suggests that these fibers gradually die back over time, Dr. Goldstein notes. However, more study is needed to determine what causes the fibers to die.

The NINDS is a component of the National Institutes of Health in Bethesda, Maryland, and is the nation's primary supporter of biomedical research on the brain and nervous system.

Reference

Goldstein DS, Holmes CS, Dendi R, Bruce SR, Li S-T. "Orthostatic Hypotension from Sympathetic Denervation in Parkinson's Disease." *Neurology*, April 23, 2002, Vol. 58, No. 8., pp. 1247–55.

Embryonic Mouse Stem Cells Reduce Symptoms in Model for Parkinson Disease

Embryonic mouse stem cells transformed into neurons in a lab dish and then transplanted into a rat model for Parkinson disease (PD) form functional connections and reduce disease symptoms, a new study shows. The finding suggests that embryonic stem (ES) cells may ultimately be useful for treating PD and other brain diseases.

The study is one of the first to show that ES cells can develop into neurons that function in the brain, according to senior author Ronald McKay, Ph.D., of the National Institute of Neurological Disorders and Stroke (NINDS).[1] The report appears in the June 20, 2002, advance online publication of *Nature*. A second study in *Nature*,[2] led by Catherine Verfaillie, M.D., at the University of Minnesota in Minneapolis, shows that bone marrow–derived cells called mesenchymal stem cells have many of the characteristics of ES cells.

Dr. McKay and his colleagues added a gene called Nurr1 to cultured mouse ES cells and exposed them to a series of growth factors that caused them to develop into neurons. Nurr1 helps neural precursor cells differentiate, or change, into neurons that produce the neurotransmitter dopamine. The loss of dopamine-producing neurons is a central feature of PD. To see if the ES cell-derived neurons would survive and function in animals, the researchers transplanted the neurons into rats that were missing the dopamine-producing cells on one side of their brains. These rats have parkinsonian symptoms on one side of their bodies. A similar group of rats received transplants of ES cells without the Nurr1 gene, and a third group received sham operations.

The researchers found that the grafted cells established functional connections with surrounding brain cells and began to release dopamine. The rats that received the Nurr1-positive cells showed significant improvements in symptoms during several behavioral tests. Rats that received cells without the Nurr1 gene showed some improvement in parkinsonian symptoms, but less than rats that received cells with the gene. Since undifferentiated ES cells sometimes multiply out of control and form tumors, the researchers measured the number of cells in the grafts at several time points after the transplants. The number of cells in the grafted areas appeared to stabilize by four weeks after the transplants, and none of the rats developed tumors.

"Dr. McKay's experiments further our understanding of the potential of stem cells to develop into differentiated neurons," says Audrey S. Penn, M.D., acting director of NINDS. "They provide proof of principle that we can start with embryonic stem cells and end up with dopamine neurons that are useful in a model for Parkinson's disease."

Previous studies have shown that neural precursor cells (which are more limited in their potential than ES cells) can grow into neurons that reduce symptoms when transplanted into an animal model of PD. However, neural precursor cells generate dopamine-producing neurons in culture for only short periods, while ES cells can proliferate extensively and may provide an unlimited source of dopamine neurons, Dr. McKay says.

In this study, Dr. McKay's group used a system that allowed them to manipulate the cells at every point until they were transplanted. "Every step of the way is controlled—we are not just putting cells into the brain," says Dr. McKay. The ability to isolate cells with specific properties for transplantation is an important part of their result, he adds. "We now know that we can start with ES cells and end with dopamine neurons. We do not know if we can make dopamine neurons by starting with any other cell type," he says. "It's as if, leaving New York, you have instructions to drive to Washington that will get you there in four and a half hours. It's possible that if you start in Chicago or Minneapolis you might get to Washington, but if you don't have instructions from that location you don't know how long it will take. We have developed the instructions that get us from ES cells to dopamine neurons."

While the results suggest that ES cell-derived neurons may be useful for treating PD and other neurological diseases, they are still preliminary, Dr. McKay says. Researchers need much more information about how the cells interact with the host brain and about their safety before similar strategies can be tested in humans. He and his colleagues are planning studies to address these questions.

The NINDS is a component of the National Institutes of Health in Bethesda, Maryland, and is the nation's primary supporter of biomedical research on the brain and nervous system.

References

1. Kim JH, Auerbach JM, Rodriguez-Gomez JA, Velasco I, Gavin D, Lumelsky N, Lee S-H, Nguyen J, Sanchez-Pernaute R, Bankiewicz K, McKay R. "Dopamine neurons derived from

embryonic stem cells function in an animal model of Parkinson's disease." *Nature*, advance online publication, June 20, 2002, DOI: 10.1038/nature00900.

2. Jiang Y, Balkrishna NJ, Reinhardt RL, Schwartz RE, Keene CD, Ortiz-Gonzalez XR, Reyes M, Lenvik T, Lund T, Blackstad M, Du J, Aldrich S, Lisberg A, Low WC, Largaespada DA, Verfaillie CM. "Pluripotency of mesenchymal stem cells derived from adult bone marrow." *Nature*, advance online publication, June 20, 2002, DOI: 10.1038/nature00870.

Study Suggests Coenzyme Q10 Slows Functional Decline in Parkinson Disease

Results of the first placebo-controlled, multicenter clinical trial of the compound coenzyme Q10 suggest that it can slow disease progression in patients with early-stage Parkinson disease (PD). While the results must be confirmed in a larger study, they provide hope that this compound may ultimately provide a new way of treating PD.

The phase II study, led by Clifford Shults, M.D., of the University of California, San Diego (UCSD) School of Medicine, looked at a total of eighty PD patients at ten centers across the country to determine if coenzyme Q10 is safe and if it can slow the rate of functional decline. The study was funded by the National Institute of Neurological Disorders and Stroke (NINDS) and appears in the October 15, 2002, issue of the *Archives of Neurology*.[1]

"This trial suggested that coenzyme Q10 can slow the rate of deterioration in Parkinson's disease," says Dr. Shults. "However, before the compound is used widely, the results need to be confirmed in a larger group of patients."

PD is a chronic, progressive neurological disease that affects about five hundred thousand people in the United States. It results from the loss of brain cells that produce the neurotransmitter dopamine and causes tremor, stiffness of the limbs and trunk, impaired balance and coordination, and slowing of movements. Patients also sometimes develop other symptoms, including difficulty swallowing, disturbed sleep, and emotional problems. PD usually affects people over the age of fifty, but it can affect younger people as well. While levodopa and other drugs can ease the symptoms of PD, none of the current treatments has been shown to slow the course of the disease.

The investigators believe coenzyme Q10 works by improving the function of mitochondria, the "powerhouses" that produce energy in cells. Coenzyme Q10 is an important link in the chain of chemical reactions that produces this energy. It also is a potent antioxidant—a chemical that "mops up" potentially harmful chemicals generated during normal metabolism. Previous studies carried out by Dr. Shults, Richard Haas, M.D., of UCSD, and Flint Beal, M.D., of Cornell University have shown that coenzyme Q10 levels in mitochondria from PD patients are reduced and that mitochondrial function in these patients is impaired. Animal studies have shown that coenzyme Q10 can protect the area of the brain that is damaged in PD. Dr. Shults and colleagues also conducted a pilot study with PD patients that showed that consumption of up to 800 mg/day of coenzyme Q10 was well tolerated and significantly increased the level of coenzyme Q10 in the blood.

All of the patients who took part in the new study had the three primary features of PD—tremor, stiffness, and slowed movements—and had been diagnosed with the disease within five years of the time they were enrolled. After an initial screening and baseline blood tests, the patients were randomly divided into four groups. Three of the groups received coenzyme Q10 at three different doses (300 mg/day, 600 mg/day, and 1,200 mg/day), along with vitamin E, while a fourth group received a matching placebo that contained vitamin E alone. Each participant received a clinical evaluation one month later and every four months for a total of sixteen months or until the investigator determined that the patient needed treatment with levodopa. None of the participants or the study investigators knew which treatment each patient had received until the study ended.

The investigators found that most side effects of coenzyme Q10 were mild, and none of the patients required a reduction of their dose. The percentage of people receiving coenzyme Q10 who reported side effects was not significantly different from that of the placebo group. During the study period, the group that received the largest dose of coenzyme Q10 (1,200 mg/day) had 44 percent less decline in mental function, motor (movement) function, and ability to carry out activities of daily living, such as feeding or dressing themselves. The greatest effect was on activities of daily living. The groups that received 300 mg/day and 600 mg/day developed slightly less disability than the placebo group, but the effects were less than those in the group that received the highest dosage of coenzyme Q10.

The groups that received coenzyme Q10 also had significant increases in the level of coenzyme Q10 in their blood and a significant increase in energy-producing reactions within their mitochondria.

The results of this study suggest that doses of coenzyme Q10 as high as 1,200 mg/day are safe and may be more effective than lower doses, says Dr. Shults. The findings are consistent with those of a recently published study of patients with early Huntington disease—another degenerative neurological disorder—that showed slightly less functional decline in groups that received 600 mg/day of coenzyme Q10.

The new study also used an efficient phase II clinical trial design—developed by biostatistician David Oakes, Ph.D., of the University of Rochester, and other study investigators—which should be useful for testing other drugs that might slow the progression of PD, says Dr. Shults. The design allowed the researchers to study the effects of three doses plus a placebo in less than three years, and to obtain useful data about the compound's effectiveness.

Dr. Shults and his colleagues strongly caution patients against taking coenzyme Q10 until a larger, definitive trial can be conducted. Because coenzyme Q10 is classified as a dietary supplement, it is not regulated by the U.S. Food and Drug Administration. The versions of the supplement sold in stores may differ, they may not contain potentially beneficial amounts of the compound, and taking coenzyme Q10 over a number of years may be costly, says Dr. Shults. In addition, the current study included only a small number of patients, and the findings may not extend to people in later stages of PD or to those who are at risk but have not been diagnosed with the disorder, he notes. Finally, if many people begin taking coenzyme Q10 because of these early results, it might make it impossible for investigators to find enough patients to carry out definitive studies of the compound's effectiveness and the proper dosages, since patients must not be taking any treatments in order to be considered for enrollment in a definitive trial.

The investigators are now planning a larger clinical trial that will examine the effects of 1,200 mg/day of coenzyme Q10, and possibly a higher dose as well, in a larger number of patients.

The NINDS is a component of the National Institutes of Health in Bethesda, Maryland, and is the nation's primary supporter of biomedical research on the brain and nervous system.

Reference

1. Shults CW, Oakes D, Kieburtz K, Beal F, Haas R, Plumb S, Juncos JL, Nutt J, Shoulson I, Carter J, Kompoliti K, Perlmutter JS, Reich S, Stern M, Watts RL, Kurlan R, Molho E, Harrison M, Lew M, and the Parkinson Study Group. "Effects of coenzyme Q10 in early Parkinson disease: evidence of

slowing of the functional decline." *Archives of Neurology*, October 2002, Vol. 59, No. 10, pp. 1541–50.

New Findings about Parkinson Disease: Coffee and Hormones Don't Mix

Several large studies have shown that caffeine intake is associated with a reduced risk of developing Parkinson disease (PD) in men, but studies in women have been inconclusive. A new study shows that hormone therapy is a possible explanation for the different effects of caffeine on PD risk in men and women.

"We hoped to find something that would explain the effect of caffeine on PD risk in men and the lack of an effect in women," says lead author Alberto Ascherio, M.D., Dr.P.H., of the Harvard School of Public Health. "Hormones seemed like a possible factor in this case."

Ascherio and his colleagues found combining coffee and hormones significantly increases women's risk of developing PD, even though each factor alone has previously been found to protect against PD. The study shows that postmenopausal women who took hormone replacement therapy (HRT) and drank more than five cups of coffee per day (heavy coffee drinkers) were one and a half times more likely to develop PD than heavy coffee drinkers who didn't take HRT.

Taking coffee out of the equation, HRT seemed to have a protective effect against PD; these results support those of earlier studies. Women who drank little or no coffee and took HRT had 65 percent less risk of developing PD than light coffee drinkers who didn't take HRT. The study was funded in part by the National Institute of Neurological Disorders and Stroke and appears in the March 11, 2003, issue of *Neurology*.[1]

The researchers studied survey data from more than seventy-seven thousand nurses who participated in the Nurses' Health Study, a comprehensive twenty-year study designed to take a closer look at women's health.[2] One hundred fifty-four women in this group were diagnosed with PD during the study. Overall, there was no difference in disease incidence between women who were and weren't using HRT. However, when caffeine consumption was factored in, HRT made a big difference in PD risk.

Among women taking HRT, the increased risk of PD was confined to women who drank more than five cups of coffee per day. Drinking small amounts of coffee per day did not appear to affect the risk of PD in these women. Women who did not take hormones who drank less than half a cup of coffee per day had a PD risk similar to that of men, Dr. Ascherio says.

The type of hormones and the duration of use did not seem to affect outcomes. The researchers note that they controlled for possible effects of cigarette smoking, which has repeatedly been shown to be associated with a decreased risk of PD.

Dr. Ascherio says these results could explain the inconsistencies researchers have seen in the caffeine-PD association in women. He says it also lends further credibility to the argument that caffeine may have a protective effect against PD. "Now we know that when you take hormones out of the equation, caffeine has the same effect on women as it does in men," says Dr. Ascherio. "To me, this is very compelling."

While this study may help researchers build a more solid case for caffeine's relationship with PD, women should not read too much into it. "Women should not change their habits or stop taking hormones because of this study," Dr. Ascherio says. "We need more studies so we can take a closer look at the relationship and mechanisms involved."

Researchers say that while caffeine is clearly associated with PD in some way, they lack convincing evidence that caffeine actually prevents the disease. "Association does not equal causality," says co-author Michael Schwarzschild, M.D., Ph.D., of Harvard Medical School and Massachusetts General Hospital.

The mechanism by which caffeine affects PD remains a riddle. In animal models, researchers have shown that caffeine can prevent the loss of dopamine-producing nerve cells seen in PD, but researchers still don't know how this occurs. Dr. Schwarzschild says the protective effect could be related to caffeine's ability to block a particular receptor in the brain. How such a blockade might protect nerve cells remains unknown, he adds.

The effect of estrogen on the relationship between caffeine and PD is even harder to explain. "There are several possible explanations, all of which need to be tested," says Dr. Schwarzschild. Estrogen is known to have neuroprotective effects in PD, so there is a chance that estrogen and caffeine are competing and therefore canceling out each other's effect, he says. Another theory is that estrogen could in some way interfere with how caffeine is broken down in the body. To begin testing these theories, researchers are now studying whether the protective effects of caffeine differ in male and female animal models.

Dr. Ascherio stresses the need to confirm the findings of this study in larger prospective studies of PD in women.

Many other researchers continue to probe the complex differences in PD risk between men and women. In a recent study appearing in the March 2003 issue of the journal *Movement Disorders*,[3] researchers at the Mayo Clinic in Rochester, Minnesota, found that environmental factors may play a greater role in the development of PD in men than in women, and that genetic factors may have a greater influence on the disease in women than in men.

The researchers suggest that more men, especially of older generations, have been exposed in the workforce to environmental factors, such as pesticides, industrial chemicals, and head injuries. On the other hand, they found that women require a stronger genetic susceptibility to develop PD. The researchers also affirmed previous findings that estrogen reduces the risk of developing PD. The Mayo Clinic study was also funded in part by NINDS.

References

1. Ascherio A, Chen H, Schwarzschild MA, Zhang SM, Colditz GA, Speizer FE. "Caffeine, postmenopausal estrogen, and risk of Parkinson's disease," *Neurology*, March 11, 2003, pp. 790–95.

2. Colditz GA, Manson JE, Hankinson SE. "The Nurses' Health Study: 20-year contribution to the understanding of health among women," *Journal of Women's Health*, 1997; vol. 6, pp. 49–62.

3. Maraganore D, de Andrade M, Lesnick TG, Farrer MJ, Bower JH, Hardy JA, Rocca WA. "Complex interactions in Parkinson's disease: A two-phased approach." *Movement Disorders*, April 2003; vol. 18, Issue 4; online early view at http://www3.interscience.wiley.com/cgi-bin/fulltext/104084206/FILE?TPL=ftx_start.

Yeast Model Yields Insight into Parkinson Disease

Scientists who developed the first yeast model of Parkinson disease (PD) have been able to describe the mechanisms of an important gene's role in the disease. Tiago Fleming Outeiro, Ph.D., and Susan Lindquist, Ph.D., of the Whitehead Institute for Biomedical Research in Cambridge, Massachusetts, studied the gene's actions under normal conditions and under abnormal conditions to learn how and when the gene's product, alpha-synuclein, becomes harmful to surrounding cells. The scientists created a yeast model that expresses the alpha-synuclein gene, which has been implicated in PD. Yeast models are often used in the study of genetic diseases because they offer researchers a simple system that allows them to clarify how genes work.

The National Institute of Neurological Disorders and Stroke, part of the National Institutes of Health, funded the study, which appears in the December 5, 2003, issue of *Science*.

The alpha-synuclein protein, which is found broadly in the brain, has been implicated in several neurodegenerative disorders. Sometimes a mutation or a misfolding of the protein causes the problems; other times there are too many copies of the normal gene. A study earlier this year reported that patients with a rare familial form of PD had too many normal copies of the alpha-synuclein gene, which resulted in a buildup of protein inside brain cells, causing the symptoms of PD.

Drs. Outeiro and Lindquist conducted their study by creating one yeast that expresses wild type synuclein, using the normal gene, and another yeast that expresses two mutant forms, using a mutated version of the gene found in patients with PD.

One theory for the cause of PD is that an aging brain no longer has the capacity to cope with accumulating or misfolding proteins. A normal healthy brain has the ability to clear out excess or mutant proteins through a process known as the quality control system. In the yeast model of PD, when the scientists doubled the expression of the alpha-synuclein gene it "profoundly changed" the fate of the yeast's quality control system, and alpha-synuclein appeared in large clumps of cells (inclusion bodies). This did not happen when they studied the actions of a single copy of the wild type synuclein. These inclusion bodies have a toxic effect that causes cell death and neurodegeneration.

"Just a twofold difference in expression was sufficient to cause a catastrophic change in behavior," the scientists report in their paper.

"These changes may give insight into important changes that happen when alpha-synuclein is overexpressed in Parkinson's patients," said Diane Murphy, Ph.D., a program director at the NINDS. "Dr. Lindquist is well known for her studies of yeast models of prion disease, and we are delighted she has extended her research to the important field of Parkinson's disease."

PD is the second most common neurodegenerative disease after Alzheimer's disease and is thought to affect five hundred thousand Americans.

Reference

Outeiro, TF, and Lindquist, S, "Yeast Cells Provide Insight into Alpha-Synuclein Biology and Pathobiology," *Science*, Vol. 302, pp. 1772–75.

Part Five

Other Brain Disorders

Chapter 20

Cerebral Palsy

Introduction

In the 1860s, an English surgeon named William Little wrote the first medical descriptions of a puzzling disorder that struck children in the first years of life, causing stiff, spastic muscles in their legs and, to a lesser degree, their arms. These children had difficulty grasping objects, crawling, and walking. They did not get better as they grew up nor did they become worse. Their condition, which was called Little's disease for many years, is now known as spastic diplegia. It is just one of several disorders that affect control of movement and are grouped together under the term cerebral palsy.

Because it seemed that many of these children were born following premature or complicated deliveries, Little suggested their condition resulted from a lack of oxygen during birth. This oxygen shortage damaged sensitive brain tissues controlling movement, he proposed. Yet in 1897 the famous psychiatrist Sigmund Freud disagreed. Noting that children with cerebral palsy often had other problems such as mental retardation, visual disturbances, and seizures, Freud suggested that the disorder might sometimes have roots earlier in life, during the brain's development in the womb. "Difficult birth, in certain cases," he wrote, "is merely a symptom of deeper effects that influence the development of the fetus."

Excerpted from "Cerebral Palsy: Hope through Research," National Institute of Neurological Disorders and Stroke, National Institutes of Health, NIH Publication Number 93-159, updated October 2004.

461

Despite Freud's observation, the belief that birth complications cause most cases of cerebral palsy was widespread among physicians, families, and even medical researchers until very recently. In the 1980s, however, scientists analyzed extensive data from a government study of more than thirty-five thousand births and were surprised to discover that such complications account for only a fraction of cases—probably less than 10 percent. In most cases of cerebral palsy, no cause of the factors explored could be found. These findings from the National Institute of Neurological Disorders and Stroke (NINSD) perinatal study have profoundly altered medical theories about cerebral palsy and have spurred today's researchers to explore alternative causes.

At the same time, biomedical research has also led to significant changes in understanding, diagnosing, and treating persons with cerebral palsy. Risk factors not previously recognized have been identified, notably intrauterine exposure to infection and disorders of coagulation, and others are under investigation. Identification of infants with cerebral palsy very early in life gives youngsters the best opportunity to receive treatment for sensory disabilities and for prevention of contractures. Biomedical research has led to improved diagnostic techniques such as advanced brain imaging and modern gait analysis. Certain conditions known to cause cerebral palsy, such as rubella (German measles) and jaundice, can now be prevented or treated. Physical, psychological, and behavioral therapy that assist with such skills as movement and speech and foster social and emotional development can help children who have cerebral palsy to achieve and succeed. Medications, surgery, and braces can often improve nerve and muscle coordination, help treat associated medical problems, and either prevent or correct deformities.

Much of the research to improve medical understanding of cerebral palsy has been supported by NINDS, one of the federal government's National Institutes of Health. The NINDS is America's leading supporter of biomedical research into cerebral palsy and other neurological disorders. Through this chapter, the NINDS hopes to help the more than 4,500 American babies and infants diagnosed each year, their families, and others concerned about cerebral palsy benefit from these research results.

What Is Cerebral Palsy?

Cerebral palsy is an umbrella-like term used to describe a group of chronic disorders impairing control of movement that appear in the first few years of life and generally do not worsen over time. The term cerebral refers to the brain's two halves, or hemispheres, and palsy describes any disorder that impairs control of body movement. Thus, these disorders are not caused by problems in the muscles or nerves. Instead, faulty development or damage to motor areas in the brain disrupts the brain's ability to adequately control movement and posture.

Symptoms of cerebral palsy lie along a spectrum of varying severity. An individual with cerebral palsy may have difficulty with fine motor tasks, such as writing or cutting with scissors; experience trouble with maintaining balance and walking; or be affected by involuntary movements, such as uncontrollable writhing motion of the hands or drooling. The symptoms differ from one person to the next, and may even change over time in the individual. Some people with cerebral palsy are also affected by other medical disorders, including seizures or mental impairment. Contrary to common belief, however, cerebral palsy does not always cause profound handicap. While a child with severe cerebral palsy might be unable to walk and need extensive, lifelong care, a child with mild cerebral palsy might only be slightly awkward and require no special assistance. Cerebral palsy is not contagious nor is it usually inherited from one generation to the next. At this time it cannot be cured, although scientific research continues to yield improved treatments and methods of prevention.

How Many People Have This Disorder?

The United Cerebral Palsy Associations estimate that more than five hundred thousand Americans have cerebral palsy. Despite advances in preventing and treating certain causes of cerebral palsy, the number of children and adults it affects has remained essentially unchanged or perhaps risen slightly over the past thirty years. This is partly because more critically premature and frail infants are surviving through improved intensive care. Unfortunately, many of these infants have developmental problems of the nervous system or suffer neurological damage. Research is under way to improve care for these infants, as in ongoing studies of technology to alleviate troubled breathing and trials of drugs to prevent bleeding in the brain before or soon after birth.

What Are the Different Forms?

Spastic diplegia, the disorder first described by Dr. Little in the 1860s, is only one of several disorders called cerebral palsy. Today doctors classify cerebral palsy into four broad categories—spastic, athetoid, ataxic, and mixed forms—according to the type of movement disturbance.

Spastic Cerebral Palsy

In this form of cerebral palsy, which affects 70 to 80 percent of patients, the muscles are stiffly and permanently contracted. Doctors will often describe which type of spastic cerebral palsy a patient has based on which limbs are affected. The names given to these types combine a Latin description of affected limbs with the term plegia or paresis, meaning paralyzed or weak.

When both legs are affected by spasticity, they may turn in and cross at the knees. As these individuals walk, their legs move awkwardly and stiffly and nearly touch at the knees. This causes a characteristic walking rhythm, known as the scissors gait.

Individuals with spastic hemiparesis may also experience hemiparetic tremors, in which uncontrollable shaking affects the limbs on one side of the body. If these tremors are severe, they can seriously impair movement.

Athetoid, or Dyskinetic, Cerebral Palsy

This form of cerebral palsy is characterized by uncontrolled, slow, writhing movements. These abnormal movements usually affect the hands, feet, arms, or legs, and, in some cases, the muscles of the face and tongue, causing grimacing or drooling. The movements often increase during periods of emotional stress and disappear during sleep. Patients may also have problems coordinating the muscle movements needed for speech, a condition known as dysarthria. Athetoid cerebral palsy affects about 10 to 20 percent of patients.

Ataxic Cerebral Palsy

This rare form affects the sense of balance and depth perception. Affected persons often have poor coordination; walk unsteadily with a wide-based gait, placing their feet unusually far apart; and experience difficulty when attempting quick or precise movements, such as writing or buttoning a shirt. They may also have intention tremor. In this form of tremor, beginning a voluntary movement, such as reaching for a book, causes a trembling that affects the body part being used and that worsens as the individual gets nearer to the desired object.

The ataxic form affects an estimated 5 to 10 percent of cerebral palsy patients.

Mixed Forms

It is common for patients to have symptoms of more than one of the previous three forms. The most common mixed form includes spasticity and athetoid movements, but other combinations are also possible.

What Other Medical Disorders Are Associated with Cerebral Palsy?

Many individuals who have cerebral palsy have no associated medical disorders. However, disorders that involve the brain and impair its motor function can also cause seizures and impair an individual's intellectual development, attentiveness to the outside world, activity and behavior, and vision and hearing. Medical disorders associated with cerebral palsy include:

- **Mental impairment:** About one-third of children who have cerebral palsy are mildly intellectually impaired, one-third are moderately or severely impaired, and the remaining third are intellectually normal. Mental impairment is even more common among children with spastic quadriplegia.

- **Seizures or epilepsy:** As many as half of all children with cerebral palsy have seizures. During a seizure, the normal, orderly pattern of electrical activity in the brain is disrupted by uncontrolled bursts of electricity. When seizures recur without a direct trigger, such as fever, the condition is called epilepsy. In the person who has cerebral palsy and epilepsy, this disruption may be spread throughout the brain and cause varied symptoms all over the body—as in tonic-clonic seizures—or may be confined to just one part of the brain and cause more specific symptoms—as in partial seizures. Tonic-clonic seizures generally cause patients to cry out and are followed by loss of consciousness, twitching of both legs and arms, convulsive body movements, and loss of bladder control. Partial seizures are classified as simple or complex. In simple partial seizures, the individual has localized symptoms, such as muscle twitches, chewing movements, and numbness or tingling. In complex partial seizures, the individual may hallucinate, stagger, perform automatic and purposeless movements, or experience impaired consciousness or confusion.

- **Growth problems:** A syndrome called failure to thrive is common in children with moderate-to-severe cerebral palsy, especially those with spastic quadriparesis. Failure to thrive is a general term physicians use to describe children who seem to lag behind in growth and development despite having enough food. In babies, this lag usually takes the form of too little weight gain; in young children, it can appear as abnormal shortness; in teenagers, it may appear as a combination of shortness and lack of sexual development. Failure to thrive probably has several causes, including, in particular, poor nutrition and damage to the brain centers controlling growth and development. In addition, the muscles and limbs affected by cerebral palsy tend to be smaller than normal. This is especially noticeable in some patients with spastic hemiplegia, because limbs on the affected side of the body may not grow as quickly or as large as those on the more normal side. This condition usually affects the hand and foot most severely. Since the involved foot in hemiplegia is often smaller than the unaffected foot even among patients who walk, this size difference is probably not due to lack of use. Scientists believe the problem is more likely to result from disruption of the complex process responsible for normal body growth.

- **Impaired vision or hearing:** A large number of children with cerebral palsy have strabismus, a condition in which the eyes are not aligned because of differences in the left and right eye muscles. In an adult, this condition causes double vision. In children, however, the brain often adapts to the condition by ignoring signals from one of the misaligned eyes. Untreated, this can lead to very poor vision in one eye and can interfere with certain visual skills, such as judging distance. In some cases, physicians may recommend surgery to correct strabismus. Children with hemiparesis may have hemianopia, which is defective vision or blindness that impairs the normal field of vision of one eye. For example, when hemianopia affects the right eye, a child looking straight ahead might have perfect vision except on the far right. In homonymous hemianopia, the impairment affects the same part of the visual field of both eyes. Impaired hearing is also more frequent among those with cerebral palsy than in the general population.

- **Abnormal sensation and perception:** Some children with cerebral palsy have impaired ability to feel simple sensations like touch and pain. They may also have stereognosia, or difficulty perceiving and identifying objects using the sense of touch. A child with stereognosia, for example, would have trouble identifying a hard ball, sponge, or other object placed in his hand without looking at the object.

What Causes Cerebral Palsy?

Cerebral palsy is not one disease with a single cause, like chicken pox or measles. It is a group of disorders with similar problems in control of movement, but probably with different causes. When physicians try to uncover the cause of cerebral palsy in an individual child, they look at the form of cerebral palsy, the mother's and child's medical history, and onset of the disorder.

In the United States, about 10 to 20 percent of children who have cerebral palsy acquire the disorder after birth. (The figures are higher in underdeveloped countries.) Acquired cerebral palsy results from brain damage in the first few months or years of life and can follow brain infections, such as bacterial meningitis or viral encephalitis, or results from head injury—most often from a motor vehicle accident, a fall, or child abuse.

Congenital cerebral palsy, on the other hand, is present at birth, although it may not be detected for months. In most cases, the cause of congenital cerebral palsy is unknown. Thanks to research, however, scientists have pinpointed some specific events during pregnancy or around the time of birth that can damage motor centers in the developing brain. Some of these causes of congenital cerebral palsy include:

- **Infections during pregnancy:** German measles, or rubella, is caused by a virus that can infect pregnant women and, therefore, the fetus in the uterus, and cause damage to the developing nervous system. Other infections that can cause brain injury in the developing fetus include cytomegalovirus and toxoplasmosis. There is relatively recent evidence that placental and perhaps other maternal infection can be associated with cerebral palsy.

- **Jaundice in the infant:** Bile pigments, compounds that are normally found in small amounts in the bloodstream, are produced when blood cells are destroyed. When many blood cells are destroyed in a short time, as in the condition called Rh incompatibility, the yellow-colored pigments can build up and cause jaundice. Severe, untreated jaundice can damage brain cells.

- **Rh incompatibility:** In this blood condition, the mother's body produces immune cells called antibodies that destroy the fetus's blood cells, leading to a form of jaundice in the newborn.

- **Severe oxygen shortage in the brain or trauma to the head during labor and delivery:** The newborn infant's blood is specially equipped to compensate for low levels of oxygen, and asphyxia (lack of oxygen caused by interruption in breathing or poor oxygen supply) is common in babies during the stresses of labor and delivery. Yet if asphyxia severely lowers the supply of oxygen to the infant's brain for lengthy periods, the child may develop brain damage called hypoxic-ischemic encephalopathy. A significant proportion of babies with this type of brain damage die, and others may develop cerebral palsy, which is then often accompanied by mental impairment and seizures. In the past, physicians and scientists attributed most cases of cerebral palsy to asphyxia or other complications during birth if they could not identify another cause. However, extensive research by NINDS scientists and others has shown that very few babies who experience asphyxia during birth develop encephalopathy soon after birth. Research also shows that a large proportion of babies who experience asphyxia do not grow up to have cerebral palsy or other neurological disorders. Birth complications including asphyxia are now estimated to account for about 6 percent of congenital cerebral palsy cases.

- **Stroke:** Coagulation disorders in mothers or infants can produce stroke in the fetus or newborn baby. Bleeding in the brain has several causes—including broken blood vessels in the brain, clogged blood vessels, or abnormal blood cells—and is one form of stroke. Although strokes are better known for their effects on older adults, they can also occur in the fetus during pregnancy or the newborn around the time of birth, damaging brain tissue and causing neurological problems. Ongoing research is testing potential treatments that may one day help prevent stroke in fetuses and newborns.

What Are the Risk Factors?

Research scientists have examined thousands of expectant mothers, followed them through childbirth, and monitored their children's early neurological development. As a result, they have uncovered certain characteristics, called risk factors, that increase the possibility that a child will later be diagnosed with cerebral palsy:

- **Breech presentation:** Babies with cerebral palsy are more likely to present feet first, instead of head first, at the beginning of labor.

- **Complicated labor and delivery:** Vascular or respiratory problems of the baby during labor and delivery may sometimes be the first sign that a baby has suffered brain damage or that a baby's brain has not developed normally. Such complications can cause permanent brain damage.

- **Low Apgar score:** The Apgar score (named for anesthesiologist Virginia Apgar) is a numbered rating that reflects a newborn's condition. To determine an Apgar score, doctors periodically check the baby's heart rate, breathing, muscle tone, reflexes, and skin color in the first minutes after birth. They then assign points; the higher the score, the more normal the baby's condition. A low score at ten to twenty minutes after delivery is often considered an important sign of potential problems.

- **Low birth weight and premature birth:** The risk of cerebral palsy is higher among babies who weigh less than 2500 grams (5 lbs., 7 ½ oz.) at birth and among babies who are born less than thirty-seven weeks into pregnancy. This risk increases as birth weight falls.

- **Multiple births:** Twins, triplets, and other multiple births are linked to an increased risk of cerebral palsy.

- **Nervous system malformations:** Some babies born with cerebral palsy have visible signs of nervous system malformation, such as an abnormally small head (microcephaly). This suggests that problems occurred in the development of the nervous system while the baby was in the womb.

- **Maternal bleeding or severe proteinuria late in pregnancy:** Vaginal bleeding during the sixth to ninth months of pregnancy and severe proteinuria (the presence of excess proteins in the urine) are linked to a higher risk of having a baby with cerebral palsy.

- **Maternal hyperthyroidism, mental retardation, or seizures:** Mothers with any of these conditions are slightly more likely to have a child with cerebral palsy.

- **Seizures in the newborn:** An infant who has seizures faces a higher risk of being diagnosed, later in childhood, with cerebral palsy.

Knowing these warning signs helps doctors keep a close eye on children who face a higher risk for long-term problems in the nervous system. However, parents should not become too alarmed if their child has one or more of these factors. Most such children do not have and do not develop cerebral palsy.

Can Cerebral Palsy Be Prevented?

Several of the causes of cerebral palsy that have been identified through research are preventable or treatable:

- Head injury can be prevented by regular use of child safety seats when driving in a car and helmets during bicycle rides, and elimination of child abuse. In addition, common sense measures around the household—like close supervision during bathing and keeping poisons out of reach—can reduce the risk of accidental injury.

- Jaundice of newborn infants can be treated with phototherapy. In phototherapy, babies are exposed to special blue lights that break down bile pigments, preventing them from building up and threatening the brain. In the few cases in which this treatment is not enough, physicians can correct the condition with a special form of blood transfusion.

- Rh incompatibility is easily identified by a simple blood test routinely performed on expectant mothers and, if indicated, expectant fathers. This incompatibility in blood types does not usually cause problems during a woman's first pregnancy, since the mother's body generally does not produce the unwanted antibodies until after delivery. In most cases, a special serum given after each childbirth can prevent the unwanted production of antibodies. In unusual cases, such as when a pregnant woman develops the antibodies during her first pregnancy or antibody production is not prevented, doctors can help minimize problems by closely watching the developing baby and, when needed, performing a transfusion to the baby while in the womb or an exchange transfusion (in which a large volume of the baby's blood is removed and replaced) after birth.

- Rubella, or German measles, can be prevented if women are vaccinated against this disease before becoming pregnant.

In addition, it is always good to work toward a healthy pregnancy through regular prenatal care and good nutrition and by eliminating smoking, alcohol consumption, and drug abuse. Despite the best efforts of parents and physicians, however, children will still be born with cerebral palsy. Since in most cases the cause of cerebral palsy is unknown, little can currently be done to prevent it. As investigators learn more about the causes of cerebral palsy through basic and clinical research, doctors and parents will be better equipped to help prevent this disorder.

What Are the Early Signs?

Early signs of cerebral palsy usually appear before three years of age, and parents are often the first to suspect that their infant is not developing motor skills normally. Infants with cerebral palsy are frequently slow to reach developmental milestones, such as learning to roll over, sit, crawl, smile, or walk. This is sometimes called developmental delay.

Some affected children have abnormal muscle tone. Decreased muscle tone is called hypotonia; the baby may seem flaccid and relaxed, even floppy. Increased muscle tone is called hypertonia, and the baby may seem stiff or rigid. In some cases, the baby has an early period of hypotonia that progresses to hypertonia after the first two to three months of life. Affected children may also have unusual posture or favor one side of their body.

Parents who are concerned about their baby's development for any reason should contact their physician, who can help distinguish normal variation in development from a developmental disorder.

How Is Cerebral Palsy Diagnosed?

Doctors diagnose cerebral palsy by testing an infant's motor skills and looking carefully at the infant's medical history. In addition to checking for those symptoms described previously—slow development, abnormal muscle tone, and unusual posture—a physician also tests the infant's reflexes and looks for early development of hand preference.

Reflexes are movements that the body makes automatically in response to a specific cue. For example, if a newborn baby is held on its back and tilted so the legs are above its head, the baby will automatically extend its arms in a gesture, called the Moro reflex, that looks like an embrace. Babies normally lose this reflex after they reach six months, but those with cerebral palsy may retain it for abnormally long periods. This is just one of several reflexes that a physician can check.

Doctors can also look for hand preference—a tendency to use either the right or left hand more often. When the doctor holds an object in front and to the side of the infant, an infant with hand preference will use the favored hand to reach for the object, even when it is held closer to the opposite hand. During the first twelve months of life, babies do not usually show hand preference. However infants with spastic hemiplegia, in particular, may develop a preference much earlier, since the hand on the unaffected side of their body is stronger and more useful.

The next step in diagnosing cerebral palsy is to rule out other disorders that can cause movement problems. Most important, doctors must determine that the child's condition is not getting worse. Although its symptoms may change over time, cerebral palsy by definition is not progressive. If a child is continuously losing motor skills, the problem more likely springs from elsewhere—including genetic diseases, muscle diseases, disorders of metabolism, or tumors in the nervous system. The child's medical history, special diagnostic tests, and, in some cases, repeated check-ups can help confirm that other disorders are not at fault.

The doctor may also order specialized tests to learn more about the possible cause of cerebral palsy. One such test is computed tomography, or CT, a sophisticated imaging technique that uses x-rays and a computer to create an anatomical picture of the brain's tissues and structures. A CT scan may reveal brain areas that are underdeveloped, abnormal cysts (sacs that are often filled with liquid) in the brain, or other physical problems. With the information from CT scans, doctors may be better equipped to judge the long-term outlook for an affected child.

Magnetic resonance imaging, or MRI, is a relatively new brain imaging technique that is rapidly gaining widespread use for identifying brain disorders. This technique uses a magnetic field and radio waves, rather than x-rays. MRI gives better pictures of structures or abnormal areas located near bone than CT does.

A third test that can expose problems in brain tissues is ultrasonography. This technique bounces sound waves off the brain and uses the pattern of echoes to form a picture, or sonogram, of its structures.

Ultrasonography can be used in infants before the bones of the skull harden and close. Although it is less precise than CT and MRI scanning, this technique can detect cysts and structures in the brain, is less expensive, and does not require long periods of immobility.

Finally, physicians may want to look for other conditions that are linked to cerebral palsy, including seizure disorders, mental impairment, and vision or hearing problems.

When the doctor suspects a seizure disorder, an electroencephalogram, or EEG, may be ordered. An EEG uses special patches called electrodes placed on the scalp to record the natural electrical currents inside the brain. This recording can help the doctor see telltale patterns in the brain's electrical activity that suggest a seizure disorder.

Intelligence tests are often used to determine if a child with cerebral palsy is mentally impaired. Sometimes, however, a child's intelligence may be underestimated because problems with movement, sensation, or speech due to cerebral palsy make it difficult for him or her to perform well on these tests.

If problems with vision are suspected, the doctor may refer the patient to an ophthalmologist for examination; if hearing impairment seems likely, an otologist may be called in.

Identifying these accompanying conditions is important and is becoming more accurate as ongoing research yields advances that make diagnosis easier. Many of these conditions can then be addressed through specific treatments, improving the long-term outlook for those with cerebral palsy.

How Is Cerebral Palsy Managed?

Cerebral palsy cannot be cured, but treatment can often improve a child's capabilities. In fact, progress due to medical research now means that many patients can enjoy near-normal lives if their neurological problems are properly managed. There is no standard therapy that works for all patients. Instead, the physician must work with a team of health care professionals first to identify a child's unique needs and impairments and then to create an individual treatment plan that addresses them.

Some approaches that can be included in this plan are drugs to control seizures and muscle spasms, special braces to compensate for muscle imbalance, surgery, mechanical aids to help overcome impairments, counseling for emotional and psychological needs, and physical, occupational, speech, and behavioral therapy. In general, the earlier treatment begins, the better chance a child has of overcoming developmental disabilities or learning new ways to accomplish difficult tasks.

The members of the treatment team for a child with cerebral palsy should be knowledgeable professionals with a wide range of specialties. A typical treatment team might include:

- a physician, such as a pediatrician, a pediatric neurologist, or a pediatric physiatrist, trained to help developmentally disabled children. This physician, often the leader of the treatment team, works to synthesize the professional advice of all team members into a comprehensive treatment plan, implements treatments, and follows the patient's progress over a number of years.

- an orthopedist, a surgeon who specializes in treating the bones, muscles, tendons, and other parts of the body's skeletal system. An orthopedist might be called on to predict, diagnose, or treat muscle problems associated with cerebral palsy.

- a physical therapist, who designs and implements special exercise programs to improve movement and strength.

- an occupational therapist, who can help patients learn skills for day-to-day living, school, and work.

- a speech and language pathologist, who specializes in diagnosing and treating communication problems.

- a social worker, who can help patients and their families locate community assistance and education programs.

- a psychologist, who helps patients and their families cope with the special stresses and demands of cerebral palsy. In some cases, psychologists may also oversee therapy to modify unhelpful or destructive behaviors or habits.

- an educator, who may play an especially important role when mental impairment or learning disabilities present a challenge to education.

Individuals who have cerebral palsy and their family or caregivers are also key members of the treatment team, and they should be intimately involved in all steps of planning, making decisions, and applying treatments. Studies have shown that family support and personal determination are two of the most important predictors of which individuals who have cerebral palsy will achieve long-term goals.

Too often, however, physicians and parents may focus primarily on an individual symptom—especially the inability to walk. While mastering specific skills is an important focus of treatment on a day-to-day basis, the ultimate goal is to help individuals grow to adulthood and have maximum independence in society. In the words of one physician, "After all, the real point of walking is to get from point A to point B. Even if a child needs a wheelchair, what's important is that they're able to achieve this goal."

What Specific Treatments Are Available?

Physical, Behavioral, and Other Therapies

Therapy—whether for movement, speech, or practical tasks—is a cornerstone of cerebral palsy treatment. The skills a two-year-old needs to explore the world are very different from those that a child needs in the classroom or a young adult needs to become independent. Cerebral palsy therapy should be tailored to reflect these changing demands.

Physical therapy usually begins in the first few years of life, soon after the diagnosis is made. Physical therapy programs use specific sets of exercises to work toward two important goals: preventing the weakening or deterioration of muscles that can follow lack of use (called disuse atrophy) and avoiding contracture, in which muscles become fixed in a rigid, abnormal position.

Contracture is one of the most common and serious complications of cerebral palsy. Normally, a child whose bones are growing stretches the body's muscles and tendons through running and walking and other daily activities. This ensures that muscles will grow at the same rate. Yet in children with cerebral palsy, spasticity prevents this stretching and, as a result, muscles do not grow fast enough to keep up with lengthening bones. The resulting contracture can disrupt balance and trigger loss of previous abilities. Physical therapy alone, or in combination with special braces (sometimes called orthotic devices), works to prevent this complication by stretching spastic muscles. For example, if a child has spastic hamstrings (tendons located behind the knee), the therapist and parents should encourage the child to sit with the legs extended to stretch them.

A third goal of some physical therapy programs is to improve the child's motor development. A widespread program of physical therapy that works toward this goal is the Bobath technique, named for a husband and wife team who pioneered this approach in England. This program is based on the idea that the primitive reflexes retained by many children with cerebral palsy present major roadblocks to learning voluntary control. A therapist using the Bobath technique tries to counteract these reflexes by positioning the child in an opposing movement. So, for example, if a child with cerebral palsy normally keeps his arm flexed, the therapist would repeatedly extend it.

A second such approach to physical therapy is "patterning," which is based on the principle that motor skills should be taught in more or less the same sequence that they develop normally. In this controversial approach, the therapist guides the child with movement problems along the path of normal motor development. For example, the child is first taught elementary movements like pulling himself to a standing position and crawling before he is taught to walk—regardless of his age. Some experts and organizations, including the American Academy of Pediatrics, have expressed strong reservations about the patterning approach, because studies have not documented its value.

Physical therapy is usually just one element of an infant development program that also includes efforts to provide a varied and stimulating environment. Like all children, the child with cerebral palsy needs new experiences and interactions with the world around him or her in order to learn. Stimulation programs can bring this valuable experience to the child who is physically unable to explore.

As the child with cerebral palsy approaches school age, the emphasis of therapy shifts away from early motor development. Efforts now focus on preparing the child for the classroom, helping the child master activities of daily living, and maximizing the child's ability to communicate.

Physical therapy can now help the child with cerebral palsy prepare for the classroom by improving his or her ability to sit, move independently or in a wheelchair, or perform precise tasks, such as writing. In occupational therapy, the therapist works with the child to develop such skills as feeding, dressing, or using the bathroom. This can help reduce demands on caregivers and boost self-reliance and self-esteem. For the many children who have difficulty communicating, speech therapy works to identify specific difficulties and overcome them through a program of exercises. For example, if a child has difficulty saying words that begin with "b," the therapist may suggest daily practice with a list of "b" words, increasing their difficulty as each list is mastered. Speech therapy can also work to help the child learn to use special communication devices, such as a computer with voice synthesizers.

Behavioral therapy provides yet another avenue to increase a child's abilities. This therapy, which uses psychological theory and techniques, can complement physical, speech, or occupational therapy. For example, behavioral therapy might include hiding a toy inside a box to reward a child for learning to reach into the box with his weaker hand. Likewise, a child learning to say his "b" words might be given a balloon for mastering the word. In other cases, therapists may try to discourage unhelpful or destructive behaviors, such as hair pulling or biting, by selectively presenting a child with rewards and praise during other, more positive activities.

As a child with cerebral palsy grows older, the need for and types of therapy and other support services will continue to change. Continuing physical therapy addresses movement problems and is supplemented by vocational training, recreation and leisure programs, and special education when necessary. Counseling for emotional and psychological challenges may be needed at any age, but is often most critical during adolescence. Depending on their physical and intellectual abilities, adults may need attendant care, living accommodations, transportation, or employment opportunities.

Regardless of the patient's age and which forms of therapy are used, treatment does not end when the patient leaves the office or treatment center. In fact, most of the work is often done at home. The therapist functions as a coach, providing parents and patients with the strategy and drills that can help improve performance at home, at school, and in the world. As research continues, doctors and parents can expect new forms of therapy and better information about which forms of therapy are most effective for individuals with cerebral palsy.

Drug Therapy

Physicians usually prescribe drugs for those who have seizures associated with cerebral palsy, and these medications are very effective in preventing seizures in many patients. In general, the drugs given to individual patients are chosen based on the type of seizures, since no one drug controls all types. However, different people with the same type of seizure may do better on different drugs, and some individuals may need a combination of two or more drugs to achieve good seizure control.

Drugs are also sometimes used to control spasticity, particularly following surgery. The three medications that are used most often are diazepam, which acts as a general relaxant of the brain and body;

baclofen, which blocks signals sent from the spinal cord to contract the muscles; and dantrolene, which interferes with the process of muscle contraction. Given by mouth, these drugs can reduce spasticity for short periods, but their value for long-term control of spasticity has not been clearly demonstrated. They may also trigger significant side effects, such as drowsiness, and their long-term effects on the developing nervous system are largely unknown. One possible solution to avoid such side effects may lie in current research to explore new routes for delivering these drugs.

Patients with athetoid cerebral palsy may sometimes be given drugs that help reduce abnormal movements. Most often, the prescribed drug belongs to a group of chemicals called anticholinergics that work by reducing the activity of acetylcholine. Acetylcholine is a chemical messenger that helps some brain cells communicate and that triggers muscle contraction. Anticholinergic drugs include trihexyphenidyl, benztropine, and procyclidine hydrochloride.

Occasionally, physicians may use alcohol "washes"—or injections of alcohol into a muscle—to reduce spasticity for a short period. This technique is most often used when physicians want to correct a developing contracture. Injecting alcohol into a muscle that is too short weakens the muscle for several weeks and gives physicians time to work on lengthening the muscle through bracing, therapy, or casts. In some cases, if the contracture is detected early enough, this technique may avert the need for surgery.

Surgery

Surgery is often recommended when contractures are severe enough to cause movement problems. In the operating room, surgeons can lengthen muscles and tendons that are proportionately too short. First, however, they must determine the exact muscles at fault, since lengthening the wrong muscle could make the problem worse.

Finding problem muscles that need correction can be a difficult task. To walk two strides with a normal gait, it takes more than thirty major muscles working at exactly the right time and exactly the right force. A problem in any one muscle can cause abnormal gait. Furthermore, the natural adjustments the body makes to compensate for muscle problems can be misleading. A new tool that enables doctors to spot gait abnormalities, pinpoint problem muscles, and separate real problems from compensation is called gait analysis. Gait analysis combines cameras that record the patient while walking, computers that analyze each portion of the patient's gait, force plates that detect when feet touch the ground, and a special recording technique that detects muscle activity (known as electromyography). Using these data, doctors are better equipped to intervene and correct significant problems. They can also use gait analysis to check surgical results.

Because lengthening a muscle makes it weaker, surgery for contractures is usually followed by months of recovery. For this reason, doctors try to fix all of the affected muscles at once when it is possible or, if more than one surgical procedure is unavoidable, they may try to schedule operations close together.

A second surgical technique, known as selective dorsal root rhizotomy, aims to reduce spasticity in the legs by reducing the amount of stimulation that reaches leg muscles via nerves. In the procedure, doctors try to locate and selectively sever overactivated nerves controlling leg muscles. Although there is scientific controversy over how selective this technique actually is, recent research results suggest it can reduce spasticity in some patients, particularly those who have spastic diplegia. Ongoing research is evaluating this surgery's effectiveness.

Experimental surgical techniques include chronic cerebellar stimulation and stereotaxic thalamotomy. In chronic cerebellar stimulation, electrodes are implanted on the surface of the cerebellum—the part of the brain responsible for coordinating movement—and are used to stimulate certain cerebellar nerves. While it was hoped that this technique would decrease spasticity and improve motor function, results of this invasive procedure have been mixed. Some studies have reported improvements in spasticity and function, while others have not.

Stereotaxic thalamotomy involves precise cutting of parts of the thalamus, which serves as the brain's relay station for messages from the muscles and sensory organs. This has been shown effective only for reducing hemiparetic tremors.

Mechanical Aids

Whether they are as humble as Velcro shoes or as advanced as computerized communication devices, special machines and gadgets in the home, school, and workplace can help the child or adult with cerebral palsy overcome limitations.

The computer is probably the most dramatic example of a new device that can make a difference in the lives of those with cerebral palsy. For example, a child who is unable to speak or write but can make head movements may be able to learn to control a computer using a special light pointer that attaches to a headband. Equipped with a computer and voice synthesizer, this child could communicate with others. In other cases, technology has led to new versions of old devices, such as the traditional wheelchair and its modern offspring that runs on electricity.

Many such devices are products of engineering research supported by private foundations and other groups.

What Other Major Problems Are Associated with Cerebral Palsy?

Poor control of the muscles of the throat, mouth, and tongue sometimes leads to drooling. Drooling can cause severe skin irritation and, because it is socially unacceptable, can lead to further isolation of affected children from their peers. Although numerous treatments for drooling have been tested over the years, there is no one treatment that always helps. Drugs called anticholinergics can reduce the flow of saliva but may cause significant side effects, such as mouth dryness and poor digestion. Surgery, while sometimes effective, carries the risk of complications, including worsening of swallowing problems. Some patients benefit from a technique called biofeedback that can tell them when they are drooling or having difficulty controlling muscles that close the mouth. This kind of therapy is most likely to work if the patient has a mental age of more than two or three years, is motivated to control drooling, and understands that drooling is not socially acceptable.

Difficulty with eating and swallowing—also triggered by motor problems in the mouth—can cause poor nutrition. Poor nutrition, in turn, may make the individual more vulnerable to infections and cause or aggravate "failure to thrive"—a lag in growth and development that is common among those with cerebral palsy. To make swallowing easier, the caregiver may want to prepare semisolid food, such as strained vegetables and fruits. Proper position, such as sitting up while eating or drinking and extending the individual's neck away from the body to reduce the risk of choking, is also helpful. In severe cases of swallowing problems and malnutrition, physicians may recommend tube feeding, in which a tube delivers food and nutrients down the throat and into the stomach, or gastrostomy, in which a surgical opening allows a tube to be placed directly into the stomach.

A common complication is incontinence, caused by faulty control over the muscles that keep the bladder closed. Incontinence can take the form of bed-wetting (also known as enuresis), uncontrolled urination during physical activities (or stress incontinence), or slow leaking of urine from the bladder. Possible medical treatments for incontinence include special exercises, biofeedback, prescription drugs, surgery, or surgically implanted devices to replace or aid muscles. Specially designed undergarments are also available.

What Research Is Being Done?

Investigators from many arenas of medicine and health are using their expertise to help improve treatment and prevention of cerebral palsy. Much of their work is supported through the National Institute of Neurological Disorders and Stroke (NINDS), the National Institute of Child Health and Human Development, other agencies within the federal government, nonprofit groups such as the United Cerebral Palsy Research Foundation, and private institutions.

The ultimate hope for overcoming cerebral palsy lies with prevention. In order to prevent cerebral palsy, however, scientists must first understand the complex process of normal brain development and what can make this process go awry.

Between early pregnancy and the first months of life, one cell divides to form first a handful of cells, and then hundreds, millions, and, eventually, billions of cells. Some of these cells specialize to become brain cells. These brain cells specialize into different types and migrate to their appropriate site in the brain. They send out branches to form crucial connections with other brain cells. Ultimately, the most complex entity known to us is created: a human brain with its billions of interconnected neurons.

Mounting evidence is pointing investigators toward this intricate process in the womb for clues about cerebral palsy. For example, a group of researchers has recently observed that more than one-third of children who have cerebral palsy also have missing enamel on certain teeth. This tooth defect can be traced to problems in the early months of fetal development, suggesting that a disruption at this period in development might be linked both to this tooth defect and to cerebral palsy.

As a result of this and other research, many scientists now believe that a significant number of children develop cerebral palsy because of mishaps early in brain development. They are examining how brain cells specialize, how they know where to migrate, and how they form the right connections—and they are looking for preventable factors that can disrupt this process before or after birth.

Scientists are also scrutinizing other events—such as bleeding in the brain, seizures, and breathing and circulation problems—that

481

threaten the brain of the newborn baby. Through this research, they hope to learn how these hazards can damage the newborn's brain and to develop new methods for prevention.

Some newborn infants, for example, have life-threatening problems with breathing and blood circulation. A recently introduced treatment to help these infants is extracorporeal membrane oxygenation, in which blood is routed from the patient to a special machine that takes over the lungs' task of removing carbon dioxide and adding oxygen. Although this technique can dramatically help many such infants, some scientists have observed that a substantial fraction of treated children later experience long-term neurological problems, including developmental delay and cerebral palsy. Investigators are studying infants through pregnancy, delivery, birth, and infancy, and are tracking those who undergo this treatment. By observing them at all stages of development, scientists can learn whether their problems developed before birth, result from the same breathing problems that made them candidates for the treatment, or spring from errors in the treatment itself. Once this is determined, they may be able to correct any existing problems or develop new treatment methods to prevent brain damage.

Other scientists are exploring how brain insults like hypoxic-ischemic encephalopathy (brain damage from a shortage of oxygen or blood flow), bleeding in the brain, and seizures can cause the abnormal release of brain chemicals and trigger brain damage. For example, research has shown that bleeding in the brain unleashes dangerously high amounts of a brain chemical called glutamate. While glutamate is normally used in the brain for communication, too much glutamate overstimulates the brain's cells and causes a cycle of destruction. Scientists are now looking closely at glutamate to detect how its release harms brain tissue and spreads the damage from stroke. By learning how brain chemicals that normally help us function can hurt the brain, scientists may be equipped to develop new drugs that block their harmful effects.

In related research, some investigators are already conducting studies to learn if certain drugs can help prevent neonatal stroke. Several of these drugs seem promising because they appear to reduce the excess production of potentially dangerous chemicals in the brain and may help control brain blood flow and volume. Earlier research has linked sudden changes in blood flow and volume to stroke in the newborn.

Low birth weight itself is also the subject of extensive research. In spite of improvements in health care for some pregnant women, the incidence of low birth-weight babies born each year in the United States remains at about 7 ½ percent. Some scientists currently investigating this serious health problem are working to understand how infections, hormonal problems, and genetic factors may increase a woman's chances of giving birth prematurely. They are also conducting more applied research that could yield: (1) new drugs that can safely delay labor, (2) new devices to further improve medical care for premature infants, and (3) new insight into how smoking and alcohol consumption can disrupt fetal development.

While this research offers hope for preventing cerebral palsy in the future, ongoing research to improve treatment brightens the outlook for those who must face the challenges of cerebral palsy today. An important thrust of such research is the evaluation of treatments already in use so that physicians and parents have the information they need to choose the best therapy. A good example of this effort is an ongoing NINDS-supported study that promises to yield new information about which patients are most likely to benefit from selective dorsal root rhizotomy, a recently introduced surgery that is becoming increasingly in demand for reduction of spasticity.

Similarly, although physical therapy programs are a popular and widespread approach to managing cerebral palsy, little scientific evidence exists to help physicians, other health professionals, and parents determine how well physical therapy works or to choose the best approach among many. Current research on cerebral palsy aims to provide this information through careful studies that compare the abilities of children who have had physical and other therapy with those who have not.

As part of this effort, scientists are working to create new measures to judge the effectiveness of treatment, as in ongoing research to precisely identify the specific brain areas responsible for movement. Using magnetic pulses, researchers can locate brain areas that control specific actions, such as raising an arm or lifting a leg, and construct detailed maps. By comparing charts made before and after therapy among children who have cerebral palsy, researchers may gain new insights into how therapy affects the brain's organization, and new data about its effectiveness.

Investigators are also working to develop new drugs—and new ways of using existing drugs—to help relieve cerebral palsy's symptoms. In one such set of studies, early research results suggest that doctors may improve the effectiveness of the anti-spasticity drug called baclofen by giving the drug through spinal injections, rather than by mouth. In addition, scientists are also exploring the use of tiny implanted pumps that deliver a constant supply of anti-spasticity drugs into the fluid around the spinal cord, in the hope of improving these drugs' effectiveness and reducing side effects, such as drowsiness.

Other experimental drug development efforts are exploring the use of minute amounts of the familiar toxin called botulinum. Ingested in large amounts, this toxin is responsible for botulism poisoning, in which the body's muscles become paralyzed. Injected in tiny amounts, however, this toxin has shown early promise in reducing spasticity in specific muscles.

A large research effort is also directed at producing more effective, nontoxic drugs to control seizures. Through its Antiepileptic Drug Development Program, the NINDS screens new compounds developed by industrial and university laboratories around the world for toxicity and anticonvulsant activity and coordinates clinical studies of efficacy and safety. To date, this program has screened more than thirteen thousand compounds and, as a result, five new antiepileptic drugs—carbamazepine, clonazepam, valproate, clorazepate, and felbamate—have been approved for marketing. A new project within the program is exploring how the structure of a given anti-seizure medication relates to its effectiveness. If successful, this project may enable scientists to design better anti-seizure medications more quickly and cheaply.

As researchers continue to explore new treatments for cerebral palsy and to expand our knowledge of brain development, we can expect significant medical advances to prevent cerebral palsy and many other disorders that strike in early life.

Research Update: June 2000

Research conducted and supported by the National Institute of Neurological Disorders and Stroke (NINDS) continuously seeks to uncover new clues about cerebral palsy (CP). Investigators from the NINDS and the California Birth Defects Monitoring Program (CBDMP) presented data suggesting that very low birth weight babies have a decreased incidence of CP when their mothers are treated with magnesium sulfate soon before giving birth. The results of this study, which were based on observations of a group of children born in four northern California counties, were published in the February 1995 issue of *Pediatrics*.[1]

Low birth weight babies are one hundred times more likely to develop CP than normal birth weight infants. If further research confirms the study's findings, use of magnesium sulfate may prevent 25 percent of the cases of CP in the approximately fifty-two thousand low birth weight babies born each year in the United States.

Magnesium is a natural compound that is responsible for numerous chemical processes within the body and brain. Obstetricians in the United States often administer magnesium sulfate, an inexpensive form of the compound, to pregnant women to prevent preterm labor and high blood pressure brought on by pregnancy. The drug, administered intravenously in the hospital, is considered safe when given under medical supervision.

Scientists speculate that magnesium may play a role in brain development and possibly prevent bleeding inside the brains of preterm infants. Previous research has shown that magnesium may protect against brain bleeding in very premature infants. Animal studies have demonstrated that magnesium given after a traumatic brain injury can reduce the severity of brain damage.

Despite these encouraging research findings, pregnant women should not change their magnesium intake because the effects of high doses have not yet been studied and the possible risks and benefits are not known.

Researchers caution that more research will be required to establish a definitive relationship between the drug and prevention of the disorder. Clinical trials now under way, one of them a collaboration between the NINDS and the National Institute of Child Health and Human Development, are evaluating magnesium for the prevention of cerebral palsy in prematurely born babies.

Reference

1. Nelson KB, and Grether JK. Can magnesium sulfate reduce the risk of cerebral palsy in very low birthweight infants? *Pediatrics*, February 1995, vol. 95, no. 2, page 263.

Chapter 21

Headache

For two years, Jim suffered the excruciating pain of cluster headaches. Night after night he paced the floor, the pain driving him to constant motion. He was only forty-eight years old when the clusters forced him to quit his job as a systems analyst. One year later, his headaches are controlled. The credit for Jim's recovery belongs to the medical staff of a headache clinic. Physicians there applied the latest research findings on headache, and prescribed for Jim a combination of new drugs.

Joan was a victim of frequent migraine. Her headaches lasted two days. Nauseous and weak, she stayed in the dark until each attack was over. Today, although migraine still interferes with her life, she has fewer attacks and less severe headaches than before. A specialist prescribed an antimigraine program for Joan that included improved drug therapy, a new diet, and relaxation training.

An avid reader, Peggy couldn't put down the new mystery thriller. After four hours of reading slumped in bed, she knew she had overdone it. Her tensed head and neck muscles felt as if they were being squeezed between two giant hands. For Peggy, however, the muscle-contraction headache and neck pain were soon relieved by a hot shower and aspirin.

Understanding why headaches occur and improving headache treatment are among the research goals of the National Institute of

Excerpted from "Headache: Hope through Research," National Institute of Neurological Disorders and Stroke, National Institutes of Health, NIH Publication Number 02-158, updated November 2004.

Neurological Disorders and Stroke (NINDS). As the leading supporter of brain research in the federal government, the NINDS also supports and conducts studies to improve the diagnosis of headaches and to find ways to prevent them.

Why does it hurt?

What hurts when you have a headache? The bones of the skull and tissues of the brain itself never hurt, because they lack pain-sensitive nerve fibers. Several areas of the head can hurt, including a network of nerves that extends over the scalp and certain nerves in the face, mouth, and throat. Also sensitive to pain, because they contain delicate nerve fibers, are the muscles of the head and blood vessels found along the surface and at the base of the brain.

The ends of these pain-sensitive nerves, called nociceptors, can be stimulated by stress, muscular tension, dilated blood vessels, and other triggers of headache. Once stimulated, a nociceptor sends a message up the length of the nerve fiber to the nerve cells in the brain, signaling that a part of the body hurts. The message is determined by the location of the nociceptor. A person who suddenly realizes "My toe hurts," is responding to nociceptors in the foot that have been stimulated by the stubbing of a toe.

A number of chemicals help transmit pain-related information to the brain. Some of these chemicals are natural painkilling proteins called endorphins, Greek for "the morphine within." One theory suggests that people who suffer from severe headache and other types of chronic pain have lower levels of endorphins than people who are generally pain free.

When should you see a physician?

Not all headaches require medical attention. Some result from missed meals or occasional muscle tension and are easily remedied. Yet some types of headache are signals of more serious disorders, and call for prompt medical care. These include:

- Sudden, severe headache
- Sudden, severe headache associated with a stiff neck
- Headache associated with fever
- Headache associated with convulsions
- Headache accompanied by confusion or loss of consciousness
- Headache following a blow on the head

- Headache associated with pain in the eye or ear
- Persistent headache in a person who was previously headache free
- Recurring headache in children
- Headache that interferes with normal life

A headache sufferer usually seeks help from a family practitioner. If the problem is not relieved by standard treatments, the patient may then be referred to a specialist—perhaps an internist or neurologist. Additional referrals may be made to psychologists.

What tests are used to diagnose headache?

Diagnosing a headache is like playing Twenty Questions. Experts agree that a detailed question-and-answer session with a patient can often produce enough information for a diagnosis. Many types of headaches have clear-cut symptoms that fall into an easily recognizable pattern.

Patients may be asked: How often do you have headaches? Where is the pain? How long do the headaches last? When did you first develop headaches? The patient's sleep habits and family and work situations may also be probed.

Most physicians will also obtain a full medical history from the patient, inquiring about past head trauma or surgery, eye strain, sinus problems, dental problems, difficulties with opening and closing of the jaw, and the use of medications. This may be enough to suggest strongly that the patient has migraine or cluster headaches. A complete and careful physical and neurological examination will exclude many possibilities and the suspicion of aneurysm, meningitis, or certain brain tumors. A blood test may be ordered to screen for thyroid disease, anemia, or infections that might cause a headache.

A test called an electroencephalogram (EEG) may be given to measure brain activity. EEG's can indicate a malfunction in the brain, but they cannot usually pinpoint a problem that might be causing a headache. A physician may suggest that a patient with unusual headaches undergo a computed tomographic (CT) scan or a magnetic resonance imaging (MRI) scan. The scans enable the physician to distinguish, for example, between a bleeding blood vessel in the brain and a brain tumor, and are important diagnostic tools in cases of headache associated with brain lesions or other serious disease. CT scans produce x-ray images of the brain that show structures or variations in the density of different types of tissue. MRI scans use magnetic fields and radio waves to produce an image that provides information about the structure and biochemistry of the brain.

If an aneurysm—an abnormal ballooning of a blood vessel—is suspected, a physician may order a CT scan to examine for blood and then an angiogram. In this test, a special fluid that can be seen on an x-ray is injected into the patient and carried in the bloodstream to the brain to reveal any abnormalities in the blood vessels there.

A physician analyzes the results of all these diagnostic tests along with a patient's medical history and examination in order to arrive at a diagnosis.

Headaches are diagnosed as

- Vascular
- Muscle contraction (tension)
- Traction
- Inflammatory

Vascular headaches—a group that includes the well-known migraine—are so named because they are thought to involve abnormal function of the brain's blood vessels or vascular system. Muscle contraction headaches appear to involve the tightening or tensing of facial and neck muscles. Traction and inflammatory headaches are symptoms of other disorders, ranging from stroke to sinus infection. Some people have more than one type of headache.

What are migraine headaches?

The most common type of vascular headache is migraine. Migraine headaches are usually characterized by severe pain on one or both sides of the head, an upset stomach, and at times disturbed vision.

Former basketball star Kareem Abdul-Jabbar remembers experiencing his first migraine at age fourteen. The pain was unlike the discomfort of his previous mild headaches.

"When I got this one I thought, 'This is a headache,'" he says. "The pain was intense and I felt nausea and a great sensitivity to light. All I could think about was when it would stop. I sat in a dark room for an hour and it passed."

Symptoms of Migraine: Abdul-Jabbar's sensitivity to light is a standard symptom of the two most prevalent types of migraine-caused headache: classic and common.

The major difference between the two types is the appearance of neurological symptoms ten to thirty minutes before a classic migraine attack. These symptoms are called an aura. The person may see flashing lights or zigzag lines, or may temporarily lose vision. Other classic symptoms include speech difficulty, weakness of an arm or leg, tingling of the face or hands, and confusion.

The pain of a classic migraine headache may be described as intense, throbbing, or pounding and is felt in the forehead, temple, ear, jaw, or around the eye. Classic migraine starts on one side of the head but may eventually spread to the other side. An attack lasts one to two pain-wracked days.

Common migraine—a term that reflects the disorder's greater occurrence in the general population—is not preceded by an aura. Yet some people experience a variety of vague symptoms beforehand, including mental fuzziness, mood changes, fatigue, and unusual retention of fluids. During the headache phase of a common migraine, a person may have diarrhea and increased urination, as well as nausea and vomiting. Common migraine pain can last three or four days.

Both classic and common migraine can strike as often as several times a week, or as rarely as once every few years. Both types can occur at any time. Some people, however, experience migraines at predictable times—for example, near the days of menstruation or every Saturday morning after a stressful week of work.

The Migraine Process: Research scientists are unclear about the precise cause of migraine headaches. There seems to be general agreement, however, that a key element is blood flow changes in the brain. People who get migraine headaches appear to have blood vessels that overreact to various triggers.

Scientists have devised one theory of migraine that explains these blood flow changes and also certain biochemical changes that may be involved in the headache process. According to this theory, the nervous system responds to a trigger such as stress by causing a spasm of the nerve-rich arteries at the base of the brain. The spasm closes down or constricts several arteries supplying blood to the brain, including the scalp artery and the carotid or neck arteries.

As these arteries constrict, the flow of blood to the brain is reduced. At the same time, blood-clotting particles called platelets clump together—a process that is believed to release a chemical called serotonin. Serotonin acts as a powerful constrictor of arteries, further reducing the blood supply to the brain.

Reduced blood flow decreases the brain's supply of oxygen. Symptoms signaling a headache, such as distorted vision or speech, may then result, similar to symptoms of stroke.

Reacting to the reduced oxygen supply, certain arteries within the brain open wider to meet the brain's energy needs. This widening or dilation spreads, finally affecting the neck and scalp arteries. The dilation of these arteries triggers the release of pain-producing substances called prostaglandins from various tissues and blood cells. Chemicals that cause inflammation and swelling, and substances that increase sensitivity to pain, are also released. The circulation of these chemicals and the dilation of the scalp arteries stimulate the pain-sensitive nociceptors. The result, according to this theory: a throbbing pain in the head.

Women and Migraine: Although males and females seem to be equally affected by migraine, the condition is more common in adult women. Both sexes may develop migraine in infancy, but most often the disorder begins between the ages of five and thirty-five.

The relationship between female hormones and migraine is still unclear. Women may have "menstrual migraine"—headaches around the time of their menstrual period—which may disappear during pregnancy. Other women develop migraine for the first time when they are pregnant. Some are first affected after menopause.

The effect of oral contraceptives on headaches is perplexing. Scientists report that some women with migraine who take birth control pills experience more frequent and severe attacks. However, a small percentage of women have fewer and less severe migraine headaches when they take birth control pills. Normal women who do not suffer from headaches may develop migraines as a side effect when they use oral contraceptives. Investigators around the world are studying hormonal changes in women with migraine in the hope of identifying the specific ways these naturally occurring chemicals cause headaches.

Triggers of Headache: Although many sufferers have a family history of migraine, the exact hereditary nature of this condition is still unknown. People who get migraines are thought to have an inherited abnormality in the regulation of blood vessels.

"It's like a cocked gun with a hair trigger," explains one specialist. "A person is born with a potential for migraine and the headache is triggered by things that are really not so terrible."

These triggers include stress and other normal emotions, as well as biological and environmental conditions. Fatigue, glaring or flickering lights, changes in the weather, and certain foods can set off migraine.

It may seem hard to believe that eating such seemingly harmless foods as yogurt, nuts, and lima beans can result in a painful migraine headache. However, some scientists believe that these foods and several others contain chemical substances, such as tyramine, that constrict arteries—the first step of the migraine process. Other scientists believe that foods cause headaches by setting off an allergic reaction in susceptible people.

While a food-triggered migraine usually occurs soon after eating, other triggers may not cause immediate pain. Scientists report that people can develop migraine not only during a period of stress but also afterward when their vascular systems are still reacting. For example, migraines that wake people up in the middle of the night are believed to result from a delayed reaction to stress.

Other Forms of Migraine: In addition to classic and common, migraine headache can take several other forms:

- Patients with **hemiplegic migraine** have temporary paralysis on one side of the body, a condition known as hemiplegia. Some people may experience vision problems and vertigo—a feeling that the world is spinning. These symptoms begin ten to ninety minutes before the onset of headache pain.

- In **ophthalmoplegic migraine**, the pain is around the eye and is associated with a droopy eyelid, double vision, and other problems with vision.

- **Basilar artery migraine** involves a disturbance of a major brain artery at the base of the brain. Preheadache symptoms include vertigo, double vision, and poor muscular coordination. This type of migraine occurs primarily in adolescent and young adult women and is often associated with the menstrual cycle.

- **Benign exertional headache** is brought on by running, lifting, coughing, sneezing, or bending. The headache begins at the onset of activity, and pain rarely lasts more than several minutes.

- **Status migrainosus** is a rare and severe type of migraine that can last seventy-two hours or longer. The pain and nausea are so intense that people who have this type of headache must be hospitalized. The use of certain drugs can trigger status migrainosus. Neurologists report that many of their status migrainosus patients were depressed and anxious before they experienced headache attacks.

493

- **Headache-free migraine** is characterized by such migraine symptoms as visual problems, nausea, vomiting, constipation, or diarrhea. Patients, however, do not experience head pain. Headache specialists have suggested that unexplained pain in a particular part of the body, fever, and dizziness could also be possible types of headache-free migraine.

How is migraine headache treated?

During the Stone Age, pieces of a headache sufferer's skull were cut away with flint instruments to relieve pain. Another unpleasant remedy used in the British Isles around the ninth century involved drinking "the juice of elderseed, cow's brain, and goat's dung dissolved in vinegar." Fortunately, today's headache patients are spared such drastic measures.

Drug therapy, biofeedback training, stress reduction, and elimination of certain foods from the diet are the most common methods of preventing and controlling migraine and other vascular headaches. Joan, the migraine sufferer, was helped by treatment with a combination of an antimigraine drug and diet control.

Regular exercise, such as swimming or vigorous walking, can also reduce the frequency and severity of migraine headaches. Joan found that whirlpool and yoga baths helped her relax.

During a migraine headache, temporary relief can sometimes be obtained by applying cold packs to the head or by pressing on the bulging artery found in front of the ear on the painful side of the head.

Drug Therapy: There are two ways to approach the treatment of migraine headache with drugs: prevent the attacks, or relieve symptoms after the headache occurs.

For infrequent migraine, drugs can be taken at the first sign of a headache in order to stop it or to at least ease the pain. People who get occasional mild migraine may benefit by taking aspirin or acetaminophen at the start of an attack. Aspirin raises a person's tolerance to pain and also discourages clumping of blood platelets. Small amounts of caffeine may be useful if taken in the early stages of migraine. Yet for most migraine sufferers who get moderate to severe headaches, and for all cluster headache patients (see section "Besides Migraine, What Are Other Types of Vascular Headaches?"), stronger drugs may be necessary to control the pain.

Several drugs for the prevention of migraine have been developed in recent years, including serotonin agonists that mimic the action of this key brain chemical. One of the most commonly used drugs for the relief of classic and common migraine symptoms is sumatriptan, which binds to serotonin receptors. For optimal benefit, the drug is taken during the early stages of an attack. If a migraine has been in progress for about an hour after the drug is taken, a repeat dose can be given.

Physicians caution that sumatriptan should not be taken by people who have angina pectoris, basilar migraine, severe hypertension, or vascular or liver disease.

Another migraine drug is ergotamine tartrate, a vasoconstrictor that helps counteract the painful dilation stage of the headache. Other drugs that constrict dilated blood vessels or help reduce blood vessel inflammation also are available.

For headaches that occur three or more times a month, preventive treatment is usually recommended. Drugs used to prevent classic and common migraine include methysergide maleate, which counteracts blood vessel constriction; propranolol hydrochloride, which stops blood vessel dilation; amitriptyline, an antidepressant; valproic acid, an anticonvulsant; and verapamil, a calcium channel blocker.

Antidepressants called MAO inhibitors also prevent migraine. These drugs block an enzyme called monoamine oxidase that normally helps nerve cells absorb the artery-constricting brain chemical serotonin. MAO inhibitors can have potentially serious side effects—particularly if taken while ingesting foods or beverages that contain tyramine, a substance that constricts arteries.

Many antimigraine drugs can have adverse side effects. Yet like most medicines, they are relatively safe when used carefully and under a physician's supervision. To avoid long-term side effects of preventive medications, headache specialists advise patients to reduce the dosage of these drugs and then stop taking them as soon as possible.

Biofeedback and Relaxation Training: Drug therapy for migraine is often combined with biofeedback and relaxation training. Biofeedback refers to a technique that can give people better control over such body function indicators as blood pressure, heart rate, temperature, muscle tension, and brain waves. Thermal biofeedback allows a patient to consciously raise hand temperature. Some patients who are able to increase hand temperature can reduce the number and intensity of migraines. The mechanisms underlying these self-regulation treatments are being studied by research scientists.

"To succeed in biofeedback," says a headache specialist, "you must be able to concentrate and you must be motivated to get well."

A patient learning thermal biofeedback wears a device that transmits the temperature of an index finger or hand to a monitor. While the patient tries to warm his hands, the monitor provides feedback either on a gauge that shows the temperature reading or by emitting a sound or beep that increases in intensity as the temperature increases. The patient is not told how to raise hand temperature, but is given suggestions such as "Imagine your hands feel very warm and heavy."

"I have a good imagination," says one headache sufferer who traded in her medication for thermal biofeedback. The technique decreased the number and severity of headaches she experienced.

In another type of biofeedback called electromyographic or EMG training, the patient learns to control muscle tension in the face, neck, and shoulders.

Either kind of biofeedback may be combined with relaxation training, during which patients learn to relax the mind and body.

Biofeedback can be practiced at home with a portable monitor. Yet the ultimate goal of treatment is to wean the patient from the machine. The patient can then use biofeedback anywhere at the first sign of a headache.

The Antimigraine Diet: Scientists estimate that a small percentage of migraine sufferers will benefit from a treatment program focused solely on eliminating headache-provoking foods and beverages.

Other migraine patients may be helped by a diet to prevent low blood sugar. Low blood sugar, or hypoglycemia, can cause headache. This condition can occur after a period without food: overnight, for example, or when a meal is skipped. People who wake up in the morning with a headache may be reacting to the low blood sugar caused by the lack of food overnight.

Treatment for headaches caused by low blood sugar consists of scheduling smaller, more frequent meals for the patient. A special diet designed to stabilize the body's sugar-regulating system is sometimes recommended.

For the same reason, many specialists also recommend that migraine patients avoid oversleeping on weekends. Sleeping late can change the body's normal blood sugar level and lead to a headache.

Besides migraine, what are other types of vascular headaches?

After migraine, the most common type of vascular headache is the toxic headache produced by fever. Pneumonia, measles, mumps, and tonsillitis are among the diseases that can cause severe toxic vascular headaches. Toxic headaches can also result from the presence of foreign chemicals in the body. Other kinds of vascular headaches include "clusters," which cause repeated episodes of intense pain, and headaches resulting from a rise in blood pressure.

Chemical Culprits: Repeated exposure to nitrite compounds can result in a dull, pounding headache that may be accompanied by a flushed face. Nitrite, which dilates blood vessels, is found in such products as heart medicine and dynamite, but is also used as a chemical to preserve meat. Hot dogs and other processed meats containing sodium nitrite can cause headaches.

Eating foods prepared with monosodium glutamate (MSG) can result in headache. Soy sauce, meat tenderizer, and a variety of packaged foods contain this chemical that is touted as a flavor enhancer.

Headache can also result from exposure to poisons, even common household varieties like insecticides, carbon tetrachloride, and lead. Children who ingest flakes of lead paint may develop headaches. So may anyone who has contact with lead batteries or lead-glazed pottery.

Artists and industrial workers may experience headaches after exposure to materials that contain chemical solvents. These solvents, like benzene, are found in turpentine, spray adhesives, rubber cement, and inks.

Drugs such as amphetamines can cause headaches as a side effect. Another type of drug-related headache occurs during withdrawal from long-term therapy with the antimigraine drug ergotamine tartrate.

Jokes are often made about alcohol hangovers but the headache associated with "the morning after" is no laughing matter. Fortunately, there are several suggested treatments for the pain. The hangover headache may also be reduced by taking honey, which speeds alcohol metabolism, or caffeine, a constrictor of dilated arteries. Caffeine, however, can cause headaches as well as cure them. Heavy coffee drinkers often get headaches when they try to break the caffeine habit.

Cluster Headaches: Cluster headaches, named for their repeated occurrence over weeks or months at roughly the same time of day or night in clusters, begin as a minor pain around one eye, eventually spreading to that side of the face. The pain quickly intensifies, compelling the victim to pace the floor or rock in a chair. "You can't lie down, you're fidgety," explains a cluster patient. "The pain is unbearable."

Other symptoms include a stuffed and runny nose and a droopy eyelid over a red and tearing eye.

Cluster headaches last between thirty and forty-five minutes. Yet the relief people feel at the end of an attack is usually mixed with dread as they await a recurrence. Clusters may mysteriously disappear for months or years. Many people have cluster bouts during the spring and fall. At their worst, chronic cluster headaches can last continuously for years.

Cluster attacks can strike at any age but usually start between the ages of twenty and forty. Unlike migraine, cluster headaches are more common in men and do not run in families.

Studies of cluster patients show that they are likely to have hazel eyes and that they tend to be heavy smokers and drinkers. Paradoxically, both nicotine, which constricts arteries, and alcohol, which dilates them, trigger cluster headaches. The exact connection between these substances and cluster attacks is not known.

Despite a cluster headache's distinguishing characteristics, its relative infrequency and similarity to such disorders as sinusitis can lead to misdiagnosis. Some cluster patients have had tooth extractions, sinus surgery, or psychiatric treatment in futile efforts to cure their pain.

Research studies have turned up several clues as to the cause of cluster headache, but no answers. One clue is found in the thermograms of untreated cluster patients, which show a "cold spot" of reduced blood flow above the eye.

The sudden start and brief duration of cluster headaches can make them difficult to treat; however, research scientists have identified several effective drugs for these headaches. The antimigraine drug sumatriptan can subdue a cluster, if taken at the first sign of an attack. Injections of dihydroergotamine, a form of ergotamine tartrate, are sometimes used to treat clusters. Corticosteroids also can be used, either orally or by intramuscular injection.

Some cluster patients can prevent attacks by taking propranolol, methysergide, valproic acid, verapamil, or lithium carbonate.

Another option that works for some cluster patients is rapid inhalation of pure oxygen through a mask for five to fifteen minutes. The oxygen seems to ease the pain of cluster headache by reducing blood flow to the brain.

In chronic cases of cluster headache, certain facial nerves may be surgically cut or destroyed to provide relief. These procedures have had limited success. Some cluster patients have had facial nerves cut only to have them regenerate years later.

Painful Pressure: Chronic high blood pressure can cause headache, as can rapid rises in blood pressure like those experienced during anger, vigorous exercise, or sexual excitement.

The severe "orgasmic headache" occurs right before orgasm and is believed to be a vascular headache. Since sudden rupture of a cerebral blood vessel can occur, this type of headache should be evaluated by a doctor.

What are muscle-contraction headaches?

It's 5:00 P.M. and your boss has just asked you to prepare a twenty-page briefing paper. Due date: tomorrow. You're angry and tired and the more you think about the assignment, the tenser you become. Your teeth clench, your brow wrinkles, and soon you have a splitting tension headache.

Tension headache is named not only for the role of stress in triggering the pain, but also for the contraction of neck, face, and scalp muscles brought on by stressful events. Tension headache is a severe but temporary form of muscle-contraction headache. The pain is mild to moderate and feels like pressure is being applied to the head or neck. The headache usually disappears after the period of stress is over. Ninety percent of all headaches are classified as tension/muscle contraction headaches.

By contrast, chronic muscle-contraction headaches can last for weeks, months, and sometimes years. The pain of these headaches is often described as a tight band around the head or a feeling that the head and neck are in a cast. "It feels like somebody is tightening a giant vise around my head," says one patient. The pain is steady, and is usually felt on both sides of the head. Chronic muscle-contraction headaches can cause sore scalps—even combing one's hair can be painful.

In the past, many scientists believed that the primary cause of the pain of muscle-contraction headache was sustained muscle tension. However, a growing number of authorities now believe that a far more complex mechanism is responsible.

Occasionally, muscle-contraction headaches will be accompanied by nausea, vomiting, and blurred vision, but there is no pre-headache syndrome as with migraine. Muscle-contraction headaches have not been linked to hormones or foods, as has migraine, nor is there a strong hereditary connection.

Research has shown that for many people, chronic muscle-contraction headaches are caused by depression and anxiety. These people tend to get their headaches in the early morning or evening when conflicts in the office or home are anticipated.

Emotional factors are not the only triggers of muscle-contraction headaches. Certain physical postures that tense head and neck muscles—such as holding one's chin down while reading—can lead to head and neck pain. So can prolonged writing under poor light, or holding a phone between the shoulder and ear, or even gum-chewing.

More serious problems that can cause muscle-contraction headaches include degenerative arthritis of the neck and temporomandibular joint dysfunction, or TMD. TMD is a disorder of the joint between the temporal bone (above the ear) and the mandible or lower jawbone. The disorder results from poor bite and jaw clenching.

Treatment for muscle-contraction headache varies. The first consideration is to treat any specific disorder or disease that may be causing the headache. For example, arthritis of the neck is treated with anti-inflammatory medication and TMD may be helped by corrective devices for the mouth and jaw.

Acute tension headaches not associated with a disease are treated with analgesics like aspirin and acetaminophen. Stronger analgesics, such as propoxyphene and codeine, are sometimes prescribed. As prolonged use of these drugs can lead to dependence, patients taking them should have periodic medical checkups and follow their physicians' instructions carefully.

Nondrug therapy for chronic muscle-contraction headaches includes biofeedback, relaxation training, and counseling. A technique called cognitive restructuring teaches people to change their attitudes and responses to stress. Patients might be encouraged, for example, to imagine that they are coping successfully with a stressful situation. In progressive relaxation therapy, patients are taught to first tense and then relax individual muscle groups. Finally, the patient tries to relax his or her whole body. Many people imagine a peaceful scene—such as lying on the beach or by a beautiful lake. Passive relaxation does not involve tensing of muscles. Instead, patients are encouraged to focus on different muscles, suggesting that they relax. Some people might think to themselves, *Relax* or *My muscles feel warm*.

People with chronic muscle-contraction headaches my also be helped by taking antidepressants or MAO inhibitors. Mixed muscle-contraction and migraine headaches are sometimes treated with barbiturate compounds, which slow down nerve function in the brain and spinal cord.

People who suffer infrequent muscle-contraction headaches may benefit from a hot shower or moist heat applied to the back of the neck. Cervical collars are sometimes recommended as an aid to good posture.

Physical therapy, massage, and gentle exercise of the neck may also be helpful.

When is headache a warning of a more serious condition?

Like other types of pain, headaches can serve as warning signals of more serious disorders. This is particularly true for headaches caused by traction or inflammation.

Traction headaches can occur if the pain-sensitive parts of the head are pulled, stretched, or displaced, as, for example, when eye muscles are tensed to compensate for eyestrain. Headaches caused by inflammation include those related to meningitis as well as those resulting from diseases of the sinuses, spine, neck, ears, and teeth. Ear and tooth infections and glaucoma can cause headaches. In oral and dental disorders, headache is experienced as pain in the entire head, including the face. These headaches are treated by curing the underlying problem. This may involve surgery, antibiotics, or other drugs.

Characteristics of the various types of more serious traction and inflammatory headaches vary by disorder:

- **Brain tumor:** Brain tumors are diagnosed in about eleven thousand people every year. As they grow, these tumors sometimes cause headache by pushing on the outer layer of nerve tissue that covers the brain or by pressing against pain-sensitive blood vessel walls. Headache resulting from a brain tumor may be periodic or continuous. Typically, it feels like a strong pressure is being applied to the head. The pain is relieved when the tumor is treated by surgery, radiation, or chemotherapy.

- **Stroke:** Headache may accompany several conditions that can lead to stroke, including hypertension or high blood pressure, arteriosclerosis, and heart disease. Headaches are also associated with completed stroke, when brain cells die from lack of sufficient oxygen. Many stroke-related headaches can be prevented by careful management of the patient's condition through diet, exercise, and medication. Mild to moderate headaches are associated with transient ischemic attacks (TIA's), sometimes called "mini-strokes," which result from a temporary lack of blood supply to the brain. The head pain occurs near the clot or lesion that blocks blood flow. The similarity between migraine and symptoms of TIA can cause problems in diagnosis. The rare person under age forty who suffers a TIA may be misdiagnosed as having migraine; similarly, TIA-prone older patients who suffer migraine may be misdiagnosed as having stroke-related headaches.

- **Spinal tap:** About one-fourth of the people who undergo a lumbar puncture or spinal tap develop a headache. Many scientists believe these headaches result from leakage of the cerebrospinal fluid that flows through pain-sensitive membranes around the brain and down to the spinal cord. The fluid, they suggest, drains through the tiny hole created by the spinal tap needle, causing the membranes to rub painfully against the bony skull. Since headache pain occurs only when the patient stands up, the "cure" is to remain lying down until the headache runs its course—anywhere from a few hours to several days.

- **Head trauma:** Headaches may develop after a blow to the head, either immediately or months later. There is little relationship between the severity of the trauma and the intensity of headache pain. In most cases, the cause of the headache is not known. Occasionally the cause is ruptured blood vessels that result in an accumulation of blood called a hematoma. This mass of blood can displace brain tissue and cause headaches as well as weakness, confusion, memory loss, and seizures. Hematomas can be drained to produce rapid relief of symptoms.

- **Temporal arteritis:** Arteritis, an inflammation of certain arteries in the head, primarily affects people over age fifty. Symptoms include throbbing headache, fever, and loss of appetite. Some patients experience blurring or loss of vision. Prompt treatment with corticosteroid drugs helps to relieve symptoms.

- **Meningitis and encephalitis headaches** are caused by infections of meninges—the brain's outer covering—and in encephalitis, inflammation of the brain itself.

- **Trigeminal neuralgia:** Trigeminal neuralgia, or tic douloureux, results from a disorder of the trigeminal nerve. This nerve supplies the face, teeth, mouth, and nasal cavity with feeling and also enables the mouth muscles to chew. Symptoms are headache and intense facial pain that comes in short, excruciating jabs set off by the slightest touch to or movement of trigger points in the face or mouth. People with trigeminal neuralgia often fear brushing their teeth or chewing on the side of the mouth that is affected. Many trigeminal neuralgia patients are controlled with drugs, including carbamazepine. Patients who do not respond to drugs may be helped by surgery on the trigeminal nerve.

- **Sinus infection:** In a condition called acute sinusitis, a viral or bacterial infection of the upper respiratory tract spreads to the membrane that lines the sinus cavities. When one or more of these cavities are filled with fluid from the inflammation, they become painful. Treatment of acute sinusitis includes antibiotics, analgesics, and decongestants. Chronic sinusitis may be caused by an allergy to such irritants as dust, ragweed, animal hair, and smoke. Research scientists disagree about whether chronic sinusitis triggers headache.

What causes headache in children?

Like adults, children experience the infections, trauma, and stresses that can lead to headaches. In fact, research shows that as young people enter adolescence and encounter the stresses of puberty and secondary school, the frequency of headache increases.

Migraine headaches often begin in childhood or adolescence. According to recent surveys, as many as half of all schoolchildren experience some type of headache.

Children with migraine often have nausea and excessive vomiting. Some children have periodic vomiting, but no headache—the so-called abdominal migraine. Research scientists have found that these children usually develop headaches when they are older.

Physicians have many drugs to treat migraine in children. Different classes that may be tried include analgesics, antiemetics, anticonvulsants, beta-blockers, and sedatives. A diet may also be prescribed to protect the child from foods that trigger headache. Sometimes psychological counseling or even psychiatric treatment for the child and the parents is recommended.

Childhood headache can be a sign of depression. Parents should alert the family pediatrician if a child develops headaches along with other symptoms such as a change in mood or sleep habits. Antidepressant medication and psychotherapy are effective treatments for childhood depression and related headache.

Conclusion

If you suffer from headaches and none of the standard treatments help, do not despair. Some people find that their headaches disappear once they deal with a troubled marriage, pass their certifying board exams, or resolve some other stressful problem. Others find that if they control their psychological reaction to stress, the headaches disappear.

"I had migraines for several years," says one woman, "and then they went away. I think it was because I lowered my personal goals in life. Today, even though I have one hundred things to do at night, I don't worry about it. I learned to say no."

For those who cannot say no, or who get headaches anyway, today's headache research offers hope. The work of NINDS-supported scientists around the world promises to improve our understanding of this complex disorder and provide better tools to treat it.

Chapter 22

Hydrocephalus

What is hydrocephalus?

The term *hydrocephalus* is derived from the Greek words "hydro," meaning water, and "cephalus," meaning head. As its name implies, it is a condition in which the primary characteristic is excessive accumulation of fluid in the brain. Although hydrocephalus was once known as "water on the brain," the "water" is actually cerebrospinal fluid (CSF)—a clear fluid surrounding the brain and spinal cord. The excessive accumulation of CSF results in an abnormal dilation of the spaces in the brain called ventricles. This dilation causes potentially harmful pressure on the tissues of the brain.

The ventricular system is made up of four ventricles connected by narrow pathways. Normally, CSF flows through the ventricles, exits into cisterns (closed spaces that serve as reservoirs) at the base of the brain, bathes the surfaces of the brain and spinal cord, and then is absorbed into the bloodstream.

CSF has three important life-sustaining functions: (1) to keep the brain tissue buoyant, acting as a cushion or "shock absorber"; (2) to act as the vehicle for delivering nutrients to the brain and removing waste; and (3) to flow between the cranium and spine to compensate for changes in intracranial blood volume (the amount of blood within the brain).

Excerpted from "Hydrocephalus Fact Sheet," National Institute of Neurological Disorders and Stroke, National Institutes of Health, NIH Publication Number 99-385, updated November 2004.

505

The balance between production and absorption of CSF is critically important. Ideally, the fluid is almost completely absorbed into the bloodstream as it circulates; however, there are circumstances that, when present, will prevent or disturb the production or absorption of CSF, or that will inhibit its normal flow. When this balance is disturbed, hydrocephalus is the result.

What are the different types of hydrocephalus?

Hydrocephalus may be congenital or acquired. Congenital hydrocephalus is present at birth, and may be caused by either environmental influences during fetal development or genetic predisposition. Acquired hydrocephalus develops at the time of birth or at some point afterward. This type of hydrocephalus can affect individuals of all ages and may be caused by injury or disease.

Hydrocephalus may also be communicating or noncommunicating. Communicating hydrocephalus occurs when the flow of CSF is blocked after it exits from the ventricles. This form is called communicating because the CSF can still flow between the ventricles, which remain open. Noncommunicating hydrocephalus—also called "obstructive" hydrocephalus—occurs when the flow of CSF is blocked along one or more of the narrow pathways connecting the ventricles. One of the most common causes of hydrocephalus is "aqueductal stenosis." In this case, hydrocephalus results from a narrowing of the aqueduct of Sylvius, a small passageway between the third and fourth ventricles in the middle of the brain.

There are two other forms of hydrocephalus that do not fit distinctly into the categories mentioned above and primarily affect adults: hydrocephalus ex-vacuo and normal pressure hydrocephalus.

Hydrocephalus ex-vacuo occurs when there is damage to the brain caused by stroke or traumatic injury. In these cases, there may be actual shrinkage (atrophy or wasting) of brain tissue. Normal pressure hydrocephalus commonly occurs in the elderly and is characterized by many of the same symptoms associated with other conditions that occur more often in the elderly, such as memory loss, dementia, gait disorder, urinary incontinence, and a general slowing of activity.

Who gets this disorder?

Incidence and prevalence data are difficult to establish as there is no existing national registry or database of people with hydrocephalus and closely associated disorders; however, hydrocephalus is believed to affect approximately one in every five hundred children. At present, most of these cases are diagnosed prenatally, at the time of delivery, or in early childhood. Advances in diagnostic imaging technology allow more accurate diagnoses in individuals with atypical presentations, including adults with conditions such as normal pressure hydrocephalus.

What causes hydrocephalus?

The causes of hydrocephalus are not all well understood. Hydrocephalus may result from genetic inheritance (aqueductal stenosis) or developmental disorders such as those associated with neural tube defects including spina bifida and encephalocele. Other possible causes include complications of premature birth such as intraventricular hemorrhage, diseases such as meningitis, tumors, traumatic head injury, or subarachnoid hemorrhage blocking the exit from the ventricles to the cisterns and eliminating the cisterns themselves.

What are the symptoms?

Symptoms of hydrocephalus vary with age, disease progression, and individual differences in tolerance to CSF. For example, an infant's ability to tolerate CSF pressure differs from an adult's. The infant skull can expand to accommodate the buildup of CSF because the sutures (the fibrous joints that connect the bones of the skull) have not yet closed.

In infancy, the most obvious indication of hydrocephalus is often the rapid increase in head circumference or an unusually large head size. Other symptoms may include vomiting, sleepiness, irritability, downward deviation of the eyes (also called "sunsetting"), and seizures.

Older children and adults may experience different symptoms because their skulls cannot expand to accommodate the buildup of CSF. In older children or adults, symptoms may include headache followed by vomiting, nausea, papilledema (swelling of the optic disk which is part of the optic nerve), blurred vision, diplopia (double vision), sunsetting of the eyes, problems with balance, poor coordination, gait disturbance, urinary incontinence, slowing or loss of development, lethargy, drowsiness, irritability, or other changes in personality or cognition including memory loss.

The symptoms described in this section account for the most typical ways in which progressive hydrocephalus manifests itself; it is, however, important to remember that symptoms vary significantly from individual to individual.

How is hydrocephalus diagnosed?

Hydrocephalus is diagnosed through clinical neurological evaluation and by using cranial imaging techniques such as ultrasonography, computed tomography (CT), magnetic resonance imaging (MRI), or pressure-monitoring techniques. A physician selects the appropriate diagnostic tool based on the patient's age, clinical presentation, and the presence of known or suspected abnormalities of the brain or spinal cord.

What is the current treatment?

Hydrocephalus is most often treated with the surgical placement of a shunt system. This system diverts the flow of CSF from a site within the central nervous system (CNS) to another area of the body where it can be absorbed as part of the circulatory process.

A shunt is a flexible but sturdy silastic tube. A shunt system consists of the shunt, a catheter, and a valve. One end of the catheter is placed in the CNS—most usually within a ventricle inside the brain, but also potentially within a cyst or in a site close to the spinal cord. The other end of the catheter is commonly placed within the peritoneal (abdominal) cavity, but may also be placed at other sites within the body such as a chamber of the heart or a cavity in the lung where the CSF can drain and be absorbed. A valve located along the catheter maintains one-way flow and regulates the rate of CSF flow.

A limited number of patients can be treated with an alternative procedure called third ventriculostomy. In this procedure, a neuro-endoscope—a small camera designed to visualize small and difficult to reach surgical areas—allows a doctor to view the ventricular surface using fiber optic technology. The scope is guided into position so that a small hole can be made in the floor of the third ventricle, allowing the CSF to bypass the obstruction and flow toward the site of resorption around the surface of the brain.

What are the possible complications of a shunt system?

Shunt systems are not perfect devices. Complications may include mechanical failure, infections, obstructions, and the need to lengthen or replace the catheter. Generally, shunt systems require monitoring and regular medical follow-up. When complications do occur, usually the shunt system will require some type of revision.

Some complications can lead to other problems such as overdraining or underdraining. Overdraining occurs when the shunt allows CSF to drain from the ventricles more quickly than it is produced. This overdraining can cause the ventricles to collapse, tearing blood vessels and causing headache, hemorrhage (subdural hematoma), or slit-like ventricles (slit ventricle syndrome). Underdraining occurs when CSF is not removed quickly enough and the symptoms of hydrocephalus recur (see "What are the symptoms of hydrocephalus?"). In addition to the common symptoms of hydrocephalus, infections from a shunt may also produce symptoms such as a low-grade fever, soreness of the neck or shoulder muscles, and redness or tenderness along the shunt tract. When there is reason to suspect that a shunt system is not functioning properly (for example, if the symptoms of hydrocephalus return), medical attention should be sought immediately.

What is the prognosis?

The prognosis for patients diagnosed with hydrocephalus is difficult to predict, although there is some correlation between the specific cause of the hydrocephalus and the patient's outcome. Prognosis is further complicated by the presence of associated disorders, the timeliness of diagnosis, and the success of treatment. The degree to which decompression (relief of CSF pressure or buildup) following shunt surgery can minimize or reverse damage to the brain is not well understood.

Affected individuals and their families should be aware that hydrocephalus poses risks to both cognitive and physical development. However, many children diagnosed with the disorder benefit from rehabilitation therapies and educational interventions, and go on to lead normal lives with few limitations. Treatment by an interdisciplinary team of medical professionals, rehabilitation specialists, and educational experts is critical to a positive outcome.

Treatment of patients with hydrocephalus is life saving and life sustaining. Left untreated, progressive hydrocephalus is, with rare exceptions, fatal.

What research is being done?

Within the federal government, the leading supporter of research on hydrocephalus is the National Institute of Neurological Disorders and Stroke (NINDS). The NINDS, a part of the National Institutes of Health (NIH), is responsible for supporting and conducting research on the brain and the central nervous system. NINDS conducts research in its laboratories at NIH and also supports studies through grants to major medical institutions across the country.

One NINDS-supported study examined cognitive development, academic achievement, and behavioral adjustment in children with hydrocephalus. With further research, investigators hope to shed new light on the influence of hydrocephalus on development as well as the more general issue of the effect of early brain injury.

The NINDS also conducts and supports a wide range of fundamental studies that explore the complex mechanisms of normal brain development. The knowledge gained from these studies provides the foundation for understanding how this process can go awry and, thus, offers hope for new means to treat and prevent developmental brain disorders such as hydrocephalus.

Chapter 23

Narcolepsy

What is narcolepsy?

Narcolepsy is a chronic neurological disorder caused by the brain's inability to regulate sleep-wake cycles normally. At various times throughout the day, people with narcolepsy experience fleeting urges to sleep. If the urge becomes overwhelming, patients fall asleep for periods lasting from a few seconds to several minutes. In rare cases, some people may remain asleep for an hour or longer.

Narcoleptic sleep episodes can occur at any time, and thus frequently prove profoundly disabling. People may involuntarily fall asleep while at work or at school, when having a conversation, playing a game, or eating a meal, or, most dangerously, when driving an automobile or operating other types of potentially hazardous machinery. In addition to daytime sleepiness, three other major symptoms frequently characterize narcolepsy: cataplexy, or the sudden loss of voluntary muscle tone; vivid hallucinations during sleep onset or upon awakening; and brief episodes of total paralysis at the beginning or end of sleep.

Contrary to common beliefs, people with narcolepsy do not spend a substantially greater proportion of their time asleep during a twenty-four-hour period than do normal sleepers. In addition to daytime drowsiness and involuntary sleep episodes, most patients also

Excerpted from "Narcolepsy Fact Sheet," National Institute of Neurological Disorders and Stroke, National Institutes of Health, NIH Publication Number 03-1637, updated October 2004.

experience frequent awakenings during nighttime sleep. For these reasons, narcolepsy is considered to be a disorder of the normal boundaries between the sleeping and waking states.

For most adults, a normal night's sleep lasts about eight hours and is composed of four to six separate sleep cycles. A sleep cycle is defined by a segment of non-rapid eye movement (NREM) sleep followed by a period of rapid eye movement (REM) sleep. The NREM segment can be further divided into stages according to the size and frequency of brain waves. REM sleep, in contrast, is accompanied by bursts of rapid eye movement (hence the acronym REM sleep) along with sharply heightened brain activity and temporary paralysis of the muscles that control posture and body movement. When subjects are awakened from sleep, they report that they were "having a dream" more often if they have been in REM sleep than if they have been in NREM sleep. Transitions from NREM to REM sleep are governed by interactions among groups of neurons (nerve cells) in certain parts of the brain.

Scientists now believe that narcolepsy results from disease processes affecting brain mechanisms that regulate REM sleep. For normal sleepers a typical sleep cycle is about 100–110 minutes long, beginning with NREM sleep and transitioning to REM sleep after 80–100 minutes. However, people with narcolepsy frequently enter REM sleep within a few minutes of falling asleep.

Who gets narcolepsy?

Narcolepsy is not rare, but it is an underrecognized and underdiagnosed condition. According to current estimates, the disorder affects about 1 in every 2,000 Americans—a total of more than 135,000 individuals. After obstructive sleep apnea and restless legs syndrome, narcolepsy is the third most frequently diagnosed primary sleep disorder found in patients seeking treatment at sleep clinics. Yet the exact prevalence rate remains uncertain, and the disorder may affect a larger segment of the population than currently estimated.

Narcolepsy appears throughout the world in every racial and ethnic group, affecting males and females equally. Yet prevalence rates vary among populations. Compared to the U.S. population, for example, the prevalence rate is substantially lower in Israel (about 1 per 500,000) and considerably higher in Japan (about 1 per 600).

Most cases of narcolepsy are sporadic—that is, the disorder occurs independently in individuals without strong evidence of being inherited. Yet familial clusters are known to occur. Up to 10 percent of patients diagnosed with narcolepsy with cataplexy report having a close relative with the same symptoms. Genetic factors alone are not sufficient to cause narcolepsy. Other factors—such as infection, immune system dysfunction, trauma, hormonal changes, or stress—may also be present before the disease develops. Thus, while close relatives of people with narcolepsy have a statistically higher risk of developing the disorder than do members of the general population, that risk remains low in comparison to diseases that are purely genetic in origin.

What are the symptoms?

People with narcolepsy experience highly individualized patterns of REM sleep disturbances that tend to begin subtly and may change dramatically over time. The most common major symptom, other than excessive daytime sleepiness (EDS), is cataplexy, which occurs in about 70 percent of all patients. Sleep paralysis and hallucinations are somewhat less common. Only 10 to 25 percent of patients, however, display all four of these major symptoms during the course of their illness.

Excessive Daytime Sleepiness: EDS, the symptom most consistently experienced by almost all patients, is usually the first to become clinically apparent. Generally, EDS interferes with normal activities on a daily basis, whether or not patients have sufficient sleep at night. People with EDS describe it as a persistent sense of mental cloudiness, a lack of energy, a depressed mood, or extreme exhaustion. Many find that they have great difficulty maintaining their concentration while at school or work. Some experience memory lapses. Many find it nearly impossible to stay alert in passive situations, as when listening to lectures or watching television. People tend to awaken from such unavoidable sleeps feeling refreshed and finding that their feelings of drowsiness and fatigue subside for an hour or two.

Involuntary sleep episodes are sometimes very brief, lasting no more than seconds at a time. As many as 40 percent of all people with narcolepsy are prone to automatic behavior during such "microsleeps." They fall asleep for a few seconds while performing a task but continue carrying it through to completion without any apparent interruption. During these episodes, people are usually engaged in habitual, essentially "second nature" activities such as taking notes in class, typing, or driving. They cannot recall their actions, and their performance is almost always impaired during a microsleep. Their handwriting may, for example, degenerate into an illegible scrawl, or they may store items in bizarre locations and then forget where they placed them. If an episode occurs while driving, patients may get lost or have an accident.

Cataplexy: Cataplexy is a sudden loss of muscle tone that leads to feelings of weakness and a loss of voluntary muscle control. Attacks can occur at any time during the waking period, with patients usually experiencing their first episodes several weeks or months after the onset of EDS. Yet in about 10 percent of all cases, cataplexy is the first symptom to appear and can be misdiagnosed as a manifestation of a seizure disorder. Cataplectic attacks vary in duration and severity. The loss of muscle tone can be barely perceptible, involving no more than a momentary sense of slight weakness in a limited number of muscles, such as mild drooping of the eyelids. The most severe attacks result in a complete loss of tone in all voluntary muscles, leading to total physical collapse in which patients are unable to move, speak, or keep their eyes open. Yet even during the most severe episodes, people remain fully conscious, a characteristic that distinguishes cataplexy from seizure disorders. Although cataplexy can occur spontaneously, it is more often triggered by sudden, strong emotions such as fear, anger, stress, excitement, or humor. Laughter is reportedly the most frequent trigger.

The loss of muscle tone during a cataplectic episode resembles the interruption of muscle activity that naturally occurs during REM sleep. A group of neurons in the brainstem ceases activity during REM sleep, inhibiting muscle movement. Using an animal model, scientists have recently learned that this same group of neurons becomes inactive during cataplectic attacks, a discovery that provides a clue to at least one of the neurological abnormalities contributing to human narcoleptic symptoms.

Sleep Paralysis: The temporary inability to move or speak while falling asleep or waking up also parallels REM-induced inhibitions of voluntary muscle activity. This natural inhibition usually goes unnoticed by people who experience normal sleep because it occurs only when they are fully asleep and entering the REM stage at the appropriate time in the sleep cycle. Experiencing sleep paralysis resembles undergoing a cataplectic attack affecting the entire body. As with cataplexy, people remain fully conscious. Cataplexy and sleep paralysis are frightening events, especially when first experienced. Shocked by suddenly being unable to move, many patients fear that they may be permanently paralyzed or even dying. However, even when severe, cataplexy and sleep paralysis do not result in permanent dysfunction. After episodes end, people rapidly recover their full capacity to move and speak.

Hallucinations: Hallucinations can accompany sleep paralysis or can occur in isolation when people are falling asleep or waking up. Referred to as hypnagogic hallucinations when accompanying sleep onset and as hypnopompic hallucinations when occurring during awakening, these delusional experiences are unusually vivid and frequently frightening. Most often, the content is primarily visual, but any of the other senses can be involved. These hallucinations represent another intrusion of an element of REM sleep—dreaming—into the wakeful state.

When do symptoms appear?

In most cases, symptoms first appear when people are between the ages of ten and twenty-five but narcolepsy can become clinically apparent at virtually any age. Many patients first experience symptoms between the ages of thirty-five and forty-five. A smaller number initially manifest the disorder around the ages of fifty to fifty-five. Narcolepsy can also develop early in life, probably more frequently than is generally recognized. For example, three-year-old children have been diagnosed with the disorder. Whatever the age of onset, patients find that the symptoms tend to get worse over the two to three decades after the first symptoms appear. Many older patients find that some daytime symptoms decrease in severity after age sixty.

Narcoleptic symptoms, especially EDS, often prove more severe when the disorder develops early in life rather than during the adult years. Experts have also begun to recognize that narcolepsy sometimes contributes to certain childhood behavioral problems, such as attention-deficit hyperactivity disorder, and must be addressed before the behavioral problem can be resolved. If left undiagnosed and untreated, narcolepsy can pose special problems for children and adolescents, interfering with their psychological, social, and cognitive development and undermining their ability to succeed at school. For some young people, feelings of low self-esteem due to poor academic performance may persist into adulthood.

What causes narcolepsy?

The cause of narcolepsy remains unknown but during the past decade, scientists have made considerable progress in understanding its pathogenesis and in identifying genes strongly associated with the disorder. Researchers have also discovered abnormalities in various parts of the brain involved in regulating REM sleep that appear to contribute to symptom development. Experts now believe it is likely that—similar to many other complex, chronic neurological diseases— narcolepsy involves multiple factors interacting to cause neurological dysfunction and REM sleep disturbances.

A number of variant forms (alleles) of genes located in a region of chromosome 6 known as the HLA complex have proved to be strongly, although not invariably, associated with narcolepsy. The HLA complex comprises a large number of interrelated genes that regulate key aspects of immune-system function. The majority of people diagnosed with narcolepsy are known to have specific variants in certain HLA genes. However, these variations are neither necessary nor sufficient to cause the disorder. Some people with narcolepsy do not have the variant genes, while many people in the general population without narcolepsy do possess these variant genes. Thus it appears that specific variations in HLA genes increase an individual's predisposition to develop the disorder—possibly through a yet-undiscovered route involving changes in immune system function—when other causative factors are present.

Many other genes besides those making up the HLA complex may contribute to the development of narcolepsy. Groups of neurons in several parts of the brainstem and the central brain, including the thalamus and hypothalamus, interact to control sleep. Large numbers of genes on different chromosomes control these neurons' activities, any of which could contribute to development of the disease. Scientists studying narcolepsy in dogs have identified a mutation in a gene on chromosome 12 that appears to contribute to the disorder. This mutated gene disrupts the processing of a special class of neurotransmitters called hypocretins (also known as orexins) that are produced by neurons located in the hypothalamus. Neurotransmitters are special proteins that neurons produce to communicate with each other and to regulate biological processes. The neurons that produce hypocretins are active during wakefulness, and research suggests that they keep the brain systems needed for wakefulness from shutting down unexpectedly. Mice born without functioning hypocretin genes develop many symptoms of narcolepsy.

Except in rare cases, narcolepsy in humans is not associated with mutations of the hypocretin gene. However, scientists have found that brains from humans with narcolepsy often contain greatly reduced numbers of hypocretin-producing neurons. Certain HLA subtypes may increase susceptibility to an immune attack on hypocretin neurons in the hypothalamus, leading to degeneration of neurons in the hypocretin system. Other factors also may interfere with proper functioning of this system. The hypocretins regulate appetite and feeding behavior in addition to controlling sleep. Therefore, the loss of hypocretin-producing neurons may explain not only how narcolepsy develops in some people, but also why people with narcolepsy have higher rates of obesity compared to the general population.

Other factors appear to play important roles in the development of narcolepsy. Some rare cases are known to result from traumatic injuries to parts of the brain involved in REM sleep or from tumor growth and other disease processes in the same regions. Infections, exposure to toxins, dietary factors, stress, hormonal changes such as those occurring during puberty or menopause, and alterations in a person's sleep schedule are just a few of the many factors that may exert direct or indirect effects on the brain, thereby possibly contributing to disease development.

How is narcolepsy diagnosed?

Narcolepsy is not definitively diagnosed in most patients until ten to fifteen years after the first symptoms appear. This unusually long lag-time is due to several factors, including the disorder's subtle onset and the variability of symptoms. As important, however, is the fact that the public is largely unfamiliar with the disorder, as are many health professionals. When symptoms initially develop, people often do not recognize that they are experiencing the onset of a distinct neurological disorder and thus fail to seek medical treatment.

A clinical examination and exhaustive medical history are essential for diagnosis and treatment. However, none of the major symptoms is exclusive to narcolepsy. EDS—the most common of all narcoleptic symptoms—can result from a wide range of medical conditions, including other sleep disorders such as sleep apnea, various viral or bacterial infections, mood disorders such as depression, and painful chronic illnesses such as congestive heart failure and rheumatoid arthritis that disrupt normal sleep patterns. Various medications can also lead to EDS, as can consumption of caffeine, alcohol, and nicotine. Finally, sleep deprivation has become one of the most common causes of EDS among Americans.

This lack of specificity greatly increases the difficulty of arriving at an accurate diagnosis based on a consideration of symptoms alone. Thus, a battery of specialized tests, which can be performed in a sleep disorders clinic, is usually required before a diagnosis can be established.

Two tests in particular are considered essential in confirming a diagnosis of narcolepsy: the polysomnogram (PSG) and the multiple sleep latency test (MSLT). The PSG is an overnight test that takes continuous multiple measurements while a patient is asleep to document abnormalities in the sleep cycle. It records heart and respiratory rates, electrical activity in the brain through electroencephalography (EEG), and nerve activity in muscles through electromyography (EMG). A PSG can help reveal whether REM sleep occurs at abnormal times in the sleep cycle and can eliminate the possibility that an individual's symptoms result from another condition.

The MSLT is performed during the day to measure a person's tendency to fall asleep and to determine whether isolated elements of REM sleep intrude at inappropriate times during the waking hours. As part of the test, an individual is asked to take four or five short naps usually scheduled two hours apart over the course of a day. As the name suggests, the sleep latency test measures the amount of time it takes for a person to fall asleep. Because sleep latency periods are normally ten minutes or longer, a latency period of five minutes or less is considered suggestive of narcolepsy. The MSLT also measures heart and respiratory rates, records nerve activity in muscles, and pinpoints the occurrence of abnormally timed REM episodes through EEG recordings. If a person enters REM sleep either at the beginning or within a few minutes of sleep onset during at least two of the scheduled naps, this is also considered a positive indication of narcolepsy.

What treatments are available?

Narcolepsy cannot yet be cured. But EDS and cataplexy, the most disabling symptoms of the disorder, can be controlled in most patients with drug treatment. Often the treatment regimen is modified as symptoms change.

For decades, doctors have used central nervous system stimulants—amphetamines such as methylphenidate, dextroamphetamine, methamphetamine, and pemoline—to alleviate EDS and reduce the incidence of sleep attacks. For most patients these medications are generally quite effective at reducing daytime drowsiness and improving levels of alertness. However, they are associated with a wide array of undesirable side effects so their use must be carefully monitored. Common side effects include irritability and nervousness, shakiness, disturbances in heart rhythm, stomach upset, nighttime sleep disruption, and anorexia. Patients may also develop tolerance with long-term use, leading to the need for increased dosages to maintain effectiveness. In addition, doctors should be careful when prescribing these drugs and patients should be careful using them because the potential for abuse is high with any amphetamine.

In 1999, the FDA approved a new non-amphetamine wake-promoting drug called modafinil for the treatment of EDS. In clinical trials, modafinil proved to be effective in alleviating EDS while producing fewer, less serious side effects than do amphetamines. Headache is the most commonly reported adverse effect. Long-term use of modafinil does not appear to lead to tolerance.

Two classes of antidepressant drugs have proved effective in controlling cataplexy in many patients: tricyclics (including imipramine, desipramine, clomipramine, and protriptyline) and selective serotonin reuptake inhibitors (including fluoxetine and sertraline). In general, antidepressants produce fewer adverse effects than do amphetamines. Yet troublesome side effects still occur in some patients, including impotence, high blood pressure, and heart rhythm irregularities.

What behavioral strategies help people cope with symptoms?

None of the currently available medications enables people with narcolepsy to consistently maintain a fully normal state of alertness. Thus, drug therapy should be supplemented by various behavioral strategies according to the needs of the individual patient.

To gain greater control over their symptoms, many patients take short, regularly scheduled naps at times when they tend to feel sleepiest. Adults can often negotiate with employers to modify their work schedules so they can take naps when necessary and perform their most demanding tasks when they are most alert. The Americans with Disabilities Act requires employers to provide reasonable accommodations for all employees with disabilities. Children and adolescents with narcolepsy can be similarly accommodated through modifying class schedules and informing school personnel of special needs, including medication requirements during the school day.

Improving the quality of nighttime sleep can combat EDS and help relieve persistent feelings of fatigue. Among the most important common-sense measures patients can take to enhance sleep quality are: (1) maintaining a regular sleep schedule; (2) avoiding alcohol and caffeine-containing beverages for several hours before bedtime; (3) avoiding smoking, especially at night; (4) maintaining a comfortable, adequately warmed bedroom environment; and (5) engaging in relaxing activities such as a warm bath before bedtime. Exercising for at least twenty minutes per day at least four or five hours before bedtime also improves sleep quality and can help people with narcolepsy avoid gaining excess weight.

Safety precautions, particularly when driving, are of paramount importance for all persons with narcolepsy. Although the disorder, in itself, is not fatal, EDS and cataplexy can lead to serious injury or death if left uncontrolled. Suddenly falling asleep or losing muscle control can transform actions that are ordinarily safe, such as walking down a long flight of stairs, into hazards. People with untreated narcoleptic symptoms are involved in automobile accidents roughly ten times more frequently than the general population. However, accident rates are normal among patients who have received appropriate medication.

Finally, patient support groups frequently prove extremely beneficial because people with narcolepsy may become socially isolated due to embarrassment about their symptoms. Many patients also attempt to avoid experiencing strong emotions, since humor, excitement, and other intense feelings can trigger cataplectic attacks. Moreover, because of the widespread lack of public knowledge about the disorder, people with narcolepsy are too often unfairly judged to be lazy, unintelligent, undisciplined, or unmotivated. Such stigmatization often increases the tendency toward self-imposed isolation. The empathy and understanding that support groups offer people can be crucial to their overall sense of wellbeing and provide them with a network of social contacts who can offer practical help and emotional support.

What research is being done?

Within the federal government, the National Institute of Neurological Disorders and Stroke (NINDS), a component of the National Institutes of Health (NIH), has primary responsibility for sponsoring research on neurological disorders. As part of its mission, the NINDS supports research on narcolepsy and other sleep disorders with a neurological basis through grants to major medical institutions across the country.

Within the National Heart, Lung, and Blood Institute, also a component of the NIH, the National Center on Sleep Disorders Research (NCSDR) coordinates federal government sleep research activities and shares information with private and nonprofit groups. NCSDR staff also promote doctoral and postdoctoral training programs, and educate the public and health care professionals about sleep disorders.

NINDS-sponsored researchers are conducting studies devoted to further clarifying the wide range of genetic factors—both HLA genes and non-HLA genes—that may cause narcolepsy. Other scientists are conducting investigations using animal models to identify neurotransmitters other than the hypocretins that may contribute to disease development. A greater understanding of the complex genetic and biochemical bases of narcolepsy will eventually lead to the formulation of new therapies to control symptoms and may lead to a cure. Researchers are also investigating the modes of action of wake-promoting compounds to widen the range of available therapeutic options.

Scientists have long suspected that abnormal immunological processes may be an important element in the cause of narcolepsy, but until recently clear evidence supporting this suspicion has been lacking. NINDS-sponsored scientists have recently uncovered evidence demonstrating the presence of unusual, possibly pathological, forms of immunological activity in narcoleptic dogs. These researchers are now investigating whether drugs that suppress immunological processes may interrupt the development of narcolepsy in this animal model.

Recently there has been a growing awareness that narcolepsy can develop during childhood and may contribute to the development of behavior disorders. A group of NINDS-sponsored scientists is now conducting a large epidemiological study to determine the prevalence of narcolepsy in children aged two to fourteen years who have been diagnosed with attention-deficit hyperactivity disorder.

Finally, the NINDS continues to support investigations into the basic biology of sleep, including the brain mechanisms involved in generating and regulating REM sleep. Scientists are now examining physiological processes occurring in a portion of the hindbrain called the amygdala in order to uncover novel biochemical processes underlying REM sleep. A more comprehensive understanding of the complex biology of sleep will undoubtedly further clarify the pathological processes that underlie narcolepsy and other sleep disorders.

Part Six

Additional
Help and Information

Chapter 24

Glossary of Brain-Related Terms

Absence epilepsy: Epilepsy in which the person has repeated absence seizures.

Absence seizures: The type of seizure seen in absence epilepsy, in which the person experiences a momentary loss in consciousness. The person may stare into space for several seconds and may have some twitching or jerking of muscles.

Accessible tumor: A tumor that can be reached and removed using surgical tools without unreasonable risk of severe damage.

Acetylcholine: A neurotransmitter that is important for the formation of memories. Studies have shown that levels of acetylcholine are reduced in the brains of people with Alzheimer's disease.

ACTH (adrenocorticotropic hormone): A substance that can be used to treat infantile spasms.

The terms in this glossary were excerpted from the following publications from the National Institute of Neurological Disorders and Stroke: "Multiple Sclerosis: Hope through Research" (2004); "Huntington's Disease: Hope through Research" (2004); "Traumatic Brain Injury: Hope through Research" (2004); "The Dementias: Hope through Research" (2004); "Cerebral Palsy: Hope through Research" (2004); "Stroke: Hope through Research" (2004); "Seizures and Epilepsy: Hope through Research" (2004); "Brain and Spinal Cord Tumors: Hope through Research" (2004); "Headache: Hope through Research" (2004); and "Parkinson's Disease: Hope through Research" (2004).

Acute stroke: A stage of stroke starting at the onset of symptoms and lasting for a few hours thereafter.

Agnosia: A cognitive disability characterized by ignorance of or inability to acknowledge one side of the body or one side of the visual field.

Akinesia: Decreased body movements.

Alzheimer's disease: The most common cause of dementia in people aged sixty-five and older. Nearly all brain functions, including memory, movement, language, judgment, behavior, and abstract thinking, are eventually affected.

Amyloid plaques: Unusual clumps of material found in the tissue between nerve cells, a hallmark of Alzheimer's disease.

Amyloid precursor protein: A normal brain protein that is a precursor for beta amyloid, the abnormal substance found in the characteristic amyloid plaques of Alzheimer's disease patients.

Anaplastic: Cancerous, malignant.

Aneurysm: A weak or thin spot on an artery wall that has stretched or ballooned out from the wall and filled with blood, or damage to an artery leading to pooling of blood between the layers of the blood vessel walls.

Angiography: An imaging technique that provides an x-ray picture, called an angiogram, of blood vessels.

Anoxia: An absence of oxygen supply to an organ's tissues leading to cell death.

Antibodies: Proteins made by the immune system that bind to structures (antigens) they recognize as foreign to the body.

Anticoagulants: A drug therapy used to prevent the formation of blood clots that can become lodged in cerebral arteries and cause strokes.

Antigen: A structure foreign to the body, such as a virus. The body usually responds to antigens by producing antibodies.

Antiplatelet agents: A type of anticoagulant drug therapy that prevents the formation of blood clots by preventing the accumulation of platelets that form the basis of blood clots; some common antiplatelets include aspirin and ticlopidine.

Antithrombotics: A type of anticoagulant drug therapy that prevents the formation of blood clots by inhibiting the coagulating actions of the blood protein thrombin; some common antithrombotics include warfarin and heparin.

Apgar score: A numbered score doctors use to assess a baby's physical state at the time of birth.

Aphasia: The inability to understand or create speech, writing, or language in general due to damage to the speech centers of the brain.

Apolipoprotein E: A gene that has been linked to an increased risk of Alzheimer's disease. People with a variant form of the gene, called apoE epsilon 4, have about ten times the risk of developing Alzheimer's disease.

Apoplexy: A historical, but obsolete term for a cerebral stroke, most often intracerebral hemorrhage, that was applied to any condition that involved disorientation or paralysis.

Apoptosis: Cell death that occurs naturally as part of normal development, maintenance, and renewal of tissues within an organism.

Apraxia: A movement disorder characterized by the inability to perform skilled or purposeful voluntary movements, generally caused by damage to the areas of the brain responsible for voluntary movement.

Arachnoid membrane: One of the three membranes that cover the brain; it is between the pia mater and the dura. Collectively, these three membranes form the meninges.

Arteriography: An x-ray of the carotid artery taken when a special dye is injected into the artery.

Arteriovenous malformation (AVM): A congenital disorder characterized by a complex tangled web of arteries and veins.

Asphyxia: Lack of oxygen due to trouble with breathing or poor oxygen supply in the air.

Ataxia: A condition in which the muscles fail to function in a coordinated manner.

Atherosclerosis: A blood vessel disease characterized by the buildup of plaque, or deposits of fatty substances and other matter in the inner lining of an artery.

Atonic seizures: Seizures that cause a sudden loss of muscle tone, also called drop attacks.

Aura (epileptic): Unusual sensations or movements that warn of an impending, more severe seizure. These auras are actually simple focal seizures in which the person maintains consciousness.

Aura (migraine): A symptom of classic migraine headache in which the patient sees flashing lights or zigzag lines, or may temporarily lose vision

Autoimmune disease: A disease in which the body's defense system malfunctions and attacks a part of the body itself rather than foreign matter.

Automatisms: Strange, repetitious behaviors that occur during a seizure. Automatisms may include blinks, twitches, mouth movements, or even walking in a circle.

Autosomal dominant disorder: A non-sex-linked disorder that can be inherited even if only one parent passes on the defective gene.

Basal ganglia: A region located at the base of the brain composed of four clusters of neurons, or nerve cells. This area is responsible for body movement and coordination. The neuron groups most prominently and consistently affected by Huntington Disease—the pallidum and striatum—are located here. See neuron, pallidum, striatum.

Basilar artery migraine: Migraine, occurring primarily in young women and often associated with the menstrual cycle, that involves a disturbance of a major brain artery. Symptoms include vertigo, double vision, and poor muscular coordination.

Benign: Nonmalignant or noncancerous. Often used to describe tumor cells that are similar to other normal cells, grow relatively slowly, and are confined to one location.

Benign exertional headache: Headache brought on by running, lifting, coughing, sneezing, or bending.

Benign infantile encephalopathy: A type of epilepsy syndrome that occurs in infants. It is considered benign because it does not seem to impair cognitive functions or development.

Benign neonatal convulsions: A type of epilepsy syndrome in newborns that does not seem to impair cognitive functions or development.

Beta amyloid: A protein found in the characteristic clumps of tissue (called plaques) that appear in the brains of Alzheimer's patients.

Binswanger disease: A rare form of dementia characterized by damage to small blood vessels in the white matter of the brain. This damage leads to brain lesions, loss of memory, disordered cognition, and mood changes.

Biofeedback: A technique in which patients are trained to gain some voluntary control over certain physiological conditions, such as blood pressure and muscle tension, to promote relaxation. Thermal biofeedback helps patients consciously raise hand temperature, which can sometimes reduce the number and intensity of migraines.

Biopsy: Diagnostic test in which a sample of a patient's tissue is examined for disease.

Blood-brain barrier: An elaborate meshwork of fine blood vessels and cells that filters blood reaching the central nervous system.

Bradykinesia: Gradual loss of spontaneous movement.

Brain death: An irreversible cessation of measurable brain function.

Broca's aphasia: See nonfluent aphasia.

CADASIL: A rare hereditary disorder which is linked to a type of vascular dementia. It stands for cerebral autosomal dominant arteriopathy with subcortical infarct and leukoencephalopathy.

Carotid artery: An artery, located on either side of the neck, that supplies the brain with blood.

Carotid endarterectomy: Surgery used to remove fatty deposits from the carotid arteries.

Caudate nuclei: Part of the striatum in the basal ganglia. See basal ganglia, striatum.

Celiac disease: An intolerance to wheat gluten in foods that can lead to seizures and other symptoms.

Central nervous system (CNS): The brain and spinal cord.

Central stroke pain (central pain syndrome): Pain caused by damage to an area in the thalamus. The pain is a mixture of sensations, including heat and cold, burning, tingling, numbness, and sharp stabbing and underlying aching pain.

Cerebral: Relating to the two hemispheres of the human brain.

Cerebral blood flow (CBF): The flow of blood through the arteries that lead to the brain, called the cerebrovascular system.

Cerebrospinal fluid (CSF): The fluid that bathes and protects the brain and spinal cord.

Cerebrovascular disease: A reduction in the supply of blood to the brain either by narrowing of the arteries through the buildup of plaque on the inside walls of the arteries, called stenosis, or through blockage of an artery due to a blood clot.

Cholesterol: A waxy substance, produced naturally by the liver and also found in foods, that circulates in the blood and helps maintain tissues and cell membranes. Excess cholesterol in the body can contribute to atherosclerosis and high blood pressure.

Cholinesterase inhibitors: Drugs that slow the breakdown of the neurotransmitter acetylcholine.

Chorea: Uncontrolled body movements. Chorea is derived from the Greek word for dance.

Chromosomes: The structures in cells that contain genes. They are composed of deoxyribonucleic acid (DNA) and proteins and, under a microscope, appear as rod-like structures. See deoxyribonucleic acid (DNA), gene.

Clonic seizures: Seizures that cause repeated jerking movements of muscles on both sides of the body.

Closed head injury: An injury that occurs when the head suddenly and violently hits an object but the object does not break through the skull.

Clipping: Surgical procedure for treatment of brain aneurysms, involving clamping an aneurysm from a blood vessel, surgically removing this ballooned part of the blood vessel, and closing the opening in the artery wall.

Cluster headaches: Intensely painful headaches, occurring suddenly and lasting between thirty and forty-five minutes, named for their repeated occurrence in groups or clusters. They begin as minor pain around one eye and eventually spread to that side of the face.

Cognitive training: A type of training in which patients practice tasks designed to improve mental performance. Examples include memory aids, such as mnemonics, and computerized recall devices.

Coma: A state of profound unconsciousness caused by disease, injury, or poison.

Complex focal seizures: Seizures in which only one part of the brain is affected, but the person has a change in or loss of consciousness.

Compressive cranial neuropathies: Degeneration of nerves in the brain caused by pressure on those nerves.

Computed tomography (CT): A scan that creates a series of cross-sectional x-rays of the head and brain; also called computerized axial tomography or CAT scan.

Concussion: Injury to the brain caused by a hard blow or violent shaking, causing a sudden and temporary impairment of brain function, such as a short loss of consciousness or disturbance of vision and equilibrium.

Congenital tumor: An abnormal growth present at birth.

Contracture: A condition in which muscles become fixed in a rigid, abnormal position causing distortion or deformity.

Contrecoup: A contusion caused by the shaking of the brain back and forth within the confines of the skull.

Contusion: Distinct area of swollen brain tissue mixed with blood released from broken blood vessels.

Convulsions: Sudden contractions of the muscles that may be caused by seizures.

Corpus callosotomy: Surgery that severs the corpus callosum, or network of neural connections between the right and left hemispheres of the brain.

Corpus striatum: A part of the brain that helps regulate motor activities.

Cortex: Part of the brain responsible for thought, perception, and memory.

Cortical atrophy: Degeneration of the brain's cortex (outer layer). Cortical atrophy is common in many forms of dementia and may be visible on a brain scan.

Cortical dementia: A type of dementia in which the damage primarily occurs in the brain's cortex, or outer layer.

Corticobasal degeneration: A progressive disorder characterized by nerve cell loss and atrophy in multiple areas of the brain.

Creutzfeldt-Jakob disease: A rare, degenerative, fatal brain disorder believed to be linked to an abnormal form of a protein called a prion.

Cryothalamotomy: A surgical procedure in which a supercooled probe is inserted into a part of the brain called the thalamus in order to stop tremors.

CSF fistula: A tear between two of the three membranes—the dura and arachnoid membranes—that encase the brain.

CT (computed tomography): A type of brain scan that reveals the structure of the brain.

Cytokines: Small, hormone-like proteins released by leukocytes, endothelial cells, and other cells to promote an inflammatory immune response to an injury.

Cytotoxic edema: A state of cell compromise involving influx of fluids and toxic chemicals into a cell causing subsequent swelling of the cell.

Deep vein thrombosis: Formation of a blood clot deep within a vein.

Dementia: A term for a collection of symptoms that significantly impair thinking and normal activities and relationships.

Dementia pugilistica: A form of dementia caused by head trauma such as that experienced by boxers. It is also called chronic traumatic encephalopathy or Boxer's syndrome.

Demyelination: Damage caused to myelin by recurrent attacks of inflammation. Demyelination ultimately results in nervous system scars, called plaques, which interrupt communications between the nerves and the rest of the body.

Deoxyribonucleic acid (DNA): The substance of heredity containing the genetic information necessary for cells to divide and produce proteins. DNA carries the code for every inherited characteristic of an organism. See gene.

Depressed skull fracture: A fracture occurring when pieces of broken skull press into the tissues of the brain.

Detachable coil: A platinum coil that is inserted into an artery in the thigh and strung through the arteries to the site of an aneurysm. The coil is released into the aneurysm, creating an immune response from the body. The body produces a blood clot inside the aneurysm, strengthening the artery walls and reducing the risk of rupture.

Diffuse axonal injury: See shearing.

Dihydroergotamine: A drug that is given by injection to treat cluster headaches. It is a form of the antimigraine drug ergotamine tartrate.

Dominant: A trait that is apparent even when the gene for that disorder is inherited from only one parent. See autosomal dominant disorder, recessive, gene.

Dopamine: A chemical messenger, deficient in the brains of Parkinson disease patients, that transmits impulses from one nerve cell to another.

Drop attacks: Seizures that cause sudden falls; another term for atonic seizures.

Duplex Doppler ultrasound: A diagnostic imaging technique in which an image of an artery can be formed by bouncing sound waves off the moving blood in the artery and measuring the frequency changes of the echoes.

Dura: A tough, fibrous membrane lining the brain; the outermost of the three membranes collectively called the meninges.

Dysarthria: Problems with speaking caused by difficulty moving or coordinating the muscles needed for speech.

Dyskinesias: Abnormal involuntary movements that can result from long-term use of high doses of levodopa.

Dysphagia: Trouble eating and swallowing.

Dysplasia: Areas of misplaced or abnormally formed neurons in the brain.

Early myoclonic encephalopathy: A type of epilepsy syndrome that usually includes neurological and developmental problems.

Early seizures: Seizures that occur within one week after a traumatic brain injury.

Eclampsia: A life-threatening condition that can develop in pregnant women. Its symptoms include sudden elevations of blood pressure and seizures.

Edema: The swelling of a cell that results from the influx of large amounts of water or fluid into the cell.

Electroencephalogram (EEG): A medical procedure that records patterns of electrical activity in the brain.

Electromyography (EMG): A special recording technique that detects electric activity in muscle. Patients are sometimes offered a type of biofeedback called EMG training, in which they learn to control muscle tension in the face, neck, and shoulders.

Embolic stroke: A stroke caused by an embolus.

Embolus: A free-roaming clot that usually forms in the heart.

Endorphins: Naturally occurring painkilling chemicals. Some scientists theorize that people who suffer from severe headache have lower levels of endorphins than people who are generally pain free.

Endothelial wall: A flat layer of cells that make up the innermost lining of a blood vessel.

Epidural hematoma: Bleeding into the area between the skull and the dura.

Epilepsy syndromes: Disorders with a specific set of symptoms that include epilepsy.

Ergotamine tartrate: A drug that is used to control the painful dilation stage of migraine.

Erosive gastritis: Inflammation and degeneration of the tissues of the stomach.

Excitatory amino acids: A subset of neurotransmitters; proteins released by one neuron into the space between two neurons to promote an excitatory state in the other neuron.

Excitatory neurotransmitters: Nerve signaling chemicals that increase activity in neurons.

Experimental allergic encephalomyelitis (EAE): A chronic brain and spinal cord disease similar to MS which is induced by injecting myelin basic protein into laboratory animals.

Extracranial/intracranial (EC/IC) bypass: A type of surgery that restores blood flow to a blood-deprived area of brain tissue by rerouting a healthy artery in the scalp to the area of brain tissue affected by a blocked artery.

Failure to thrive: A condition characterized by lag in physical growth and development.

Fatal familial insomnia: An inherited disease that affects a brain region called the thalamus, which is partially responsible for controlling sleep. The disease causes dementia and a progressive insomnia that eventually leads to a complete lack of sleep.

Fatigue: Tiredness that may accompany activity or may persist even without exertion.

Febrile seizures: Seizures in infants and children that are associated with a high fever.

Festination: A symptom characterized by small, quick forward steps.

Fluent aphasia: A condition in which patients display little meaning in their speech even though they speak in complete sentences. Also called Wernicke or motor aphasia.

Focal seizures: Seizures that occur in just one part of the brain.

Frontal lobe epilepsy: A type of epilepsy that originates in the frontal lobe of the brain. It usually involves a cluster of short seizures with a sudden onset and termination.

Frontotemporal dementias: A group of dementias characterized by degeneration of nerve cells, especially those in the frontal and temporal lobes of the brain.

FTDP-17: One of the frontotemporal dementias, linked to a mutation in the tau gene. It is much like other types of the frontotemporal dementias but often includes psychiatric symptoms such as delusions and hallucinations.

Functional magnetic resonance imaging (fMRI): A type of imaging that measures increases in blood flow within the brain.

GABA (gamma-aminobutyric acid): An inhibitory neurotransmitter that plays a role in some types of epilepsy.

Gadolinium: A chemical compound given during MRI scans that helps distinguish new lesions from old.

Gait analysis: A technique that uses camera recording, force plates, electromyography, and computer analysis to objectively measure an individual's pattern of walking.

Gastrostomy: A surgical procedure to create an artificial opening in the stomach.

Gene: The basic unit of heredity, composed of a segment of DNA containing the code for a specific trait. See deoxyribonucleic acid (DNA).

Generalized seizures: Seizures that result from abnormal neuronal activity in many parts of the brain. These seizures may cause loss of consciousness, falls, or massive muscle spasms.

Gerstmann-Straussler-Scheinker disease: A rare, fatal hereditary disease that causes ataxia and progressive dementia.

Glasgow Coma Scale: A clinical tool used to assess the degree of consciousness and neurological functioning—and therefore severity of brain injury—by testing motor responsiveness, verbal acuity, and eye opening.

Glia: Also called neuroglia; supportive cells of the nervous system that make up the blood-brain barrier, provide nutrients and oxygen to the vital neurons, and protect the neurons from infection, toxicity, and trauma. Some examples of glia are oligodendroglia, astrocytes, and microglia.

Global aphasia: A condition in which patients suffer severe communication disabilities as a result of extensive damage to portions of the brain responsible for language.

Glutamate: Also known as glutamic acid, an amino acid that acts as an excitatory neurotransmitter in the brain.

Grand mal seizures: An older term for tonic-clonic seizures.

Hematoma: Heavy bleeding into or around the brain caused by damage to a major blood vessel in the head.

Hemianopia: Defective vision or blindness that impairs half of the normal field of vision.

Hemiparesis: Weakness on one side of the body.

Hemiparetic tremors: Uncontrollable shaking affecting the limbs on the spastic side of the body in those who have spastic hemiplegia.

Hemiplegia: Paralysis on one side of the body.

Hemiplegic migraine: A type of migraine causing temporary paralysis on one side of the body (hemiplegia)

Hemispheres: The right and left halves of the brain.

Hemorrhagic stroke: Stroke caused by bleeding out of one of the major arteries leading to the brain.

Heparin: A type of anticoagulant.

High-density lipoprotein (HDL): Also known as the good cholesterol; a compound consisting of a lipid and a protein that carries a small percentage of the total cholesterol in the blood and deposits it in the liver.

Hippocampus: A brain structure important for memory and learning.

HIV-associated dementia: A dementia that results from infection with the human immunodeficiency virus (HIV) that causes AIDS. It can cause widespread destruction of the brain's white matter.

Homeostasis: A state of equilibrium or balance among various fluids and chemicals in a cell, in tissues, or in the body as a whole.

Human leukocyte antigens (HLAs): Antigens, tolerated by the body, that correspond to genes that govern immune responses.

Huntington disease: A degenerative hereditary disorder caused by a faulty gene for a protein called huntington. The disease causes degeneration in many regions of the brain and spinal cord and patients eventually develop severe dementia.

Hydrocephalus: Abnormal accumulation of cerebrospinal fluid within the skull.

Hypermetabolism: A condition in which the body produces too much heat energy.

Hypertension (high blood pressure): Characterized by persistently high arterial blood pressure defined as a measurement greater than or equal to 140 mm/Hg systolic pressure over 90 mm/Hg diastolic pressure.

Hypertonia: Increased tone.

Hypothyroidism: Decreased production of thyroid hormone leading to low metabolic rate, weight gain, chronic drowsiness, dry skin and hair, and fluid accumulation and retention in connective tissues.

Hypotonia: Decreased tone.

Hypoxia: A state of decreased oxygen delivery to a cell so that the oxygen falls below normal levels; see anoxia.

Hypoxic-ischemic encephalopathy: Brain damage caused by poor blood flow or insufficient oxygen supply to the brain.

Idiopathic epilepsy: Epilepsy with an unknown cause.

Immediate seizures: Seizures that occur within twenty-four hours of a traumatic brain injury.

Immunoglobulin G (IgG): An antibody-containing substance produced by human plasma cells in diseased central nervous system plaques. Levels of IgG are increased in the cerebrospinal fluid of most multiple sclerosis patients.

Immunosuppression: Suppression of immune system functions. Many medications under investigation for the treatment of multiple sclerosis are immunosuppressants.

Inaccessible or inoperable tumor: A tumor that cannot be reached surgically without unreasonable risk of severe damage to nearby tissue.

Incidence: The extent or frequency of an occurrence; the number of specific new events in a given period of time.

Infantile spasms: Clusters of seizures that usually begin before the age of six months. During these seizures the infant may bend and cry out.

Infarct: An area of tissue that is dead or dying because of a loss of blood supply.

Infarction: A sudden loss of blood supply to tissue, causing the formation of an infarct.

Inflammatory headache: A headache that is a symptom of another disorder, such as sinus infection, and is treated by curing the underlying problem.

Inhibitory neurotransmitters: Nerve signaling chemicals that decrease activity in neurons.

Interferons: Cytokines belonging to a family of antiviral proteins that occur naturally in the body. Gamma interferon is produced by immune system cells, enhances T-cell recognition of antigens, and causes worsening of multiple sclerosis symptoms. Alpha and beta interferon probably exert a suppressive effect on the immune system and may be beneficial in the treatment of multiple sclerosis.

Interleukins: A group of cytokine-related proteins secreted by leukocytes and involved in the inflammatory immune response of the ischemic cascade.

Intracerebral hematoma: Bleeding within the brain caused by damage to a major blood vessel.

Intracerebral hemorrhage: Occurs when a vessel within the brain leaks blood into the brain.

Intracranial pressure: Buildup of pressure in the brain as a result of injury.

Intractable: About 20 percent of people with epilepsy will continue to experience seizures even with the best available treatment.

Ion channels: Molecular "gates" that control the flow of ions in and out of cells and regulate neuron signaling.

Ischemia: A loss of blood flow to tissue, caused by an obstruction of the blood vessel, usually in the form of plaque stenosis or a blood clot.

Ischemic cascade: A series of events lasting for several hours to several days following initial ischemia that results in extensive cell death and tissue damage beyond the area of tissue originally affected by the initial lack of blood flow.

Ischemic penumbra: Areas of damaged, but still living, brain cells arranged in a patchwork pattern around areas of dead brain cells.

Ischemic stroke: Stroke caused by the formation of a clot that blocks blood flow through an artery to the brain.

Jaundice: A blood disorder caused by the abnormal buildup of bile pigments in the bloodstream.

Juvenile myoclonic epilepsy: A type of epilepsy characterized by sudden myoclonic jerks that usually begins in childhood or adolescence.

Ketogenic diet: A strict diet rich in fats and low in carbohydrates that causes the body to break down fats instead of carbohydrates to survive.

Kindling: A phenomenon in which a small change in neuronal activity, if it is repeated, can eventually lead to full-blown epilepsy.

Lacunar infarction: Occlusion of a small artery in the brain resulting in a small area of dead brain tissue, called a lacunar infarct; often caused by stenosis of the small arteries, called small vessel disease.

Lafora disease: A severe, progressive form of epilepsy that begins in childhood and has been linked to a gene that helps to break down carbohydrates.

Large vessel disease: Stenosis in large arteries of the cerebrovascular system.

Lennox-Gastaut syndrome: A type of epilepsy that begins in childhood and usually causes several different kinds of seizures, including absence seizures.

Lesion: An abnormal change in the structure of an organ due to disease or injury.

Lesionectomy: Removal of a specific brain lesion.

Leukocytes: Blood proteins involved in the inflammatory immune response of the ischemic cascade.

Lewy body dementia: One of the most common types of progressive dementia, characterized by the presence of abnormal structures called Lewy bodies in the brain. In many ways the symptoms of this disease overlap with those of Alzheimer's disease.

Lipoprotein: Small globules of cholesterol covered by a layer of protein; produced by the liver.

Lobectomy: Removal of a lobe of the brain.

Locked-in syndrome: A condition in which a patient is aware and awake, but cannot move or communicate due to complete paralysis of the body.

Low-density lipoprotein (LDL): Also known as the bad cholesterol; a compound consisting of a lipid and a protein that carries the majority of the total cholesterol in the blood and deposits the excess along the inside of arterial walls.

Lumbar puncture: A diagnostic procedure in which a sample of cerebrospinal fluid is removed from the spinal cord using a needle.

Magnetic resonance angiography (MRA): An imaging technique involving injection of a contrast dye into a blood vessel and using magnetic resonance techniques to create an image of the flowing blood through the vessel; often used to detect stenosis of the brain arteries inside the skull.

Magnetic resonance imaging (MRI): An imaging technique that uses radiowaves, magnetic fields, and computer analysis to create a picture of body tissues and structures.

Magnetic resonance spectroscopy (MRS): A type of brain scan that can detect abnormalities in the brain's biochemical processes.

Magnetoencephalogram (MEG): A type of brain scan that detects the magnetic signals generated by neurons to allow doctors to monitor brain activity at different points in the brain over time, revealing different brain functions.

Malignant: Harmful, cancerous. Often used to describe tumor cells that are very different from normal cells, grow relatively quickly, and can easily spread to other locations.

Marker: A piece of DNA that lies on the chromosome so close to a gene that the two are inherited together. Like a signpost, markers are used during genetic testing and research to locate the nearby presence of a gene. See chromosome, deoxyribonucleic acid (DNA).

Meninges: Membranes that cover the brain and spinal cord.

Meningitis: Inflammation of the three membranes that envelop the brain and spinal cord, collectively known as the meninges; the meninges include the dura, pia mater, and arachnoid.

Metabolized: Broken down or otherwise transformed by the body.

Metastatic tumors: Tumors caused by cancerous cells that have spread from other parts of the body.

Migraine: A vascular headache believed to be caused by blood flow changes and certain chemical changes in the brain leading to a cascade of events—including constriction of arteries supplying blood to the brain and the release of certain brain chemicals—that result in severe head pain, stomach upset, and visual disturbances.

Mild cognitive impairment: A condition associated with impairments in understanding and memory not severe enough to be diagnosed as dementia, but more pronounced than those associated with normal aging.

Mini-Mental State Examination: A test used to assess cognitive skills in people with suspected dementia. The test examines orientation, memory, and attention, as well as the ability to name objects, follow verbal and written commands, write a sentence spontaneously, and copy a complex shape.

Mitochondria: Microscopic, energy-producing bodies within cells that are the cells' "power plants."

Motor aphasia: See nonfluent aphasia.

Multi-infarct dementia: A type of vascular dementia caused by numerous small strokes in the brain.

Multiple sub-pial transection: A type of operation in which surgeons make a series of cuts in the brain that are designed to prevent seizures from spreading into other parts of the brain while leaving the person's normal abilities intact.

Muscle-contraction headaches: Headaches caused primarily by sustained muscle tension or, possibly, by restricted blood flow to the brain. Two forms of muscle-contraction headache are tension headache, induced by stress, and chronic muscle-contraction headache, which can last for extended periods, involves steady pain, and is usually felt on both sides of the head.

Mutation: In genetics, any defect in a gene. See gene.

Myelin basic protein (MBP): A major component of myelin. When myelin breakdown occurs (as in multiple sclerosis), MBP can often be found in abnormally high levels in the patient's cerebrospinal fluid. When injected into laboratory animals, MBP induces experimental allergic encephalomyelitis, a chronic brain and spinal cord disease similar to multiple sclerosis.

Myelin: A fatty covering insulating nerve cell fibers in the brain and spinal cord, myelin facilitates the smooth, high-speed transmission of electrochemical messages between these components of the central nervous system and the rest of the body. In multiple sclerosis, myelin is damaged through a process known as demyelination, which results in distorted or blocked signals.

Myelogram: A diagnostic test that uses injected dye and x-rays to create a picture of the spinal cord.

Myoclonic seizures: Seizures that cause sudden jerks or twitches, especially in the upper body, arms, or legs.

Myoclonus: A condition in which muscles or portions of muscles contract involuntarily in a jerky fashion.

Near-infrared spectroscopy: A technique that can detect oxygen levels in brain tissue.

Necrosis: A form of cell death resulting from anoxia, trauma, or any other form of irreversible damage to the cell; involves the release of toxic cellular material into the intercellular space, poisoning surrounding cells.

Neocortical epilepsy: Epilepsy that originates in the brain's cortex, or outer layer. Seizures can be either focal or generalized, and may cause strange sensations, hallucinations, or emotional changes.

Neonatal hemorrhage: Bleeding of brain blood vessels in the newborn.

Neoplasms: New, abnormal growths in the body.

Neural stem cells: Cells found only in adult neural tissue that can develop into several different cell types in the central nervous system.

Neurocysticercosis: A parasitic infection of the brain that can cause seizures.

Neuroexcitation: The electrical activation of cells in the brain; neuroexcitation is part of the normal functioning of the brain or can also be the result of abnormal activity related to an injury.

Neurofibrillary tangles: Bundles of twisted filaments found within neurons, and a characteristic feature found in the brains of Alzheimer's patients. These tangles are largely made up of a protein called tau.

Neuron: Greek word for a nerve cell, the basic impulse-conducting unit of the nervous system. Nerve cells communicate with other cells through an electrochemical process called neurotransmission. Consists of a cell body, an axon, and dendrites.

Neuroprotective agents: Medications that protect the brain from secondary injury caused by stroke.

Neurotransmitter: A type of chemical, such as acetylcholine, that transmits signals from one neuron to another. People with Alzheimer's disease have reduced supplies of acetylcholine.

Nociceptors: The endings of pain-sensitive nerves that, when stimulated by stress, muscular tension, dilated blood vessels, or other triggers, send messages up the nerve fibers to nerve cells in the brain, signaling that a part of the body hurts.

Nonconvulsive: Any type of seizure that does not include violent muscle contractions.

Nonepileptic events: Any phenomena that look like seizures but do not result from abnormal brain activity. Nonepileptic events may include psychogenic seizures or symptoms of medical conditions such as sleep disorders, Tourette syndrome, or cardiac arrhythmia.

Nonfluent aphasia: A condition in which patients have trouble recalling words and speaking in complete sentences. Also called Broca's or motor aphasia.

Oligodendrocytes: A type of support cell in the brain that produces myelin, the fatty sheath that surrounds and insulates axons.

On-off effect: A change in the patient's condition, with sometimes rapid fluctuations between uncontrolled movements and normal movement, usually occurring after long-term use of levodopa and probably caused by changes in the ability to respond to this drug.

Ophthalmoplegic migraine: A form of migraine felt around the eye and associated with a droopy eyelid, double vision, and other sight problems.

Optic neuritis: An inflammatory disorder of the optic nerve that usually occurs in only one eye and causes visual loss and sometimes blindness. It is generally temporary.

Organic brain syndrome: A term that refers to physical disorders (not psychiatric in origin) that impair mental functions.

Orthotic devices: Special devices, such as splints or braces, used to treat problems of the muscles, ligaments, or bones of the skeletal system.

Oxygen-free radicals: Toxic chemicals released during the process of cellular respiration and released in excessive amounts during necrosis of a cell; involved in secondary cell death associated with the ischemic cascade.

Pallidotomy: A surgical procedure in which a part of the brain called the globus pallidus is lesioned in order to improve symptoms of tremor, rigidity, and bradykinesia.

Pallidum: Part of the basal ganglia of the brain. The pallidum is composed of the globus pallidus and the ventral pallidum. See basal ganglia.

Palsy: Paralysis, or problems in the control of voluntary movement.

Paresis or plegia: Weakness or paralysis. In cerebral palsy, these terms are typically combined with another phrase that describes the distribution of paralysis and weakness, e.g., paraparesis.

Paresthesias: Abnormal sensations such as numbness, prickling, or "pins and needles."

Parkinsonism: A term referring to a group of conditions that are characterized by four typical symptoms—tremor, rigidity, postural instability, and bradykinesia.

Parkinson's dementia: A secondary dementia that sometimes occurs in people with advanced Parkinson's disease, which is primarily a movement disorder. Many Parkinson's patients have the characteristic amyloid plaques and neurofibrillary tangles found in Alzheimer's disease, but it is not yet clear if the diseases are linked.

Partial seizures: Another term used to describe focal seizures, those that occur in just one part of the brain.

Penetrating head injury: A brain injury in which an object pierces the skull and enters the brain tissue.

Persistent vegetative state: An ongoing state of severely impaired consciousness, in which the patient is incapable of voluntary motion.

Petit mal seizures: An older term for absence seizures.

Photosensitive epilepsy: Epilepsy with seizures triggered by flickering or flashing lights. It also may be called photic epilepsy or photogenic epilepsy.

Pick's disease: A type of frontotemporal dementia where certain nerve cells become abnormal and swollen before they die. The brains of people with Pick's disease have abnormal structures, called Pick bodies, inside the neurons. The symptoms are very similar to those of Alzheimer's disease.

Plaque: Fatty cholesterol deposits found along the inside of artery walls that lead to atherosclerosis and stenosis of the arteries.

Plaques: patchy areas of inflammation and demyelination typical of multiple sclerosis, plaques disrupt or block nerve signals that would normally pass through the regions affected by the plaques; unusual clumps of material found between the tissues of the brain in Alzheimer's disease. See also amyloid plaques.

Plasticity: The ability to be formed or molded; in reference to the brain, the ability to adapt to deficits and injury.

Platelets: Structures found in blood that are known primarily for their role in blood coagulation.

Pneumocephalus: A condition in which air or gas is trapped within the intracranial cavity.

Positron emission tomography (PET): A tool used to diagnose brain functions and disorders. PET produces three-dimensional, colored images of chemicals or substances functioning within the body. These images are called PET scans. PET shows brain function, in contrast to CT or MRI, which show brain structure.

Post-concussion syndrome (PCS): A complex, poorly understood problem that may cause headache after head injury; in most cases, patients cannot remember the event that caused the concussion and a variable period of time prior to the injury.

Post-traumatic amnesia (PTA): A state of acute confusion due to a traumatic brain injury, marked by difficulty with perception, thinking, remembering, and concentration; during this acute stage, patients often cannot form new memories.

Post-traumatic dementia: A dementia brought on by a single traumatic brain injury. It is much like dementia pugilistica, but usually also includes long-term memory problems.

Post-traumatic epilepsy: Recurrent seizures occurring more than one week after a traumatic brain injury.

Postural instability: Impaired balance and coordination, often causing patients to lean forward or backward and to fall easily.

Prednisone: A drug that can be used to treat infantile spasms.

Presenilin 1 and 2: Proteins produced by genes that influence susceptibility to early-onset Alzheimer's disease.

Prevalence: The number of cases of a disease that are present in a particular population at a given time.

Primary dementia: A dementia, such as Alzheimer's disease, that is not the result of another disease.

Primary progressive aphasia: A type of frontotemporal dementia resulting in deficits in language functions. Many, but not all, people with this type of aphasia eventually develop symptoms of dementia.

Primary tumors: As opposed to metastatic tumors, these are abnormal growths that originate in the location where they are diagnosed.

Prognosis: The likely outcome of a situation, especially for an individual with a disease.

Progressive dementia: A dementia that gets worse over time, gradually interfering with more and more cognitive abilities.

Progressive epilepsy: Epilepsy in which seizures or the person's cognitive abilities get worse over time.

Progressive myoclonus epilepsy: A type of epilepsy that has been linked to an abnormality in the gene that codes for a protein called cystatin B. This protein regulates enzymes that break down other proteins.

Prosodic dysfunction: Problems with speech intonation or inflection.

Prostaglandins: Naturally occurring pain-producing substances thought to be implicated in migraine attacks. Their release is triggered by the dilation of arteries. Prostaglandins are extremely potent chemicals involved in a diverse group of physiological processes.

Pruning: Process whereby an injury destroys an important neural network in children, and another less useful neural network that would have eventually died takes over the responsibilities of the damaged network.

Psychogenic seizure: A type of nonepileptic event that is caused by psychological factors.

Putamen: An area of the brain that decreases in size as a result of the damage produced by Huntington disease.

Rasmussen's encephalitis: A progressive type of epilepsy in which half of the brain shows continual inflammation.

Receptors: Proteins that serve as recognition sites on cells and cause a response in the body when stimulated by chemicals called neurotransmitters. They act as on-and-off switches for the next nerve cell. See neuron, neurotransmitters.

Recessive: A trait that is apparent only when the gene or genes for it are inherited from both parents. See dominant, gene.

Recombinant tissue plasminogen activator (rt-PA): A genetically engineered form of t-PA, a thrombolytic, anti-clotting substance made naturally by the body.

Reflexes: Movements that the body makes automatically in response to a specific cue.

Retrobulbar neuritis: An inflammatory disorder of the optic nerve that is usually temporary. It causes rapid loss of vision and may cause pain upon moving the eye.

Retropulsion: The tendency to step backward if bumped from the front or upon initiating walking, usually seen in patients who tend to lean backward because of problems with balance.

Rh incompatibility: A blood condition in which antibodies in a pregnant woman's blood can attack fetal blood cells, impairing the fetus's supply of oxygen and nutrients.

Rigidity: A symptom of the disease in which muscles feel stiff and display resistance to movement even when another person tries to move the affected part of the body, such as an arm.

Rubella: Also known as German measles, rubella is a viral infection that can damage the nervous system in the developing fetus.

Secondary dementia: A dementia that occurs as a consequence of another disease or an injury.

Seizure focus: An area of the brain where seizures originate.

Seizure threshold: A term that refers to a person's susceptibility to seizures.

Seizure triggers: Phenomena that trigger seizures in some people. Seizure triggers do not cause epilepsy but can lead to first seizures or cause breakthrough seizures in people who otherwise experience good seizure control with their medication.

Seizures: Abnormal activity of nerve cells in the brain causing strange sensations, emotions, and behavior, or sometimes convulsions, muscle spasms, and loss of consciousness.

Selective dorsal root rhizotomy: A surgical procedure in which selected nerves are severed to reduce spasticity in the legs.

Senile chorea: A relatively mild and rare disorder found in elderly adults and characterized by choreic movements.

Senile dementia: An outdated term that reflects the formerly wide-spread belief that dementia was a normal part of aging. The word senile is derived from a Latin term that means, roughly, "old age. "

Sensory aphasia: See fluent aphasia.

Serotonin: A key neurotransmitter that acts as a powerful constric-tor of arteries, reducing the blood supply to the brain and contribut-ing to the pain of headache.

Shaken baby syndrome: A severe form of head injury that occurs when an infant or small child is shaken forcibly enough to cause the brain to bounce against the skull; the degree of brain damage depends on the extent and duration of the shaking. Minor symptoms include irritability, lethargy, tremors, or vomiting; major symptoms include seizures, coma, stupor, or death.

Shearing (or diffuse axonal injury): Damage to individual neu-rons resulting in disruption of neural networks and the breakdown of overall communication among neurons in the brain.

Simple focal seizures: Seizures that affect only one part of the brain. People experiencing simple focal seizures remain conscious but may experience unusual feelings or sensations.

Single photon emission computed tomography (SPECT): A type of brain scan sometimes used to locate seizure foci in the brain.

Sinusitis: An infection, either viral or bacterial, of the sinus cavities. The infection leads to inflammation of these cavities, causing pain and sometimes headache.

Small vessel disease: A cerebrovascular disease defined by stenosis in small arteries of the brain.

Spastic diplegia: A form of cerebral palsy in which both arms and both legs are affected, the legs being more severely affected.

Spastic hemiplegia (or hemiparesis): A form of cerebral palsy in which spasticity affects the arm and leg on one side of the body.

Spastic paraplegia (or paraparesis): A form of cerebral palsy in which spasticity affects both legs but the arms are relatively or completely spared.

Spastic quadriplegia (or quadriparesis): A form of cerebral palsy in which all four limbs are affected equally.

Spasticity: Abnormal, involuntary stiffness or contraction of the body's muscles.

Status epilepticus: A potentially life-threatening condition in which a seizure is abnormally prolonged. Although there is no strict definition for the time at which a seizure turns into status epilepticus, most people agree that any seizure lasting longer than five minutes should, for practical purposes, be treated as though it was status epilepticus.

Status migrainosus: A rare, sustained, and severe type of migraine, characterized by intense pain and nausea and often leading to hospitalization of the patient.

Stenosis: Narrowing of an artery due to the buildup of plaque on the inside wall of the artery.

Stereognosia: Difficulty perceiving and identifying objects using the sense of touch.

Stereotyped: Similar every time. In epilepsy this refers to the symptoms an individual person has, and the progression of those symptoms.

Strabismus: Misalignment of the eyes.

Striatum: Part of the basal ganglia of the brain. The striatum is composed of the caudate nucleus, putamen, and ventral striatum. See basal ganglia, caudate nuclei.

Stroke belt: An area of the southeastern United States with the highest stroke mortality rate in the country.

Stroke buckle: Three southeastern states, North Carolina, South Carolina, and Georgia, that have an extremely high stroke mortality rate.

Stupor: A state of impaired consciousness in which the patient is unresponsive but can be aroused briefly by a strong stimulus.

Subarachnoid hemorrhage: Bleeding within the meninges, or outer membranes, of the brain into the clear fluid that surrounds the brain.

Subcortical dementia: Dementia that affects parts of the brain below the outer brain layer, or cortex.

Subdural hematoma: Bleeding confined to the area between the dura and the arachnoid membranes.

Subdural hygroma: A buildup of protein-rich fluid in the area between the dura and the arachnoid membranes, usually caused by a tear in the arachnoid membrane.

Substance-induced persisting dementia: Dementia caused by abuse of substances such as alcohol and recreational drugs that persists even after the substance abuse has ended.

Substantia nigra: Movement-control center in the brain where loss of dopamine-producing nerve cells triggers the symptoms of Parkinson's disease; substantia nigra means "black substance," so called because the cells in this area are dark.

Sudden unexplained death: Death that occurs suddenly for no discernible reason. Epilepsy increases the risk of sudden unexplained death about twofold.

Sumatriptan: A commonly used migraine drug that binds to receptors for the neurotransmitter serotonin.

Syndrome of inappropriate secretion of antidiuretic hormone (SIADH): A condition in which excessive secretion of antidiuretic hormone leads to a sodium deficiency in the blood and abnormally concentrated urine; symptoms include weakness, lethargy, confusion, coma, seizures, or death if left untreated.

T cells: Immune system cells that develop in the thymus gland. Findings suggest that T cells are implicated in myelin destruction.

Tau protein: A protein that helps the functioning of microtubules, which are part of the cell's structural support and help to deliver substances throughout the cell. In Alzheimer's disease, tau is changed in a way that causes it to twist into pairs of helical filaments that collect into tangles.

Temporal lobe epilepsy: The most common epilepsy syndrome with focal seizures.

Temporal lobe resection: A type of surgery for temporal lobe epilepsy in which all or part of the affected temporal lobe of the brain is removed.

Temporomandibular joint dysfunction: A disorder of the joint between the temporal bone (above the ear) and the lower jaw bone that can cause muscle-contraction headaches.

Thermography: A technique sometimes used for diagnosing headache in which an infrared camera converts skin temperature into a color picture, called a thermogram, with different degrees of heat appearing as different colors.

Thrombolytics: Drugs used to treat an ongoing, acute ischemic stroke by dissolving the blood clot causing the stroke and thereby restoring blood flow through the artery.

Thrombosis or thrombus: The formation of a blood clot at the site of an injury.

Thrombotic stroke: A stroke caused by thrombosis.

Tic douloureux: See trigeminal neuralgia

Tissue necrosis factors: Chemicals released by leukocytes and other cells that cause secondary cell death during the inflammatory immune response associated with the ischemic cascade.

Tonic seizures: Seizures that cause stiffening of muscles of the body, generally those in the back, legs, and arms.

Tonic-clonic seizures: Seizures that cause a mixture of symptoms, including loss of consciousness, stiffening of the body, and repeated jerks of the arms and legs. In the past these seizures were sometimes referred to as grand mal seizures.

Total serum cholesterol: A combined measurement of a person's high-density lipoprotein (HDL) and low-density lipoprotein (LDL).

t-PA: See recombinant tissue plasminogen activator.

Traction headaches: Headaches caused by pulling or stretching pain in sensitive parts of the head, as, for example, when eye muscles are tensed to compensate for eyestrain.

Trait: Any genetically determined characteristic. See dominant, gene, recessive.

Transcranial magnetic stimulation (TMS): A procedure that uses a strong magnet held outside the head to influence brain activity. This is an experimental treatment for seizures.

Transgenic mice: Mice that receive injections of foreign genes during the embryonic stage of development. Their cells then follow the "instructions" of the foreign genes, resulting in the development of a certain trait or characteristic. Transgenic mice can serve as an animal model of a certain disease, telling researchers how genes work in specific cells.

Transient ischemic attack (TIA): A short-lived stroke that lasts from a few minutes up to twenty-four hours; often called a mini-stroke.

Transmissible spongiform encephalopathies: Part of a family of human and animal diseases in which brains become filled with holes resembling sponges when examined under a microscope. Creutzfeldt-Jakob disease is the most common of the known transmissible spongiform encephalopathies.

Transverse myelitis: An acute spinal cord disorder causing sudden low back pain and muscle weakness and abnormal sensory sensations in the lower extremities. Transverse myelitis often remits spontaneously; however, severe or long-lasting cases may lead to permanent disability.

Tremor: Shakiness or trembling, often in a hand, which in Parkinson disease is usually most apparent when the affected part is at rest.

Trigeminal neuralgia: A condition resulting from a disorder of the trigeminal nerve. Symptoms are headache and intense facial pain that comes in short, excruciating jabs.

Ultrasonography: A technique that bounces sound waves off of tissues and structures and uses the pattern of echoes to form an image, called a sonogram.

Vascular dementia: A type of dementia caused by brain damage from cerebrovascular or cardiovascular problems, usually strokes. It accounts for up to 20 percent of all dementias.

Vascular headaches: Headaches caused by abnormal function of the brain's blood vessels or vascular system. Migraine is a type of vascular headache.

Vasodilators: Medications that increase blood flow to the brain by expanding or dilating blood vessels.

Vasospasm: A dangerous side effect of subarachnoid hemorrhage in which the blood vessels in the subarachnoid space constrict erratically, cutting off blood flow.

Vegetative state: A condition in which patients are unconscious and unaware of their surroundings, but continue to have a sleep/wake cycle and can have periods of alertness.

Ventricles: Cavities within the brain that are filled with cerebrospinal fluid. In Huntington disease, tissue loss causes enlargement of the ventricles.

Ventriculostomy: A surgical procedure that drains cerebrospinal fluid from the brain by creating an opening in one of the small cavities called ventricles.

Vertebral artery: An artery on either side of the neck; see carotid artery.

Warfarin: A commonly used anticoagulant, also known as Coumadin®.

Wearing-off effect: The tendency, following long-term levodopa treatment, for each dose of the drug to be effective for shorter and shorter periods.

Wernicke aphasia: See fluent aphasia.

White matter: Nerve fibers that are the site of MS lesions and underlie the gray matter of the brain and spinal cord.

Chapter 25

Brain Disorders: Resources for Information and Support

General Information

Brain Resources and Information Network (BRAIN)

National Institute of Neurological Disorders and Stroke
P.O. Box 5801
Bethesda, MD 20824
Toll-Free: (800) 352-9424
Phone: (301) 496-5751
Website: http://www.ninds.nih.gov

Centers for Disease Control and Prevention (CDC)

U.S. Department of Health and Human Services
1600 Clifton Road, N.E.
Atlanta, GA 30333
Toll-Free: 800-311-3435
Phone: 404-639-3311/
404-639-3543
Website: http://www.cdc.gov
E-mail: inquiry@cdc.gov

The information in this chapter was compiled from various sources deemed accurate. All contact information was verified and updated in November 2004. Inclusion does not imply endorsement. This list is intended to serve as a starting point for information gathering; it is not comprehensive.

557

**National Institute
on Disability and
Rehabilitation
Research (NIDRR)**
U.S. Department of Education
Office of Special Education and
Rehabilitative Services
400 Maryland Ave., S.W.
Washington, DC 20202
Phone: 202-205-5465
TTY: (202) 245-7316
Website: http://www.ed.gov/
about/offices/list/osers/nidrr

**National Organization for
Rare Disorders (NORD)**
P.O. Box 1968
55 Kenosia Avenue
Danbury, CT 06813-1968
Phone: Tel: 203-744-0100/Voice
Mail 800-999-NORD (6673)
Fax: 203-798-2291
Website: http://www.rare
diseases.org
E-mail: orphan@rarediseases
.org

**National Rehabilitation
Information Center (NARIC)**
4200 Forbes Boulevard
Suite 202
Lanham, MD 20706-4829
Toll-Free: 800-346-2742
Phone: 301-459-5900
TTY: 301-459-5984
Fax: 301-562-2401
Website: http://www.naric.com
E-mail: naricinfo@heitech
services.com

**U.S. Food and Drug
Administration (FDA)**
U.S. Department of Health and
Human Services
5600 Fishers Lane
CDER-HFD-240
Rockville, MD 20857
Toll-Free: 888-INFO-FDA (463-
6332)
Phone: 301-827-4573
Website: http://www.fda.gov

Caregiver Support

**C-Mac Informational
Services/Caregiver News
(For Alzheimer's Type
Dementia Caregivers)**
271 Cedar Lane
East Meadow, NY 11554-2720
Phone: 516-481-6682
Fax: 516-486-7820
Website: http://www.caregiver
news.org
E-mail: caregiver_cmi@
hotmail.com

Family Caregiver Alliance
690 Market Street
Suite 600
San Francisco, CA 94104
Toll-Free: 800-445-8106
Phone: 415-434-3388
Fax: 415-434-3508
Website: http://
www.caregiver.org
E-mail: info@caregiver.org

National Family Caregivers Association

10400 Connecticut Avenue,
Suite 500
Kensington, MD 20895-3944
Toll-Free: 800-896-3650
Phone: 301-942-6430
Fax: 301-942-2302
Website: http://www.nfcacares
.org
E-mail: info@nfcacares.org

National Hospice and Palliative Care Organization / National Hospice Foundation

1700 Diagonal Road
Suite 625
Alexandria, VA 22314
Helpline: 800-658-8898
Phone: 703-837-1500
Fax: 703-837-1233
Website: http://www.nhpco.org
E-mail: info@nhpco.org

National Respite Network and Resource Center

800 Eastowne Drive
Suite 105
Chapel Hill, NC 27514
Toll-Free: 800-7-RELIEF (773-5433)
Phone: 919-490-5577
Fax: 919-490-4905
TDD: 919-490-5577
Website: http://www.archrespite
.org

Well Spouse Foundation

63 West Main Street
Suite H
Freehold, NJ 07728
Toll-Free: 800-838-0879
Phone: 732-577-8899
Fax: 732-577-8644
Website: http://www.wellspouse
.org
E-mail: info@wellspouse.org

Amyotrophic Lateral Sclerosis

ALS Association (ALSA)

27001 Agoura Road
Suite 150
Calabasas Hills, CA 91301-5104
Toll-Free: 800-782-4747
Phone: 818-880-9007
Fax: 818-880-9006
Website: http://www.alsa.org
E-mail: info@alsa-national.org

ALS Digest

Website: http://www.alslinks
.com/currentdigest.htm
E-mail: als@alslinks.com

ALS March of Faces—Moe's ALS Kids' page

Website: http://www.march-of-faces.org/KIDS/moe7.html

ALS Resource Page

Website: http://www.alslinks
.com

Baylor College of Medicine
Department of Neurology
One Baylor Plaza
Houston, TX 77030
Website: http://www.bcm.tmc
.edu/neurol/struct/als/als1.html

Les Turner ALS Foundation
8142 North Lawndale Avenue
Skokie, IL 60076-3322
Toll-Free: 888-ALS-1107
Phone: 847-679-3311
Fax: 847-679-9109
Website: http://www.
lesturnerals.org
E-mail: info@lesturnerals.org

Muscular Dystrophy Association
3300 East Sunrise Drive
Tucson, AZ 85718-3208
Toll-Free: 800-572-1717
Phone: 520-529-2000
Fax: 520-529-5300
Website: http://www.mdausa.org
E-mail: mda@mdausa.org

Project ALS
511 Avenue of the Americas
Suite 341
New York, NY 10011
Toll-Free: 800-603-0270
Phone: 212-969-0329
Fax: 212-337-9915
Website: http://www.projectals
.org
E-mail: info@projectals.org

Alzheimer's and Other Dementias

Alzheimer's Association
225 North Michigan Avenue
17th Floor
Chicago, IL 60601-7633
Toll-Free: 800-272-3900
Phone: 312-335-8700
Fax: 312-335-1110
Website: http://www.alz.org
E-mail: info@alz.org

Alzheimer's Disease Education and Referral Center (ADEAR)
P.O. Box 8250
Silver Spring, MD 20907-8250
Toll-Free: 800-438-4380
Phone: 301-495-3311
Fax: 301-495-3334
Website: http://www.alzheimers
.org
E-mail: adear@alzheimers.org

Alzheimer's Foundation of America
322 Eighth Avenue
6th Floor
New York, NY 10001
Phone: 866-AFA-8484 (232-8484)
Fax: 646-638-1546
Website: http://www.alzfdn.org
E-mail: info@alzfdn.org

American Health Assistance Foundation
22512 Gateway Center Drive
Clarksburg, MD 20871
Toll-Free: 800-437-AHAF (2423)
Phone: 301-948-3244
Fax: 301-258-9454
Website: http://www.ahaf.org
E-mail: info@ahaf.org

Association for Frontotemporal Dementias (AFTD)
P.O. Box 7191
St. David's, PA 19087-7191
Website: http://www.FTD-Picks.org
E-mail: info@ftd-picks.org

Children of Aging Parents
1609 Woodbourne Road
Suite 302A
Levittown, PA 19057
Toll-Free: 800-227-7294
Website: http://www.caps4caregivers.org

Institute for the Study of Aging
1414 Avenue of the Americas,
Suite 4600
New York, NY 10019
Phone: 212-935-2402
Fax: 212-935-2408
Website: http://www.aging-institute.org
E-mail: hfillit@aging-institute.org

National Institute of Mental Health (NIMH)
National Institutes of Health, DHHS
6001 Executive Blvd.
Rm. 8184, MSC 9663
Bethesda, MD 20892-9663
Toll-Free: 866-615-NIMH (6464)
Phone: 301-443-4513
TTY: 301-443-8431
Fax: 301-443-4279
Website: http://www.nimh.nih.gov
E-mail: nimhinfo@nih.gov

National Institute on Aging Information Center
Building 31, Room 5C27
31 Center Drive, MSC 2292
Gaithersburg, MD 20892
Toll-Free: 800-222-2225
TTY: 800-222-4225 (TTY)
Fax: 301-589-3014
Website: http://www.nia.nih.gov

Simon Foundation for Continence
Box 835-F
Wilmette, IL 60091
Toll-Free: 800-237-SIMON
Phone: 847-864-3913
Fax: 847-864-9758
Website: http://www.simonfoundation.org
E-mail: simoninfo@simonfoundation.org

Brain Tumors

American Brain Tumor Association (ABTA)
2720 River Road
Suite 146
Des Plaines, IL 60018-4110
Toll-Free: 800-886-2282
Phone: 847-827-9910
Fax: 847-827-9918
Website: http://www.abta.org
E-mail: info@abta.org

American Cancer Society
National Home Office
1599 Clifton Road, NE
Atlanta, GA 30329-4251
Toll-Free: 800-ACS-2345 (227-2345)
Website: http://www.cancer.org

Brain Tumor Society
124 Watertown Street
Suite 3H
Watertown, MA 02472-2500
Toll-Free: 800-770-TBTS (8287)
Phone: 617-924-9997
Fax: 617-924-9998
Website: http://www.tbts.org
E-mail: info@tbts.org

Children's Brain Tumor Foundation
274 Madison Avenue
Suite 1301
New York, NY 10016
Toll-Free: 866-CBT-HOPE (228-4673)
Phone: 212-448-9494
Fax: 212-448-1022
Website: http://www.cbtf.org
E-mail: info@cbtf.org

National Brain Tumor Foundation (NBTF)
22 Battery Street
Suite 612
San Francisco, CA 94111-5520
Toll-Free: 800-934-CURE (2873)
Phone: 415-834-9970
Fax: 415-834-9980
Website: http://www.braintumor.org
E-mail: nbtf@braintumor.org

National Cancer Institute
Office of Cancer Communications
Building 31
Room 10A-03
Bethesda, MD 20892-2580
Toll-Free: 800-4-CANCER (800-422-6237)
Website: http://www.cancernet.nci.nih.gov
E-mail: cancergovstaff@mail.nih.gov

Cerebral Palsy

Children's Hemiplegia and Stroke Association (CHASA)
4101 West Green Oaks Blvd.
Suite 305
PMB #149
Arlington, TX 76016
Phone: 817-492-4325
Website: http://www.hemikids.org
E-mail: info437@chasa.org

Easter Seals
230 West Monroe Street
Suite 1800
Chicago, IL 60606-4802
Toll-Free: 800-221-6827
Phone: 312-726-6200
Fax: 312-726-1494
TTY: 312-726-4258
Website: http://www.easter-seals
.org
E-mail: info@easter-seals.org

March of Dimes Birth
Defects Foundation
1275 Mamaroneck Avenue
White Plains, NY 10605
Toll-Free: 888-MODIMES (663-
4637)
Phone: 914-428-7100
Fax: 914-428-8203
Website: http://www.
marchofdimes.com
E-mail: askus@marchofdimes
.com

United Cerebral Palsy
(UCP)
1600 L Street NW
Suite 700
Washington, DC 20036
Toll-Free: 800-USA-5UCP (872-
5827)
Phone: 202-776-0406
Fax: 202-776-0414
TTY: 202-973-7197
Website: http://www.ucp.org
E-mail: national@ucp.org

Creutzfeldt-Jakob Disease

CJD Aware!
213 3rd Street NE
Hickory, NC 28601-5124
Phone: 828-324-0751
Fax: 828-324-6486
E-mail: cjdaware@iwon.com

Creutzfeldt-Jakob (CJD)
Foundation Inc.
P.O. Box 5312
Akron, OH 44334
Toll-Free: 800-659-1991
Phone: 330-665-5590
Fax: 330-668-2474
Website: http://www.cjd
foundation.org
E-mail: crjakob@aol.com

Epilepsy and Seizures

Charlie Foundation (An
Epilepsy Resource)
1223 Wilshire Boulevard
Suite 815
Santa Monica, CA 90403
Toll-Free: 800-FOR-KETO (367-
5386)
Phone: 310-395-6751
Fax: 310-393-1978
Website: http://www.charlie
foundation.org

Citizens United for
Research in Epilepsy (CURE)
730 N. Franklin St., Suite 404
Chicago, IL 60610
Phone: 312-255-1801
Fax: 312-255-1809
Website: http://www
.CUREepilepsy.org
E-mail: info@cureepilepsy.org

Epilepsy Foundation
4351 Garden City Drive
Landover, MD 20785-7223
Toll-Free: 800-EFA-1000 (332-1000)
Phone: 301-459-3700
Website: http://www.epilepsy
foundation.org

Epilepsy Institute
257 Park Avenue South
Suite 302
New York, NY 10010
Phone: 212-677-8550
Fax: 212-677-5825
Website: http://www.epilepsy
institute.org

Parents Against Childhood Epilepsy (PACE)
7 East 85th Street
Suite A3
New York, NY 10028
Phone: 212-665-PACE (7223)
Fax: 212-327-3075
Website: http://www.paceusa.org
E-mail: pacenyemail@aol.com

Headaches

American Council for Headache Education
19 Mantua Road
Mt. Royal, NJ 08061
Toll-Free: 800-255-ACHE (255-2243)
Phone: 856-423-0258
Fax: 856-423-0082
Website: http://www.achenet.org
E-mail: achehq@talley.com

National Headache Foundation
820 N. Orleans
Suite 217
Chicago, IL 60610-3132
Toll-Free: 888-NHF-5552 (643-5552)
Phone: 773-388-6399
Fax: 773-525-7357
Website: http://www.headaches
.org
E-mail: info@headaches.org

Huntington Disease

Huntington's Disease Society of America
158 West 29th Street
7th Floor
New York, NY 10001-5300
Toll-Free: 800-345-HDSA (4372)
Phone: 212-242-1968
Fax: 212-239-3430
Website: http://www.hdsa.org
E-mail: hdsainfo@hdsa.org

Hereditary Disease Foundation
3960 Broadway
6th Floor
New York, NY 10032
Phone: 212-928-2121
Fax: 212-928-2172
Website: http://
www.hdfoundation.org
E-mail: cures@hdfoundation
.org

Hydrocephalus

Guardians of Hydrocephalus Research Foundation
2618 Avenue Z
Brooklyn, NY 11235-2023
Phone: 718-743-GHRF (4473)
Fax: 718-743-1171
Website: http://ghrf.Homestead
.com/ghrf.html
E-mail: GHRF2618@aol.com

Hydrocephalus Association
870 Market Street
Suite 705
San Francisco, CA 94102
Toll-Free: 888-598-3789
Phone: 415-732-7040
Fax: 415-732-7044
Website: http://www.hydroassoc
.org
E-mail: info@hydroassoc.org

Hydrocephalus Support Group, Inc.
P.O. Box 4236
Chesterfield, MO 63006-4236
Phone: 636-532-8228
E-mail: hydrodb@earthlink.net

National Hydrocephalus Foundation
12413 Centralia Road
Lakewood, CA 90715-1653
Toll-Free: 888-857-3434
Phone: 562-402-3523
Fax: 562-924-6666
Website: http://nhfonline.org
E-mail: hydrobrat@earthlink.net

Multiple Sclerosis

American Autoimmune Related Diseases Association
22100 Gratiot Avenue
East Detroit, MI 48201-2227
Toll-Free: 800-598-4668
Phone: 586-776-3900
Fax: 586-776-3903
Website: http://www.aarda.org
E-mail: aarda@aol.com

Boston Cure Project for MS
300 Fifth Avenue
Waltham, MA 02451
Phone: 781-487-0008
Fax: 781-487-0009
Website: http://
www.bostoncure.org
E-mail: info@bostoncure.org

International Essential Tremor Foundation
P.O. Box 14005
Lenexa, KS 66285-4005
Toll-Free: 888-387-3667
Phone: 913-341-3880
Fax: 913-341-1296
Website: http://www.essential
tremor.org
E-mail: staff@essentialtremor.org

Multiple Sclerosis Association of America
706 Haddonfield Road
Cherry Hill, NJ 08002
Toll-Free: 800-532-7667
Phone: 856-488-4500
Fax: 856-661-9797
Website: http://www.msaa.com
E-mail: webmaster@msaa.com

Multiple Sclerosis Foundation

6350 North Andrews Avenue
Ft. Lauderdale, FL 33309-2130
Toll-Free: 888-MSFocus (673-6287)
Phone: 954-776-6805
Fax: 954-351-0630
Website: http://www.msfocus.org
E-mail: support@msfocus.org

National Ataxia Foundation (NAF)

2600 Fernbrook Lane
Suite 119
Minneapolis, MN 55447-4752
Phone: 763-553-0020
Fax: 763-553-0167
Website: http://www.ataxia.org
E-mail: naf@ataxia.org

National Multiple Sclerosis Society

733 Third Avenue
6th Floor
New York, NY 10017-3288
Toll-Free: 800-344-4867 (FIGHTMS)
Phone: 212-986-3240
Fax: 212-986-7981
Website: http://www.nationalmssociety.org
E-mail: nat@nmss.org

Parkinson Disease

American Parkinson Disease Association

1250 Hylan Blvd.
Suite 4B
Staten Island, NY 10305-1946
Toll-Free: 800-223-2732 (California: 800-908-2732)
Phone: 718-981-8001
Fax: 718-981-4399
Website: http://www.apdaparkinson.org
E-mail: apda@apdaparkinson.org

Michael J. Fox Foundation for Parkinson's Research

Grand Central Station
P.O. Box 4777
New York, NY 10163
Toll-Free: 800-708-7644
Phone: 212-509-0995
Website: http://www.michaeljfox.org

National Parkinson Foundation

1501 N.W. 9th Avenue
Bob Hope Research Center
Miami, FL 33136-1494
Toll-Free: 800-327-4545 (Florida: 800-433-7022)
Phone: 305-243-6666
Fax: 305-243-5595
Website: http://www.parkinson.org
E-mail: contact@parkinson.org

Parkinson's Action Network (PAN)

1000 Vermont Ave. N.W.
Suite 900
Washington, DC 20005
Toll-Free: 800-850-4726
Phone: 202-842-4101 (California: 707-544-1994)
Fax: 202-842-4105
Website: http://www
.parkinsonsaction.org
E-mail: info@parkinsonsaction
.org

Parkinson's Disease Foundation (PDF)

710 West 168th Street
New York, NY 10032-9982
Toll-Free: 800-457-6676
Phone: 212-923-4700
Fax: 212-923-4778
Website: http://www
.parkinsons-foundation.org
E-mail: info@pdf.org

Parkinson's Institute

1170 Morse Avenue
Sunnyvale, CA 94089-1605
Toll-Free: 800-786-2958
Phone: 408-734-2800
Fax: 408-734-8522
Website: http://www
.parkinsonsinstitute.org
E-mail: outreach@parkinsons
institute.org

Worldwide Education & Awareness for Movement Disorders (WE MOVE)

204 West 84th Street
New York, NY 10024
Toll-Free: 800-437-MOV2 (6682)
Phone: 212-875-8312
Fax: 212-875-8389
Website: http://www.wemove.org
E-mail: wemove@wemove.org

Stroke and Aneurysm

American Speech Language Hearing Association (ASHA)

10801 Rockville Pike
Rockville, MD 20852-3279
Toll-Free: 800-638-8255
Phone: 301-897-5700
Fax: 301-571-0457
Website: http://www.asha.org
E-mail: actioncenter@asha.org

American Stroke Association: A Division of American Heart Association

7272 Greenville Avenue
Dallas, TX 75231-4596
Toll-Free: 1-888-4STROKE (478-7653)
Fax: 214-706-5231
Website: http://www
.strokeassociation.org
E-mail: strokeassociation@
heart.org

Brain Aneurysm Foundation
12 Clarendon Street
Boston, MA 02116
Phone: 617-723-3870
Fax: 617-723-8672
Website: http://www.bafound.org
E-mail: information@bafound
.org

Children's Hemiplegia and Stroke Association (CHASA)
4101 West Green Oaks Blvd.
PMB #149, Suite 305
Arlington, TX 76016
Phone: 817-492-4325
Website: http://www.hemikids
.org
E-mail: info437@chasa.org

Hazel K. Goddess Fund for Stroke Research in Women
785 Park Avenue
New York, NY 10021-3552
Phone: 212-734-8067
Fax: 212-288-2160
Website: http://www
.thegoddessfund.org
E-mail: info@thegoddessfund.org

National Aphasia Association
7 Dey St., Suite 600
New York, NY 10007
Toll-Free: 800-922-4NAA (4622)
Phone: 212-267-2814
Fax: 212-267-2812
Website: http://www.aphasia.org
E-mail: naa@aphasia.org

National Stroke Association
9707 East Easter Lane
Englewood, CO 80112-3747
Toll-Free: 800-STROKES (787-6537)
Phone: 303-649-9299
Fax: 303-649-1328
Website: http://www.stroke.org
E-mail: info@stroke.org

Traumatic Brain Injury

Acoustic Neuroma Association
600 Peachtree Parkway, Suite 108
Cumming, GA 30041-6899
Phone: 770-205-8211
Fax: 770-205-0239
Website: http://www.anausa.org
E-mail: anausa@aol.com

Brain Injury Association
8201 Greensboro Drive, Suite 611
McLean, VA 22102
Toll-Free: 800-444-6443
Phone: 703-761-0750
Fax: 703-761-0755
Website: http://www.biausa.org
E-mail: FamilyHelpline@
biausa.org

Brain Trauma Foundation
523 East 72nd Street, 8th Floor
New York, NY 10021
Phone: 212-772-0608
Fax: 212-772-0357
Website: http://www
.braintrauma.org
E-mail: info@braintrauma.org

Index

Index

Page numbers followed by 'n' indicate a footnote. Page numbers in *italics* indicate a table or illustration.

A

AAASPS *see* African American Antiplatelet Stroke Prevention Study
AANS *see* American Association of Neurological Surgeons
absence epilepsy
  defined 525
  described 252–53
absence seizures
  defined 525
  described 252
  first aid 310
ABTA *see* American Brain Tumor Association
accessible tumor, defined 525
acetaminophen 412, *413*
acetazolamide 302
acetylcholine
  defined 525
  dementia 357
  described *21*
  seizures 250

Acoustic Neuroma Association, contact information 568
acrylonitrile, brain tumors 142
ACTH *see* adrenocorticotropic hormone
action potentials, described 17–18
acute stroke, defined 526
acyclovir 177
A.D.A.M., Inc., publications
  brain abscess 170n
  cerebral angiography 27n
  computed tomography 31n
  electroencephalogram 35n
  electromyography 39n
  isotope study 47n
  nerve conduction velocity 42n
ADEAR *see* Alzheimer's Disease Education and Referral Center
adrenocorticotropic hormone (ACTH)
  defined 525
  multiple sclerosis 405–6
African American Antiplatelet Stroke Prevention Study (AAASPS) 101
AFTD *see* Association for Fronto-temporal Dementias
age factor
  atrial fibrillation 82
  brain tumors 141
  dementia 349, 351
  epilepsy 287–92

age factor, continued
  frontotemporal dementias 341–42
  Huntington disease 371–72
  hypoxia 201
  multiple sclerosis 395
  stroke risk 80
  vascular dementia 339
agnosia, defined 526
Aguilar, M. 415n
akinesia
  defined 526
  described 371
akinetic mutism, described 232
alcohol abuse, stroke risk 86
alcohol use
  dementia 352
  headache 497
  Parkinson disease 439
Alexander disease 347
alpha interferon
  described 539
  multiple sclerosis 406
alpha-synuclein 456–57
ALS see amyotrophic lateral sclerosis
ALSA see ALS Association
ALS Association (ALSA), contact
  information 559
ALS Digest, contact information 559
ALS March of Faces - Moe's ALS
  Kids' Page, Web site address 559
ALS Resource Page, Web site address
  559
alternative therapies, multiple
  sclerosis 410–11
Alzheimer, Alois 335
Alzheimer's Association, contact
  information 560
Alzheimer's disease
  defined 526
  described 337–39
  research 362–66
  traumatic brain injury 219
Alzheimer's Disease Education and
  Referral Center (ADEAR), contact
  information 560
Alzheimer's Foundation of America,
  contact information 560
amantadine 412, 413
amantadine hydrochloride 438

American Association of Neurological
  Surgeons (AANS), brain anatomy
  publication 3n
American Autoimmune Related
  Diseases Association, contact
  information 565
American Brain Tumor Association
  (ABTA), contact information 562
American Cancer Society, contact
  information 562
American Council for Headache
  Education, contact information 564
American Health Assistance
  Foundation, contact information
  561
American Heart Association,
  angioplasty publication 108n
American Parkinson Disease
  Association, contact information
  566
American Speech Language Hearing
  Association (ASHA), contact
  information 567
American Stroke Association, contact
  information 567
aminopyridine 408
amitriptyline 495
amphetamines 439, 497, 518–19
amphotericin B 165–66
amplification of risk, described 81
amyloid angiopathy, described 339
amyloid plaques
  defined 526
  dementia 345
amyloid precursor protein
  defined 526
  dementia 350
amyotrophic lateral sclerosis (ALS)
  overview 316–24
  research 323–24, 325–33
"Amyotrophic Lateral Sclerosis Fact
  Sheet" (NINDS) 316n
anaplastic, defined 526
"Anatomy of the Brain" (AANS) 3n
aneurysms
  defined 526
  overview 124–33
  stroke 76, 129
  surgical procedures 90–91

angiogram
  brain tumors 143
  coma 236
angiography, defined 526
angioplasty, stroke research 108–9
"Angioplasty Clears Clogged Brain
  Arteries" (American Heart Association) 108n
animal studies
  amyotrophic lateral sclerosis 327–29
  epilepsy 248, 270
  Huntington disease 382–83, 384
  minocycline 325–26
  multiple sclerosis 408, 427–29
  Parkinson disease 445–46, 449–50
  stroke 97–98
anoxia
  defined 526
  dementia 348–49
  stroke 97–98
antibiotic medications
  brain abscess 172
  encephalitis 178
  meningitis 160
antibodies, defined 526
anticoagulants
  defined 526
  described 88–89
  stroke research 108
  see also heparin; warfarin
Anticonvulsant Screening Program
  (ASP) 269
antidepressant medications
  migraine 495
  multiple sclerosis 412, *413*
  narcolepsy 520
antiepileptic medications
  birth control 276
  cerebral palsy 484
  described 258–59
  elderly 289–92
  pregnancy 278
antigens, defined 526
antiplatelet agents
  defined 526–27
  described 88
antithrombotics
  defined 527
  described 88

Apgar score
  cerebral palsy 469
  defined 527
aphasia
  defined 527
  dementia 342
  described 11
apolipoprotein E
  defined 527
  dementia 350
apoplexy
  defined 527
  described 72
  see also stroke
apoptosis, defined 527
apraxia, defined 527
Aqueduct of Sylvius, described 6
arachnoid, described 5
arachnoid membrane
  defined 527
  stroke 76
arboviral encephalitis 174, 178–88
Aricept (donepezil) 357, 358
Artane (trihexyphenidyl) 439
arterial blood gas, coma 235
arteriography
  defined 527
  stroke 79
arteriovenous malformation (AVM)
  defined 527
  stroke 76
arteritis, headache 502
ASA *see* atrial septal aneurysm
Ascherio, Alberto 454–55
ASHA *see* American Speech Language Hearing Association
ASP *see* Anticonvulsant Screening
  Program
asphyxia, defined 527
aspirin 88–89, 101, 412, *413*
assistive devices, cerebral palsy
  479–80
Association for Frontotemporal
  Dementias (AFTD), contact
  information 561
astrocytes
  blood-brain barrier 16
  described 4, 16
astrocytoma, described 140

astroglia, described 4
ataxia, defined 527
ataxic cerebral palsy, described 464–65
atherosclerosis
  cholesterol 83–85
  defined 528
  dementia 352
  described 75
  tobacco use 86
athetoid cerebral palsy, described 464
atonic seizures
  defined 528
  described 252
atorvastatin 428–29
atrial fibrillation
  stroke risk 82–83
  warfarin 89
atrial septal aneurysm (ASA), stroke
  83
aura (epileptic)
  defined 528
  described 251
aura (migraine), defined 528
autoimmune disease, defined 528
automatisms, defined 528
autosomal dominant disorder, defined
  528
AVM *see* arteriovenous malformation
Avonex (beta interferon) 406, 416,
  419
axons
  described 14
  multiple sclerosis 420, 426
  neurons 18–19
azathioprine 407

B

baclofen 411, *413*, 478
bad cholesterol *see* low-density
  lipoprotein (LDL) cholesterol
balloon angioplasty
  carotid arteries 26
  stroke research 108–9
basal ganglia, defined 528
basilar artery migraine
  defined 528
  described 493

Batten disease 346
Baylor College of Medicine, contact
  information 560
Beal, Flint 452
behavioral problems
  epilepsy 264
  traumatic brain injury 218
behavioral therapy
  cerebral palsy 477
  dementia 357
benign, defined 528
benign exertional headache
  defined 528
  described 493
benign infantile
  encephalopathy
  defined 529
  described 254
benign neonatal convulsions
  defined 529
  described 254
benzodiazepines 178, 439
benztropine 439
benztropine mesylate 439
beta amyloid
  defined 529
  dementia 350–51
beta-hydroxybutyrate (BHB) 263
beta interferon
  described 539
  multiple sclerosis 406, 416, 419
betamethasone 405
Betaseron (beta interferon) 406, 416,
  419
BHB *see* beta-hydroxybutyrate
Binswanger's disease
  defined 529
  described 340
biofeedback
  defined 529
  migraine 495–96
biopsy
  brain tumors 144
  defined 529
"Birth Control" (Epilepsy Ontario)
  274n
blood-brain barrier
  defined 529
  described 16–17

blood clots
  stroke 74–75, 83
  stroke research 112–14
"Bone Marrow Generates New
  Neurons in Human Brains"
  (NINDS) 61n
bone marrow transplantation
  clinical trial 61–63
  multiple sclerosis 407
Boston Cure for MS, contact
  information 565
botulinum 484
bovine spongiform encephalopathy
  (BSE) 345
boxer's syndrome, defined 533
bradykinesia
  defined 529
  Parkinson disease 435
BRAIN *see* Brain Resources and
  Information Network
brain
  described 136–38
  overview 3–12
"Brain Abscess" (A.D.A.M., Inc.) 170n
brain abscess, overview 170–73
"Brain and Spinal Cord Tumors:
  Hope through Research" (NINDS)
  525n
Brain Aneurysm Foundation, contact
  information 568
brain aneurysms
  described 129–30
  overview 124–33
brain attack *see* stroke
brain death
  cerebellum 10
  defined 529
  described 232
  overview 65–67
  traumatic brain injury 213
brain disorders, diagnostic tests
  24–52
brain infections *see* brain abscess;
  cysticercosis; encephalitis; meningitis
Brain Injury Association
  coma publication 229n
  contact information 568
"Brain Produces New Cells in
  Multiple Sclerosis" (NINDS) 426n

Brain Resources and Information
  Network (BRAIN), contact
  information 557
brain stem, described 10, 138
brain stem glioma, described 140
Brain Trauma Foundation, contact
  information 568
brain tumors
  cell types 4
  dementia 348
  headache 51
  metastasis 154–58
  overview 136–53
  ventricular system 6
Brain Tumor Society, contact
  information 562
*The Brain: Understanding Neuro-
  biology through the Study of
  Addiction* (BSCS) 13n
Broca's aphasia
  defined 529
  described 11
  traumatic brain injury 529
Broca's area, described 8, 11
bromocriptine 439
BSCS, neurobiology publication 13n
butyrophenones 439

C

CADASIL *see* cerebral autosomal dominant arteriopathy with subcortical
  infarct and leukoencephalopathy
caffeine
  headache 497
  Parkinson disease 454–56
calcium channel blockers, stroke 89
calcium ion influx, traumatic brain
  injury 222–23
Campbell, Morgan S. III 114–15
cancer, described 138
carbamazepine 276, *413*
carbidopa 438
caregivers
  dementia 361–62
  Huntington disease 378–79
  hypoxia 202–3
carotenoids, stroke research 121–22

carotid artery, defined 529
carotid endarterectomy
  defined 529
  described 26, 89–90
Carotid Occlusion Surgery Study
  (COSS) 102–3
Carotid Revascularization Endarterectomy *versus* Stenting Trial
  (CREST) 102
carotid ultrasound, overview 24–27
caspases 351
cataplexy 513, 514
catheters
  cerebral angiography 27–28, 126
  positron emission tomography 48
  stroke research 114–16
CAT scan *see* computed tomography
caudate nuclei, defined 529
CBF *see* cerebral blood flow
celiac disease
  defined 530
  epilepsy 249
cell body, described 13
cell death
  Huntington disease 383–84
  Parkinson disease 437
  stroke 106–7
Centers for Disease Control and
  Prevention (CDC)
  contact information 557
  publications
    arboviral encephalitides 174n
    cysticercosis 189n
    meningitis 160n
    trichinellosis 193n
central nervous system (CNS)
  defined 530
  described 4
central pain syndrome, defined 530
central stroke pain, defined 530
cerebellum, described 9–10, 137
cerebral, defined 530
cerebral abscess *see* brain abscess
cerebral aneurysms *see* brain
  aneurysms
cerebral angiography
  brain aneurysm 126
  overview 27–30
  traumatic brain injury 213

"Cerebral Angiography" (A.D.A.M.,
  Inc.) 27n
cerebral autosomal dominant
  arteriopathy with subcortical
  infarct and leukoencephalopathy
  (CADASIL)
  defined 529
  described 87–88, 340
cerebral blood flow (CBF), defined
  530
cerebral palsy
  overview 461–85
  research 481–85
"Cerebral Palsy: Hope through
  Research" (NINDS) 461n, 525n
cerebrospinal fluid (CSF)
  defined 530
  described 5–6
  hydrocephalus 505–9
  stroke 76
  ventricular system 6
cerebrovascular disease
  defined 530
  described 72–73
cerebrum, described 6–8, 137
Chance, Phillip 332–33
Charlie Foundation, contact information 563
CHASA *see* Children's Hemiplegia
  and Stroke Association
chemical signals, neurons 17–19
chemotherapy, brain tumors 149
children
  amyotrophic lateral sclerosis 332–33
  cerebral angiography 28
  cerebral palsy 461–85
  cochlear implants 162–64
  computed tomography 31
  dementia 346–47
  electroencephalogram 36
  electromyography 39
  febrile seizures 304–8
  Huntington disease 371–72
  ketogenic diet 300–302
  migraine 503
  nerve conduction velocity 42
  positron emission tomography 48
  shaken baby syndrome 238–41
  stroke 95–96

Children of Aging Parents, contact information 561
Children's Brain Tumor Foundation, contact information 562
Children's Health Act (2000) 225
Children's Hemiplegia and Stroke Association (CHASA), contact information 562, 568
chlorprothixene 439
cholesterol
  defined 530
  dementia 352, 359
  stroke 75, 83–85
  see also high-density lipoprotein (HDL) cholesterol; low-density lipoprotein (LDL) cholesterol
cholesterol-lowering medications, stroke research 116–18, 120–21
cholinesterase inhibitors
  defined 530
  dementia 341, 357, 358
chorea
  defined 530
  described 368
chromosomes, defined 530
chronic cerebellar stimulation 479
chronic traumatic encephalopathy, defined 533
cimetidine 439
Cipro 439
Citizens United for Research in Epilepsy (CURE), contact information 563
CJD *see* Creutzfeldt-Jakob disease
CJD Aware!, contact information 563
cladribine 407
clinical trials
  amyotrophic lateral sclerosis 320
  aneurysm 103
  brain aneurysms 127–28, 133
  carotid occlusion 102–3
  constraint-induced therapy 104
  dementia 365
  epilepsy 271
  estrogen 95, 101
  extracranial/intracranial (EC/IC) bypass 90
  hormone therapy 58–60
  Huntington disease 385, 387–90

clinical trials, continued
  magnesium 105
  Parkinson disease 442, 451–53
  stents 102
  stroke 98–105
  stroke prevention 88–89, 101
  stroke recovery 102
  subarachnoid aneurysm 133
  subcortical stroke 104–5
  traumatic brain injury 225
  vagus nerve stimulation 296
  warfarin *vs.* aspirin 100–101, 103, 104
clipping
  brain aneurysm 127–28, 130–31
  defined 531
  described 90–91
clonazepam 358, 411, *413*
clonic seizures
  defined 530
  described 252
clopidogrel 88, 104, 105
closed head injury, defined 530
clozapine 341
clumping, described 363, 390–91
cluster headaches
  defined 531
  described 497–98
C-Mac Informational Services/ Caregiver News, contact information 558
CNS *see* central nervous system
CNS abscess *see* brain abscess
cochlear implants, bacterial meningitis 162–64
"Cochlear Implants and Bacterial Meningitis" (FDA) 160n
codeine 412, *413*
Coenzyme Q10 387–89, 451–53
Cogentin (benztropine) 439
Cognex (tacrine) 357
cognitive defects
  dementia 349
  epilepsy 253–54
  stroke 93
  traumatic brain injury 217
cognitive function
  described 58
  multiple sclerosis 402–3

cognitive training
    defined 531
    dementia 356
coil embolization, brain aneurysm
    127
coma
    defined 531
    hypoxia 200–201
    overview 229–37
    see also Glasgow Coma Scale
"Coma" (Brain Injury Association)
    229n
complex focal seizures
    defined 531
    described 251
    first aid 310
compressive cranial neuropathies,
    defined 531
computed tomography (CT scan)
    brain aneurysms 126
    brain tumors 143
    cerebral palsy 472
    coma 236
    concussion 227
    defined 531, 532
    dementia 354
    encephalitis 177
    epilepsy 257
    headache 489
    Huntington disease 373–74
    hydrocephalus 508
    hypoxia 201
    overview 31–35
    stroke 78
    traumatic brain injury 211, 213
Comtan (entacapone) 439
concussion
    defined 531
    overview 226–28
"Concussion" (Mueller; Oro) 226n
congenital tumor, defined 531
contracture, defined 531
contrecoup, defined 531
contusion, defined 531
convulsions, defined 531
cooling therapy
    multiple sclerosis 420–25
    stroke research 110–12
Copaxone (copolymer I) 408

Copaxone (glatiramer acetate) 419
copolymer I 408
corkscrew device, stroke research
    112–14
corpus callosotomy
    defined 532
    epilepsy 262
corpus striatum, defined 532
cortex, defined 532
cortical atrophy
    defined 532
    described 354
cortical dementia
    defined 532
    described 337
corticobasal degeneration
    defined 532
    described 343–44
COSS *see* Carotid Occlusion Surgery
    Study
Coumadin (warfarin) 88, 555
CRAG test, cryptococcal meningitis
    165
cranial computed tomography scan,
    overview 31–35
"Cranial CT Scan" (A.D.A.M., Inc.) 31n
cranial nerves, described 10, 11, *12*
craniopharyngioma, described 140
cranium, described 5
CREST *see* Carotid Revascularization
    Endarterectomy *versus* Stenting
    Trial
Creutzfeldt-Jakob disease (CJD)
    defined 532
    described 344–45, 554
Creutzfeldt-Jakob (CJD) Foundation
    Inc., contact information 563
cryothalamotomy, defined 532
"Cryptococcal Meningitis" (University
    of New Mexico) 160n
cryptococcal meningitis, overview
    164–66
CSF *see* cerebrospinal fluid
CSF fistula
    defined 532
    traumatic brain injury 214
CT scan *see* computed tomography
CURE *see* Citizens United for
    Research in Epilepsy

cyclophosphamide 407
cyclosporine 407
Cylert (pemoline) 412, *413*
cystamine 390–91
cystatin B 249
cysticercosis, overview 189–92
"Cysticercosis Fact Sheet" (CDC)
 189n
cytokines
 defined 532
 described 539
 multiple sclerosis 409–10
cytotoxic edema, defined 532
Cytoxan (cyclophosphamide) 407

D

Daclizumab 429–31
Dandy, Walter 130
Dantrium (dantrolene) 411, *413*
dantrolene 411, *413*, 478
DBS *see* deep brain stimulation
deep brain stimulation (DBS), overview 54–57
"Deep Brain Stimulation: Pacemakers for the Brain" (Medtronic, Inc.)
 54n
deep vein thrombosis, defined 532
deer ticks, encephalitis 179, 185
DeJong, Allan 239–40
delirium, dementia 349
dementia
 defined 532
 described 58–59
 overview 335–66
 traumatic brain injury 219–20
 see also Alzheimer's disease; cortical
  dementia; dementia pugilistica;
  frontotemporal dementias; HIV-
  associated dementia; Lewy body
  dementia; multi-infarct dementia; Parkinson's dementia; post-
  traumatic dementia; primary
  dementia; progressive dementia;
  secondary dementias; senile dementia; subcortical dementia;
  substance-induced persisting dementia; vascular dementia

dementia pugilistica
 defined 533
 described 343
 traumatic brain injury 219–20
"The Dementias: Hope through
 Research" (NINDS) 335n, 525n
demyelination, defined 533
dendrites
 described 14
 Huntington disease 383–84
deoxyribonucleic acid (DNA)
 defined 533
 Huntington disease 368–70
Depo-Provera (medroxyprogesterone)
 276
deprenyl 439
depressed skull fracture, defined 533
depression, dementia 349
detachable coil, defined 533
developmental delay, described 471
dexamethasone 405
dextroamphetamine 518
diabetes mellitus
 dementia 352, 359
 metabolic syndrome 118–19
 stroke risk 85
Diamox (acetazolamide) 302
diazepam 411, *413*
diet and nutrition
 amyotrophic lateral sclerosis 321–22
 brain aneurysms 130
 dementia 347
 epilepsy 263
 migraine 496
 multiple sclerosis 410
 Parkinson disease 441–42
 stroke research 121–22
diffuse axonal injury, defined 550
 see also shearing
digital subtraction angiography
 (DSI), described 28
dihydroergotamine
 defined 533
 described 498
Dilantin (phenytoin) 276
Disipal (orphenadrine) 439
diuretic medications, encephalitis 178
DNA *see* deoxyribonucleic acid
dominant, defined 533

donepezil 357, 358
dopamine
  defined 533
  described *21*
  Parkinson disease 449 438–39
  traumatic brain injury 224
Doppler, Christian 24–25
Doppler Effect, described 24–25
Doppler ultrasound
  stroke 79
  traumatic brain injury 213
"Doubling Up: Researchers Combine
  a Common Dietary Supplement
  with an Antibiotic to Treat Lou
  Gehrig's Disease" (NINDS) 325n
Down syndrome, dementia 353
drop attacks
  defined 533
  described 253
drug abuse, blood-brain barrier 17
DSI *see* digital subtraction angiography
duplex Doppler ultrasound, defined
  533
dura
  defined 534
  described 5
dura mater, described 5
dysarthria
  defined 534
  traumatic brain injury 218
dyskinesias
  defined 534
  Parkinson disease 438
dyskinetic cerebral palsy, described 464
dysphagia, defined 534
dysplasia
  defined 534
  epilepsy 249
dystonia, Huntington disease 377

E

EAE *see* experimental allergic
  encephalomyelitis
early myoclonic encephalopathy
  defined 534
  described 254
early seizures, defined 534

eastern equine encephalitis (EEE)
  179–80, 182–83
Easter Seals, contact information 563
EC bypass *see* extracranial bypass
EC/IC *see* extracranial/intracranial
  (EC/IC) bypass surgery
eclampsia
  defined 534
  described 256
edema
  defined 534
  stroke 98
EEE *see* eastern equine encephalitis
EEG *see* electroencephalogram
"EEG" (A.D.A.M., Inc.) 35n
Elam, Jennifer Stine 331
Eldepryl (deprenyl) 439
electrical signals, neurons 17–19
electrical stimulation, cerebrum 7–8
electroencephalogram (EEG)
  cerebral palsy 473
  coma 235
  defined 534
  dementia 355
  encephalitis 177
  epilepsy 256
  headache 489
  hypoxia 201
  narcolepsy 518
  overview 35–38
  traumatic brain injury 213
electrolytes, coma 235
"Electromyography" (A.D.A.M., Inc.) 39n
electromyography (EMG)
  amyotrophic lateral sclerosis 319
  defined 534
  narcolepsy 518
  overview 39–41
Elkins, William 111
embolic stroke
  defined 534
  described 75
embolus
  defined 534
  described 75
"Embryonic Mouse Stem Cells
  Reduce Symptoms in Model for
  Parkinson's Disease" (NINDS) 443n
EMG *see* electromyography

emotional deficits
  stroke 93
  traumatic brain injury 218
encephalitis
  headache 502
  overview 174–88
"Encephalitis"
  (Healthcommunities.com, Inc.) 174n
endarterectomy
  defined 541
  described 26, 89–90
  stroke 79
endorphins
  defined 534
  headache 488
endothelial wall, defined 534
endovascular coiling, brain aneurysms 127, 131–32
entacapone 439
environmental factors
  brain tumors 142
  Parkinson disease 437
ependymal cells, described 4
ependymoma, described 140
epidural hematoma, defined 534
epilepsy
  cerebral palsy 465–66
  elderly 287–92
  overview 246–73
  women 274–86
  see also absence epilepsy; frontal lobe
    epilepsy; idiopathic epilepsy;
    juvenile myoclonic epilepsy; neo-
    cortical epilepsy; photosensitive
    epilepsy; progressive epilepsy;
    progressive myoclonus epilepsy
Epilepsy Association Australia,
  seizures first aid publication 309n
Epilepsy Foundation, contact information 564
Epilepsy Institute, contact information 564
Epilepsy Ontario, publications
  elderly epilepsy 287n
  epilepsy 274n
  vagus nerve stimulation 293n
Epilepsy Project, publications
  psychogenic seizures 303n
  seizures first aid 309n

epilepsy syndromes, defined 535
ergotamine tartrate
  defined 535
  migraine 495, 497
erosive gastritis, defined 535
estrogen
  clinical trial 58–60
  dementia 363
  Parkinson disease 454–56
  stroke 94–95
ethnic factors
  multiple sclerosis 398
  stroke risk 80
evoked potentials (EP), hypoxia 201
excessive daytime sleepiness,
  described 513–14
excitatory amino acids, defined 535
excitatory neurotransmitters
  defined 535
  described 19
  Parkinson disease 437
EXCITE *see* Extremity Constrain-
  Induced Therapy Evaluation
excitotoxicity, described 96
Exelon (rivastigmine) 357
exercise
  dementia 360
  Parkinson disease 441
experimental allergic encephalomyelitis (EAE), defined 535
extracranial bypass (EC bypass),
  defined 535
extracranial/intracranial (EC/IC)
  bypass surgery, described 89–90
Extremity Constrain-Induced
  Therapy Evaluation (EXCITE) 104

F

failure to thrive
  cerebral palsy 466, 480
  defined 535
falx, described 5
familial British dementia 345
familial Danish dementia 345
Family Caregiver Alliance
  contact information 558
  hypoxia publication 197n

Family Intervention in Recovery from Stroke Trial (FIRST) 102

FAST-MAG *see* Field Administration of Stroke Therapy Magnesium Trial

fatal familial insomnia
defined 535
described 345

fatigue, defined 535

FDA *see* US Food and Drug Administration

febrile seizures
defined 535
described 255, 304–8

"Febrile Seizures Fact Sheet" (NINDS) 303n

festination, defined 535

fibrinogen 86

Field Administration of Stroke Therapy Magnesium Trial (FAST-MAG) 105

financial considerations
multiple sclerosis 396
stroke 73
traumatic brain injury 206–7
vagus nerve stimulation 298

FIRST *see* Family Intervention in Recovery from Stroke Trial

"First Aid" (Epilepsy Association Australia) 309n

first aid, seizures 309–12

first seizures
caregivers 272
described 254–55

Fischbeck, Kenneth H. 333

fissures, described 7

fluconazole, cryptococcal meningitis 165–66

flucytosine 165

fluent aphasia, defined 535

fluoroscope
brain aneurysm 127
cerebral angiography 27

fluoxetine 377

fMRI *see* functional magnetic resonance imaging

focal seizures
defined 535
described 251

folic acid 263

Food and Drug Administration (FDA) *see* US Food and Drug Administration

Foramen of Munro, described 6

formaldehyde, brain tumors 142

Michael J. Fox Foundation for Parkinson's Research, contact information 566

fractionation, brain tumors 148

"Frequently Asked Questions about the Women's Health Initiative Memory Study (WHIMS)" (WHI) 58n

Freud, Sigmund 461–62

Friedlander, Robert 326, 327–29

frontal lobe epilepsy, defined 536

frontal lobes, described 7, 8

frontotemporal dementias
defined 536
described 341–42

FTDP-17, defined 536

functional magnetic resonance imaging (fMRI)
defined 536
dementia 355
epilepsy 257
Huntington disease 385
multiple sclerosis 404
stroke 79

G

GABA *see* gamma-aminobutyric acid

gadolinium, defined 536

gait analysis
cerebral palsy 478–79
defined 536
dementia 341

galantamine 357

gamma-aminobutyric acid (GABA)
defined 536
described *21*
epilepsy 270

gamma interferon, described 539

gamma knife surgery, described 156–57

gastrostomy, defined 536

Lou Gehrig's disease *see* amyotrophic lateral sclerosis

Gencheva, Eugenia 116–18
gender factor
  amyotrophic lateral sclerosis 317
  brain tumors 141
  stroke risk 80
generalized seizures
  defined 536
  described 252
genes
  amyotrophic lateral sclerosis 332–
    33
  defined 536
  dementia 350–51, 363
  epilepsy 249, 270
  Huntington disease 368–70
  multiple sclerosis 398–99
  narcolepsy 516
  Parkinson disease 436–37, 443–45
gene therapy
  Huntington disease 381–82
  stroke 97
German measles *see* rubella
germ cell tumor of brain, described 141
Gerstmann-Straussler-Scheinker
  disease
  defined 536
  described 345
Glasgow Coma Scale
  defined 536
  described 210–11, 237
glatiramer acetate 419
glia
  cerebrum 7
  defined 536–37
  described 16
  stroke 75, 106
glial cells *see* glia
gliomas, described 140
global aphasia, defined 537
glutamate
  amyotrophic lateral sclerosis 320
  defined 537
  dementia 357
  described *21*
  stroke 96, 107
glycine, described *21*
Hazel K. Goddess Fund for Stroke
  Research in Women, contact information 568

Goldstein, David S. 447–48
good cholesterol *see* high-density
  lipoprotein (HDL) cholesterol
Gorelick, Philip B. 117
grand mal seizures
  defined 537
  described 252
gray matter, described 7
Guardians of Hydrocephalus Research
  Foundation, contact information
  565
Guglielmi detachable coils, described
  131
gyri, described 7

H

Haemophilus influenzae type b (Hib),
  meningitis 160
HAI *see* hypoxic-anoxic injury
Haldol (haloperidol) 439
hallucinations, described 515
haloperidol 439
Harper-Bennie, Judith 420n
Hart, John 330–31
*Harvard Medical School Family
  Health Guide* (Harvard College)
  45n, 51n
HDL *see* high-density lipoprotein
headache
  overview 487–504
  triggers 492–93
headache-free migraine, described
  494
"Headache: Hope through Research"
  (NINDS) 487n, 525n
head injuries
  cerebral palsy 470
  epilepsy 250
  headache 502
  stroke risk 87
Healthcommunities.com, Inc.,
  encephalitis publication 174n
heart disease
  dementia 349
  stroke risk 82–83
The Heart of Diabetes: Understanding
  Insulin Resistance program 120

helmet-type cooling apparatus, stroke
    research 110–12
hematoma, defined 537
hemianopia
    defined 537
    described 466
hemiparesis, defined 537, 551
hemiparetic tremors, defined 537
hemiplegia, defined 537
hemiplegic migraine
    defined 537
    described 493
hemispherectomy 262
hemispheres
    defined 537
    described 6–7
    language 11
hemispherotomy 262
hemorrhagic stroke
    children 95
    defined 537
    described 75–76
heparin
    cerebral angiography 28, 88
    defined 537
    stroke therapy 88
Hereditary Disease Foundation,
    contact information 564
heredity
    amyotrophic lateral sclerosis 317,
        329–31
    brain tumors 142
    dementia 345, 350, 351–52, 363
    epilepsy 248–49, 270
    frontotemporal dementia 342
    Huntington disease 369–70
    hydrocephalus 506
    multiple sclerosis 398–99
    Parkinson disease 436–37, 443–45
    stroke 97
    stroke risk 80, 87–88
herpes simplex encephalitis 174
Hib see Haemophilus influenzae type b
high blood pressure see hypertension
high-density lipoprotein (HDL)
    cholesterol
    defined 537
    stroke 84–85
HII see hypoxic-ischemic injury

hippocampus, defined 537
HIV-associated dementia
    defined 537
    described 343
HIV disease, cryptococcal meningitis 165
HLA see human leukocyte antigens
homeostasis
    defined 538
    primary cell death 106
homocysteine 359
homonymous hemianopia 466
hormones
    epilepsy 274–77
    Parkinson disease 454–56
Horsley, Victor 130
human leukocyte antigens (HLA),
    defined 538
huntingtin 382–83, 390–91
Huntington, George 368
Huntington disease
    defined 538
    described 343
    research 380–86, 387–91
"Huntington's Disease: Hope through
    Research" (NINDS) 368n, 525n
Huntington's Disease Society of
    America, contact information 564
hydrocephalus
    defined 538
    described 6
    overview 505–10
    traumatic brain injury 214
Hydrocephalus Association, contact
    information 565
"Hydrocephalus Fact Sheet" (NINDS)
    505n
Hydrocephalus Support Group, Inc.,
    contact information 565
hypercholesterolemia 117–18
hyperfractionation, brain tumors 148
hypermetabolism, defined 538
hypertension (high blood pressure)
    alcohol abuse 86
    brain aneurysms 130
    defined 538
    dementia 359–60
    stroke 76, 81–82
hyperthyroidism, traumatic brain
    injury 216

hypertonia, defined 538
hypocretin gene 516–17
hypothalamus, described 6, 9
hypothermia therapy, stroke research 110–12
hypothyroidism, defined 538
hypotonia, described 471
hypoxia
    defined 538
    overview 197–203
    stroke 97–98
"Hypoxic-Anoxic Brain Injury" (Family Caregiver Alliance) 197n
hypoxic-anoxic injury (HAI), described 197–201
hypoxic-ischemic encephalopathy
    cerebral palsy 482
    defined 538
hypoxic-ischemic injury (HII), described 198–201

I

IC bypass *see* intracranial bypass
ICP *see* intracranial pressure
idiopathic epilepsy, defined 538
IgG *see* immunoglobulin G
IHAST *see* Intraoperative Hypothermia for Aneurysm Surgery Trial
immediate seizures, defined 538
immune response, stroke 107
immune system, multiple sclerosis 396–98, 414
immunoglobulin G (IgG), defined 538
immunosuppression
    defined 539
    multiple sclerosis 406–7
Imuran (azathioprine) 407
inaccessible tumor, defined 539
incidence, defined 539
infantile spasms, defined 539
infarction
    defined 539
    described 74
infarcts
    defined 539
    vascular dementia 339

infections
    dementia 347–48
    multiple sclerosis 398
    stroke risk 87
    traumatic brain injury 214
inflammation
    dementia 360
    multiple sclerosis 426
    stroke 107
inflammatory headache, defined 539
"Information on Arboviral Encephalitides" (CDC) 174n
inhibitory neurotransmitters
    defined 539
    described 19
inoperable tumor, defined 539
Institute for the Study of Aging, contact information 561
interferons
    defined 539
    multiple sclerosis 406, 415–19
interleukins
    defined 539
    multiple sclerosis 409–10
International Essential Tremor Foundation, contact information 565
International RadioSurgery Association (IRSA), metastatic brain tumors publication 154n
International Subarachnoid Aneurysm Trial (ISAT) 127–28, 133
intracerebral hematoma, defined 539
intracerebral hemorrhage
    defined 539
    described 76
intracranial aneurysms *see* brain aneurysms
intracranial bypass (IC bypass), defined 535
intracranial pressure (ICP)
    defined 540
    traumatic brain injury 211
intractable, defined 540
Intraoperative Hypothermia for Aneurysm Surgery Trial (IHAST) 103
"Introduction to Vagus Nerve Stimulation" (Epilepsy Ontario) 293n

ion channels
  defined 540
  epilepsy 249
ions, neurons 17–18
IRSA *see* International
  RadioSurgery Association
Isacson, Ole 446
ISAT *see* International Subarachnoid
  Aneurysm Trial
ischemia
  defined 540
  described 74
ischemic cascade
  defined 540
  described 96, 105–6
ischemic penumbra
  defined 540
  described 74
ischemic stroke
  carotenoids 121–22
  cooling helmets 110–12
  defined 540
  described 74–75
  stroke research 112, 117
isotope, positron emission
  tomography 48–49
"Isotope Study" (A.D.A.M., Inc.)
  47n

J

Japanese encephalitis 175, 186
jaundice
  cerebral palsy 467–68.470
  defined 540
juvenile myoclonic epilepsy, defined
  540

K

Karpuj, Marcela 390
ketogenic diet
  defined 540
  overview 300–302
kindling, defined 540
Klonopin (clonazepam) 411, *413*
Koroshetz, Walter J. 389

L

LaCrosse encephalitis (LAC) 179,
  181–82
lacunar infarction
  defined 540
  described 75
Lafora body disease
  defined 540
  described 346–47
Landis, Story C. 430
language deficits, stroke 93
language functions, left hemisphere 11
large vessel disease, defined 541
lateral ventricles, described 6
LDL *see* low-density lipoprotein
Lennox-Gastaut syndrome
  defined 541
  epilepsy 253
  ketogenic diet 300
  vagal nerve stimulation 299
lesion, defined 541
lesionectomy
  defined 541
  epilepsy 261
leukocytes
  defined 541
  stroke 107
leukodystrophies 347
Leustatin (cladribine) 407
levodopa 438–40, 449, 555
Lewy body dementia
  defined 541
  described 340–41
  Parkinson disease 346
  treatment 358
lifestyles
  brain aneurysms 130
  stroke risk 85–86
limbic system, described 11
Lindquist, Susan 456
Lioresal (baclofen) 411, *413*
lipids, described 84
Lipitor (atorvastatin) 428–29
lipoprotein
  defined 541
  see also high-density lipoprotein
    (HDL) cholesterol; low-density
    lipoprotein (LDL) cholesterol

lithium 377
lithium carbonate 498
Little, William 461, 463
lobectomy
  defined 541
  epilepsy 261
lobes, described 7
locked-in syndrome
  defined 541
  described 232
  traumatic brain injury 212–13
Lou Gehrig's disease *see* amyotrophic
  lateral sclerosis
low-density lipoprotein (LDL) cholesterol
  defined 541
  stroke 84–85
lumbar puncture (spinal tap)
  brain tumors 144
  defined 541
  headache 502
  overview 51–52
Luminal (phenobarbital) 276

M

Ma, Jing 121–22
macroglia, described 16
mad cow disease *see* bovine
  spongiform encephalopathy
magnesium sulfate 105
magnetic resonance angiography
  (MRA)
  defined 541
  stroke 79
magnetic resonance imaging (MRI)
  brain tumors 143
  cerebral palsy 472
  coma 236
  concussion 227–28
  defined 541
  dementia 354
  encephalitis 177
  epilepsy 257
  headache 489–90
  Huntington disease 373–74
  hydrocephalus 508
  hypoxia 201

magnetic resonance imaging (MRI),
  continued
  multiple sclerosis 403–5, 414
  overview 45–46
  stroke 78–79
  traumatic brain injury 211, 213
magnetic resonance spectroscopy
  (MRS), defined 542
magnetization transfer imaging
  (MTI), multiple sclerosis 404
magnetoencephalogram (MEG)
  defined 542
  dementia 355
  epilepsy 257
magnets, vagus nerve stimulation
  298–99
malignant, defined 542
March of Dimes Birth Defects Foundation, contact information 563
marker, defined 542
Marks, Michael P. 108–9
Martí-Fabregas, Joan 120–21
Martin, Roland 430
MBP *see* myelin basic protein
McClellan, Mark B. 163
McKay, Ronald 449–50
mechanical aids, cerebral palsy 479–80
medications
  amyotrophic lateral sclerosis 320–21
  dementia 356–58
  migraine 494–95
  Parkinson disease 438–40
  stroke therapies 88–89
  see also individual medications
medroxyprogesterone 276
Medtronic, Inc., deep brain
  stimulation publication 54n
medulla oblongata, described 10
medulloblastoma, described 140
MEG *see* magnetoencephalogram
melatonin 263
memantine 357
meninges
  defined 542
  described 5
meningioma, described 140
meningitis
  headache 502
  overview 160–69

"Meningococcal Disease" (CDC) 160n
meningococcal vaccine 166–69
"Meningococcal Vaccine: What You
  Need to Know" (CDC) 160n
menopause, epilepsy 285–86
mental impairment, cerebral palsy
  465
MERCI Retrieval System 113–14
messages, cerebrum 7–8
metabolic syndrome, stroke research
  118–20
metabolized, defined 542
metachromatic leukodystrophy 347
"Metastatic Brain Tumors" (IRSA)
  154n
metastatic tumors
  brain 154–58
  defined 542
methamphetamine 518
methotrexate 407
methylphenidate 518
methylprednisolone 405, 411, *413*
methysergide 498
methysergide maleate 495
metoclopramide 439
Mezey, Éva 61–63
microglia
  dementia 350
  described 16
midbrain, described 10
migraine headache
  aura, defined 528
  defined 542
  described 490–96
  see also basilar artery migraine;
    hemiplegic migraine; ophthal-
    moplegic migraine
mild cognitive impairment
  defined 542
  dementia 352
  described 349
minimally responsive state, described
  231
Mini-Mental State Examination
  (MMSE)
  defined 542
  described 354
mini-stroke *see* transient ischemic
  attack

minocycline 325–26, 327–29
"Minocycline Delays Onset and Slows
  Progression of ALS in Mice"
  (NINDS) 325n
Mirapex (pramipexole) 439
"Misbehaving Molecules:
  3-Dimensional Pictures of ALS
  Mutant Proteins Support Two
  Major Theories about How the
  Disease is Caused" (NINDS) 325n
mitochondria
  amyotrophic lateral sclerosis (ALS)
    325–26
  defined 543
  Parkinson disease 437
mitochondrial myopathies 347
mitoxantrone 407, 419
MMSE *see* Mini-Mental State
  Examination
modafinil 519
monoclonal antibodies, multiple
  sclerosis 407
monosodium glutamate (MSG) 497
mosquitoes, encephalitis 174, 179–88
motor aphasia, defined 543
MRA *see* magnetic resonance
  angiography
MRI *see* magnetic resonance imaging
MRS *see* magnetic resonance
  spectroscopy
MSG *see* monosodium glutamate
MTI *see* magnetization transfer
  imaging
mucopolysaccharidosis III 347
Mueller, D.M. 226n
multi-infarct dementia
  defined 543
  described 339
multiple sclerosis (MS)
  cooling 420–25
  dementia 346
  interferons 539
  myelin breakdown 543
  overview 394–415
  research 426–31
  treatment safety issues 415–19
  *Multiple Sclerosis and Cooling,
    Third Edition* (Roberts; Harper-
    Bennie) 420n

Multiple Sclerosis Association of
America, contact information 565
Multiple Sclerosis Foundation,
contact information 566
"Multiple Sclerosis: Hope through
Research" (NINDS) 394n, 525n
"Multiple Sclerosis Treatment: Some
Safety Issues to Keep in Mind"
(American Academy of Neurology)
415n
multiple subpial transection
defined 543
epilepsy 261–62
Murphy, Diane 457
Murray Valley encephalitis 175, 188
muscle-contraction headaches
defined 543
described 499–501
muscles, amyotrophic lateral sclerosis
316–18
Muscular Dystrophy Association,
contact information 560
mutations, defined 543
myelin
defined 543
dementia 340, 363
multiple sclerosis 394, 395, 408,
420, 426
myelin basic protein (MBP), defined
543
myelin sheaths, described 16
myelogram
brain tumors 144
defined 543
myoclonic seizures
defined 543
described 252
myoclonus
defined 543
Huntington disease 371
treatment 358
Mysoline (primidone) 276

N

Nadkarni, Vinay 112
NAF *see* National Ataxia Foundation
Najarian, Robert M. 118–20

Namenda (memantine) 357
narcolepsy, overview 511–21
"Narcolepsy Fact Sheet" (NINDS) 511n
NARIC *see* National Rehabilitation
Information Center
National Aphasia Association, contact
information 568
National Ataxia Foundation (NAF),
contact information 566
National Brain Tumor Foundation
(NBTF), contact information 562
National Cancer Institute (NCI)
brain tumors publication 136n
contact information 562
National Family Caregiver Associa-
tion, contact information 559
National Headache Foundation,
contact information 564
National Hospice and Palliative Care
Organization/National Hospice Foundation, contact information 559
National Hydrocephalus Foundation,
contact information 565
National Institute of Mental Health
(NIMH), contact information 561
National Institute of Neurological
Disorders and Stroke (NINDS),
publications
amyotrophic lateral sclerosis 316n
amyotrophic lateral sclerosis
research 325n
bone marrow study 61n
brain tumors 525n
cerebral palsy 461n
dementias 335n
epilepsy 246n
febrile seizures 303n
headache 487n
Huntington disease 368n
Huntington disease research 387n
hydrocephalus 505n
multiple sclerosis 394n
multiple sclerosis research 426n
narcolepsy 511n
Parkinson disease 525n
Parkinson disease research 443n
seizures 246n
stroke 72n
traumatic brain injury 206n

National Institute on Aging Information Center, contact information 561

National Institute on Disability and Rehabilitation Research (NIDRR), contact information 558

National Multiple Sclerosis Society, contact information 566

National Organization for Rare Disorders (NORD), contact information 558

National Parkinson Foundation, contact information 566

National Rehabilitation Information Center (NARIC), contact information 558

National Respite Network and Resource Center, contact information 559

National Stroke Association, contact information 568

Navane (thiothixene) 439

NBTF *see* National Brain Tumor Foundation

NCV *see* nerve conduction velocity

near-infrared spectroscopy, defined 544

neck injuries, stroke risk 87

necrosis, defined 544

Neisseria meningitidis, meningitis 160, 161–62

neocortical epilepsy
    defined 544
    described 253

neonatal hemorrhage, defined 544

neoplasms, defined 544

neprilysin 365

nerve cells *see* neurons

"Nerve Conduction Velocity" (A.D.A.M., Inc.) 42n

nerve conduction velocity (NCV)
    amyotrophic lateral sclerosis 319
    overview 42–44

nervous system, described 4

neural stem cells
    defined 544
    traumatic brain injury 224

neurocysticercosis
    defined 544
    described 189, 190
    epilepsy 249

neurodegeneration with brain iron accumulation 347

neuroexcitation, defined 544

neurofibrillary tangles
    defined 544
    dementia 345

NeuroFlo 114–15

neuroglia
    defined 536–37
    described 4

neurons
    amyotrophic lateral sclerosis 316
    cerebrum 7
    defined 544
    depicted *14, 15*
    described 4, 13–15
    epilepsy 246, 249, 270
    Huntington disease 369
    multiple sclerosis 426
    signals 17–19
    stroke 106

neuroprotectants, described 89

neuroprotection, described 96

neuroprotective agents, defined 544

neurotransmitters
    amyotrophic lateral sclerosis 320
    defined 544
    epilepsy 269–70
    neurons 18–19

"New Findings about Parkinson's Disease: Coffee and Hormones Don't Mix" (NINDS) 443n

"New Horizons for Seniors Living with Epilepsy" (Epilepsy Ontario) 274n, 287

NIDRR *see* National Institute on Disability and Rehabilitation Research

Niemann-Pick disease, dementia 346

NIH Stroke Scale
    described 78
    stroke research 115

NIMH *see* National Institute of Mental Health

nimodipine 89

NINDS *see* National Institute of Neurological Disorders and Stroke

nociceptors
    defined 544–45
    headache 488, 492

nonconvulsive, defined 545
nonepileptic events
  defined 545
  described 255–56
nonepileptic seizures, overview 303–8
nonfluent aphasia, defined 545
nonsteroidal anti-inflammatory drugs
  (NSAID), dementia 360
NORD *see* National Organization for
  Rare Disorders
norepinephrine, described *21*
normal pressure hydrocephalus 346
nortriptyline 377
Novantrone (mitoxantrone) 407, 419,
  429
Nyenhuis, David 116, 118

O

Oakes, David 453
occipital lobes, described 7, 8
occupational therapy
  brain tumor recovery 152
  cerebral palsy 474
  Parkinson disease 442
  stroke recovery 91, *91*
olanzapine 341
"Old Drug, New Use: New
  Research Shows Common
  Cholesterol-Lowering Drug
  Reduces Multiple Sclerosis
  Symptoms in Mice" (NINDS) 426n
oligodendrocytes
  defined 545
  described 16
  multiple sclerosis 426–27
oligodendroglia, described 4
oligodendroglioma, described 140
Oliver, Eugene J. 389
olivopontocerebellar atrophy 346
on-off effect, defined 545
ophthalmoplegic migraine
  defined 545
  described 493
optic neuritis, defined 545
oral contraceptives
  epilepsy 275–76, 279
  stroke 94–95

organic brain syndrome, defined 545
  see also senile dementia
orgasmic headache 499
Oro, J.J. 226n
orphenadrine 439
orthostatic hypotension 447–48
orthotic devices, defined 545
osteoporosis, epilepsy 286
Outeiro, Tiago Fleming 456
oxygen-free radicals, defined 545

P

PACE *see* Parents Against Childhood
  Epilepsy
pain
  stroke 93–94
  traumatic brain injury 215
pallidotomy, defined 545
pallidum, defined 546
palsy, defined 546
  see also cerebral palsy
PAN *see* Parkinson's Action Network
papaverine *413*
paralysis, stroke 92
paraparesis, defined 551
"Parenting Concerns" (Epilepsy
  Ontario) 274n
Parents Against Childhood Epilepsy
  (PACE), contact information 564
paresis, defined 546
paresthesias, defined 546
parietal lobes, described 7, 9
Parkinson disease
  deep brain stimulation 54–57
  dementia 345–46
  overview 434–42
  research 443–57
  traumatic brain injury 219
"Parkinsonian Symptoms Decrease in
  Rats Given Stem Cell Transplants"
  (NINDS) 443n
Parkinsonism, defined 546
Parkinson's Action Network (PAN),
  contact information 567
Parkinson's dementia, defined 546
"Parkinson's Disease: An Overview"
  (PDF) 434n

Parkinson's Disease Foundation (PDF)
  contact information 567
  Parkinson disease publication 434n
"Parkinson's Disease: Hope through
  Research" (NINDS) 525n
Parkinson's Institute, contact information 567
Parlodel (bromocriptine) 439
partial seizures, defined 546
patent foramen ovale (PFO), stroke 83
pathologists, described 4
"A Patient's Guide to Carotid Ultrasound" (Rundek; Sacco) 24n
PCS *see* post-concussive syndrome
PDF *see* Parkinson's Disease Foundation
pemoline 412, *413*, 518
penetrating head injury, defined 546
penicillin 167
peptide therapy, multiple sclerosis
  408–9
pergolide 439
Pericak-Vance, Margaret A. 443, 445
periosteum, described 5
peripheral nervous system, described 4
Permax (pergolide) 439
persistent vegetative state (PVS)
  defined 546
  described 231
  traumatic brain injury 212
  see also vegetative state
petit mal seizures
  defined 546
  described 252
PET scan *see* positron emission
  tomography
PFO *see* patent foramen ovale
phenobarbital 276
phenol 411
phenothiazines 439
phenytoin 276
photosensitive epilepsy
  defined 546
  described 250
physical therapy
  amyotrophic lateral sclerosis 321
  brain tumor recovery 152
  cerebral palsy 474, 475–77
  Parkinson disease 442
  stroke recovery 91, *91*

pia mater
  described 5
  stroke 76
Pick's disease
  defined 546
  described 342
pineal gland, described 9
pineal region tumor, described 141
pituitary fossa, described 9
pituitary gland, hypothalamus 9
plaque
  atherosclerosis 75, 84
  carotid ultrasound 25–26
  defined 546, 547
plasma homocysteine, dementia 352
plasmapheresis, multiple sclerosis 407
plasticity, defined 547
platelets, defined 547
plegia, defined 546
pneumocephalus, defined 547
poison
  dementia 348
  seizures 250
pons, described 10
positron emission tomography (PET scan)
  coma 236
  defined 547
  dementia 355
  Huntington disease 374, 385
  overview 47–50
post-concussive syndrome (PCS),
  defined 547
post-traumatic amnesia (PTA),
  defined 547
post-traumatic dementia
  defined 547
  traumatic brain injury 220
postural instability, defined 547
Powassan encephalitis 175, 179, 185
pramipexole 439
prednisolone 405
prednisone
  defined 547
  described 405
pregnancy
  cerebral palsy 467–70
  eclampsia 256
  epilepsy 266–68, 270–71, 274, 277–79
  stroke 94–95

"Pregnancy" (Epilepsy Ontario) 274n
premotor cortex, described 8
presenile dementia with motor
  neuron disease 346
presenilins
  defined 547
  dementia 350
presynaptic terminals, described 14–15
prevalence, defined 548
primary dementia
  defined 548
  described 337
primary encephalitis, described 174–75
primary progressive aphasia
  defined 548
  described 342
primary tumors, defined 548
primidone 276
procyclidine 439
progestin, clinical trial 58–60
prognosis, defined 548
progressive dementia
  defined 548
  described 337
progressive epilepsy, defined 548
progressive myoclonus epilepsy,
  defined 548
Project ALS, contact information 560
propranolol 498
propranolol hydrochloride 495
prosodic dysfunction
  defined 548
  traumatic brain injury 218
prostaglandins
  defined 548
  migraine headaches 492
protein antigen feeding, multiple
  sclerosis 409
proton beam radiation therapy, brain
  tumors 148
pruning, defined 548
psychiatric therapy, stroke recovery
  91, 92
psychogenic seizures
  defined 548
  described 255, 303–4
"Psychogenic Seizures" (Epilepsy
  Project) 303n

psychological therapy, stroke recovery
  91, 92
PTA see post-traumatic amnesia
putamen, defined 548
PVS see persistent vegetative state

Q

quadriparesis, defined 551

R

racial factor
  brain tumors 141
  stroke risk 80
radiation therapy, brain tumors 142,
  148–49, 155–56
radiosurgery, brain tumors 156–57
Rancho Los Amigos Scale, described
  237
Rankin scale, stroke research 116
Rasmussen's encephalitis
  defined 549
  described 253, 347
Rebif (beta interferon) 406, 416, 419
rebound effect, alcohol use 86
receptors
  defined 549
  molecules 20
  neurons 18–19
recessive, defined 549
recombinant tissue plasminogen
  activator (rt-PA)
  defined 549
  described 89
recurrent stroke, described 77
reductase inhibitors, cholesterol
  levels 85
reflexes, defined 549
Reglan (metoclopramide) 439
rehabilitation therapy
  stroke 91–92
  traumatic brain injury 220–21
relapsing-remitting multiple sclerosis
  399
relaxation therapy, migraine 495–96
remacemide 387–89

Reminyl (galantamine) 357
remyelination
  described 410
  multiple sclerosis 426–27
Requip (ropinirole) 439
"Researchers Find Genetic Links for
  Late-Onset Parkinson's Disease"
  (NINDS) 443n
resting membrane potentials,
  described 17–18
reticular activating system, described
  10
retrobulbar neuritis, defined 549
retropulsion, defined 549
Rh incompatibility
  cerebral palsy 468, 470
  defined 549
ribavirin 177
rigidity
  defined 549
  Parkinson disease 435
Rilutek (riluzole) 320–21
riluzole 320–21, 326
risk factors
  cerebral palsy 468–70
  encephalitis 175–76
  traumatic brain injury 208
rivastigmine 357
Roberts, Adam 420n
ropinirole 439
rt-PA *see* recombinant tissue
  plasminogen activator
rubella (German measles)
  cerebral palsy 471
  defined 549
Rundek, Tanja 24n

S

Sacco, Ralph L. 24n
St. Louis encephalitis (SLE) 179–80,
  184–85
Sandimmune (cyclosporine) 407
Sanfilippo syndrome 347
Schilder's disease 347
Schwann cells, described 16
Schwannoma, described 140
Schwarzschild, Michael 455

"Scientists Identify Potential
  New Treatment for Huntington's
  Disease" (NINDS) 387n
Scott, William K. 444
secondary dementias
  defined 549
  described 337, 345–46
secondary encephalitis, described 175
Secondary Prevention of Small
  Subcortical Strokes (SPS3) 104–5
secondary-progressive multiple
  sclerosis 399
second opinions, brain tumors 145–46
seizure focus, defined 549
seizures
  cerebral palsy 465–66
  children 96
  defined 550
  elderly 287–92
  epilepsy 246–73
  first aid 309–12
  nonepileptic 303–8
  see also clonic seizures; complex
    focal seizures; early seizures;
    febrile seizures; focal seizures;
    generalized seizures; grand mal
    seizures; immediate seizures;
    myoclonic seizures; partial sei-
    zures; petit mal seizures; tonic-
    clonic seizures; tonic seizures
"Seizures and Epilepsy: Hope
  through Research" (NINDS) 246n,
  525n
"Seizures in Airplanes" (Epilepsy
  Project) 309n
"Seizures in Water" (Epilepsy Project)
  309n
seizure threshold, defined 549
seizure triggers, defined 549–50
selective dorsal root rhizotomy
  defined 550
  described 479, 483
Selegiline 439
senataxin gene 332–33
"Senataxin Gene Linked to Juvenile-
  Onset ALS" (NINDS) 325n
senile chorea
  defined 550
  described 372

senile dementia
  defined 550
  described 335–36
senility *see* senile dementia
senses, described 3
sensory aphasia *see* fluent aphasia
Serbinenko, Fjodor A. 131
serotonin
  defined 550
  described *21*
  migraine headaches 491, 494
sertraline 377
SES *see* socioeconomic status
sexual relationships
  epilepsy 282–85
  multiple sclerosis 413
"Sexual Relationships" (Epilepsy Ontario) 274n
shaken baby syndrome
  defined 550
  overview 238–41
shearing, defined 550
Shults, Clifford 451
SIADH *see* syndrome of inappropriate secretion of antidiuretic hormone
sickle cell anemia, stroke 95
side effects
  brain tumor treatments 149–51, 155
  cerebral palsy medications 478
  fluconazole 166
  Parkinson disease medications 440
  vagus nerve stimulation 296
Simon Foundation for Continence, contact information 561
simple focus seizures
  defined 550
  described 251
Sinemet (carbidopa) 438, 439
Sinemet (levodopa) 439
single-infarct dementia, described 340
single photon emission computed tomography (SPECT scan)
  coma 237
  defined 550
  dementia 355
  epilepsy 257
  traumatic brain injury 213

sinus infection, headache 503
sinusitis, defined 550
skull, described 5
skull fractures, traumatic brain injury 214–15
SLE *see* St. Louis encephalitis
sleep deprivation
  epilepsy 250
  narcolepsy 511–21
sleep paralysis, described 514–15
"Small Trial Shows Daclizumab Add-On Therapy Improves Multiple Sclerosis Outcome" (NINDS) 426n
small vessel disease, defined 551
smoking cessation, brain aneurysms 130
socioeconomic status (SES), stroke risk 81
SOD1 *see* superoxide dismutase 1
sodium valproate 358
Solu-Medrol (methylprednisolone) 411, *413*
soma, described 13
Soni, Deepa 129n
SPAF *see* Stroke Prevention in Atrial Fibrillation
spastic cerebral palsy, described 464
spastic diplegia, defined 551
spastic hemiplegia, defined 551
spasticity, defined 551
spastic paraplegia, defined 551
spastic quadriplegia, defined 551
SPECT scan *see* single photon emission computed tomography
speech functions
  left hemisphere 11
  traumatic brain injury 218
speech therapy
  amyotrophic lateral sclerosis 321–22
  brain tumor recovery 152
  cerebral palsy 474
  Parkinson disease 442
  stroke recovery *91*, 91–92
spinal tap *see* lumbar puncture
SPS3 *see* Secondary Prevention of Small Subcortical Strokes
Stalevo (carbidopa, levodopa, entacapone) 438

Starkman, Sidney 113–14
statin medications
  cholesterol levels 85
  dementia 363
  multiple sclerosis 427–29
  stroke research 120–21
statistics
  amyotrophic lateral sclerosis 317
  brain aneurysms 124–25
  cerebral palsy 463
  encephalitis 175
  Huntington disease 368
  hypertension 81–82
  meningococcal disease 166
  multiple sclerosis 395
  narcolepsy 512–13
  recurrent stroke 77
  traumatic brain injury 206–7
status epilepticus
  defined 551
  described 268–69
status migrainosus
  defined 551
  described 493
stem cells
  clinical trial 61–63
  Parkinson disease 445–46, 449–50
stenosis
  defined 551
  described 75
  stroke 79
  stroke research 109
stents
  carotid arteries 26
  stroke research 108–9
stereognosia
  defined 551
  described 467
stereotactic radiation therapy, brain
  tumors 148
stereotaxic thalamotomy 479
stereotyped, defined 551
steroids, multiple sclerosis 405–6
strabismus
  defined 551
  described 466
Streptococcus pneumoniae,
  meningitis 160, 162, 164
striatum, defined 551

stroke
  carotid ultrasound 25–26
  cerebral palsy 468
  described 73–74
  headache 501–2
  overview 72–107
  research 96–98, 108–22
  risk factors 79–88
  symptoms 74, 77
  therapies 88–92
  types, described 74–77
  vascular dementia 339
  see also acute stroke; embolic
    stroke; hemorrhagic stroke;
    ischemic stroke; thrombotic
    stroke; transient ischemic
    attack
stroke belt
  defined 552
  described 81
stroke buckle, defined 552
"Stroke: Hope through Research"
  (NINDS) 72n, 525n
Stroke Prevention in Atrial
  Fibrillation (SPAF) 88–89
"Study Finds Widespread
  Sympathetic Nerve Damage in
  Parkinson's Disease" (NINDS) 443n
"Study Suggests Coenzyme Q10
  Slows Functional Decline in
  Parkinson's Disease" (NINDS) 443n
stupor
  defined 552
  traumatic brain injury 212
subarachnoid hemorrhage
  brain aneurysms 124
  defined 552
  described 76
  pregnancy 94
subarachnoid space, described 5
subcortical dementia
  defined 552
  described 337
subdural hematoma
  defined 552
  dementia 348
subdural hygroma, defined 552
subdural space, described 5
substance abuse, stroke risk 86

substance-induced persisting
dementia, defined 552
substantia nigra, defined 552
sudden unexplained death
defined 552
described 269
sulci, described 7
sumatriptan
defined 552
headache 498
migraine 495
superoxide dismutase 1 (SOD1) 317,
319–20, 326, 330–31
support groups, Parkinson disease
441
surgical procedures
angioplasty 108–9
brain abscess 172–73
brain aneurysm treatment 126–28
brain tumors 147–48, 155–56
carotid endarterectomy 26, 90–91,
529
cerebral palsy 478–79
corpus callosotomy 262
deep brain stimulation 54–57
epilepsy 258–62
extracranial/intracranial (EC/IC)
bypass 89–90
hemispherectomy 262
hemispherotomy 262
lesionectomy 261, 541
lobectomy 261, 541
multiple subpial transection 261–62
pallidotomy 545
Parkinson disease 440–41
selective dorsal root rhizotomy 550
stroke risk 83
stroke therapies 89–91
ventriculostomy 555
see also biopsy
Symmetrel (amantadine) 412, *413*
Symmetrel (amantadine hydrochloride) 438
sympathetic nervous system 447–48
synapse
depicted *15*
described *20*
synaptic cleft, described 14
synaptic space, described 14

syndrome of inappropriate secretion
of antidiuretic hormone (SIADH)
defined 552
traumatic brain injury 216
synucleinopathies, described 341

T

tacrine 357
taeniasis 189
tangles, dementia 345, 351
tapeworm 189–92
Taractan (chlorprothixene) 439
Tasmar (tolcapone) 439
tau protein
defined 553
dementia 351
Parkinson disease 444
T-cells
defined 553
multiple sclerosis 397, 409–10, 414
Tegretol (carbamazepine) 276
telomerase 362
temporal lobe epilepsy (TLS),
described 253
temporal lobe resection
defined 553
epilepsy 261
temporal lobes, described 7, 8
temporomandibular joint dysfunction,
defined 553
tentorium, described 5
tests
amyotrophic lateral sclerosis 318–19
brain abscess 171–72
brain aneurysms 126
brain disorders 24–52
brain tumors 143–44
carotid ultrasound 24–27
cerebral angiography 27–30
cerebral palsy 471–73
coma 235–37
concussion 227–28
cranial computed tomography scan
31–35
cryptococcal meningitis 165
dementia 353–56
electroencephalogram 35–38

tests, continued
  electromyography 39–41
  encephalitis 177, 180–81
  epilepsy 256–57
  headache 489–90
  Huntington disease 374–77
  hydrocephalus 508
  hypoxia 201
  lumbar puncture 51–52
  magnetic resonance imaging 45–46
  Mini-Mental State Examination
    542
  multiple sclerosis 403–5
  narcolepsy 517–18
  nerve conduction velocity 42–44
  positron emission tomography 47–50
  stroke 78–79
  see also individual tests
thalamus, described 6, 9
thermography, defined 553
thiothixene 439
thioxanthenes 439
three-dimensional conformal radiation therapy, brain tumors 148
thrombolytic agents, described 89
thrombolytics, defined 553
thrombolytic therapy, stroke 78
thrombosis
  defined 553
  described 75
thrombotic stroke
  defined 553
  described 75
thrombus, defined 553
TIA *see* transient ischemic attack
tic douloureux *see* trigeminal
  neuralgia
ticks, encephalitis 175, 178–79,
  186–87
ticlopidine 88, 101
tissue necrosis factors, defined 553
tissue plasminogen activator (t-PA),
  stroke research 113
tizanidine 411, *413*
TLE *see* temporal lobe epilepsy
TMS *see* transcranial magnetic
  stimulation
TOAST *see* Trial of Org 10127 in
  Acute Stroke Treatment

tobacco use
  dementia 352
  epilepsy 250
  stroke risk 85–86
  vagus nerve stimulation 296
tolcapone 439
tonic-clonic seizures
  defined 553–54
  described 252
  first aid 309–10
tonic seizures
  defined 553
  described 252
Topamax (topiramate) 276, 302
topiramate 276, 302
total serum cholesterol, defined 554
t-PA *see* recombinant tissue
  plasminogen activator; tissue
  plasminogen activator
traction headaches, defined 554
trait, defined 554
transcranial magnetic stimulation
  (TMS)
  defined 554
  epilepsy 263
  stroke 98
transgenic mice, defined 554
transient ischemic attack (TIA)
  clinical trials 101
  defined 554
  dementia 355
  described 76–77
  headache 501–2
transmissible spongiform
  encephalopathies
  Creutzfeldt-Jakob disease 344–45
  defined 554
transverse myelitis, defined 554
Trapp, Bruce D. 426–27
traumatic brain injury (TBI), overview 206–25
"Traumatic Brain Injury: Hope through
  Research" (NINDS) 206n, 525n
"Treatment Options for Cerebral
  Aneurysms" (Soni) 129n
tremor
  defined 554
  multiple sclerosis 413
  Parkinson disease 434–35

"Trial Drugs for Huntington's
Disease Inconclusive in Slowing
Disease" (NINDS) 387n
Trial of Org 10127 in Acute Stroke
Treatment (TOAST) 89
trichinellosis, overview 193–95
"Trichinellosis Fact Sheet" (CDC)
193n
trichinosis 193–95
trigeminal neuralgia
defined 555
headache 502–3
tumors
brain 136–53
grades 139
see also accessible tumor;
congenital tumor; inaccessible
tumor; inoperable tumor; metastatic tumors; primary tumors
Les Turner ALS Foundation, contact
information 560

U

UCP *see* United Cerebral Palsy
UHDRS *see* Unified HD Rating Scale
ultrasonography
cerebral palsy 472–73
defined 555
ultrasound
described 24
stroke 79
Unified HD Rating Scale (UHDRS) 371
United Cerebral Palsy (UCP), contact
information 563
University of New Mexico, cryptococcal meningitis publication 160n
US Food and Drug Administration
(FDA)
cochlear implants publication 160n
contact information 558

V

vaccinations
cochlear implants 164
meningococcal disease 166–69

vaccines
encephalitis 180
multiple sclerosis 408
vagus nerve stimulation
described 262–63
overview 293–99
Valium (diazepam) 411, *413*
valproic acid 495, 498
Vance, Jeffrey M. 444
vascular cognitive impairment-
no dementia (VCIND), stroke
research 117
vascular dementia
defined 555
described 339–40
treatment 357–58
vascular headaches
defined 555
described 490, 496–97
vasoconstrictors, described 86
vasodilators
defined 555
stroke 96–97
vasospasms, defined 555
VCIND *see* vascular cognitive
impairment-no dementia
vegetative state
defined 555
described 230–31
traumatic brain injury 212
see also persistent vegetative state
Venezuelan equine encephalitis 175,
185–86
ventricles, defined 555
ventricular system, described 6
ventriculostomy, defined 555
VEP *see* visual evoked potential
verapamil 495, 498
vertebral artery, defined 555
vesicles, described 18–19
vinyl chloride, brain tumors 142
viral meningitis, described 160
Virazole (ribavirin) 177
visual cortex, described 8
visual evoked potential (VEP) 404
VITAL *see* Vitamins to Slow
Alzheimer's Disease
Vitamins to Slow Alzheimer's Disease
(VITAL) 365

W

Waldmann, Thomas 431
Wang, Huan 110–11
WARCEF *see* Warfarin *versus* Aspirin in Reduced Cardiac Ejection Fraction
warfarin
  clinical trials 100–101, 103, 104
  defined 555
  described 88
Warfarin *versus* Aspirin for Intracranial Arterial Stenosis (WASID) 103
Warfarin *versus* Aspirin in Reduced Cardiac Ejection Fraction (WARCEF) 104
Warfarin *versus* Aspirin Recurrent Stroke Study (WARSS) 100–101
WARSS *see* Warfarin *versus* Aspirin Recurrent Stroke Study
WASID *see* Warfarin *versus* Aspirin for Intracranial Arterial Stenosis
WBRT *see* whole brain radiation therapy
wearing-off effect, defined 555
WEE *see* western equine encephalitis
Well Spouse Foundation, contact information 559
WE MOVE *see* Worldwide Education and Awareness for Movement Disorders
Wepfer, Johann Jacob 72
Wernicke's aphasia
  described 11
  traumatic brain injury 11
  see also fluent aphasia
Wernicke's area, described 8, 11
WEST *see* Women's Estrogen for Stroke Trial
western equine encephalitis (WEE) 179–80, 183–84
West Nile virus (WNV) 187–88
"What You Need to Know about Brain Tumors" (NCI) 136n
WHI *see* Women's Health Initiative

WHIMS *see* Women's Health Initiative Memory Study
white matter
  defined 556
  described 7
  multiple sclerosis 394
whole brain radiation therapy (WBRT), described 155–56
Wilson's disease 346
WNV *see* West Nile virus
women
  brain aneurysms 125
  migraine headaches 492
  stroke 94–95
Women's Estrogen for Stroke Trial (WEST) 101
Women's Health Initiative (WHI), memory study publication 58n
Women's Health Initiative Memory Study (WHIMS) 58–60
Worldwide Education and Awareness for Movement Disorders (WE MOVE), contact information 567

X

x-rays
  brain tumors 143
  coma 235
  multiple sclerosis 407
  traumatic brain injury 211

Y

Yamada, Kentaro 110–11
"Yeast Model Yields Insight into Parkinson's Disease" (NINDS) 443n

Z

Zamvil, Scott 428–29
Zanaflex (tizanidine) 411, *413*
Zenapax (Daclizumab) 429–31
Zovirax (acyclovir) 177

Health Reference Series
COMPLETE CATALOG

Adolescent Health Sourcebook

Basic Consumer Health Information about Common Medical, Mental, and Emotional Concerns in Adolescents, Including Facts about Acne, Body Piercing, Mononucleosis, Nutrition, Eating Disorders, Stress, Depression, Behavior Problems, Peer Pressure, Violence, Gangs, Drug Use, Puberty, Sexuality, Pregnancy, Learning Disabilities, and More

Along with a Glossary of Terms and Other Resources for Further Help and Information

Edited by Chad T. Kimball. 658 pages. 2002. 0-7808-0248-9. $78.

"It is written in clear, nontechnical language aimed at general readers. . . . Recommended for public libraries, community colleges, and other agencies serving health care consumers."
— *American Reference Books Annual, 2003*

"Recommended for school and public libraries. Parents and professionals dealing with teens will appreciate the easy-to-follow format and the clearly written text. This could become a 'must have' for every high school teacher." — *E-Streams, Jan '03*

"A good starting point for information related to common medical, mental, and emotional concerns of adolescents." — *School Library Journal, Nov '02*

"This book provides accurate information in an easy to access format. It addresses topics that parents and caregivers might not be aware of and provides practical, useable information." — *Doody's Health Sciences Book Review Journal, Sep-Oct '02*

"Recommended reference source."
— *Booklist, American Library Association, Sep '02*

AIDS Sourcebook, 3rd Edition

Basic Consumer Health Information about Acquired Immune Deficiency Syndrome (AIDS) and Human Immunodeficiency Virus (HIV) Infection, Including Facts about Transmission, Prevention, Diagnosis, Treatment, Opportunistic Infections, and Other Complications, with a Section for Women and Children, Including Details about Associated Gynecological Concerns, Pregnancy, and Pediatric Care

Along with Updated Statistical Information, Reports on Current Research Initiatives, a Glossary, and Directories of Internet, Hotline, and Other Resources

Edited by Dawn D. Matthews. 664 pages. 2003. 0-7808-0631-X. $78.

ALSO AVAILABLE: AIDS Sourcebook, 1st Edition. Edited by Karen Bellenir and Peter D. Dresser. 831 pages. 1995. 0-7808-0031-1. $78.

AIDS Sourcebook, 2nd Edition. Edited by Karen Bellenir. 751 pages. 1999. 0-7808-0225-X. $78.

"The 3rd edition of the *AIDS Sourcebook*, part of Omnigraphics' *Health Reference Series*, is a welcome update. . . . This resource is highly recommended for academic and public libraries."
— *American Reference Books Annual, 2004*

"Excellent sourcebook. This continues to be a highly recommended book. There is no other book that provides as much information as this book provides."
— *AIDS Book Review Journal, Dec-Jan 2000*

"Recommended reference source."
— *Booklist, American Library Association, Dec '99*

"A solid text for college-level health libraries."
— *The Bookwatch, Aug '99*

Cited in *Reference Sources for Small and Medium-Sized Libraries, American Library Association, 1999*

Alcoholism Sourcebook

Basic Consumer Health Information about the Physical and Mental Consequences of Alcohol Abuse, Including Liver Disease, Pancreatitis, Wernicke-Korsakoff Syndrome (Alcoholic Dementia), Fetal Alcohol Syndrome, Heart Disease, Kidney Disorders, Gastrointestinal Problems, and Immune System Compromise and Featuring Facts about Addiction, Detoxification, Alcohol Withdrawal, Recovery, and the Maintenance of Sobriety

Along with a Glossary and Directories of Resources for Further Help and Information

Edited by Karen Bellenir. 613 pages. 2000. 0-7808-0325-6. $78.

"This title is one of the few reference works on alcoholism for general readers. For some readers this will be a welcome complement to the many self-help books on the market. Recommended for collections serving general readers and consumer health collections."
— *E-Streams, Mar '01*

"This book is an excellent choice for public and academic libraries."
— *American Reference Books Annual, 2001*

"Recommended reference source."
— *Booklist, American Library Association, Dec '00*

"Presents a wealth of information on alcohol use and abuse and its effects on the body and mind, treatment, and prevention." — *SciTech Book News, Dec '00*

"Important new health guide which packs in the latest consumer information about the problems of alcoholism." — *Reviewer's Bookwatch, Nov '00*

SEE ALSO Drug Abuse Sourcebook, Substance Abuse Sourcebook

Allergies Sourcebook, 2nd Edition

Basic Consumer Health Information about Allergic Disorders, Triggers, Reactions, and Related Symptoms, Including Anaphylaxis, Rhinitis, Sinusitis, Asthma, Dermatitis, Conjunctivitis, and Multiple Chemical Sensitivity

Along with Tips on Diagnosis, Prevention, and Treatment, Statistical Data, a Glossary, and a Directory of Sources for Further Help and Information

Edited by Annemarie S. Muth. 598 pages. 2002. 0-7808-0376-0. $78.

ALSO AVAILABLE: Allergies Sourcebook, 1st Edition. Edited by Allan R. Cook. 611 pages. 1997. 0-7808-0036-2. $78.

"This book brings a great deal of useful material together. . . . This is an excellent addition to public and consumer health library collections."
— *American Reference Books Annual, 2003*

"This second edition would be useful to laypersons with little or advanced knowledge of the subject matter. This book would also serve as a resource for nursing and other health care professions students. It would be useful in public, academic, and hospital libraries with consumer health collections." — *E-Streams, Jul '02*

Alternative Medicine Sourcebook, 2nd Edition

Basic Consumer Health Information about Alternative and Complementary Medical Practices, Including Acupuncture, Chiropractic, Herbal Medicine, Homeopathy, Naturopathic Medicine, Mind-Body Interventions, Ayurveda, and Other Non-Western Medical Traditions

Along with Facts about such Specific Therapies as Massage Therapy, Aromatherapy, Qigong, Hypnosis, Prayer, Dance, and Art Therapies, a Glossary, and Resources for Further Information

Edited by Dawn D. Matthews. 618 pages. 2002. 0-7808-0605-0. $78.

ALSO AVAILABLE: Alternative Medicine Sourcebook, 1st Edition. Edited by Allan R. Cook. 737 pages. 1999. 0-7808-0200-4. $78.

"Recommended for public, high school, and academic libraries that have consumer health collections. Hospital libraries that also serve the public will find this to be a useful resource." — *E-Streams, Feb '03*

"Recommended reference source."
—*Booklist, American Library Association, Jan '03*

"An important alternate health reference."
—*MBR Bookwatch, Oct '02*

"A great addition to the reference collection of every type of library." — *American Reference Books Annual, 2000*

Alzheimer's Disease Sourcebook, 3rd Edition

Basic Consumer Health Information about Alzheimer's Disease, Other Dementias, and Related Disorders, Including Multi-Infarct Dementia, AIDS Dementia Complex, Dementia with Lewy Bodies, Huntington's Disease, Wernicke-Korsakoff Syndrome (Alcohol-Reated Dementia), Delirium, and Confusional States

Along with Information for People Newly Diagnosed with Alzheimer's Disease and Caregivers, Reports Detailing Current Research Efforts in Prevention, Diagnosis, and Treatment, Facts about Long-Term Care Issues, and Listings of Sources for Additional Information

Edited by Karen Bellenir. 645 pages. 2003. 0-7808-0666-2. $78.

ALSO AVAILABLE: Alzheimer's, Stroke & 29 Other Neurological Disorders Sourcebook, 1st Edition. Edited by Frank E. Bair. 579 pages. 1993. 1-55888-748-2. $78.

ALSO AVAILABLE: Alzheimer's Disease Sourcebook, 2nd Edition. Edited by Karen Bellenir. 524 pages. 1999. 0-7808-0223-3. $78.

"This very informative and valuable tool will be a great addition to any library serving consumers, students and health care workers."
—*American Reference Books Annual, 2004*

"This is a valuable resource for people affected by dementias such as Alzheimer's. It is easy to navigate and includes important information and resources."
— *Doody's Review Service, Feb. 2004*

"Recommended reference source."
— *Booklist, American Library Association, Oct '99*

SEE ALSO Brain Disorders Sourcebook

Arthritis Sourcebook, 2nd Edition

Basic Consumer Health Information about Osteoarthritis, Rheumatoid Arthritis, Other Rheumatic Disorders, Infectious Forms of Arthritis, and Diseases with Symptoms Linked to Arthritis, Featuring Facts about Diagnosis, Pain Management, and Surgical Therapies

Along with Coping Strategies, Research Updates, a Glossary, and Resources for Additional Help and Information

Edited by Amy L. Sutton. 593 pages. 2004. 0-7808-0667-0. $78.

ALSO AVAILABLE: Arthritis Sourcebook, 1st Edition. Edited by Allan R. Cook. 550 pages. 1998. 0-7808-0201-2. $78.

". . . accessible to the layperson."
—*Reference and Research Book News, Feb '99*

Asthma Sourcebook

Basic Consumer Health Information about Asthma, Including Symptoms, Traditional and Nontraditional Remedies, Treatment Advances, Quality-of-Life Aids, Medical Research Updates, and the Role of Allergies, Exercise, Age, the Environment, and Genetics in the Development of Asthma

Along with Statistical Data, a Glossary, and Directories of Support Groups, and Other Resources for Further Information

Edited by Annemarie S. Muth. 628 pages. 2000. 0-7808-0381-7. $78.

"**A worthwhile reference acquisition for public libraries and academic medical libraries whose readers desire a quick introduction to the wide range of asthma information.**" — *Choice, Association of College & Research Libraries, Jun '01*

"**Recommended reference source.**"
— *Booklist, American Library Association, Feb '01*

"**Highly recommended.**" — *The Bookwatch, Jan '01*

"**There is much good information for patients and their families who deal with asthma daily.**"
— *American Medical Writers Association Journal, Winter '01*

"**This informative text is recommended for consumer health collections in public, secondary school, and community college libraries and the libraries of universities with a large undergraduate population.**"
— *American Reference Books Annual, 2001*

■

Attention Deficit Disorder Sourcebook

Basic Consumer Health Information about Attention Deficit/Hyperactivity Disorder in Children and Adults, Including Facts about Causes, Symptoms, Diagnostic Criteria, and Treatment Options Such as Medications, Behavior Therapy, Coaching, and Homeopathy

Along with Reports on Current Research Initiatives, Legal Issues, and Government Regulations, and Featuring a Glossary of Related Terms, Internet Resources, and a List of Additional Reading Material

Edited by Dawn D. Matthews. 470 pages. 2002. 0-7808-0624-7. $78.

"**Recommended reference source.**"
— *Booklist, American Library Association, Jan '03*

"**This book is recommended for all school libraries and the reference or consumer health sections of public libraries.**" — *American Reference Books Annual, 2003*

■

Back & Neck Sourcebook, 2nd Edition

Basic Consumer Health Information about Spinal Pain, Spinal Cord Injuries, and Related Disorders, Such as Degenerative Disk Disease, Osteoarthritis, Scoliosis, Sciatica, Spina Bifida, and Spinal Stenosis, and Featuring Facts about Maintaining Spinal Health, Self-Care, Pain Management, Rehabilitative Care, Chiro-

practic Care, Spinal Surgeries, and Complementary Therapies

Along with Suggestions for Preventing Back and Neck Pain, a Glossary of Related Terms, and a Directory of Resources

Edited by Amy L. Sutton. 633 pages. 2004. 0-7808-0738-3 $78.

ALSO AVAILABLE: *Back & Neck Disorders Sourcebook, 1st Edition.* Edited by Karen Bellenir. 548 pages. 1997. 0-7808-0202-0. $78.

"**The strength of this work is its basic, easy-to-read format. Recommended.**"
— *Reference and User Services Quarterly, American Library Association, Winter '97*

■

Blood & Circulatory Disorders Sourcebook, 2nd Edition

Basic Consumer Health Information about the Blood and Circulatory System and Related Disorders, Such as Anemia and Other Hemoglobin Diseases, Cancer of the Blood and Associated Bone Marrow Disorders, Clotting and Bleeding Problems, and Conditions That Affect the Veins, Blood Vessels, and Arteries, Including Facts about the Donation and Transplantation of Bone Marrow, Stem Cells, and Blood and Tips for Keeping the Blood and Circulatory System Healthy

Along with a Glossary of Related Terms and Resources for Additional Help and Information

Edited by Amy L. Sutton. 650 pages. 2005. 0-7808-0746-4. $78.

ALSO AVAILABLE: *Blood and Circulatory Disorders Sourcebook, 1st Edition.* Edited by Karen Bellenir and Linda M. Shin. 554 pages. 1998. 0-7808-0203-9. $78.

"**Recommended reference source.**"
— *Booklist, American Library Association, Feb '99*

"**An important reference sourcebook written in simple language for everyday, non-technical users.** "
— *Reviewer's Bookwatch, Jan '99*

■

Brain Disorders Sourcebook, 2nd Edition

Basic Consumer Health Information about Acquired and Traumatic Brain Injuries, Infections of the Brain, Epilepsy and Seizure Disorders, Cerebral Palsy, and Degenerative Neurological Disorders, Including Amyotrophic Lateral Sclerosis (ALS), Dementias, Multiple Sclerosis, and More

Along with Information on the Brain's Structure and Function, Treatment and Rehabilitation Options, Reports on Current Research Initiatives, a Glossary of Terms Related to Brain Disorders and Injuries, and a Directory of Sources for Further Help and Information

Edited by Sandra J. Judd. 625 pages. 2005. 0-7808-0744-8. $78.

ALSO AVAILABLE: *Brain Disorders Sourcebook, 1st Edition.* Edited by Karen Bellenir. 481 pages. 1999. 0-7808-0229-2. $78.

SEE ALSO *Alzheimer's Disease Sourcebook*

■

Breast Cancer Sourcebook, 2nd Edition

Basic Consumer Health Information about Breast Cancer, Including Facts about Risk Factors, Prevention, Screening and Diagnostic Methods, Treatment Options, Complementary and Alternative Therapies, Post-Treatment Concerns, Clinical Trials, Special Risk Populations, and New Developments in Breast Cancer Research

Along with Breast Cancer Statistics, a Glossary of Related Terms, and a Directory of Resources for Additional Help and Information

Edited by Sandra J. Judd. 595 pages. 2004. 0-7808-0668-9. $78.

ALSO AVAILABLE: *Breast Cancer Sourcebook, 1st Edition.* Edited by Edward J. Prucha and Karen Bellenir. 580 pages. 2001. 0-7808-0244-6. $78.

SEE ALSO *Cancer Sourcebook for Women, Women's Health Concerns Sourcebook*

■

Breastfeeding Sourcebook

Basic Consumer Health Information about the Benefits of Breastmilk, Preparing to Breastfeed, Breastfeeding as a Baby Grows, Nutrition, and More, Including Information on Special Situations and Concerns Such as Mastitis, Illness, Medications, Allergies, Multiple Births, Prematurity, Special Needs, and Adoption

Along with a Glossary and Resources for Additional Help and Information

Edited by Jenni Lynn Colson. 388 pages. 2002. 0-7808-0332-9. $78.

SEE ALSO *Pregnancy & Birth Sourcebook*

■

Burns Sourcebook

Basic Consumer Health Information about Various Types of Burns and Scalds, Including Flame, Heat, Cold, Electrical, Chemical, and Sun Burns

Along with Information on Short-Term and Long-Term Treatments, Tissue Reconstruction, Plastic Surgery, Prevention Suggestions, and First Aid

Edited by Allan R. Cook. 604 pages. 1999. 0-7808-0204-7. $78.

SEE ALSO *Skin Disorders Sourcebook*

■

Cancer Sourcebook, 4th Edition

Basic Consumer Health Information about Major Forms and Stages of Cancer, Featuring Facts about Head and Neck Cancers, Lung Cancers, Gastrointestinal Cancers, Genitourinary Cancers, Lymphomas, Blood Cell Cancers, Endocrine Cancers, Skin Cancers, Bone Cancers, Sarcomas, and Others, and Including Information about Cancer Treatments and Therapies, Identifying and Reducing Cancer Risks, and Strategies for Coping with Cancer and the Side Effects of Treatment

Along with a Cancer Glossary, Statistical and Demographic Data, and a Directory of Sources for Additional Help and Information

Edited by Karen Bellenir. 1,119 pages. 2003. 0-7808-0633-6. $78.

ALSO AVAILABLE: *Cancer Sourcebook, 1st Edition.* Edited by Frank E. Bair. 932 pages. 1990. 1-55888-888-8. $78.

New Cancer Sourcebook, 2nd Edition. Edited by Allan R. Cook. 1,313 pages. 1996. 0-7808-0041-9. $78.

Cancer Sourcebook, 3rd Edition. Edited by Edward J. Prucha. 1,069 pages. 2000. 0-7808-0227-6. $78.

"With cancer being the second leading cause of death for Americans, a prodigious work such as this one, which locates centrally so much cancer-related information, is clearly an asset to this nation's citizens and others." —Journal of the National Medical Association, 2004

"This title is recommended for health sciences and public libraries with consumer health collections." —E-Streams, Feb '01

". . . can be effectively used by cancer patients and their families who are looking for answers in a language they can understand. Public and hospital libraries should have it on their shelves." —American Reference Books Annual, 2001

"Recommended reference source." —Booklist, American Library Association, Dec '00

Cited in Reference Sources for Small and Medium-Sized Libraries, American Library Association, 1999

"The amount of factual and useful information is extensive. The writing is very clear, geared to general readers. Recommended for all levels." —Choice, Association of College & Research Libraries, Jan '97

SEE ALSO Breast Cancer Sourcebook, Cancer Sourcebook for Women, Pediatric Cancer Sourcebook, Prostate Cancer Sourcebook

■

Cancer Sourcebook for Women, 2nd Edition

Basic Consumer Health Information about Gynecologic Cancers and Related Concerns, Including Cervical Cancer, Endometrial Cancer, Gestational Trophoblastic Tumor, Ovarian Cancer, Uterine Cancer, Vaginal Cancer, Vulvar Cancer, Breast Cancer, and Common Non-Cancerous Uterine Conditions, with Facts about Cancer Risk Factors, Screening and Prevention, Treatment Options, and Reports on Current Research Initiatives

Along with a Glossary of Cancer Terms and a Directory of Resources for Additional Help and Information

Edited by Karen Bellenir. 604 pages. 2002. 0-7808-0226-8. $78.

ALSO AVAILABLE: Cancer Sourcebook for Women, 1st Edition. Edited by Allan R. Cook and Peter D. Dresser. 524 pages. 1996. 0-7808-0076-1. $78.

"An excellent addition to collections in public, consumer health, and women's health libraries." —American Reference Books Annual, 2003

"Overall, the information is excellent, and complex topics are clearly explained. As a reference book for the consumer it is a valuable resource to assist them to make informed decisions about cancer and its treatments." —Cancer Forum, Nov '02

"Highly recommended for academic and medical reference collections." —Library Bookwatch, Sep '02

"This is a highly recommended book for any public or consumer library, being reader friendly and containing accurate and helpful information." —E-Streams, Aug '02

"Recommended reference source." —Booklist, American Library Association, Jul '02

SEE ALSO Breast Cancer Sourcebook, Women's Health Concerns Sourcebook

■

Cardiovascular Diseases & Disorders Sourcebook, 3rd Edition

Basic Consumer Health Information about Heart and Vascular Diseases and Disorders, Such as Angina, Heart Attacks, Arrhythmias, Cardiomyopathy, Valve Disease, Atherosclerosis, and Aneurysms, with Information about Managing Cardiovascular Risk Factors and Maintaining Heart Health, Medications and Procedures Used to Treat Cardiovascular Disorders, and Concerns of Special Significance to Women

long with Reports on Current Research Initiatives, a Glossary of Related Medical Terms, and a Directory of Sources for Further Help and Information

Edited by Sandra J. Judd. 713 pages. 2005. 0-7808-0739-1. $78.

ALSO AVAILABLE: Heart Diseases & Disorders Sourcebook, 2nd Edition. Edited by Karen Bellenir. 612 pages. 2000. 0-7808-0238-1. $78.

Cardiovascular Diseases & Disorders Sourcebook, 1st Edition. Edited by Karen Bellenir and Peter D. Dresser. 683 pages. 1995. 0-7808-0032-X. $78.

"This work stands out as an imminently accessible resource for the general public. It is recommended for the reference and circulating shelves of school, public, and academic libraries." —American Reference Books Annual, 2001

"Recommended reference source." —Booklist, American Library Association, Dec '00

"Provides comprehensive coverage of matters related to the heart. This title is recommended for health sciences and public libraries with consumer health collections." —E-Streams, Oct '00

SEE ALSO Healthy Heart Sourcebook for Women

■

Caregiving Sourcebook

Basic Consumer Health Information for Caregivers, Including a Profile of Caregivers, Caregiving Responsibilities and Concerns, Tips for Specific Conditions, Care Environments, and the Effects of Caregiving

Along with Facts about Legal Issues, Financial Information, and Future Planning, a Glossary, and a Listing of Additional Resources

Edited by Joyce Brennfleck Shannon. 600 pages. 2001. 0-7808-0331-0. $78.

■

Child Abuse Sourcebook

Basic Consumer Health Information about the Physical, Sexual, and Emotional Abuse of Children, with Additional Facts about Neglect, Munchausen Syndrome by Proxy (MSBP), Shaken Baby Syndrome, and Controversial Issues Related to Child Abuse, Such as Withholding Medical Care, Corporal Punishment, and Child Maltreatment in Youth Sports, and Featuring Facts about Child Protective Services, Foster Care, Adoption, Parenting Challenges, and Other Abuse Prevention Efforts

Along with a Glossary of Related Terms and Resources for Additional Help and Information

Edited by Dawn D. Matthews. 620 pages. 2004. 0-7808-0705-7. $78.

■

Childhood Diseases & Disorders Sourcebook

Basic Consumer Health Information about Medical Problems Often Encountered in Pre-Adolescent Children, Including Respiratory Tract Ailments, Ear Infections, Sore Throats, Disorders of the Skin and Scalp, Digestive and Genitourinary Diseases, Infectious Diseases, Inflammatory Disorders, Chronic Physical and Developmental Disorders, Allergies, and More

Along with Information about Diagnostic Tests, Common Childhood Surgeries, and Frequently Used Medications, with a Glossary of Important Terms and Resource Directory

Edited by Chad T. Kimball. 662 pages. 2003. 0-7808-0458-9. $78.

■

Colds, Flu & Other Common Ailments Sourcebook

Basic Consumer Health Information about Common Ailments and Injuries, Including Colds, Coughs, the Flu, Sinus Problems, Headaches, Fever, Nausea and Vomiting, Menstrual Cramps, Diarrhea, Constipation, Hemorrhoids, Back Pain, Dandruff, Dry and Itchy Skin, Cuts, Scrapes, Sprains, Bruises, and More

Along with Information about Prevention, Self-Care, Choosing a Doctor, Over-the-Counter Medications, Folk Remedies, and Alternative Therapies, and Including a Glossary of Important Terms and a Directory of Resources for Further Help and Information

Edited by Chad T. Kimball. 638 pages. 2001. 0-7808-0435-X. $78.

■

Communication Disorders Sourcebook

Basic Information about Deafness and Hearing Loss, Speech and Language Disorders, Voice Disorders, Balance and Vestibular Disorders, and Disorders of Smell, Taste, and Touch

Edited by Linda M. Ross. 533 pages. 1996. 0-7808-0077-X. $78.

■

Congenital Disorders Sourcebook

Basic Information about Disorders Acquired during Gestation, Including Spina Bifida, Hydrocephalus, Cerebral Palsy, Heart Defects, Craniofacial Abnormalities, Fetal Alcohol Syndrome, and More

Along with Current Treatment Options and Statistical Data

Edited by Karen Bellenir. 607 pages. 1997. 0-7808-0205-5. $78.

SEE ALSO Pregnancy & Birth Sourcebook

■

Consumer Issues in Health Care Sourcebook

Basic Information about Health Care Fundamentals and Related Consumer Issues, Including Exams and Screening Tests, Physician Specialties, Choosing a Doctor, Using Prescription and Over-the-Counter Medications Safely, Avoiding Health Scams, Managing Common Health Risks in the Home, Care Options for Chronically or Terminally Ill Patients, and a List of Resources for Obtaining Help and Further Information

Edited by Karen Bellenir. 618 pages. 1998. 0-7808-0221-7. $78.

Contagious Diseases Sourcebook

Basic Consumer Health Information about Infectious Diseases Spread by Person-to-Person Contact through Direct Touch, Airborne Transmission, Sexual Contact, or Contact with Blood or Other Body Fluids, Including Hepatitis, Herpes, Influenza, Lice, Measles, Mumps, Pinworm, Ringworm, Severe Acute Respiratory Syndrome (SARS), Streptococcal Infections, Tuberculosis, and Others

Along with Facts about Disease Transmission, Antimicrobial Resistance, and Vaccines, with a Glossary and Directories of Resources for More Information

Edited by Karen Bellenir. 643 pages. 2004. 0-7808-0736-7. $78.

Contagious & Non-Contagious Infectious Diseases Sourcebook

Basic Information about Contagious Diseases like Measles, Polio, Hepatitis B, and Infectious Mononucleosis, and Non-Contagious Infectious Diseases like Tetanus and Toxic Shock Syndrome, and Diseases Occurring as Secondary Infections Such as Shingles and Reye Syndrome

Along with Vaccination, Prevention, and Treatment Information, and a Section Describing Emerging Infectious Disease Threats

Edited by Karen Bellenir and Peter D. Dresser. 566 pages. 1996. 0-7808-0075-3. $78.

Death & Dying Sourcebook

Basic Consumer Health Information for the Layperson about End-of-Life Care and Related Ethical and Legal Issues, Including Chief Causes of Death, Autopsies, Pain Management for the Terminally Ill, Life Support Systems, Insurance, Euthanasia, Assisted Suicide, Hospice Programs, Living Wills, Funeral Planning, Counseling, Mourning, Organ Donation, and Physician Training

Along with Statistical Data, a Glossary, and Listings of Sources for Further Help and Information

Edited by Annemarie S. Muth. 641 pages. 1999. 0-7808-0230-6. $78.

Dental Care & Oral Health Sourcebook, 2nd Edition

Basic Consumer Health Information about Dental Care, Including Oral Hygiene, Dental Visits, Pain Management, Cavities, Crowns, Bridges, Dental Implants, and Fillings, and Other Oral Health Concerns, Such as Gum Disease, Bad Breath, Dry Mouth, Genetic and Developmental Abnormalities, Oral Cancers, Orthodontics, and Temporomandibular Disorders

Along with Updates on Current Research in Oral Health, a Glossary, a Directory of Dental and Oral Health Organizations, and Resources for People with Dental and Oral Health Disorders

Edited by Amy L. Sutton. 609 pages. 2003. 0-7808-0634-4. $78.

ALSO AVAILABLE: *Oral Health Sourcebook, 1st Edition.* Edited by Allan R. Cook. 558 pages. 1997. 0-7808-0082-6. $78.

Depression Sourcebook

Basic Consumer Health Information about Unipolar Depression, Bipolar Disorder, Postpartum Depression, Seasonal Affective Disorder, and Other Types of Depression in Children, Adolescents, Women, Men, the Elderly, and Other Selected Populations

Along with Facts about Causes, Risk Factors, Diagnostic Criteria, Treatment Options, Coping Strategies, Suicide Prevention, a Glossary, and a Directory of Sources for Additional Help and Information

Edited by Karen Belleni. 602 pages. 2002. 0-7808-0611-5. $78.

*"**Depression Sourcebook** is of a very high standard. Its purpose, which is to serve as a reference source to the lay reader, is very well served."*
— *Journal of the National Medical Association, 2004*

"Invaluable reference for public and school library collections alike." — *Library Bookwatch, Apr '03*

"Recommended for purchase."
— *American Reference Books Annual, 2003*

◼

Diabetes Sourcebook, 3rd Edition

Basic Consumer Health Information about Type 1 Diabetes (Insulin-Dependent or Juvenile-Onset Diabetes), Type 2 Diabetes (Noninsulin-Dependent or Adult-Onset Diabetes), Gestational Diabetes, Impaired Glucose Tolerance (IGT), and Related Complications, Such as Amputation, Eye Disease, Gum Disease, Nerve Damage, and End-Stage Renal Disease, Including Facts about Insulin, Oral Diabetes Medications, Blood Sugar Testing, and the Role of Exercise and Nutrition in the Control of Diabetes

Along with a Glossary and Resources for Further Help and Information

Edited by Dawn D. Matthews. 622 pages. 2003. 0-7808-0629-8. $78.

ALSO AVAILABLE: *Diabetes Sourcebook, 1st Edition.* Edited by Karen Bellenir and Peter D. Dresser. 827 pages. 1994. 1-55888-751-2. $78.

Diabetes Sourcebook, 2nd Edition. Edited by Karen Bellenir. 688 pages. 1998. 0-7808-0224-1. $78.

"This edition is even more helpful than earlier versions. . . . It is a truly valuable tool for anyone seeking readable and authoritative information on diabetes."
— *American Reference Books Annual, 2004*

"An invaluable reference." — *Library Journal, May '00*

Selected as one of the 250 "Best Health Sciences Books of 1999." — *Doody's Rating Service, Mar-Apr 2000*

"Provides useful information for the general public."
— *Healthlines, University of Michigan Health Management Research Center, Sep/Oct '99*

". . . provides reliable mainstream medical information . . . belongs on the shelves of any library with a consumer health collection." — *E-Streams, Sep '99*

"Recommended reference source."
— *Booklist, American Library Association, Feb '99*

◼

Diet & Nutrition Sourcebook, 2nd Edition

Basic Consumer Health Information about Dietary Guidelines, Recommended Daily Intake Values, Vitamins, Minerals, Fiber, Fat, Weight Control, Dietary Supplements, and Food Additives

Along with Special Sections on Nutrition Needs throughout Life and Nutrition for People with Such Specific Medical Concerns as Allergies, High Blood Cholesterol, Hypertension, Diabetes, Celiac Disease, Seizure Disorders, Phenylketonuria (PKU), Cancer, and

Eating Disorders, and Including Reports on Current Nutrition Research and Source Listings for Additional Help and Information

Edited by Karen Bellenir. 650 pages. 1999. 0-7808-0228-4. $78.

ALSO AVAILABLE: *Diet & Nutrition Sourcebook, 1st Edition.* Edited by Dan R. Harris. 662 pages. 1996. 0-7808-0084-2. $78.

"This book is an excellent source of basic diet and nutrition information." — *Booklist Health Sciences Supplement, American Library Association, Dec '00*

"This reference document should be in any public library, but it would be a very good guide for beginning students in the health sciences. If the other books in this publisher's series are as good as this, they should all be in the health sciences collections."
— *American Reference Books Annual, 2000*

"This book is an excellent general nutrition reference for consumers who desire to take an active role in their health care for prevention. Consumers of all ages who select this book can feel confident they are receiving current and accurate information." — *Journal of Nutrition for the Elderly, Vol. 19, No. 4, '00*

"Recommended reference source."
— *Booklist, American Library Association, Dec '99*

SEE ALSO *Digestive Diseases & Disorders Sourcebook, Eating Disorders Sourcebook, Gastrointestinal Diseases & Disorders Sourcebook, Vegetarian Sourcebook*

◼

Digestive Diseases & Disorders Sourcebook

Basic Consumer Health Information about Diseases and Disorders that Impact the Upper and Lower Digestive System, Including Celiac Disease, Constipation, Crohn's Disease, Cyclic Vomiting Syndrome, Diarrhea, Diverticulosis and Diverticulitis, Gallstones, Heartburn, Hemorrhoids, Hernias, Indigestion (Dyspepsia), Irritable Bowel Syndrome, Lactose Intolerance, Ulcers, and More

Along with Information about Medications and Other Treatments, Tips for Maintaining a Healthy Digestive Tract, a Glossary, and Directory of Digestive Diseases Organizations

Edited by Karen Bellenir. 335 pages. 2000. 0-7808-0327-2. $78.

"This title would be an excellent addition to all public or patient-research libraries."
— *American Reference Books Annual, 2001*

"This title is recommended for public, hospital, and health sciences libraries with consumer health collections." — *E-Streams, Jul-Aug '00*

"Recommended reference source."
— *Booklist, American Library Association, May '00*

SEE ALSO *Diet & Nutrition Sourcebook, Eating Disorders Sourcebook, Gastrointestinal Diseases & Disorders Sourcebook*

Disabilities Sourcebook

Basic Consumer Health Information about Physical and Psychiatric Disabilities, Including Descriptions of Major Causes of Disability, Assistive and Adaptive Aids, Workplace Issues, and Accessibility Concerns

Along with Information about the Americans with Disabilities Act, a Glossary, and Resources for Additional Help and Information

Edited by Dawn D. Matthews. 616 pages. 2000. 0-7808-0389-2. $78.

"It is a must for libraries with a consumer health section." — *American Reference Books Annual 2002*

"A much needed addition to the Omnigraphics *Health Reference Series.* A current reference work to provide people with disabilities, their families, caregivers or those who work with them, a broad range of information in one volume, has not been available until now.... It is recommended for all public and academic library reference collections." — *E-Streams, May '01*

"An excellent source book in easy-to-read format covering many current topics; highly recommended for all libraries." — *Choice, Association of College and Research Libraries, Jan '01*

"Recommended reference source." — *Booklist, American Library Association, Jul '00*

■

Domestic Violence Sourcebook, 2nd Edition

Basic Consumer Health Information about the Causes and Consequences of Abusive Relationships, Including Physical Violence, Sexual Assault, Battery, Stalking, and Emotional Abuse, and Facts about the Effects of Violence on Women, Men, Young Adults, and the Elderly, with Reports about Domestic Violence in Selected Populations, and Featuring Facts about Medical Care, Victim Assistance and Protection, Prevention Strategies, Mental Health Services, and Legal Issues

Along with a Glossary of Related Terms and Resources for Additional Help and Information

Edited by Dawn D. Matthews. 628 pages. 2004. 0-7808-0669-7. $78.

ALSO AVAILABLE: Domestic Violence & Child Abuse Sourcebook, 1st Edition. Edited by Helene Henderson. 1,064 pages. 2001. 0-7808-0235-7. $78.

"Interested lay persons should find the book extremely beneficial.... A copy of *Domestic Violence and Child Abuse Sourcebook* should be in every public library in the United States." — *Social Science & Medicine, No. 56, 2003*

"This is important information. The Web has many resources but this sourcebook fills an important societal need. I am not aware of any other resources of this type." — *Doody's Review Service, Sep '01*

"Recommended for all libraries, scholars, and practitioners." — *Choice, Association of College & Research Libraries, Jul '01*

"Recommended reference source." — *Booklist, American Library Association, Apr '01*

"Important pick for college-level health reference libraries." — *The Bookwatch, Mar '01*

"Because this problem is so widespread and because this book includes a lot of issues within one volume, this work is recommended for all public libraries." — *American Reference Books Annual, 2001*

■

Drug Abuse Sourcebook, 2nd Edition

Basic Consumer Health Information about Illicit Substances of Abuse and the Misuse of Prescription and Over-the-Counter Medications, Including Depressants, Hallucinogens, Inhalants, Marijuana, Stimulants, and Anabolic Steroids

Along with Facts about Related Health Risks, Treatment Programs, Prevention Programs, a Glossary of Abuse and Addiction Terms, a Glossary of Drug-Related Street Terms, and a Directory of Resources for More Information

Edited by Catherine Ginther. 607 pages. 2004. 0-7808-0740-5. $78.

ALSO AVAILABLE: Drug Abuse Sourcebook, 1st Edition. Edited by Karen Bellenir. 629 pages. 2000. 0-7808-0242-X. $78.

"Containing a wealth of information.... This resource belongs in libraries that serve a lower-division undergraduate or community college clientele as well as the general public." — *Choice, Association of College and Research Libraries, Jun '01*

"Recommended reference source." — *Booklist, American Library Association, Feb '01*

"Highly recommended." — *The Bookwatch, Jan '01*

"Even though there is a plethora of books on drug abuse, this volume is recommended for school, public, and college libraries." — *American Reference Books Annual, 2001*

SEE ALSO Alcoholism Sourcebook, Substance Abuse Sourcebook

■

Ear, Nose & Throat Disorders Sourcebook

Basic Information about Disorders of the Ears, Nose, Sinus Cavities, Pharynx, and Larynx, Including Ear Infections, Tinnitus, Vestibular Disorders, Allergic and Non-Allergic Rhinitis, Sore Throats, Tonsillitis, and Cancers That Affect the Ears, Nose, Sinuses, and Throat

Along with Reports on Current Research Initiatives, a Glossary of Related Medical Terms, and a Directory of Sources for Further Help and Information

Edited by Karen Bellenir and Linda M. Shin. 576 pages. 1998. 0-7808-0206-3. $78.

"Overall, this sourcebook is helpful for the consumer seeking information on ENT issues. It is recommended for public libraries."
—*American Reference Books Annual, 1999*

"Recommended reference source."
—*Booklist, American Library Association, Dec '98*

■

Eating Disorders Sourcebook

Basic Consumer Health Information about Eating Disorders, Including Information about Anorexia Nervosa, Bulimia Nervosa, Binge Eating, Body Dysmorphic Disorder, Pica, Laxative Abuse, and Night Eating Syndrome

Along with Information about Causes, Adverse Effects, and Treatment and Prevention Issues, and Featuring a Section on Concerns Specific to Children and Adolescents, a Glossary, and Resources for Further Help and Information

Edited by Dawn D. Matthews. 322 pages. 2001. 0-7808-0335-3. $78.

"Recommended for health science libraries that are open to the public, as well as hospital libraries. This book is a good resource for the consumer who is concerned about eating disorders." —*E-Streams, Mar '02*

"This volume is another convenient collection of excerpted articles. Recommended for school and public library patrons; lower-division undergraduates; and two-year technical program students." —*Choice, Association of College & Research Libraries, Jan '02*

"Recommended reference source." —*Booklist, American Library Association, Oct '01*

SEE ALSO Diet & Nutrition Sourcebook, Digestive Diseases & Disorders Sourcebook, Gastrointestinal Diseases & Disorders Sourcebook

■

Emergency Medical Services Sourcebook

Basic Consumer Health Information about Preventing, Preparing for, and Managing Emergency Situations, When and Who to Call for Help, What to Expect in the Emergency Room, the Emergency Medical Team, Patient Issues, and Current Topics in Emergency Medicine

Along with Statistical Data, a Glossary, and Sources of Additional Help and Information

Edited by Jenni Lynn Colson. 494 pages. 2002. 0-7808-0420-1. $78.

"Handy and convenient for home, public, school, and college libraries. Recommended."
—*Choice, Association of College and Research Libraries, Apr '03*

"This reference can provide the consumer with answers to most questions about emergency care in the United States, or it will direct them to a resource where the answer can be found."
—*American Reference Books Annual, 2003*

"Recommended reference source."
—*Booklist, American Library Association, Feb '03*

Endocrine & Metabolic Disorders Sourcebook

Basic Information for the Layperson about Pancreatic and Insulin-Related Disorders Such as Pancreatitis, Diabetes, and Hypoglycemia; Adrenal Gland Disorders Such as Cushing's Syndrome, Addison's Disease, and Congenital Adrenal Hyperplasia; Pituitary Gland Disorders Such as Growth Hormone Deficiency, Acromegaly, and Pituitary Tumors; Thyroid Disorders Such as Hypothyroidism, Graves' Disease, Hashimoto's Disease, and Goiter; Hyperparathyroidism; and Other Diseases and Syndromes of Hormone Imbalance or Metabolic Dysfunction

Along with Reports on Current Research Initiatives

Edited by Linda M. Shin. 574 pages. 1998. 0-7808-0207-1. $78.

"Omnigraphics has produced another needed resource for health information consumers."
—*American Reference Books Annual, 2000*

"Recommended reference source."
—*Booklist, American Library Association, Dec '98*

■

Environmental Health Sourcebook, 2nd Edition

Basic Consumer Health Information about the Environment and Its Effect on Human Health, Including the Effects of Air Pollution, Water Pollution, Hazardous Chemicals, Food Hazards, Radiation Hazards, Biological Agents, Household Hazards, Such as Radon, Asbestos, Carbon Monoxide, and Mold, and Information about Associated Diseases and Disorders, Including Cancer, Allergies, Respiratory Problems, and Skin Disorders

Along with Information about Environmental Concerns for Specific Populations, a Glossary of Related Terms, and Resources for Further Help and Information

Edited by Dawn D. Matthews. 673 pages. 2003. 0-7808-0632-8. $78.

ALSO AVAILABLE: Environmentally Induced Disorders Sourcebook, 1st Edition. Edited by Allan R. Cook. 620 pages. 1997. 0-7808-0083-4. $78.

"This recently updated edition continues the level of quality and the reputation of the numerous other volumes in Omnigraphics' *Health Reference Series*."
—*American Reference Books Annual, 2004*

"Recommended reference source."
—*Booklist, American Library Association, Sep '98*

"This book will be a useful addition to anyone's library." —*Choice Health Sciences Supplement, Association of College and Research Libraries, May '98*

". . . a good survey of numerous environmentally induced physical disorders . . . a useful addition to anyone's library."
—*Doody's Health Sciences Book Reviews, Jan '98*

". . . provide[s] introductory information from the best authorities around. Since this volume covers topics that potentially affect everyone, it will surely be one of the most frequently consulted volumes in the *Health Reference Series*." —*Rettig on Reference, Nov '97*

Environmentally Induced Disorders Sourcebook, 1st Edition

SEE Environmental Health Sourcebook, 2nd Edition

Ethnic Diseases Sourcebook

Basic Consumer Health Information for Ethnic and Racial Minority Groups in the United States, Including General Health Indicators and Behaviors, Ethnic Diseases, Genetic Testing, the Impact of Chronic Diseases, Women's Health, Mental Health Issues, and Preventive Health Care Services

Along with a Glossary and a Listing of Additional Resources

Edited by Joyce Brennfleck Shannon. 664 pages. 2001. 0-7808-0336-1. $78.

"Recommended for health sciences libraries where public health programs are a priority."

—E-Streams, Jan '02

"Not many books have been written on this topic to date, and the Ethnic Diseases Sourcebook is a strong addition to the list. It will be an important introductory resource for health consumers, students, health care personnel, and social scientists. It is recommended for public, academic, and large hospital libraries."

—American Reference Books Annual 2002

"Recommended reference source."

—Booklist, American Library Association, Oct '01

"Will prove valuable to any library seeking to maintain a current, comprehensive reference collection of health resources.... An excellent source of health information about genetic disorders which affect particular ethnic and racial minorities in the U.S."

—The Bookwatch, Aug '01

Eye Care Sourcebook, 2nd Edition

Basic Consumer Health Information about Eye Care and Eye Disorders, Including Facts about the Diagnosis, Prevention, and Treatment of Common Refractive Problems Such as Myopia, Hyperopia, Astigmatism, and Presbyopia, and Eye Diseases, Including Glaucoma, Cataract, Age-Related Macular Degeneration, and Diabetic Retinopathy

Along with a Section on Vision Correction and Refractive Surgeries, Including LASIK and LASEK, a Glossary, and Directories of Resources for Additional Help and Information

Edited by Amy L. Sutton. 543 pages. 2003. 0-7808-0635-2. $78.

ALSO AVAILABLE: Ophthalmic Disorders Sourcebook, 1st Edition. Edited by Linda M. Ross. 631 pages. 1996. 0-7808-0081-8. $78.

". . . a solid reference tool for eye care and a valuable addition to a collection."

—American Reference Books Annual, 2004

Family Planning Sourcebook

Basic Consumer Health Information about Planning for Pregnancy and Contraception, Including Traditional Methods, Barrier Methods, Hormonal Methods, Permanent Methods, Future Methods, Emergency Contraception, and Birth Control Choices for Women at Each Stage of Life

Along with Statistics, a Glossary, and Sources of Additional Information

Edited by Amy Marcaccio Keyzer. 520 pages. 2001. 0-7808-0379-5. $78.

"Recommended for public, health, and undergraduate libraries as part of the circulating collection."

—E-Streams, Mar '02

"Information is presented in an unbiased, readable manner, and the sourcebook will certainly be a necessary addition to those public and high school libraries where Internet access is restricted or otherwise problematic."

—American Reference Books Annual 2002

"Recommended reference source."

—Booklist, American Library Association, Oct '01

"Will prove valuable to any library seeking to maintain a current, comprehensive reference collection of health resources.... Excellent reference."

—The Bookwatch, Aug '01

SEE ALSO Pregnancy & Birth Sourcebook

Fitness & Exercise Sourcebook, 2nd Edition

Basic Consumer Health Information about the Fundamentals of Fitness and Exercise, Including How to Begin and Maintain a Fitness Program, Fitness as a Lifestyle, the Link between Fitness and Diet, Advice for Specific Groups of People, Exercise as It Relates to Specific Medical Conditions, and Recent Research in Fitness and Exercise

Along with a Glossary of Important Terms and Resources for Additional Help and Information

Edited by Kristen M. Gledhill. 646 pages. 2001. 0-7808-0334-5. $78.

ALSO AVAILABLE: Fitness & Exercise Sourcebook, 1st Edition. Edited by Dan R. Harris. 663 pages. 1996. 0-7808-0186-5. $78.

"This work is recommended for all general reference collections."

—American Reference Books Annual 2002

"Highly recommended for public, consumer, and school grades fourth through college."

—E-Streams, Nov '01

"Recommended reference source." —Booklist, American Library Association, Oct '01

"The information appears quite comprehensive and is considered reliable.... This second edition is a welcomed addition to the series."

—Doody's Review Service, Sep '01

"This reference is a valuable choice for those who desire a broad source of information on exercise, fitness, and chronic-disease prevention through a healthy lifestyle." —*American Medical Writers Association Journal, Fall '01*

"Will prove valuable to any library seeking to maintain a current, comprehensive reference collection of health resources. . . . Excellent reference."
— *The Bookwatch, Aug '01*

■

Food & Animal Borne Diseases Sourcebook

Basic Information about Diseases That Can Be Spread to Humans through the Ingestion of Contaminated Food or Water or by Contact with Infected Animals and Insects, Such as Botulism, E. Coli, Hepatitis A, Trichinosis, Lyme Disease, and Rabies

Along with Information Regarding Prevention and Treatment Methods, and Including a Special Section for International Travelers Describing Diseases Such as Cholera, Malaria, Travelers' Diarrhea, and Yellow Fever, and Offering Recommendations for Avoiding Illness

Edited by Karen Bellenir and Peter D. Dresser. 535 pages. 1995. 0-7808-0033-8. $78.

"Targeting general readers and providing them with a single, comprehensive source of information on selected topics, this book continues, with the excellent caliber of its predecessors, to catalog topical information on health matters of general interest. Readable and thorough, this valuable resource is highly recommended for all libraries."
— *Academic Library Book Review, Summer '96*

"A comprehensive collection of authoritative information." — *Emergency Medical Services, Oct '95*

■

Food Safety Sourcebook

Basic Consumer Health Information about the Safe Handling of Meat, Poultry, Seafood, Eggs, Fruit Juices, and Other Food Items, and Facts about Pesticides, Drinking Water, Food Safety Overseas, and the Onset, Duration, and Symptoms of Foodborne Illnesses, Including Types of Pathogenic Bacteria, Parasitic Protozoa, Worms, Viruses, and Natural Toxins

Along with the Role of the Consumer, the Food Handler, and the Government in Food Safety; a Glossary, and Resources for Additional Help and Information

Edited by Dawn D. Matthews. 339 pages. 1999. 0-7808-0326-4. $78.

"This book is recommended for public libraries and universities with home economic and food science programs." — *E-Streams, Nov '00*

"Recommended reference source."
— *Booklist, American Library Association, May '00*

"This book takes the complex issues of food safety and foodborne pathogens and presents them in an easily understood manner. [It does] an excellent job of covering a large and often confusing topic."
— *American Reference Books Annual, 2000*

Forensic Medicine Sourcebook

Basic Consumer Information for the Layperson about Forensic Medicine, Including Crime Scene Investigation, Evidence Collection and Analysis, Expert Testimony, Computer-Aided Criminal Identification, Digital Imaging in the Courtroom, DNA Profiling, Accident Reconstruction, Autopsies, Ballistics, Drugs and Explosives Detection, Latent Fingerprints, Product Tampering, and Questioned Document Examination

Along with Statistical Data, a Glossary of Forensics Terminology, and Listings of Sources for Further Help and Information

Edited by Annemarie S. Muth. 574 pages. 1999. 0-7808-0232-2. $78.

"Given the expected widespread interest in its content and its easy to read style, this book is recommended for most public and all college and university libraries."
— *E-Streams, Feb '01*

"Recommended for public libraries."
—*Reference & User Services Quarterly, American Library Association, Spring 2000*

"Recommended reference source."
—*Booklist, American Library Association, Feb '00*

"A wealth of information, useful statistics, references are up-to-date and extremely complete. This wonderful collection of data will help students who are interested in a career in any type of forensic field. It is a great resource for attorneys who need information about types of expert witnesses needed in a particular case. It also offers useful information for fiction and nonfiction writers whose work involves a crime. A fascinating compilation. All levels." — *Choice, Association of College and Research Libraries, Jan 2000*

"There are several items that make this book attractive to consumers who are seeking certain forensic data. . . . This is a useful current source for those seeking general forensic medical answers."
—*American Reference Books Annual, 2000*

■

Gastrointestinal Diseases & Disorders Sourcebook

Basic Information about Gastroesophageal Reflux Disease (Heartburn), Ulcers, Diverticulosis, Irritable Bowel Syndrome, Crohn's Disease, Ulcerative Colitis, Diarrhea, Constipation, Lactose Intolerance, Hemorrhoids, Hepatitis, Cirrhosis, and Other Digestive Problems, Featuring Statistics, Descriptions of Symptoms, and Current Treatment Methods of Interest for Persons Living with Upper and Lower Gastrointestinal Maladies

Edited by Linda M. Ross. 413 pages. 1996. 0-7808-0078-8. $78.

". . . very readable form. The successful editorial work that brought this material together into a useful and understandable reference makes accessible to all readers information that can help them more effectively understand and obtain help for digestive tract problems."
— *Choice, Association of College & Research Libraries, Feb '97*

SEE ALSO *Diet & Nutrition Sourcebook, Digestive Diseases & Disorders, Eating Disorders Sourcebook*

■

Genetic Disorders Sourcebook, 3rd Edition

Basic Consumer Health Information about Hereditary Diseases and Disorders, Including Facts about the Human Genome, Genetic Inheritance Patterns, Disorders Associated with Specific Genes, Such as Sickle Cell Disease, Hemophilia, and Cystic Fibrosis, Chromosome Disorders, Such as Down Syndrome, Fragile X Syndrome, and Turner Syndrome, and Complex Diseases and Disorders Resulting from the Interaction of Environmental and Genetic Factors, Such as Allergies, Cancer, and Obesity

Along with Facts about Genetic Testing, Suggestions for Parents of Children with Special Needs, Reports on Current Research Initiatives, a Glossary of Genetic Terminology, and Resources for Additional Help and Information

Edited by Karen Bellenir. 777 pages. 2004. 0-7808-0742-1. $78.

ALSO AVAILABLE: Genetic Disorders Sourcebook, 1st Edition. Edited by Karen Bellenir. 642 pages. 1996. 0-7808-0034-6. $78.

Genetic Disorders Sourcebook, 2nd Edition. Edited by Kathy Massimini. 768 pages. 2001. 0-7808-0241-1. $78.

"Recommended for public libraries and medical and hospital libraries with consumer health collections."
— *E-Streams, May '01*

"Recommended reference source."
— *Booklist, American Library Association, Apr '01*

"Important pick for college-level health reference libraries." — *The Bookwatch, Mar '01*

"Provides essential medical information to both the general public and those diagnosed with a serious or fatal genetic disease or disorder." — *Choice, Association of College and Research Libraries, Jan '97*

■

Head Trauma Sourcebook

Basic Information for the Layperson about Open-Head and Closed-Head Injuries, Treatment Advances, Recovery, and Rehabilitation

Along with Reports on Current Research Initiatives

Edited by Karen Bellenir. 414 pages. 1997. 0-7808-0208-X. $78.

■

Headache Sourcebook

Basic Consumer Health Information about Migraine, Tension, Cluster, Rebound and Other Types of Headaches, with Facts about the Cause and Prevention of Headaches, the Effects of Stress and the Environment, Headaches during Pregnancy and Menopause, and Childhood Headaches

Along with a Glossary and Other Resources for Additional Help and Information

Edited by Dawn D. Matthews. 362 pages. 2002. 0-7808-0337-X. $78.

"Highly recommended for academic and medical reference collections." — *Library Bookwatch, Sep '02*

■

Health Insurance Sourcebook

Basic Information about Managed Care Organizations, Traditional Fee-for-Service Insurance, Insurance Portability and Pre-Existing Conditions Clauses, Medicare, Medicaid, Social Security, and Military Health Care

Along with Information about Insurance Fraud

Edited by Wendy Wilcox. 530 pages. 1997. 0-7808-0222-5. $78.

"Particularly useful because it brings much of this information together in one volume. This book will be a handy reference source in the health sciences library, hospital library, college and university library, and medium to large public library."
— *Medical Reference Services Quarterly, Fall '98*

Awarded "Books of the Year Award"
— *American Journal of Nursing, 1997*

"The layout of the book is particularly helpful as it provides easy access to reference material. A most useful addition to the vast amount of information about health insurance. The use of data from U.S. government agencies is most commendable. Useful in a library or learning center for healthcare professional students."
— *Doody's Health Sciences Book Reviews, Nov '97*

■

Health Reference Series Cumulative Index 1999

A Comprehensive Index to the Individual Volumes of the Health Reference Series, Including a Subject Index, Name Index, Organization Index, and Publication Index

Along with a Master List of Acronyms and Abbreviations

Edited by Edward J. Prucha, Anne Holmes, and Robert Rudnick. 990 pages. 2000. 0-7808-0382-5. $78.

"This volume will be most helpful in libraries that have a relatively complete collection of the Health Reference Series." — *American Reference Books Annual, 2001*

"Essential for collections that hold any of the numerous *Health Reference Series* titles."
— *Choice, Association of College and Research Libraries, Nov '00*

■

Healthy Aging Sourcebook

Basic Consumer Health Information about Maintaining Health through the Aging Process, Including Advice on Nutrition, Exercise, and Sleep, Help in Making Decisions about Midlife Issues and Retirement, and

Guidance Concerning Practical and Informed Choices in Health Consumerism

Along with Data Concerning the Theories of Aging, Different Experiences in Aging by Minority Groups, and Facts about Aging Now and Aging in the Future; and Featuring a Glossary, a Guide to Consumer Help, Additional Suggested Reading, and Practical Resource Directory

Edited by Jenifer Swanson. 536 pages. 1999. 0-7808-0390-6. $78.

"Recommended reference source."
—*Booklist, American Library Association, Feb '00*

SEE ALSO Physical & Mental Issues in Aging Sourcebook

■

Healthy Children Sourcebook

Basic Consumer Health Information about the Physical and Mental Development of Children between the Ages of 3 and 12, Including Routine Health Care, Preventative Health Services, Safety and First Aid, Healthy Sleep, Dental Care, Nutrition, and Fitness, and Featuring Parenting Tips on Such Topics as Bedwetting, Choosing Day Care, Monitoring TV and Other Media, and Establishing a Foundation for Substance Abuse Prevention

Along with a Glossary of Commonly Used Pediatric Terms and Resources for Additional Help and Information.

Edited by Chad T. Kimball. 647 pages. 2003. 0-7808-0247-0. $78.

"It is hard to imagine that any other single resource exists that would provide such a comprehensive guide of timely information on health promotion and disease prevention for children aged 3 to 12."
—*American Reference Books Annual, 2004*

"The strengths of this book are many. It is clearly written, presented and structured."
—*Journal of the National Medical Association, 2004*

■

Healthy Heart Sourcebook for Women

Basic Consumer Health Information about Cardiac Issues Specific to Women, Including Facts about Major Risk Factors and Prevention, Treatment and Control Strategies, and Important Dietary Issues

Along with a Special Section Regarding the Pros and Cons of Hormone Replacement Therapy and Its Impact on Heart Health, and Additional Help, Including Recipes, a Glossary, and a Directory of Resources

Edited by Dawn D. Matthews. 336 pages. 2000. 0-7808-0329-9. $78.

"A good reference source and recommended for all public, academic, medical, and hospital libraries."
—*Medical Reference Services Quarterly, Summer '01*

"Because of the lack of information specific to women on this topic, this book is recommended for public libraries and consumer libraries."
—*American Reference Books Annual, 2001*

"Contains very important information about coronary artery disease that all women should know. The information is current and presented in an easy-to-read format. The book will make a good addition to any library."
—*American Medical Writers Association Journal, Summer '00*

"Important, basic reference."
—*Reviewer's Bookwatch, Jul '00*

SEE ALSO Heart Diseases & Disorders Sourcebook, Women's Health Concerns Sourcebook

■

Heart Diseases & Disorders Sourcebook, 2nd Edition

SEE Cardiovascular Diseases & Disorders Sourcebook, 3rd Edition

■

Household Safety Sourcebook

Basic Consumer Health Information about Household Safety, Including Information about Poisons, Chemicals, Fire, and Water Hazards in the Home

Along with Advice about the Safe Use of Home Maintenance Equipment, Choosing Toys and Nursery Furniture, Holiday and Recreation Safety, a Glossary, and Resources for Further Help and Information

Edited by Dawn D. Matthews. 606 pages. 2002. 0-7808-0338-8. $78.

"This work will be useful in public libraries with large consumer health and wellness departments."
—*American Reference Books Annual, 2003*

"As a sourcebook on household safety this book meets its mark. It is encyclopedic in scope and covers a wide range of safety issues that are commonly seen in the home."
—*E-Streams, Jul '02*

■

Hypertension Sourcebook

Basic Consumer Health Information about the Causes, Diagnosis, and Treatment of High Blood Pressure, with Facts about Consequences, Complications, and Co-Occurring Disorders, Such as Coronary Heart Disease, Diabetes, Stroke, Kidney Disease, and Hypertensive Retinopathy, and Issues in Blood Pressure Control, Including Dietary Choices, Stress Management, and Medications

Along with Reports on Current Research Initiatives and Clinical Trials, a Glossary, and Resources for Additional Help and Information

Edited by Dawn D. Matthews and Karen Bellenir. 613 pages. 2004. 0-7808-0674-3. $78.

Immune System Disorders Sourcebook

Basic Information about Lupus, Multiple Sclerosis, Guillain-Barré Syndrome, Chronic Granulomatous Disease, and More

Along with Statistical and Demographic Data and Reports on Current Research Initiatives

Edited by Allan R. Cook. 608 pages. 1997. 0-7808-0209-8. $78.

Infant & Toddler Health Sourcebook

Basic Consumer Health Information about the Physical and Mental Development of Newborns, Infants, and Toddlers, Including Neonatal Concerns, Nutrition Recommendations, Immunization Schedules, Common Pediatric Disorders, Assessments and Milestones, Safety Tips, and Advice for Parents and Other Caregivers

Along with a Glossary of Terms and Resource Listings for Additional Help

Edited by Jenifer Swanson. 585 pages. 2000. 0-7808-0246-2. $78.

"As a reference for the general public, this would be useful in any library." — *E-Streams, May '01*

"Recommended reference source."
— *Booklist, American Library Association, Feb '01*

"This is a good source for general use."
—*American Reference Books Annual, 2001*

Infectious Diseases Sourcebook

Basic Consumer Health Information about Non-Contagious Bacterial, Viral, Prion, Fungal, and Parasitic Diseases Spread by Food and Water, Insects and Animals, or Environmental Contact, Including Botulism, E. Coli, Encephalitis, Legionnaires' Disease, Lyme Disease, Malaria, Plague, Rabies, Salmonella, Tetanus, and Others, and Facts about Newly Emerging Diseases, Such as Hantavirus, Mad Cow Disease, Monkeypox, and West Nile Virus

Along with Information about Preventing Disease Transmission, the Threat of Bioterrorism, and Current Research Initiatives, with a Glossary and Directory of Resources for More Information

Edited by Karen Bellenir. 634 pages. 2004. 0-7808-0675-1. $78.

Injury & Trauma Sourcebook

Basic Consumer Health Information about the Impact of Injury, the Diagnosis and Treatment of Common and Traumatic Injuries, Emergency Care, and Specific Injuries Related to Home, Community, Workplace, Transportation, and Recreation

Along with Guidelines for Injury Prevention, a Glossary, and a Directory of Additional Resources

Edited by Joyce Brennfleck Shannon. 696 pages. 2002. 0-7808-0421-X. $78.

"This publication is the most comprehensive work of its kind about injury and trauma."
— *American Reference Books Annual, 2003*

"This sourcebook provides concise, easily readable, basic health information about injuries. . . . This book is well organized and an easy to use reference resource suitable for hospital, health sciences and public libraries with consumer health collections."
— *E-Streams, Nov '02*

"Practitioners should be aware of guides such as this in order to facilitate their use by patients and their families." — *Doody's Health Sciences Book Review Journal, Sep-Oct '02*

"Recommended reference source."
— *Booklist, American Library Association, Sep '02*

"Highly recommended for academic and medical reference collections." — *Library Bookwatch, Sep '02*

Kidney & Urinary Tract Diseases & Disorders Sourcebook

Basic Information about Kidney Stones, Urinary Incontinence, Bladder Disease, End Stage Renal Disease, Dialysis, and More

Along with Statistical and Demographic Data and Reports on Current Research Initiatives

Edited by Linda M. Ross. 602 pages. 1997. 0-7808-0079-6. $78.

Learning Disabilities Sourcebook, 2nd Edition

Basic Consumer Health Information about Learning Disabilities, Including Dyslexia, Developmental Speech and Language Disabilities, Non-Verbal Learning Disorders, Developmental Arithmetic Disorder, Developmental Writing Disorder, and Other Conditions That Impede Learning Such as Attention Deficit/ Hyperactivity Disorder, Brain Injury, Hearing Impairment, Klinefelter Syndrome, Dyspraxia, and Tourette Syndrome

Along with Facts about Educational Issues and Assistive Technology, Coping Strategies, a Glossary of Related Terms, and Resources for Further Help and Information

Edited by Dawn D. Matthews. 621 pages. 2003. 0-7808-0626-3. $78.

ALSO AVAILABLE: Learning Disabilities Sourcebook, 1st Edition. Edited by Linda M. Shin. 579 pages. 1998. 0-7808-0210-1. $78.

"The second edition of *Learning Disabilities Sourcebook* far surpasses the earlier edition in that it is more focused on information that will be useful as a consumer health resource."
—*American Reference Books Annual, 2004*

"Teachers as well as consumers will find this an essential guide to understanding various syndromes and their latest treatments. [An] invaluable reference for public and school library collections alike."
— *Library Bookwatch, Apr '03*

Named "Outstanding Reference Book of 1999."
— *New York Public Library, Feb 2000*

"An excellent candidate for inclusion in a public library reference section. It's a great source of information. Teachers will also find the book useful. Definitely worth reading."
— *Journal of Adolescent & Adult Literacy, Feb 2000*

"Readable . . . provides a solid base of information regarding successful techniques used with individuals who have learning disabilities, as well as practical suggestions for educators and family members. Clear language, concise descriptions, and pertinent information for contacting multiple resources add to the strength of this book as a useful tool." — *Choice, Association of College and Research Libraries, Feb '99*

"Recommended reference source."
— *Booklist, American Library Association, Sep '98*

"A useful resource for libraries and for those who don't have the time to identify and locate the individual publications." — *Disability Resources Monthly, Sep '98*

Leukemia Sourcebook

Basic Consumer Health Information about Adult and Childhood Leukemias, Including Acute Lymphocytic Leukemia (ALL), Chronic Lymphocytic Leukemia (CLL), Acute Myelogenous Leukemia (AML), Chronic Myelogenous Leukemia (CML), and Hairy Cell Leukemia, and Treatments Such as Chemotherapy, Radiation Therapy, Peripheral Blood Stem Cell and Marrow Transplantation, and Immunotherapy

Along with Tips for Life During and After Treatment, a Glossary, and Directories of Additional Resources

Edited by Joyce Brennfleck Shannon. 587 pages. 2003. 0-7808-0627-1. $78.

"Unlike other medical books for the layperson, . . . the language does not talk down to the reader. . . . This volume is highly recommended for all libraries."
— *American Reference Books Annual, 2004*

Liver Disorders Sourcebook

Basic Consumer Health Information about the Liver and How It Works; Liver Diseases, Including Cancer, Cirrhosis, Hepatitis, and Toxic and Drug Related Diseases; Tips for Maintaining a Healthy Liver; Laboratory Tests, Radiology Tests, and Facts about Liver Transplantation

Along with a Section on Support Groups, a Glossary, and Resource Listings

Edited by Joyce Brennfleck Shannon. 591 pages. 2000. 0-7808-0383-3. $78.

"A valuable resource."
— *American Reference Books Annual, 2001*

"This title is recommended for health sciences and public libraries with consumer health collections."
— *E-Streams, Oct '00*

"Recommended reference source."
— *Booklist, American Library Association, Jun '00*

Lung Disorders Sourcebook

Basic Consumer Health Information about Emphysema, Pneumonia, Tuberculosis, Asthma, Cystic Fibrosis, and Other Lung Disorders, Including Facts about Diagnostic Procedures, Treatment Strategies, Disease Prevention Efforts, and Such Risk Factors as Smoking, Air Pollution, and Exposure to Asbestos, Radon, and Other Agents

Along with a Glossary and Resources for Additional Help and Information

Edited by Dawn D. Matthews. 678 pages. 2002. 0-7808-0339-6. $78.

"This title is a great addition for public and school libraries because it provides concise health information on the lungs."
— *American Reference Books Annual, 2003*

"Highly recommended for academic and medical reference collections." — *Library Bookwatch, Sep '02*

Medical Tests Sourcebook, 2nd Edition

Basic Consumer Health Information about Medical Tests, Including Age-Specific Health Tests, Important Health Screenings and Exams, Home-Use Tests, Blood and Specimen Tests, Electrical Tests, Scope Tests, Genetic Testing, and Imaging Tests, Such as X-Rays, Ultrasound, Computed Tomography, Magnetic Resonance Imaging, Angiography, and Nuclear Medicine

Along with a Glossary and Directory of Additional Resources

Edited by Joyce Brennfleck Shannon. 654 pages. 2004. 0-7808-0670-0. $78.

ALSO AVAILABLE: *Medical Tests, 1st Edition.* Edited by Joyce Brennfleck Shannon. 691 pages. 1999. 0-7808-0243-8. $78.

"Recommended for hospital and health sciences libraries with consumer health collections."
— *E-Streams, Mar '00*

"This is an overall excellent reference with a wealth of general knowledge that may aid those who are reluctant to get vital tests performed."
— *Today's Librarian, Jan 2000*

"A valuable reference guide."
— *American Reference Books Annual, 2000*

Men's Health Concerns Sourcebook, 2nd Edition

Basic Consumer Health Information about the Medical and Mental Concerns of Men, Including Theories about the Shorter Male Lifespan, the Leading Causes of Death and Disability, Physical Concerns of Special Significance to Men, Reproductive and Sexual Concerns, Sexually Transmitted Diseases, Men's Mental and Emotional Health, and Lifestyle Choices That Affect Wellness, Such as Nutrition, Fitness, and Substance Use

Along with a Glossary of Related Terms and a Directory of Organizational Resources in Men's Health

Edited by Robert Aquinas McNally. 644 pages. 2004. 0-7808-0671-9. $78.

ALSO AVAILABLE: Men's Health Concerns Sourcebook, 1st Edition. Edited by Allan R. Cook. 738 pages. 1998. 0-7808-0212-8. $78.

"This comprehensive resource and the series are highly recommended."
—*American Reference Books Annual, 2000*

"Recommended reference source."
—*Booklist, American Library Association, Dec '98*

Mental Health Disorders Sourcebook, 2nd Edition

Basic Consumer Health Information about Anxiety Disorders, Depression and Other Mood Disorders, Eating Disorders, Personality Disorders, Schizophrenia, and More, Including Disease Descriptions, Treatment Options, and Reports on Current Research Initiatives

Along with Statistical Data, Tips for Maintaining Mental Health, a Glossary, and Directory of Sources for Additional Help and Information

Edited by Karen Bellenir. 605 pages. 2000. 0-7808-0240-3. $78.

ALSO AVAILABLE: Mental Health Disorders Sourcebook, 1st Edition. Edited by Karen Bellenir. 548 pages. 1995. 0-7808-0040-0. $78.

"Well organized and well written."
—*American Reference Books Annual, 2001*

"Recommended reference source."
—*Booklist, American Library Association, Jun '00*

Mental Retardation Sourcebook

Basic Consumer Health Information about Mental Retardation and Its Causes, Including Down Syndrome, Fetal Alcohol Syndrome, Fragile X Syndrome, Genetic Conditions, Injury, and Environmental Sources

Along with Preventive Strategies, Parenting Issues, Educational Implications, Health Care Needs, Employment and Economic Matters, Legal Issues, a Glossary, and a Resource Listing for Additional Help and Information

Edited by Joyce Brennfleck Shannon. 642 pages. 2000. 0-7808-0377-9. $78.

"Public libraries will find the book useful for reference and as a beginning research point for students, parents, and caregivers."
—*American Reference Books Annual, 2001*

"The strength of this work is that it compiles many basic fact sheets and addresses for further information in one volume. It is intended and suitable for the general public. This sourcebook is relevant to any collection providing health information to the general public."
— *E-Streams, Nov '00*

"From preventing retardation to parenting and family challenges, this covers health, social and legal issues and will prove an invaluable overview."
— *Reviewer's Bookwatch, Jul '00*

Movement Disorders Sourcebook

Basic Consumer Health Information about Neurological Movement Disorders, Including Essential Tremor, Parkinson's Disease, Dystonia, Cerebral Palsy, Huntington's Disease, Myasthenia Gravis, Multiple Sclerosis, and Other Early-Onset and Adult-Onset Movement Disorders, Their Symptoms and Causes, Diagnostic Tests, and Treatments

Along with Mobility and Assistive Technology Information, a Glossary, and a Directory of Additional Resources

Edited by Joyce Brennfleck Shannon. 655 pages. 2003. 0-7808-0628-X. $78.

". . . a good resource for consumers and recommended for public, community college and undergraduate libraries."
— *American Reference Books Annual, 2004*

Muscular Dystrophy Sourcebook

Basic Consumer Health Information about Congenital, Childhood-Onset, and Adult-Onset Forms of Muscular Dystrophy, Such as Duchenne, Becker, Emery-Dreifuss, Distal, Limb-Girdle, Facioscapulohumeral (FSHD), Myotonic, and Ophthalmoplegic Muscular Dystrophies, Including Facts about Diagnostic Tests, Medical and Physical Therapies, Management of Co-Occurring Conditions, and Parenting Guidelines

Along with Practical Tips for Home Care, a Glossary, and Directories of Additional Resources

Edited by Joyce Brennfleck Shannon. 577 pages. 2004. 0-7808-0676-X. $78.

Obesity Sourcebook

Basic Consumer Health Information about Diseases and Other Problems Associated with Obesity, and Including Facts about Risk Factors, Prevention Issues, and Management Approaches

Along with Statistical and Demographic Data, Information about Special Populations, Research Updates, a Glossary, and Source Listings for Further Help and Information

Edited by Wilma Caldwell and Chad T. Kimball. 376 pages. 2001. 0-7808-0333-7. $78.

"The book synthesizes the reliable medical literature on obesity into one easy-to-read and useful resource for the general public."
—*American Reference Books Annual 2002*

"This is a very useful resource book for the lay public."
—*Doody's Review Service, Nov '01*

"Well suited for the health reference collection of a public library or an academic health science library that serves the general population." —*E-Streams, Sep '01*

"Recommended reference source."
—*Booklist, American Library Association, Apr '01*

" Recommended pick both for specialty health library collections and any general consumer health reference collection." — *The Bookwatch, Apr '01*

■

Ophthalmic Disorders Sourcebook, 1st Edition

SEE Eye Care Sourcebook, 2nd Edition

■

Oral Health Sourcebook

SEE Dental Care & Oral Health Sourcebook, 2nd Ed.

■

Osteoporosis Sourcebook

Basic Consumer Health Information about Primary and Secondary Osteoporosis and Juvenile Osteoporosis and Related Conditions, Including Fibrous Dysplasia, Gaucher Disease, Hyperthyroidism, Hypophosphatasia, Myeloma, Osteopetrosis, Osteogenesis Imperfecta, and Paget's Disease

Along with Information about Risk Factors, Treatments, Traditional and Non-Traditional Pain Management, a Glossary of Related Terms, and a Directory of Resources

Edited by Allan R. Cook. 584 pages. 2001. 0-7808-0239-X. $78.

"This would be a book to be kept in a staff or patient library. The targeted audience is the layperson, but the therapist who needs a quick bit of information on a particular topic will also find the book useful."
—*Physical Therapy, Jan '02*

"This resource is recommended as a great reference source for public, health, and academic libraries, and is another triumph for the editors of Omnigraphics."
—*American Reference Books Annual 2002*

"Recommended for all public libraries and general health collections, especially those supporting patient education or consumer health programs."
—*E-Streams, Nov '01*

"Will prove valuable to any library seeking to maintain a current, comprehensive reference collection of health resources. . . . From prevention to treatment and associated conditions, this provides an excellent survey."
—*The Bookwatch, Aug '01*

"Recommended reference source."
—*Booklist, American Library Association, July '01*

SEE ALSO Women's Health Concerns Sourcebook

■

Pain Sourcebook, 2nd Edition

Basic Consumer Health Information about Specific Forms of Acute and Chronic Pain, Including Muscle and Skeletal Pain, Nerve Pain, Cancer Pain, and Disorders Characterized by Pain, Such as Fibromyalgia, Shingles, Angina, Arthritis, and Headaches

Along with Information about Pain Medications and Management Techniques, Complementary and Alternative Pain Relief Options, Tips for People Living with Chronic Pain, a Glossary, and a Directory of Sources for Further Information

Edited by Karen Bellenir. 670 pages. 2002. 0-7808-0612-3. $78.

ALSO AVAILABLE: Pain Sourcebook, 1st Edition. Edited by Allan R. Cook. 667 pages. 1997. 0-7808-0213-6. $78.

"A source of valuable information. . . . This book offers help to nonmedical people who need information about pain and pain management. It is also an excellent reference for those who participate in patient education."
—*Doody's Review Service, Sep '02*

"The text is readable, easily understood, and well indexed. This excellent volume belongs in all patient education libraries, consumer health sections of public libraries, and many personal collections."
—*American Reference Books Annual, 1999*

"A beneficial reference." — *Booklist Health Sciences Supplement, American Library Association, Oct '98*

"The information is basic in terms of scholarship and is appropriate for general readers. Written in journalistic style . . . intended for non-professionals. Quite thorough in its coverage of different pain conditions and summarizes the latest clinical information regarding pain treatment." — *Choice, Association of College and Research Libraries, Jun '98*

"Recommended reference source."
—*Booklist, American Library Association, Mar '98*

■

Pediatric Cancer Sourcebook

Basic Consumer Health Information about Leukemias, Brain Tumors, Sarcomas, Lymphomas, and Other Cancers in Infants, Children, and Adolescents, Including Descriptions of Cancers, Treatments, and Coping Strategies

Along with Suggestions for Parents, Caregivers, and Concerned Relatives, a Glossary of Cancer Terms, and Resource Listings

Edited by Edward J. Prucha. 587 pages. 1999. 0-7808-0245-4. $78.

"An excellent source of information. Recommended for public, hospital, and health science libraries with consumer health collections." — *E-Streams, Jun '00*

"Recommended reference source."
—*Booklist, American Library Association, Feb '00*

Physical & Mental Issues in Aging Sourcebook

Basic Consumer Health Information on Physical and Mental Disorders Associated with the Aging Process, Including Concerns about Cardiovascular Disease, Pulmonary Disease, Oral Health, Digestive Disorders, Musculoskeletal and Skin Disorders, Metabolic Changes, Sexual and Reproductive Issues, and Changes in Vision, Hearing, and Other Senses

Along with Data about Longevity and Causes of Death, Information on Acute and Chronic Pain, Descriptions of Mental Concerns, a Glossary of Terms, and Resource Listings for Additional Help

Edited by Jenifer Swanson. 660 pages. 1999. 0-7808-0233-0. $78.

SEE ALSO *Healthy Aging Sourcebook*

Podiatry Sourcebook

Basic Consumer Health Information about Foot Conditions, Diseases, and Injuries, Including Bunions, Corns, Calluses, Athlete's Foot, Plantar Warts, Hammertoes and Clawtoes, Clubfoot, Heel Pain, Gout, and More

Along with Facts about Foot Care, Disease Prevention, Foot Safety, Choosing a Foot Care Specialist, a Glossary of Terms, and Resource Listings for Additional Information

Edited by M. Lisa Weatherford. 380 pages. 2001. 0-7808-0215-2. $78.

Pregnancy & Birth Sourcebook, 2nd Edition

Basic Consumer Health Information about Conception and Pregnancy, Including Facts about Fertility, Infertility, Pregnancy Symptoms and Complications, Fetal Growth and Development, Labor, Delivery, and the Postpartum Period, as Well as Information about Maintaining Health and Wellness during Pregnancy and Caring for a Newborn

Along with Information about Public Health Assistance for Low-Income Pregnant Women, a Glossary, and Directories of Agencies and Organizations Providing Help and Support

Edited by Amy L. Sutton. 626 pages. 2004. 0-7808-0672-7. $78.

ALSO AVAILABLE: *Pregnancy & Birth Sourcebook, 1st Edition.* Edited by Heather E. Aldred. 737 pages. 1997. 0-7808-0216-0. $78.

SEE ALSO *Congenital Disorders Sourcebook, Family Planning Sourcebook*

Prostate Cancer Sourcebook

Basic Consumer Health Information about Prostate Cancer, Including Information about the Associated Risk Factors, Detection, Diagnosis, and Treatment of Prostate Cancer

Along with Information on Non-Malignant Prostate Conditions, and Featuring a Section Listing Support and Treatment Centers and a Glossary of Related Terms

Edited by Dawn D. Matthews. 358 pages. 2001. 0-7808-0324-8. $78.

Public Health Sourcebook

Basic Information about Government Health Agencies, Including National Health Statistics and Trends, Healthy People 2000 Program Goals and Objectives, the Centers for Disease Control and Prevention, the Food and Drug Administration, and the National Institutes of Health

Along with Full Contact Information for Each Agency

Edited by Wendy Wilcox. 698 pages. 1998. 0-7808-0220-9. $78.

Reconstructive & Cosmetic Surgery Sourcebook

Basic Consumer Health Information on Cosmetic and Reconstructive Plastic Surgery, Including Statistical Information about Different Surgical Procedures, Things to Consider Prior to Surgery, Plastic Surgery Techniques and Tools, Emotional and Psychological Considerations, and Procedure-Specific Information

Along with a Glossary of Terms and a Listing of Resources for Additional Help and Information

Edited by M. Lisa Weatherford. 374 pages. 2001. 0-7808-0214-4. $78.

"An excellent reference that addresses cosmetic and medically necessary reconstructive surgeries. . . . The style of the prose is calm and reassuring, discussing the many positive outcomes now available due to advances in surgical techniques."
— *American Reference Books Annual 2002*

"Recommended for health science libraries that are open to the public, as well as hospital libraries that are open to the patients. This book is a good resource for the consumer interested in plastic surgery."
— *E-Streams, Dec '01*

"Recommended reference source."
— *Booklist, American Library Association, July '01*

Rehabilitation Sourcebook

Basic Consumer Health Information about Rehabilitation for People Recovering from Heart Surgery, Spinal Cord Injury, Stroke, Orthopedic Impairments, Amputation, Pulmonary Impairments, Traumatic Injury, and More, Including Physical Therapy, Occupational Therapy, Speech/ Language Therapy, Massage Therapy, Dance Therapy, Art Therapy, and Recreational Therapy

Along with Information on Assistive and Adaptive Devices, a Glossary, and Resources for Additional Help and Information

Edited by Dawn D. Matthews. 531 pages. 1999. 0-7808-0236-5. $78.

"This is an excellent resource for public library reference and health collections."
— *American Reference Books Annual, 2001*

"Recommended reference source."
— *Booklist, American Library Association, May '00*

Respiratory Diseases & Disorders Sourcebook

Basic Information about Respiratory Diseases and Disorders, Including Asthma, Cystic Fibrosis, Pneumonia, the Common Cold, Influenza, and Others, Featuring Facts about the Respiratory System, Statistical and Demographic Data, Treatments, Self-Help Management Suggestions, and Current Research Initiatives

Edited by Allan R. Cook and Peter D. Dresser. 771 pages. 1995. 0-7808-0037-0. $78.

"Designed for the layperson and for patients and their families coping with respiratory illness. . . . an extensive array of information on diagnosis, treatment, management, and prevention of respiratory illnesses for the general reader."
— *Choice, Association of College and Research Libraries, Jun '96*

"A highly recommended text for all collections. It is a comforting reminder of the power of knowledge that good books carry between their covers."
— *Academic Library Book Review, Spring '96*

"A comprehensive collection of authoritative information presented in a nontechnical, humanitarian style for patients, families, and caregivers." — *Association of Operating Room Nurses, Sep/Oct '95*

SEE ALSO Lung Disorders Sourcebook

Sexually Transmitted Diseases Sourcebook, 2nd Edition

Basic Consumer Health Information about Sexually Transmitted Diseases, Including Information on the Diagnosis and Treatment of Chlamydia, Gonorrhea, Hepatitis, Herpes, HIV, Mononucleosis, Syphilis, and Others

Along with Information on Prevention, Such as Condom Use, Vaccines, and STD Education; And Featuring a Section on Issues Related to Youth and Adolescents, a Glossary, and Resources for Additional Help and Information

Edited by Dawn D. Matthews. 538 pages. 2001. 0-7808-0249-7. $78.

ALSO AVAILABLE: Sexually Transmitted Diseases Sourcebook, 1st Edition. Edited by Linda M. Ross. 550 pages. 1997. 0-7808-0217-9. $78.

"Recommended for consumer health collections in public libraries, and secondary school and community college libraries."
— *American Reference Books Annual 2002*

"Every school and public library should have a copy of this comprehensive and user-friendly reference book."
— *Choice, Association of College & Research Libraries, Sep '01*

"This is a highly recommended book. This is an especially important book for all school and public libraries." — *AIDS Book Review Journal, Jul-Aug '01*

"Recommended reference source."
— *Booklist, American Library Association, Apr '01*

"Recommended pick both for specialty health library collections and any general consumer health reference collection." — *The Bookwatch, Apr '01*

Skin Disorders Sourcebook

Basic Information about Common Skin and Scalp Conditions Caused by Aging, Allergies, Immune Reactions, Sun Exposure, Infectious Organisms, Parasites, Cosmetics, and Skin Traumas, Including Abrasions, Cuts, and Pressure Sores

Along with Information on Prevention and Treatment

Edited by Allan R. Cook. 647 pages. 1997. 0-7808-0080-X. $78.

"... comprehensive, easily read reference book."
—*Doody's Health Sciences Book Reviews, Oct '97*

SEE ALSO *Burns Sourcebook*

∎

Sleep Disorders Sourcebook, 2nd Edition

Basic Consumer Health Information about Sleep and Sleep Disorders, Including Insomnia, Sleep Apnea, Restless Legs Syndrome, Narcolepsy, Parasomnias, and Other Health Problems That Affect Sleep, Plus Facts about Diagnostic Procedures, Treatment Strategies, Sleep Medications, and Tips for Improving Sleep Quality

Along with a Glossary of Related Terms and Resources for Additional Help and Information

Edited by Amy L. Sutton. 567 pages. 2005. 0-7808-0745-6. $78.

ALSO AVAILABLE: *Sleep Disorders Sourcebook, 1st Edition.* Edited by Jenifer Swanson. 439 pages. 1998. 0-7808-0234-9. $78.

"This text will complement any home or medical library. It is user-friendly and ideal for the adult reader."
—*American Reference Books Annual, 2000*

"A useful resource that provides accurate, relevant, and accessible information on sleep to the general public. Health care providers who deal with sleep disorders patients may also find it helpful in being prepared to answer some of the questions patients ask."
—*Respiratory Care, Jul '99*

"Recommended reference source."
—*Booklist, American Library Association, Feb '99*

∎

Smoking Concerns Sourcebook

Basic Consumer Health Information about Nicotine Addiction and Smoking Cessation, Featuring Facts about the Health Effects of Tobacco Use, Including Lung and Other Cancers, Heart Disease, Stroke, and Respiratory Disorders, Such as Emphysema and Chronic Bronchitis

Along with Information about Smoking Prevention Programs, Suggestions for Achieving and Maintaining a Smoke-Free Lifestyle, Statistics about Tobacco Use, Reports on Current Research Initiatives, a Glossary of Related Terms, and Directories of Resources for Additional Help and Information

Edited by Karen Bellenir. 621 pages. 2004. 0-7808-0323-X. $78.

∎

Sports Injuries Sourcebook, 2nd Edition

Basic Consumer Health Information about the Diagnosis, Treatment, and Rehabilitation of Common Sports-Related Injuries in Children and Adults

Along with Suggestions for Conditioning and Training, Information and Prevention Tips for Injuries Frequently Associated with Specific Sports and Special Populations, a Glossary, and a Directory of Additional Resources

Edited by Joyce Brennfleck Shannon. 614 pages. 2002. 0-7808-0604-2. $78.

ALSO AVAILABLE: *Sports Injuries Sourcebook, 1st Edition.* Edited by Heather E. Aldred. 624 pages. 1999. 0-7808-0218-7. $78.

"This is an excellent reference for consumers and it is recommended for public, community college, and undergraduate libraries."
—*American Reference Books Annual, 2003*

"Recommended reference source."
—*Booklist, American Library Association, Feb '03*

∎

Stress-Related Disorders Sourcebook

Basic Consumer Health Information about Stress and Stress-Related Disorders, Including Stress Origins and Signals, Environmental Stress at Work and Home, Mental and Emotional Stress Associated with Depression, Post-Traumatic Stress Disorder, Panic Disorder, Suicide, and the Physical Effects of Stress on the Cardiovascular, Immune, and Nervous Systems

Along with Stress Management Techniques, a Glossary, and a Listing of Additional Resources

Edited by Joyce Brennfleck Shannon. 610 pages. 2002. 0-7808-0560-7. $78.

"Well written for a general readership, the *Stress-Related Disorders Sourcebook* is a useful addition to the health reference literature."
—*American Reference Books Annual, 2003*

"I am impressed by the amount of information. It offers a thorough overview of the causes and consequences of stress for the layperson. . . . A well-done and thorough reference guide for professionals and nonprofessionals alike."
—*Doody's Review Service, Dec '02*

∎

Stroke Sourcebook

Basic Consumer Health Information about Stroke, Including Ischemic, Hemorrhagic, Transient Ischemic Attack (TIA), and Pediatric Stroke, Stroke Triggers and Risks, Diagnostic Tests, Treatments, and Rehabilitation Information

Along with Stroke Prevention Guidelines, Legal and Financial Information, a Glossary, and a Directory of Additional Resources

Edited by Joyce Brennfleck Shannon. 606 pages. 2003. 0-7808-0630-1. $78.

"This volume is highly recommended and should be in every medical, hospital, and public library."
—*American Reference Books Annual, 2004*

Substance Abuse Sourcebook

Basic Health-Related Information about the Abuse of Legal and Illegal Substances Such as Alcohol, Tobacco, Prescription Drugs, Marijuana, Cocaine, and Heroin; and Including Facts about Substance Abuse Prevention Strategies, Intervention Methods, Treatment and Recovery Programs, and a Section Addressing the Special Problems Related to Substance Abuse during Pregnancy

Edited by Karen Bellenir. 573 pages. 1996. 0-7808-0038-9. $78.

"A valuable addition to any health reference section. Highly recommended."
— *The Book Report, Mar/Apr '97*

". . . a comprehensive collection of substance abuse information that's both highly readable and compact. Families and caregivers of substance abusers will find the information enlightening and helpful, while teachers, social workers and journalists should benefit from the concise format. Recommended."
— *Drug Abuse Update, Winter '96/'97*

SEE ALSO *Alcoholism Sourcebook, Drug Abuse Sourcebook*

■

Surgery Sourcebook

Basic Consumer Health Information about Inpatient and Outpatient Surgeries, Including Cardiac, Vascular, Orthopedic, Ocular, Reconstructive, Cosmetic, Gynecologic, and Ear, Nose, and Throat Procedures and More

Along with Information about Operating Room Policies and Instruments, Laser Surgery Techniques, Hospital Errors, Statistical Data, a Glossary, and Listings of Sources for Further Help and Information

Edited by Annemarie S. Muth and Karen Bellenir. 596 pages. 2002. 0-7808-0380-9. $78.

"Large public libraries and medical libraries would benefit from this material in their reference collections."
— *American Reference Books Annual, 2004*

"Invaluable reference for public and school library collections alike."
— *Library Bookwatch, Apr '03*

■

Thyroid Disorders Sourcebook

Basic Consumer Health Information about Disorders of the Thyroid and Parathyroid Glands, Including Hypothyroidism, Hyperthyroidism, Graves Disease, Hashimoto Thyroiditis, Thyroid Cancer, and Parathyroid Disorders, Featuring Facts about Symptoms, Risk Factors, Tests, and Treatments

Along with Information about the Effects of Thyroid Imbalance on Other Body Systems, Environmental Factors That Affect the Thyroid Gland, a Glossary, and a Directory of Additional Resources

Edited by Joyce Brennfleck Shannon. 600 pages. 2005. 0-7808-0745-6. $78.

Transplantation Sourcebook

Basic Consumer Health Information about Organ and Tissue Transplantation, Including Physical and Financial Preparations, Procedures and Issues Relating to Specific Solid Organ and Tissue Transplants, Rehabilitation, Pediatric Transplant Information, the Future of Transplantation, and Organ and Tissue Donation

Along with a Glossary and Listings of Additional Resources

Edited by Joyce Brennfleck Shannon. 628 pages. 2002. 0-7808-0322-1. $78.

"Along with these advances [in transplantation technology] have come a number of daunting questions for potential transplant patients, their families, and their health care providers. This reference text is the best single tool to address many of these questions. . . . It will be a much-needed addition to the reference collections in health care, academic, and large public libraries."
— *American Reference Books Annual, 2003*

"Recommended for libraries with an interest in offering consumer health information." — *E-Streams, Jul '02*

"This is a unique and valuable resource for patients facing transplantation and their families."
— *Doody's Review Service, Jun '02*

■

Traveler's Health Sourcebook

Basic Consumer Health Information for Travelers, Including Physical and Medical Preparations, Transportation Health and Safety, Essential Information about Food and Water, Sun Exposure, Insect and Snake Bites, Camping and Wilderness Medicine, and Travel with Physical or Medical Disabilities

Along with International Travel Tips, Vaccination Recommendations, Geographical Health Issues, Disease Risks, a Glossary, and a Listing of Additional Resources

Edited by Joyce Brennfleck Shannon. 613 pages. 2000. 0-7808-0384-1. $78.

"Recommended reference source."
— *Booklist, American Library Association, Feb '01*

"This book is recommended for any public library, any travel collection, and especially any collection for the physically disabled."
— *American Reference Books Annual, 2001*

■

Vegetarian Sourcebook

Basic Consumer Health Information about Vegetarian Diets, Lifestyle, and Philosophy, Including Definitions of Vegetarianism and Veganism, Tips about Adopting Vegetarianism, Creating a Vegetarian Pantry, and Meeting Nutritional Needs of Vegetarians, with Facts Regarding Vegetarianism's Effect on Pregnant and Lactating Women, Children, Athletes, and Senior Citizens

Along with a Glossary of Commonly Used Vegetarian Terms and Resources for Additional Help and Information

Edited by Chad T. Kimball. 360 pages. 2002. 0-7808-0439-2. $78.

"Organizes into one concise volume the answers to the most common questions concerning vegetarian diets and lifestyles. This title is recommended for public and secondary school libraries."   — E-Streams, Apr '03

"Invaluable reference for public and school library collections alike."   — Library Bookwatch, Apr '03

"The articles in this volume are easy to read and come from authoritative sources. The book does not necessarily support the vegetarian diet but instead provides the pros and cons of this important decision. The *Vegetarian Sourcebook* is recommended for public libraries and consumer health libraries."
          — American Reference Books Annual, 2003

Women's Health Concerns Sourcebook, 2nd Edition

Basic Consumer Health Information about the Medical and Mental Concerns of Women, Including Maintaining Health and Wellness, Gynecological Concerns, Breast Health, Sexuality and Reproductive Issues, Menopause, Cancer in Women, the Leading Causes of Death and Disability among Women, Physical Concerns of Special Significance to Women, and Women's Mental and Emotional Health

Along with a Glossary of Related Terms and Directories of Resources for Additional Help and Information

Edited by Amy L. Sutton. 748 pages. 2004. 0-7808-0673-5. $78.

ALSO AVAILABLE: *Women's Health Concerns Sourcebook, 1st Edition. Edited by Heather E. Aldred. 567 pages. 1997. 0-7808-0219-5. $78.*

"Handy compilation. There is an impressive range of diseases, devices, disorders, procedures, and other physical and emotional issues covered . . . well organized, illustrated, and indexed."   — Choice, Association of College and Research Libraries, Jan '98

SEE ALSO *Breast Cancer Sourcebook, Cancer Sourcebook for Women, Healthy Heart Sourcebook for Women, Osteoporosis Sourcebook*

Workplace Health & Safety Sourcebook

Basic Consumer Health Information about Workplace Health and Safety, Including the Effect of Workplace Hazards on the Lungs, Skin, Heart, Ears, Eyes, Brain, Reproductive Organs, Musculoskeletal System, and Other Organs and Body Parts

Along with Information about Occupational Cancer, Personal Protective Equipment, Toxic and Hazardous Chemicals, Child Labor, Stress, and Workplace Violence

Edited by Chad T. Kimball. 626 pages. 2000. 0-7808-0231-4. $78.

"As a reference for the general public, this would be useful in any library."   — E-Streams, Jun '01

"Provides helpful information for primary care physicians and other caregivers interested in occupational medicine. . . . General readers; professionals."
          — Choice, Association of College & Research Libraries, May '01

"Recommended reference source."
          — Booklist, American Library Association, Feb '01

"Highly recommended."   — The Bookwatch, Jan '01

Worldwide Health Sourcebook

Basic Information about Global Health Issues, Including Malnutrition, Reproductive Health, Disease Dispersion and Prevention, Emerging Diseases, Risky Health Behaviors, and the Leading Causes of Death

Along with Global Health Concerns for Children, Women, and the Elderly, Mental Health Issues, Research and Technology Advancements, and Economic, Environmental, and Political Health Implications, a Glossary, and a Resource Listing for Additional Help and Information

Edited by Joyce Brennfleck Shannon. 614 pages. 2001. 0-7808-0330-2. $78.

"Named an Outstanding Academic Title."
          — Choice, Association of College & Research Libraries, Jan '02

"Yet another handy but also unique compilation in the extensive Health Reference Series, this is a useful work because many of the international publications reprinted or excerpted are not readily available. Highly recommended."   — Choice, Association of College & Research Libraries, Nov '01

"Recommended reference source."
          — Booklist, American Library Association, Oct '01

Teen Health Series

Helping Young Adults Understand, Manage, and Avoid Serious Illness

Alcohol Information For Teens

Health Tips About Alcohol And Alcoholism

Including Facts about Underage Drinking, Preventing Teen Alcohol Use, Alcohol's Effects on the Brain and the Body, Alcohol Abuse Treatment, Help for Children of Alcoholics, and More

Edited by Joyce Brennfleck Shannon. 370 pages. 2005. 0-7808-0741-3. $58.

■

Asthma Information for Teens

Health Tips about Managing Asthma and Related Concerns

Including Facts about Asthma Causes, Triggers, Symptoms, Diagnosis, and Treatment

Edited by Karen Bellenir. 375 pages. 2005. 0-7808-0770-7. $58.

■

Cancer Information for Teens

Health Tips about Cancer Awareness, Prevention, Diagnosis, and Treatment

Including Facts about Frequently Occurring Cancers, Cancer Risk Factors, and Coping Strategies for Teens Fighting Cancer or Dealing with Cancer in Friends or Family Members

Edited by Wilma R. Caldwell. 428 pages. 2004. 0-7808-0678-6. $58.

■

Diet Information for Teens

Health Tips about Diet and Nutrition

Including Facts about Nutrients, Dietary Guidelines, Breakfasts, School Lunches, Snacks, Party Food, Weight Control, Eating Disorders, and More

Edited by Karen Bellenir. 399 pages. 2001. 0-7808-0441-4. $58.

"Full of helpful insights and facts throughout the book. ... An excellent resource to be placed in public libraries or even in personal collections."
—*American Reference Books Annual 2002*

"Recommended for middle and high school libraries and media centers as well as academic libraries that educate future teachers of teenagers. It is also a suitable addition to health science libraries that serve patrons who are interested in teen health promotion and education."
—*E-Streams, Oct '01*

"This comprehensive book would be beneficial to collections that need information about nutrition, dietary guidelines, meal planning, and weight control. ... This reference is so easy to use that its purchase is recommended."
—*The Book Report, Sep-Oct '01*

"This book is written in an easy to understand format describing issues that many teens face every day, and then provides thoughtful explanations so that teens can make informed decisions. This is an interesting book that provides important facts and information for today's teens."
—*Doody's Health Sciences Book Review Journal, Jul-Aug '01*

"A comprehensive compendium of diet and nutrition. The information is presented in a straightforward, plain-spoken manner. This title will be useful to those working on reports on a variety of topics, as well as to general readers concerned about their dietary health."
—*School Library Journal, Jun '01*

■

Drug Information for Teens

Health Tips about the Physical and Mental Effects of Substance Abuse

Including Facts about Alcohol, Anabolic Steroids, Club Drugs, Cocaine, Depressants, Hallucinogens, Herbal Products, Inhalants, Marijuana, Narcotics, Stimulants, Tobacco, and More

Edited by Karen Bellenir. 452 pages. 2002. 0-7808-0444-9. $58.

"A clearly written resource for general readers and researchers alike."
—*School Library Journal*

"The chapters are quick to make a connection to their teenage reading audience. The prose is straightforward and the book lends itself to spot reading. It should be useful both for practical information and for research, and it is suitable for public and school libraries."
—*American Reference Books Annual, 2003*

"Recommended reference source."
—*Booklist, American Library Association, Feb '03*

"This is an excellent resource for teens and their parents. Education about drugs and substances is key to discouraging teen drug abuse and this book provides this much needed information in a way that is interesting and factual."
—*Doody's Review Service, Dec '02*

■

Fitness Information for Teens

Health Tips about Exercise, Physical Well-Being, and Health Maintenance

Including Facts about Aerobic and Anaerobic Conditioning, Stretching, Body Shape and Body Image, Sports Training, Nutrition, and Activities for Non-Athletes

Edited by Karen Bellenir. 425 pages. 2004. 0-7808-0679-4. $58.

Mental Health Information for Teens

Health Tips about Mental Health and Mental Illness

Including Facts about Anxiety, Depression, Suicide, Eating Disorders, Obsessive-Compulsive Disorders, Panic Attacks, Phobias, Schizophrenia, and More

Edited by Karen Bellenir. 406 pages. 2001. 0-7808-0442-2. $58.

"In both language and approach, this user-friendly entry in the *Teen Health Series* is on target for teens needing information on mental health concerns." — *Booklist, American Library Association, Jan '02*

"Readers will find the material accessible and informative, with the shaded notes, facts, and embedded glossary insets adding appropriately to the already interesting and succinct presentation."
— *School Library Journal, Jan '02*

"This title is highly recommended for any library that serves adolescents and parents/caregivers of adolescents." — *E-Streams, Jan '02*

"Recommended for high school libraries and young adult collections in public libraries. Both health professionals and teenagers will find this book useful."
— *American Reference Books Annual 2002*

"This is a nice book written to enlighten the society, primarily teenagers, about common teen mental health issues. It is highly recommended to teachers and parents as well as adolescents."
— *Doody's Review Service, Dec '01*

Sexual Health Information for Teens

Health Tips about Sexual Development, Human Reproduction, and Sexually Transmitted Diseases

Including Facts about Puberty, Reproductive Health, Chlamydia, Human Papillomavirus, Pelvic Inflammatory Disease, Herpes, AIDS, Contraception, Pregnancy, and More

Edited by Deborah A. Stanley. 391 pages. 2003. 0-7808-0445-7. $58.

"This work should be included in all high school libraries and many larger public libraries. . . . highly recommended."
— *American Reference Books Annual 2004*

"Sexual Health approaches its subject with appropriate seriousness and offers easily accessible advice and information." — *School Library Journal, Feb. 2004*

Skin Health Information For Teens

Health Tips about Dermatological Concerns and Skin Cancer Risks

Including Facts about Acne, Warts, Hives, and Other Conditions and Lifestyle Choices, Such as Tanning, Tattooing, and Piercing, That Affect the Skin, Nails, Scalp, and Hair

Edited by Robert Aquinas McNally. 429 pages. 2003. 0-7808-0446-5. $58.

"This volume, as with others in the series, will be a useful addition to school and public library collections."
— *American Reference Books Annual 2004*

"This volume serves as a one-stop source and should be a necessity for any health collection."
— *Library Media Connection*

Sports Injuries Information For Teens

Health Tips about Sports Injuries and Injury Protection

Including Facts about Specific Injuries, Emergency Treatment, Rehabilitation, Sports Safety, Competition Stress, Fitness, Sports Nutrition, Steroid Risks, and More

Edited by Joyce Brennfleck Shannon. 405 pages. 2003. 0-7808-0447-3. $58.

"This work will be useful in the young adult collections of public libraries as well as high school libraries."
— *American Reference Books Annual 2004*

Suicide Information for Teens

Health Tips about Suicide Causes and Prevention

Including Facts about Depression, Risk Factors, Getting Help, Survivor Support, and More

Edited by Joyce Brennfleck Shannon. 368 pages. 2005. 0-7808-0737-5. $58.

Health Reference Series

Adolescent Health Sourcebook

AIDS Sourcebook, 3rd Edition

Alcoholism Sourcebook

Allergies Sourcebook, 2nd Edition

Alternative Medicine Sourcebook,
2nd Edition

Alzheimer's Disease Sourcebook,
3rd Edition

Arthritis Sourcebook, 2nd Edition

Asthma Sourcebook

Attention Deficit Disorder Sourcebook

Back & Neck Sourcebook, 2nd Edition

Blood & Circulatory Disorders
Sourcebook, 2nd Edition

Brain Disorders Sourcebook, 2nd Edition

Breast Cancer Sourcebook, 2nd Edition

Breastfeeding Sourcebook

Burns Sourcebook

Cancer Sourcebook, 4th Edition

Cancer Sourcebook for Women,
2nd Edition

Cardiovascular Diseases & Disorders
Sourcebook, 3rd Edition

Caregiving Sourcebook

Child Abuse Sourcebook

Childhood Diseases & Disorders
Sourcebook

Colds, Flu & Other Common Ailments
Sourcebook

Communication Disorders
Sourcebook

Congenital Disorders Sourcebook

Consumer Issues in Health Care
Sourcebook

Contagious & Non-Contagious
Infectious Diseases Sourcebook

Contagious Diseases Sourcebook

Death & Dying Sourcebook

Dental Care & Oral Health Sourcebook,
2nd Edition

Depression Sourcebook

Diabetes Sourcebook, 3rd Edition

Diet & Nutrition Sourcebook,
2nd Edition

Digestive Diseases & Disorder
Sourcebook

Disabilities Sourcebook

Domestic Violence Sourcebook,
2nd Edition

Drug Abuse Sourcebook, 2nd Edition

Ear, Nose & Throat Disorders
Sourcebook

Eating Disorders Sourcebook

Emergency Medical Services
Sourcebook

Endocrine & Metabolic Disorders
Sourcebook

Environmentally Health Sourcebook,
2nd Edition

Ethnic Diseases Sourcebook

Eye Care Sourcebook, 2nd Edition

Family Planning Sourcebook

Fitness & Exercise Sourcebook,
2nd Edition

Food & Animal Borne Diseases
Sourcebook

Food Safety Sourcebook

Forensic Medicine Sourcebook

Gastrointestinal Diseases & Disorders
Sourcebook

Genetic Disorders Sourcebook,
2nd Edition

Head Trauma Sourcebook

Headache Sourcebook

Health Insurance Sourcebook

Health Reference Series Cumulative
Index 1999

Healthy Aging Sourcebook

Healthy Children Sourcebook

Healthy Heart Sourcebook for Women